Screening Mammography

Breast Cancer Diagnosis in Asymptomatic Women

Screening Mammography

Breast Cancer Diagnosis in Asymptomatic Women

Gunilla Svane, M.D., Ph.D.
Director, Mammography Section
Department of Diagnostic Radiology
Karolinska Institute and Hospital
Stockholm, Sweden

E. James Potchen, M.D.
University Distinguished Professor
   and Chairman
Department of Radiology
Michigan State University
East Lansing, Michigan

Arlene Sierra, M.P.A.
Assistant Chairperson
Director of Clinical Services
Department of Radiology
Michigan State University
East Lansing, Michigan

Edward Azavedo, M.D., Ph.D.
Associate Director, Mammography
   Section
Department of Diagnostic Radiology
Karolinska Institute and Hospital
Stockholm, Sweden

with 695 illustrations

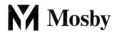 **Mosby**

St. Louis Baltimore Boston Chicago London Philadelphia Sydney Toronto

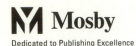

Mosby
Dedicated to Publishing Excellence

Publisher: George Stamathis
Editor: Anne Patterson
Developmental Editor: Carolyn Malik
Project Manager: Peggy Fagen
Designer: Julie Taugner

Printed in the United States of America

Mosby–Year Book, Inc.
11830 Westline Industrial Drive
St. Louis, Missouri 63146

Library of Congress Cataloging in Publication Data

Screening mammography : breast cancer diagnosis in asymptomatic women
/ Gunilla Svane ... [et al.].
   p. cm.
   Includes bibliographical references and index.
   ISBN 0-8016-6488-8
   1. Breast—Cancer—Diagnosis.   2. Breast—Radiography.   3. Medical
screening.   4. Mammography.   I. Svane, Gunilla.
   [DNLM: 1. Breast Neoplasms—diagnosis.   WP 870 S433]
   RC280.B8S4 1992
   616.99'4490757—dc20
   DNLM/DLC   92-49262
   for Library of Congress   CIP

93 94 95 96 97 CL/MY 9 8 7 6 5 4 3 2 1

*To accomplish any worthwhile endeavor requires
cooperation and understanding of others.*

*We dedicate this text to
our spouses and children,
who have surpassed all expectations
of patience and support.*

ACKNOWLEDGMENTS

Many thanks to Anne Patterson and Carolyn Malik of Mosby–Year Book, Inc., in acknowledging and supporting the concept and the importance of this text.

The orderly, and sometimes not so orderly, progression of the book's completion was achieved with the good humor and tireless efforts of several other key individuals. We appreciate the support from the entire secretarial staff, with special acknowledgment to executive secretaries Kathy Miller and Karen Keck, photographer Bud Schulz, and graphic illustrator Anne Schulz, whose roles have been paramount to completing the project.

Gunilla Svane
E. James Potchen
Arlene Sierra
Edward Azavedo

CONTENTS

A SYSTEM TO DIAGNOSE NONPALPABLE BREAST LESIONS

Effective diagnosis of early breast cancer requires that the disease be detected in the nonpalpable stage. Mammography is the only proven method to effectively screen healthy women for nonpalpable breast cancer. Most systems of breast cancer diagnosis result in producing many indeterminate mammograms. The management of those women with an indeterminate mammogram has, at times, led to unnecessary breast surgery. At the Karolinska Institute in Stockholm, a system of breast care has been designed that includes women selected for screening, specific criteria with select categories for interpretation of mammographic abnormalities, and, finally, stereotaxic fine-needle aspiration cytology to evaluate the indeterminate lesion prior to surgical biopsy. This system, when combined with knowledge of the ambient frequency of breast carcinoma in the population under study, allows us to maximize the detection rate of early breast carcinoma and minimize the false-positive interpretation of mammograms. The Karolinska system of breast cancer control has been more effective in detecting cancer at the ambient prevalence rate, without resorting to unnecessary surgical biopsies, than any other system that has been published.

To determine the frequency of breast cancer it is necessary to thoroughly review the risk factors associated with the disease. Thus, this book is designed to present an overview of the system of breast cancer diagnosis currently being used at the Karolinska Institute, in addition to a review of the evidence that supports the use of screening mammography and the risk factors associated with breast cancer. The initial chapter will review the background that brought this book to fruition. Chapter 2 is designed to present the knowledge-base required for rational interpretation of a mammographic image. This includes epidemiology, risk factors, and background information relevant to mammographic interpretation. Chapter 3 discusses the approach to imaging the breast while Chapter 4 tells how to interpret a screening mammogram. This is then followed by a review of past and current criteria used for surgical biopsies. This sequence of chapters logically leads to the rational basis and approach to stereotaxic fine-needle aspiration cytology. These materials form the background needed to understand and make the diagnosis of early breast cancer, as seen in the accompanying atlas. Hopefully, the sequence and presentation will allow the reader to become thoroughly informed about the basis for screening mammography and its application in detecting the earliest of breast cancers. Wider awareness of these techniques and approaches may potentially contribute to the usefulness of screening mammography and its ability to decrease death from breast cancer.

Chapter 1

INTRODUCTION AND OVERVIEW

"The mortality rate for carcinoma of the breast remains unchanged for the last 60 years."

G. DODD, 1988

OVERVIEW

Many books have been written about mammography and breast cancer detection. Why add an additional volume to the literature? Screening mammography should contribute to decreasing deaths from breast cancer. However, it will require more than breast imaging alone to maximize that contribution. We can better diagnose early breast cancer by using a *system* of breast cancer detection that differs from what is usually performed in the United States today. The early literature on mammography featured women who were sufficiently symptomatic to warrant a physician's request that a mammogram be performed. Most women who underwent mammograms were symptomatic, and usually it was they who discovered a lump. Mammography texts and much of the general mammography literature discusses this type of symptomatic patient. There has been, however, relatively little emphasis on the analysis of women who are totally asymptomatic at the time of their mammography examination. Screening of healthy women is where mammography's greatest impact can be made.

When we do not separate women who have symptoms from those women who ask to be screened when they are symptom free, we do not distinguish features of early breast cancer in the asymptomatic screened population from cancer features in women with a palpable mass. The difference is substantial. The symptoms of a palpable breast mass must be responded to. Usually that response includes mammography and cytologic assessment of palpable lesions.[18] Women who consider themselves healthy,

however, pursue medical evaluation differently from women who perceive symptoms that may be due to breast cancer.

We advocate that totally healthy women should present themselves for a diagnostic study to exclude disease. Such a screening process is quite different from diagnosing patients who perceive they have a medical problem, based on specific symptoms. In healthy women, the diagnostic process itself may contribute to the induction of "dis-ease." A apparently healthy woman presents herself for a screening mammogram. When the mammogram interpretation is uncertain, it suggests to the patient that she is more likely to have cancer than she thought before the mammogram. Her quality of life is then affected. Once uncertainty is created by the diagnostic system, the early resolution of this uncertainty is important. Ellman et al. have studied women's psychiatric morbidity induced by breast cancer screening results.[8] The level of anxiety was shown to be significantly higher in women with false-positive mammogram findings, who participated in routine breast screening while assuming they were disease free. Further investigation to clarify a suspicious breast lesion decreased the possibility of sustaining increasing anxiety. These authors conclude that a breast cancer screening program need not increase psychiatric morbidity if delays in follow-up examinations are kept to a minimum and women are kept well informed. The psychiatric morbidity induced by our present mammographic system of frequent false-positive mammogram findings and by prolongation of the final diagnostic process (e.g., when follow-up examinations are delayed for 6 months) causes "dis-ease." Unnecessary uncertainty or prolongation of the uncertainty beyond the time essential for proper diagnosis may cause as much "dis-ease" as could potentially be diminished by the early breast cancer diagnosis.

Many current publications on the control of breast cancer begin with the statistics of breast cancer and the wish that something different could be done to obtain an earlier diagnosis. In the first 70 years of this century, efforts to decrease the number of deaths from breast cancer emphasized alternative treatment modalities. Variations in the treatment of breast cancer are legendary. Halstead established the early paradigms of breast cancer treatment. He emphasized excision of a primary tumor and its lymphatic spread. Initially, breast cancer was thought to spread only by way of the lymphatic system, and therefore the excision of potential lymphatic reservoirs was considered to be essential to eradicate the disease. "If you can't cut it out, you can't cure it" was the battle cry. These earlier ideas produced increasingly radical surgery, leading to a common acceptance of the most radical mastectomy, including excision of the internal mammary nodes. Over the years progressive investigators have shown that radiation therapy and cosmetic breast-conserving surgery are more effective. The capacity of this combination to decrease deaths from breast cancer is equivalent to earlier more radical approaches.[10] The addition of various chemotherapy combinations continues to be a subject of extensive investigation. The major issues of breast cancer control have focused on ways in which the disease can be more easily diagnosed at an earlier stage, thereby decreasing the probability of dissemination by either lymphatic or vascular spread.

Shapiro, using data obtained from the Health Insurance Plan (HIP) of New York, was the first to systematically document that deaths from breast cancer can be decreased through medical intervention.[23] Medical intervention, as implemented in his program, meant earlier diagnosis with the use of mammography and clinical examination. Screening mammography thus became established as an effective means of decreasing mortality from breast cancer in some patients. Since these initial screening results, there has been a cacophony in the literature on the issue of screening mammography for the early detection of breast cancer. Stomper et al. have reviewed numerous series of screening mammographies.[26] They report on aggregate experiences involving a total of 238,000 women in randomized trials in which mammography was used to make the diagnosis and mortality results were reported. Stomper, quoting Shapiro's HIP study, confirmed a 22% reduction in cancer deaths 18 years later. The Swedish two-county (S-2C) study revealed a 27% reduction in 8 years. Stomper et al. also noted that the Swedish Malmo study had different outcomes. Results of the Malmo study did not show a

significant reduction in mortality at 9 years. Despite these findings, the current prospects for decreasing breast cancer mortality through combinations of early detection and breast-conserving surgical and radiation treatment are now even more promising. The value of early detection through screening has been confirmed by many investigators. Ansell et al. studied a nurse-operated breast cancer detection program in Cook County Hospital.[1] He noted that the chance of detecting of localized breast cancer was significantly greater for women whose cancer was diagnosed through the screening program (44 of 72; 61%) when compared with those whose cancer was diagnosed through referral from other clinical areas (71 of 213; 33%).

The incidence of breast cancer may be increasing. Approximately one of every nine U.S. women will someday be diagnosed with breast cancer. If each of these women were screened annually, many mammograms would result in the suspicion of cancer. After more thorough evaluation of suspicious findings and even surgical biopsy, the tests may confirm normality. These "normal women" will have gone through a series of diagnostic procedures that could significantly decrease their quality of life through increasing anxiety and concern that they may, indeed, have breast cancer. An improved system of breast cancer detection may refine the accuracy of mammographic interpretation and decrease unnecessary morbidity induced by the diagnosis of breast cancer. Clinicians may be able to decrease mortality from this disease by establishing a more effective, efficient, accurate, and humane system of diagnosis. More women may participate in a diagnostic system having these attributes. The frequency of false-positive examination results is, in part, responsible for the suboptimal acceptance of screening mammography by both physicians and their patients. Unnecessary false-positive findings limit the acceptance of the mammography procedure both in terms of patient acceptance and in the increase in societal costs of failing to decrease breast cancer mortality.

As early as 1976, Magarey recognized these issues and conveyed them in terms that can be readily appreciated today.[16] "Breast cancer mortality can be reduced by early detection and treatment. The cost, however, of diagnosis of early tumors from amongst the large number of non-malignant disorders, found as a result of public education and population screening, is likely to be prohibitive, both economically and emotionally, as long as admission to hospital for biopsy and possible immediate mastectomy remains the major diagnostic policy. An alternative policy is proposed for the management of women with breast symptoms; it avoids operation on most people and detects the smallest tumors, by means of mammography, fine-needle aspiration biopsy, large-needle biopsy, and outpatient open biopsy. Such a policy is likely to provide positive reassurance with the least emotional distress for the majority of women with breast symptoms who do not have malignant disease, and is thus likely to lead to more positive behavior in the community such as regular breast self-examination and the early reporting of breast symptoms."

We believe there is sufficient evidence to suggest that alternative approaches to the present system of breast cancer diagnosis may yield improved results—that is, earlier, more timely diagnosis—and may lead to a decrease in false-positive findings without sacrificing the capacity to detect the earliest cancers that may be curable.

This book developed from an unusual relationship, between the radiologic faculty at the Karolinska Hospital in Stockholm and the radiologic faculty at Michigan State University. This evolved from our mutual attempts to systematically improve early breast cancer diagnosis. Our efforts to understand the use of mammography in the state of Michigan resulted in studies that revealed remarkable discrepancies in the quality of mammography examination and in patient and physician compliance with the recommendations of the American Cancer Society. Our studies demonstrated that family practitioners were more likely to ensure that their patients comply than were internists.[17] Other investigators have identified a substantial problem with the quality of mammographic techniques. This was simultaneously recognized by the American College of Radiology (ACR) as it began to establish and promote an ACR accreditation process throughout the United States. The state of Michigan became acutely aware of the wide range in quality of mammography. At some established centers, mammograms were performed by untrained personnel and interpreted by general physicians who had little or no experience in the interpretation of mammograms. Many small mammography installations developed throughout the state. In some there was little attention to quality control. There were relatively few nonradiologists who recognized the importance of a high-volume mammography practice including dedicated technologists and dedicated mammographic physicians. Brown et al. and others have pointed out that the number of mammographic machines in the United States has grown explosively.[4] They estimate that there are as many as four times the number of machines that would be needed, if they were used in even a "moderately" efficient manner. Brown also points out that high-volume screening mammography practices may be the only way to decrease the cost of mammography and improve the quality of performance. He believes it would be better for society if fewer sites performed mammography, with each site performing more mammography examinations.

The Michigan mammography experience became the subject of a series of newspaper articles resulting in a political process that changed Michigan laws. A law passed requiring that mammography be performed by trained technologists, using dedicated equipment, and interpreted by competent physicians. This unique law was largely due to an increasing awareness by the public and the medical profession that breast cancer control may be improved.

Too many mammographic installations resulted in an insufficient volume at individual sites, so that the quality and experience of both the technologist and the mammographic interpreter were not maintained. Our literature review revealed that other world centers had far better results in mammographic screening than those existing in the state of Michigan.

THE KAROLINSKA SYSTEM

The Karolinska Hospital in Stockholm, Sweden, has reported on a unique system of breast cancer detection with far superior results as compared with all published reports, including results from the United States up to 1990. With no increase in false-negative findings, they were able to decrease the number of surgical biopsies per cancer found by fourfold over what is commonly seen in the United States.

In the care of breast lesions, mammography only makes a difference when nonpalpable lesions are detected. Palpable lesions require a response independent of the mammographic appearance. It is with the asymptomatic lesion that mammography makes a real contribution. In the United States the mammographic appearance is usually the only element used in deciding whether surgical biopsy is warranted in a case of suspected asymptomatic breast cancer. Obviously, in patients at higher risk (e.g., strong family history, cancer in the opposite breast), an uncertain mammogram would lead to surgical biopsy more often than when no risk factors were present in the patient. The regional variation in surgical biopsy rates seems to be independent of a scientific basis that establishes a distinction between subtle mammographic findings.

The mammographic practice at the Karolinska Institute has evolved over the past 16 years under the direction of Gunilla Svane. Over a decade ago, Edward Azavedo, with a background in cytopathology, became a radiologist and partner in developing the Karolinska system of screening mammography for the detection of nonpalpable breast cancer. The Karolinska system entails that only a limited number of radiologists read a large volume of films. At the Karolinska screening films are double read, and each radiologist reads approximately 120 to 140 mammograms per day. Of that number some 90 to 100 cases come from their screening clinic and the remainder are referrals.

Mammogram interpretation

In interpreting a mammogram, attention is paid to patterns of malignant calcification, densities above regional stromal densities, stromal retractions, and asymmetric masses of stromal density displaced from normal stroma. Other common considerations in mammographic interpretation, such as skin thickening or vascular pattern, are not considered to be as important in the diagnosis of nonpalpable cancer. Skin thickening is not characteristic of subtle nonpalpable breast cancer. When skin thickening is associated with breast cancer, the patient usually has clinical findings. Mammography is primarily used to find asymptomatic lesions within the breast. Mammographic film at the Karolinska Institute emphasizes contrast rather than the latitude needed to include skin imaging. Skin can be examined by appropriate viewing systems rather than by modifying the film and compromising film contrast.

Screening protocol

In screening mammograms, encounter forms indicate whether a case warrants additional workup. For women who are not called back, an interpretation of "normal" is definitive and conveyed without lengthy descriptions or hedging about subtle abnormalities on the films. Obviously, most films are interpreted as normal, and therefore a quick response is possible.

Some 3.87% of women are recalled for additional mammographic examinations. These women are given specific examinations designed to address questions raised by the initial mammogram. Questionable areas of calcification may undergo subsequent magnification mammograms, whereas areas of questionable tissue density or stromal retraction are addressed by obtaining additional views, such as focal compression mammography. Usually additional patient workup includes a lateral medial projection and coned-down and magnification views. For certain suspicious densities, rolled mammographic views are obtained, allowing alternative projections of breast tissue to confirm their presence.

Mammogram coding

Mammograms are coded with a classification ranging from 1 to 5 so that all parties are conversant on exactly what is being communicated (on the basis of the mammogram alone). The classification system indicates the following: code 0 indicates no breast; code 1 indicates a normal mammogram; code 2 indicates an abnormality with no suspicion of malignancy; code 3 indicates uncertainty and some suspicion concerning malignancy; code 4 indicates probable malignancy; and code 5 indicates definite malignancy. Less than 3% of screening mammograms are coded as 3, 4, or 5.

The coding process is important because it provides a structured response to subsequent tests that may indicate the need for a surgical biopsy. Mammograms that are coded as a 3 after additional workup indicate a need for cytologic assessment of the abnormality. Code 4 leads to a surgical biopsy. Code 5 abnormalities require a surgical biopsy, because they are considered to be malignant. In a patient with a code 5 mammogram, if the pathologist is unable to identify malignancy in the first surgical cutting

of the tissue, the specimen should be reexamined because malignancy is found in over 98% of these cases.

Techniques

Stereotactic fine-needle aspiration and Rotex biopsies are a hallmark of the Karolinska system. Patients whose mammographic lesions are coded as 3, 4, or 5 undergo a stereotactic fine-needle biopsy SFNB at the focus of the abnormality. The Karolinska system uses a technique in which the patient lies on a suspended table with the affected breast pendulant through an aperture at the head of the table. The radiology equipment used to perform the stereotactic images is located beneath the table. This allows for ease of operation with the technical activity being performed out of the patient's sight, thereby diminishing patient anxiety. This procedure does not require anesthesia. Most women state that pain from the procedure is less than they encounter at routine compression from mammography. Therefore the stereotactic procedure can be performed rapidly on a patient shortly after a concern is raised about a mammogram. This allows for clarification of mammographic uncertainties without the prolonged delays so often encountered when follow-up mammograms are scheduled 6 months later or even when surgical biopsies are performed within a few weeks. *An important feature of this approach is the decreased uncertainty caused by the system of screening mammography.*

At the time of the stereotactic needle biopsy, the texture of the tissue is felt and evaluated as the needle enters the lesion. This texture is then correlated with the mammographic image. Some mammograms may suggest the presence of a scar, and thus the texture of the scar will be quite different from the texture of either normal breasts or some cancers. As the needle enters the tissue, the traditional cancer texture can be appreciated, often described as the feeling of a needle entering a pear (as opposed to a tomato or an apple, which are more characteristic of a benign cyst or normal stroma). The grainy and firm sensation that is envisioned from the texture of a pear best resembles the texture found in many breast cancers at the time of needle biopsy. This clinical "feeling" of the lesion is an important addition to the diagnostic criteria of breast cancer. The classical pearlike feel when the cytology needle penetrates a lesion is an indication for surgical biopsy, independent of what results the cytology assessment yields.

Once the cytology specimen is obtained, the smear can be examined immediately in the diagnostic radiology suite to ascertain whether an adequate sample has been obtained.

The cytologic specimens are then sent to the pathology department for cytologic assessment. *The cytologic reports are returned to the radiologist, who then integrates the cytologic assessment with the risk factors, the mammographic observation, and the clinical texture of the tumor to decide whether a surgical biopsy is warranted.* Thus the decision for surgical biopsy does not depend merely on the mammographic imaging or the cytology findings alone. For nonpalpable lesions in asymptomatic women, the decision to perform a surgical biopsy is based on all available information about the lesion, the risk profile, the mammogram, the tissue texture at needle biopsy, and the pathologist's cytology report.

The cytologic report is used by *the radiologist* to complement the mammographic findings and the tissue texture at SFNB to decide whether a patient would benefit from a surgical biopsy. The *referring physician* is not presented the cytology report without the mammographic report. Rather, *the radiologist incorporates the cytologic report into an integrated assessment for presurgical diagnosis of probable breast cancer.* Integrative reporting uses the mammographic appearance with the cytologic confirmation of the presence or absence of epithelial cells (e.g., versus a report of stromal fragments). This permits the radiologist to reinterpret the mammogram based on the type of cells obtained from the area of concern. When no cells are obtained from a dense-appearing lesion suggestive of highly cellular tissue, the probability that the mammographic abnormality is due to a malignancy is diminished.

Finally, the process Karolinska radiologists use to localize small, nonpalpable cancers is different from those routinely used in the United States. In the United States it is customary to place wires in breast tissue to guide a surgeon in the removal of a nonpalpable breast lesion. At the Karolinska Institute, a system was developed in which the lesion is tattooed by injecting medical carbon suspended in an aqueous solution. The injected tract of carbon marks the lesion site and continues to the skin surface with a fine carbon dot placed on the patient's skin. The surgeon then dissects the breast tissue with minimal disruption of normal breast structures. Very small malignancies can be excised using this technique. In our experience we have been able to remove malignancies as small as 3 mm using carbon localization, without substantial disruption of adjacent normal breast tissue.

System summary

In summary, the hallmarks of the Karolinska mammography system are:
- *High-volume screening mammography*—Over 100 mammograms are interpreted per day, with separate interpretations of screening mammograms from studies of symptomatic women.
- *The discovery of nonpalpable lesions*—The Karolinska system emphasizes the discovery of such lesions, with a relative deemphasis on mammographic patterns of skin thickening or vascular patterns.
- *The use of follow-up examinations*—Patients are called back for additional views, and the Institute has

protocols to approach specific common screening mammography findings.
- *The classification of mammograms into codes*—Codes guide ultimate patient management.
- *The use of stereotactic fine-needle biopsy*—In women with suspected mammographic abnormalities, fine-needle biopsy is performed, rather than surgical biopsy or delayed follow-up mammographies.
- *The radiologist integrates the information*—The risk profile, mammographic appearance, cytology report, and texture of the lesion are combined to decide whether a patient needs a surgical biopsy. **Consistency in mammography, cytology, and lesion texture is an essential part of the radiologic diagnosis.**
- *The use of carbon localization*—Carbon localization replaces wire localization to guide surgeons to small nonpalpable breast cancers and their removal.

COMPARISON OF KAROLINSKA WITH U.S. PRACTICES

In the United States recent efforts have focused on the use of stereotactic localization with a biopsy gun or cutting needle to obtain histologic rather than cytologic samples. The Karolinska experience initially used cytologic stereotactic biopsy evaluations rather than histologic biopsies. The comparative merit of the two approaches has not been thoroughly studied. American pathologists seem to prefer the use of histologic material for the definitive diagnosis of breast cancer. Karolinska Institute cytologists have sufficient expertise to suggest that, rather than limiting their interpretation solely to histology findings, a less invasive approach may be preferred, once pathologists gain confidence in interpreting breast cytology findings.

Currently significant progress is being made in the United States with rapid diffusion of the stereotactic biopsy technique to diagnose nonpalpable breast lesions. Initially, large-core needle biopsy may be a rational intermediary approach in the United States. Ultimately, it seems that the use of fine-needle cytology and carbon localization of breast lesions would significantly decrease the invasiveness required for the early diagnosis of breast cancer. Decreasing invasive approaches to breast cancer diagnosis and the time of medical uncertainty, which is induced by the diagnostic system itself, may contribute to the increased compliance of women with the American Cancer Society's recommendations for screening mammography. The decrease in surgical biopsies affords a less costly and more humane system of early breast cancer detection than that seen in many U.S. radiology departments.

This book is intended to present the experience of the Karolinska Hospital's mammography system in relation to the United States. We hope to show that Swedish experience can be repeated. The book presents evidence from the literature to distinguish current practices in the United

States and to compare these with the Stockholm experience. What attributes of the Karolinska system can be readily transferred and applied in the United States? To answer this question it will be necessary to systematically review the problems of early breast cancer detection in asymptomatic women and to investigate the issues relating to a system of care most appropriate for the early diagnosis of breast cancer.

GOALS OF THIS PUBLICATION

This book addresses a number of problems related to the detection of early breast cancer. We emphasize the risk profile of each patient. A knowledge of risk factors is essential to properly weigh the risk in evaluating the indeterminant mammogram. We seek to identify why screening mammography works and how it can be improved. The issues raised include: Why screen at all? How does one interpret a mammogram? What are the outcomes of interpretation? What is the role of standardized reporting? What to do with a questionable mammographic finding? How long should mammogram follow-up examination intervals be? What is the role of fine-needle biopsy? What are the indications for surgical biopsies? The role of radiology, pathology, surgery, and primary care physicians working as a team is emphasized. How does this team select the most appropriate patient for an invasive diagnostic procedure? A major effort is made to examine how many surgical biopsies should be necessary to maximize cancer control.

There is great controversy over the best approach to a positive mammogram finding. The proper approach depends on what is considered to be a positive finding. The distinction between signs of relative positivity and the implications of these mammographic signs is thoroughly discussed. We explore how to best interpret a mammogram to diminish the occurrence of false-negative and false-positive mammographic interpretations.

We hope to present the problems of screening mammography and to aid the reader in distilling the massive volume of literature on the subject. We seek to better understand the merits of alternative approaches to breast cancer diagnosis. The best system for the earliest diagnosis of breast cancer remains controversial. Questions range from who should get screening examinations and how often to what aspects of the mammogram clearly warrant concern. Attention to the excessive number of surgical biopsies per cancers found is important to improve breast cancer diagnosis.

Chapter 2 discusses problems in breast cancer detection. The risk for breast cancer is put into perspective in relation to the incidence of the disease. The prevalence and incidence of breast cancer may be changing. The evidence is analyzed in terms of how more women can be cured of breast cancer and why more women are not being cured. Current treatment alternatives do not make as much

of a difference as we would like. The current prospects for increasing the cure rate depend entirely on better (and earlier) diagnosis.

The problem of earlier diagnosis must take into account the ambient frequency of the disease. Each mammogram must be interpreted with an appreciation of that woman's probability of having the disease. Most screening mammograms are normal. In postmenopausal women who are not receiving estrogen, the relatively radiolucent breast will aid in confidently interpreting the mammogram as normal. In the denser breasts of premenopausal women or postmenopausal women receiving exogenous estrogens, the normal mammogram may be more difficult to interpret.

Most breast cancers are obvious on the screening mammogram. At the Karolinska Institute over 60% of breast cancers detected at screening were classified as a 4 or 5 at the time of initial mammography. It is the subtle mammographic findings that induce uncertainty in breast cancer detection. Such uncertainty begins when a radiologist classifies a mammogram as a code 3—not definitely cancer, but warranting further diagnostic studies. The problem of early cancer and the uncertain mammogram is discussed throughout this book.

A review of evidence, including studies performed in the United States and in several other countries, shows that screening mammography really works. We discuss the evidence for advocating various mammography guidelines. We review why some physicians and women do not comply with the recommended guidelines. We seek to better understand what can be done to enhance participation in screening mammography. In the United States a major detraction to complying with the recommendation of the American Cancer Society may be the perceived cost of such compliance in relation to the anticipated benefit. An cost-and-benefit analysis is intended to clarify this issue.

Chapter 3 addresses the various diagnostic methods that have been advocated to diagnose breast cancer. The physical examination and the mammogram are the most important. Although all women should undergo routine physical evaluation to diagnose palpable, mammographically occult breast cancer, the physical examination is more relevant to symptomatic than to asymptomatic women. The characteristic of nonpalpable breast cancer is the lack of physical findings. Although this text emphasizes mammography and cytology, we briefly look at the role of ultrasound, galactography, and various other techniques that have been advocated for the early diagnosis of breast cancer.

A major portion of this book is devoted to interpreting mammograms. *Most breast cancer diagnosed on mammography is conspicuous.* A mammographically conspicuous cancer is defined as mammographic evidence of cancer that is readily obvious to most observers (Figs. 1-1 and 1-2). However, there are many subtle undetected breast cancers in which detection must be improved to maximize

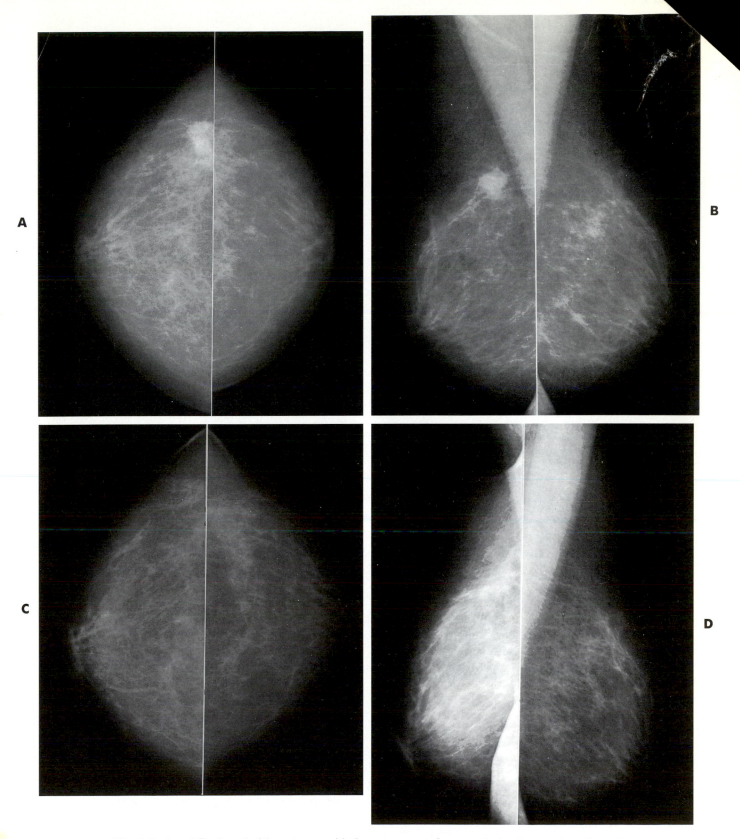

Fig. 1-1. A and **B,** A typical breast mass with the appearance of cancer. Its borders are irregular and somewhat spiculated. The breast is otherwise somewhat radiolucent. There are no abnormal calcifications. In this 55-year-old woman, whose prior mammogram yielded normal findings, this image would be coded as a 5. The patient did have invasive ductal carcinoma without axillary metastases. She underwent a lumpectomy. **C** and **D,** Subsequent radiographic films taken 2 years later reveal a residual surgical scar that is most evident in the mediolateral projection. Indeed, the craniocaudal projection does not delineate any abnormality that would warrant suspicion that this patient has had breast cancer excised by lumpectomy.

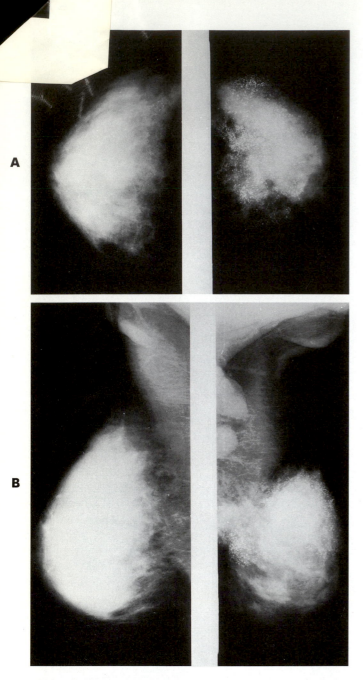

Fig. 1-2. A, A craniocaudal projection and, **B,** a mediolateral projection of a 70-year-old woman with massive microcalcifications involving the entire left breast. This is a category 5 carcinoma. Note the large lymph nodes in the left axillae. These are unusually dense breasts for a patient of this age.

the contribution of mammography. The distinction between a subtle occult breast cancer and a "normal" screening mammogram is the major issue. To understand the contribution of screening mammography we must recognize that distinction.

The U.S. medical malpractice system influences the interpretation of screening mammograms. The distinction

between a missed lesion and masked breast cancer is especially important. Serial screening mammograms may reveal a breast cancer, which in retrospect may have been detected on a prior study. This concern increases the defensive behavior of U.S. radiologists to a greater degree than is evident in Sweden. In part, the increase in false-positive mammographic interpretations seen in U.S. studies is due to this phenomenon. The excessive false-positive mammographic interpretations have a substantial negative effect on the U.S. system of screening mammography.

Screening mammography, when properly interpreted, may decrease the number of women who are subjected to unnecessary "dis-ease" by our system of breast cancer diagnosis. A review of available literature focuses on how many women should be subjected to further diagnostic tests, based on the initial mammography screening results. Once a lesion is detected, how do we establish that it is cancer? Once a mammographic pattern is thought to warrant further attention, what is the next best step? We emphasize the role of additional views and cytologic assessment of subtle mammographic findings.

Most nonpalpable lesions require a stereotactic fine-needle aspiration or biopsy. What is the evidence on the merits of alternative cytologic assessments? What are the cytologic implications of early breast cancer? Salter et al. observed that meticulous follow-up and liberal use of needle aspiration resulted in a progressive increase of the malignant-to-benign ratio, from 18% in 1970 to as high as 56% near the end of their study 9 years later.[22] This occurred while the overall hospital ratio of malignant-to-benign breast biopsies remained at 25%. They observed that *the liberal use of needle aspiration decreased unnecessary hospital admissions, while decreasing the patients' anxiety.*

U.S. radiologists more often use stereotactic core biopsy, whereas the Karolinska experience is limited to breast cytology. They do not do core biopsies. Rather, they rely on their excellent experience with cytology. Most U.S. pathologists are not as comfortable with needle aspiration breast cytology as with core-biopsy histology. In competent hands, there is no evidence that one method is better than the other in selecting patients who require surgery.

Core-biopsy histology has the advantage of portraying cellular relationships and therefore can distinguish invasive cancers from in situ lesions. However, a positive core biopsy finding still requires subsequent surgery. Core biopsies require larger needles, which usually necessitate local anesthesia. There is usually some delay in histologic preparation. When core biopsies require a scalpel to "break the skin," these biopsies are less distinguishable from open surgical biopsies. Some physicians prefer core biopsies over open surgical biopsies because the core biopsy can confirm normality without resorting to an open surgical biopsy, which has the potential to be more risky, disfiguring, and costly.

Aspiration or Rotex breast cytology is less invasive because a finer needle is used and no anesthesia is required. In experienced hands cytology sampling is quicker and has less complications than core or large-bore breast biopsies. Breast cytology can be effective in rapidly reducing the uncertainty caused by a suspicious screening mammogram.

Fox's most fascinating article, entitled "Innovation in Medical Diagnosis: The Scandinavian Curiosity," discusses the failure of the United States to apply Swedish evidence that fine-needle aspiration biopsy is most useful.[11] The procedure is rapid and inexpensive and technologically simple, yet it has found only limited—albeit increasing—acceptance in medical practice outside of Scandinavia. Fox asserts "there is reluctance among medical communities to accept subjective types of innovation. Fine needle aspiration biopsy (FNA) is a major diagnostic tool in Scandinavia. As many as 8,000 biopsies are performed in large metropolitan hospitals each year, yet this procedure has seen only limited application in the United States." Some American centers have had excellent results using fine-needle aspiration to diagnose palpable breast masses. At the Mayo Clinic, in 100 unselected patients with palpable breast masses, Grant et al. reported that fine-needle aspiration revealed a false-negative findings rate of 6%, no false-positive findings, and an accuracy of 94%.[12] Grant concludes that fine-needle aspirations add a measure of confidence in the diagnosis of benign breast lesions and provide a safeguard for preventing the misdiagnosis of malignant lesions.[12] He believes that wider use of fine-needle aspiration may expedite and reduce the cost of managing both primary and recurrent cancer. However, his study is limited to the use of fine-needle aspiration in palpable breast lesions. Similar results in nonpalpable breast lesions using stereotactically guided fine-needle aspiration could markedly enhance the use of mammography as a screening procedure in the early detection of breast cancer. Bibbo et al. used stereotactic fine-needle aspiration biopsy on nonpalpable lesions and concluded that fine-needle aspiration cytology may help to raise the low specificity yielded by mammography alone.[3] This represents a significant advance for the patient in terms of the accuracy, expedience, and reduced cost of diagnosing these lesions.

A limitation to implementing fine-needle biopsies in the United States is the availability of pathologists to interpret the stereotactic cytologies. Smeets et al. sent questionnaires to 90 pathologists in San Diego County.[24] He found that only 2% to 10% of new breast cancer cases were diagnosed either by fine-needle aspiration cytology or tru-cut needle biopsy. It is their opinion that this lack of appropriate use of cytology or large-bore needle biopsy techniques is "due mainly to the reluctance of clinicians to use the technique." They also state, however, that there is a lack of confidence among pathologists in training and interpreting aspiration cytology specimens. Pathologists were more comfortable with large-bore needle biopsies and histologic assessment. Smeets et al. believe approximately 90% of all palpable breast cancers can be diagnosed by needle biopsy techniques.[24] Cohen et al. did a similar survey on the perceptions of clinicians to fine-needle aspiration biopsy.[7] They sent surveys to clinicians at a tertiary medical center and found that fine-needle aspiration biopsy is used more often in hospitals than in private practitioners' offices for the evaluation of palpable masses. The need for experience in the hands of the individual performing the procedure is evident from the studies of Lilleng et al., in which they identified a clear relationship between the frequency of inadequate specimens and the experience in aspiration technique, as judged by the number of specimens referred by an individual physician.[15] Pamilo et al. studied the frequency of recall mammographies and their results in a series of 579 women.[19] The number of follow-up mammographies for microcalcification fell with increased physician experience. They observe that, in surgical biopsy, a finding of malignancy was highest when a radiologist undertaking the primary study performs all further examinations. Heathfield et al. express concern that the development of a widespread availability of fine-needle aspiration services will require an increasing number of pathologists and laboratories to be able to offer this service.[14] Although the technique is not inherently complicated because the number of possible conclusions is essentially limited to four (i.e., unsatisfactory, benign, suspicious, and malignant), there is an inherent hesitancy on the part of pathologists to use fine-needle aspiration cytology in the diagnosis of breast cancer.

The combination of a lack of radiologists adequately experienced and trained in stereotactic fine-needle biopsy and a lack of pathologists adequately experienced and trained in breast cytology is, in part, responsible for the limited acceptance of fine-needle aspiration as an adjunct to screening mammography in the United States. We hope that, with its additional information on the stereotaxic procedure and relevant mammographic images, this text may create a wider awareness of both how the technique is performed and when it should be used.

The cytologic assessment of mammographic abnormalities provides an opportunity for rapid insight into certain aspects of tumor biology. What do you do with the cells obtained on stereotactic fine-needle aspiration biopsy? We briefly present alternative cytochemical techniques that may be used to reveal the nature of a lesion. This is very useful to radiologists because it adds a dimension to the assessment of mammographic patterns.

For example, Fallenius et al. reported on the use of cytomorphometry and biochemical characteristics in nonpalpable breast cancer.[9] Tumors were analyzed with respect to DNA distribution pattern, steroid receptor content, and histopathologic criteria. They found no significant histomorphologic differences between nonpalpable and palpable breast cancers. However, they did observe the DNA distribution of palpable and nonpalpable tumors differed substantially. In relatively small breast cancers 90% had DNA amounts within the diploid or tetraploid regions of normal breast epithelium, whereas in palpable breast cancers only 55% were of the diploid and tetraploid type. More recent reports from the same group established that, in nonpalpable lesions, 65% were euploid and 35% were aneuploid tumors. They measured DNA distribution patterns from the cytology obtained through stereotactic fine-needle biopsy.[2] In addition, this group reported on preoperative estrogen receptor measurements in nonpalpable tumors using an immunocytochemical technique.

A screening program requires not only a valid test but an entire valid screening program.[13] The principle of the Karolinska technique is to combine the clinical findings with mammographic and cytologic assessments to determine whether patients with nonpalpable breast abnormalities warrant further diagnostic or therapeutic procedures. *The Karolinska screening diagnosis is not limited to the mammographic film alone.* In part, this difference from the standard approach used in the United States may be responsible for the better results. Hakama evaluated the approaches to test the merits of alternative breast cancer screening systems.[13] He shares our concern that one must understand the entire system rather than only one element. In evaluating a system of breast cancer screening, it is important to include the quality of mammography, the quality of the laboratory (cytology and pathology), the attendance of a screening population, and the availability of referral or treatment facilities.

Finally, this book presents an atlas of study cases from extensive clinical experience at the Karolinska Institute. A 17-year Karolinska experience includes over 9000 stereotactic fine-needle biopsies. The atlas comprises 50 routine cases obtained from one year (1989 to 1990). The diagnosis of breast cancer was made on screening mammograms in asymptomatic women with nonpalpable lesions. The patterns that result in the detection of early breast cancer become obvious as one reviews the atlas of case studies.

The major issues this book addresses are why screening mammography should be performed; how high-quality mammograms should be performed; how mammograms should be interpreted; how report results should be communicated; how follow-up care should be conducted when a mammogram is normal, questionable, or positive; and how many surgical biopsies are necessary to diagnose breast cancer. We seek to better understand how to reach a majority of women and to decrease both the morbidity induced by the diagnostic process itself and the mortality resulting from this disease.

Theory of breast cancer screening

The public health literature abounds with criteria and methods to evaluate the use of screening tests. Many authors have used the standard six criteria for the evaluation of screening tests.[6,27] These six criteria are:

1. The disease is important.
2. It has a recognizable presymptomatic stage.
3. At this stage reliable tests exist that are acceptable with regard to risk, cost, and patient discomfort.
4. Therapy in the presymptomatic stage reduces morbidity and mortality more than therapy after symptoms appear.
5. Facilities are available for the diagnosis and therapy of those persons with positive screening test results.
6. The screening program takes precedence over other needs competing for the same resource.

The detection of nonpalpable breast cancer almost ideally meets each of these criteria. Clearly the disease is important. Nonpalpable breast cancer is at the presymptomatic stage that can be detected on mammography. Mammography has been well established as a technique that can detect most nonpalpable breast cancers, and it is performed with a low risk, especially in patients over 40 years of age. The cost is potentially a burden, but can be diminished with increasing volume. There is modest patient discomfort for about 3% of patients.

The treatment in the presymptomatic stage clearly diminishes morbidity and mortality. Smaller breast cancers that are diagnosed before they are symptomatic have a higher probability of cure than do those that are larger or symptomatic. The facilities available for the diagnosis and treatment of these patients are widespread, and in the United States might even be excessive. Finally, this screening program has a demonstrated marginal use over other needs competing for the same resource. While this last issue is heavily debated because the cost per survival seems excessive, when compared with other applications of either screening or therapeutic modalities, breast cancer screening rates are seen as both effective and efficient. Each of these above issues is discussed throughout this text. However, before we get into the issues related to the appropriate application of mammography in breast cancer screening, it is worthwhile to reflect a bit on the theoretic basis for screening and how the timeliness of observation can substantially affect the probability of cure in a woman with breast cancer.

Breast cancer screening is based on the premise that finding a cancer before it would be detected without the screen will allow medical intervention to more dramatically affect the course of the disease. The importance of earlier cancer detection depends on whether there is a successful medical intervention to alter the course of the disease. It also depends on whether the cancer would have become evident within a sufficiently short time, so that the earlier diagnosis makes no real difference in the outcome of the disease. Thus an important consideration in advocating a specific screening policy is whether an earlier diagnosis allows a suitable length of time to make a difference.

Fig. 1-3 represents a theoretic model for considering these issues. In case A, the cancer would be clinically detectable at time I, II, or III. A screening mammogram would help detectability in this case. In case B, the cancer would have been detectable by a mammogram at time I and would have been clinically detectable in the interval between time I and time II. If this lesion was detected at time I, the period from time I until the lesion became clinically apparent is the "lead time." **Lead time** is defined as the time that screening detection would precede the usual case finding. Similarly, in case C a screening mammogram performed at time I would not be able to detect a cancer, although it is present in a predetectable state. This cancer

could have been detected mammographically in the interval between time I and time II.

Case D represents a situation in which the cancer is mammographically detectable at times I and II, but does not become clinically apparent until time III. This time period—from the onset of the tumor until it is detected—may lead to a **length-time bias.** Length-time bias occurs when there are a disproportionate number of slower growing tumors that may be detected on a prevalence screen, but that do not become clinically evident for a long time. This is of special concern in older women who undergo their first mammogram.

If a cancer is found, it may have been there a long time without becoming clinically significant. The older the women, the more time a cancer may have existed. On the average, breast cancers in older women may have a more indolent, slower growing course. These two factors increase the chances of a length-time bias affecting the results of breast cancer screening in the older woman. It is possible for a screening program to *overdiagnose* breast cancer that may never become clinically significant. Peeters et al. evaluated the overdiagnosis of breast cancer in the Nijmegen series.[20] They defined *overdiagnosis* as "a

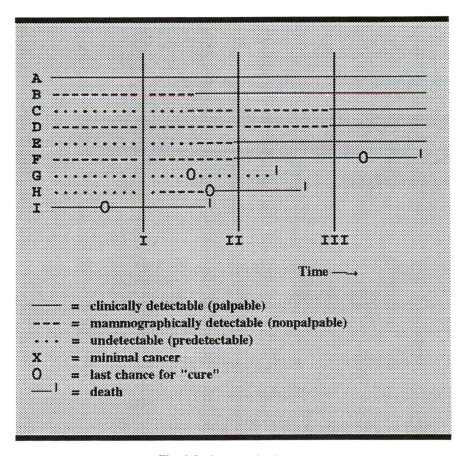

Fig. 1-3. See narrative in text.

histologically established diagnosis of invasive or intraductal breast cancer that would never have developed into a clinically manifest tumor during the patient's normal life expectancy if no screening examination had been carried out." During a 12-year period, they showed an excess of 11% in breast cancer cases in Nijmegen when compared with the neighboring city of Arnham, where no mass screening was performed. Some of these excess breast cancers were due to overdiagnosis of lesions that would never have become clinically significant. Length-time bias may affect the fatality rates in mammographically detected breast cancers when compared with controls. Clarification, adjustment, or both for length-time bias is necessary before concluding that a screening program, itself, is responsible for mortality reduction.

Case E represents a situation in which the cancer has a very short lead time compared with case D. The cancer would be mammographically detectable only during the interval between time I and time II. Thus, although it may be detected by a mammogram performed at time II, it may also be clinically evident at that time. Screening mammography may have relatively little marginal use in this situation. Case F depicts a cancer for which there is a long lead time, and it would have been possible to detect this cancer preclinically on screens performed at either time I or II. The screening detection would make no essential difference in the chance for cure because the last chance occurs after time III.

Case G represents an unusual occurrence in which a primary breast cancer is lethal without ever being mammographically detectable or showing clinical evidence of the disease in the breast. In these cases disseminated metasta-

sis of unknown origin is shown to be microscopically primary in the breast at autopsy. Case H is a similar situation in which the cancer does not clinically manifest in the breast before dissemination and death. In this case a screening mammogram may have detected a curable cancer only if it were done in the interval between times I and II. Finally, in Case I the cancer is clinically evident; however, even if it was detected at time I, it would be too late to effect a cure.

Fig. 1-4 presents the theoretical basis for early breast cancer detection. The time when cancer is considered to have first occurred is an important aspect of breast cancer screening programs. Usually the cancer has been present for a long period of time before it becomes detectable. Some investigators estimate that it takes 20 doubling times to develop the 1 million cells needed to produce a 1 mm lesion. Thirty doubling times would result in a 1 cm lesion, which may be diagnosed by palpation. Nonpalpable breast cancers are detected at about 26 to 27 doublings. Plotkin and Blankenberg estimate that the lead time possible with early mammographic detection represents only about 20% of the total lifetime of a cancer.[21] Doubling time assumptions, although interesting, are controversial. Breast cancer tends to grow in spurts. Therefore the average doubling time may have little meaning in any individual patent. Growth promoters and restrainers are obviously important to any growth rate estimate. These may vary considerably.

In point I in Fig. 1-4 the breast is normal and no cancer exists. This is true for most women during the course of their life. At point II the cancer is not diagnosable but is present within the breast. Undoubtedly, many of the can-

Time ⟶

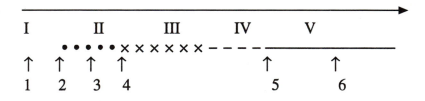

I = Normal
II = Not diagnosable
III = Diagnosable, but usually not seen
IV = Mammographically apparent
V = Symptomatic (palpable)

Fig. 1-4. See narrative in text.

cers that are subsequently identified on incidence mammograms may have been present but not diagnosable on a previous mammogram. Point III represents that period of time when cancer was diagnosable but not usually seen. These masked cancers may be hidden by normal overlying stroma. A similar sized cancer may be detected in other areas of the breast where normal stroma does not occur. At point IV, cancers are mammographically apparent, and point V represents symptomatic cancers.

A mammogram done at time 1 should be a normal mammogram. In these patients there are frequent false-positive examination results in which abnormality is suspected on the basis of the stromal pattern or calcification. These are normal variants or abnormalities caused by a benign process not related to cancer. Time 2 is the earliest detectable cancer. At times a false-positive mammogram impression may result in the fortuitous identification of cancer that would not have been detected and that may not have resulted in clinical symptoms for many years to come. These earliest of nondiagnosable cancers may occasionally be diagnosed accidentally when an abnormality appears normal on the mammogram, but is revealed as malignant by cytologic and subsequent histologic examinations. Most lobular carcinomas in situ (LCIS) and some ductal carcinomas in situ (DCIS) are found incidentally in biopsy specimens removed for what turned out to be a normal mammographic variant or a benign process. Although DCIS is considered a premalignant lesion, LCIS is a marker of risk for the subsequent development of invasive cancer somewhere in either breast. LCIS is common in women who have multicentric breast cancers. In these instances a quadrant biopsy often yields positive results for malignant cells in patients in whom the mammographic abnormality does not demonstrate suspicious areas for concern.

Time 4 is the earliest a tumor can be detected by mammogram. Early breast cancer may accidentally be found on cytologic or histologic examination, and not truly identifiable on the mammogram. In retrospect, efforts are made to define the mammographic clue that leads to their detection, although this may be fallacious. At time 5 the tumors are mammographically apparent and should be detected. Failure to detect tumors on the mammogram at this time is due to observer error or a technical inadequacy of the film itself. Technical inadequacies most often occur because the region in which the tumor is present is not included in the mammographic image. This is a special problem for tumors located posteriorly against the chest wall. At time 6 the tumor is palpable and subsequent clinical care depends on the clinical observations, not on mammographic findings. For this reason, it is said that *mammography makes its contribution in nonpalpable cancers*—palpable lesions warrant subsequent clinical care independent of normal mammogram findings. At any time the mammogram find-

ings may be normal although cancer is present. Some cancers do not appear as abnormalities on mammograms when they are diagnosed. They are diagnosed by clinical symptoms, usually as a palpable lump. These tumors could not be detected earlier by screening or in a nonpalpable state because they are not even seen on the mammogram when the lesion is palpable.

LCIS has no mammographic signs. DCIS is occasionally detected by the presence of regional density or microcalcification. Standertskjold-Nordenstam et al. found false-negative mammogram results in 3.2% of 92 breast cancers.[25] Cahill et al. found a negative mammogram finding in 9.3% of 323 consecutive patients who had surgically proven breast cancer.[5] The difficulty in accurately defining the clinically significant mammogram finding is exemplified in the studies of Young et al.[28] They analyzed the preoperative mammogram reports in 342 women with suspicious breast lumps. The false-negative mammogram results ranged from 11% to 25%, depending on how equivocally mammogram reports were interpreted. This points out the need for rigorous reporting criteria when interpreting mammograms. Without standard criteria it is impossible to reliably assess the performance of the diagnostic system.

Fig. 1-4 illustrates the effect of timing of clinical palpation, mammography, or fine-needle biopsy. Fine-needle biopsy performed at time 1 is normal, whereas at times 2 to 6 it may well be abnormal, if a sample was obtained from the area in which the cancer exists. Fine-needle biopsy may reveal cancer, although the mammogram yields normal findings. Breast cancer can be detected by mammography, palpation, or both and can be confirmed by fine-needle biopsy. There is a continuum of probable thresholds for the detection of breast cancer for each of the various diagnostic procedures. Each of the diagnostic procedures has sensitivity constraints. Cytologic examinations are the first to reveal abnormalities, if one is fortunate enough to obtain cells from an area of cancer that was totally unapparent on mammography or palpation. Mammography would be the next likely study to yield to positive results because nonpalpable lesions can be detected only on mammography.

The choice of performing a stereotactic fine-needle biopsy or waiting 6 months for subsequent confirmation of an abnormality should now be obvious. Many tumors are so slow growing that numerous follow-up examinations may be necessary to identify a cancer that could have been identified by fine-needle biopsy following the initial mammogram. A SFNB, if positive, will lead to the definitive diagnosis at an earlier time. Even if the SFNB is negative, it does not adversely affect the ability of mammographs taken in the subsequent 6 months to accurately detect cancer. The residuum from a SFNB does not distort the mammographic image. Subsequent films may lead to the affirmation of a normality or the identification of a lesion sufficiently suspicious to warrant repeat SFNB. SFNB can substantially clarify false-positive results of early mammograms. A normal SFNB in the face of a code 3 mammographic lesion would tip the balance to negate malignancy, making a surgical biopsy unnecessary at that time. A diagnostic system using the SFNB approach provides considerably more options in the management of patients than those diagnostic systems that do not use this adjunct.

REFERENCES

1. Ansell DA, Dillard J, Rothenberg M, et al: Breast cancer screening in an urban black population: a preliminary report, *Cancer* 62(2):425-428, 1988.
2. Azavedo E, Fallenius A, Svane G, Auer G: Nuclear DNA content, histological grade, and clinical course in patients with nonpalpable mammographically detected breast adenocarcinomas, *Am J Clin Oncol* 13(1):23-27, 1990.
3. Bibbo M, Scheiber M, Cajulis R, et al: Stereotaxic fine needle aspiration cytology of clinically occult malignant and premalignant breast lesions, *Acta Cytol* 32(2):193-201, 1988.
4. Brown ML, Kessler LG, Rueter FG: Is the supply of mammography machines outstripping need and demand? An economic analysis, *Ann Intern Med* 113(7):547-552, 1990.
5. Cahill CJ, Boulter PS, Gibbs NM, Price JL: Features of mammographically negative breast tumours, *Br J Surg* 68(12):882-884, 1981.
6. Carter AP, Thompson RS, Bourdeau RV, et al: A clinically effective breast cancer screening program can be cost-effective, too, *Prevent Med* 16(1):19-34, 1987.
7. Cohen MB, Miller TR, Gonzales JM, et al: Fine-needle aspiration biopsy: perceptions of physicians at an academic medical center, *Arch Pathol Lab Med* 110(9):813-817, 1986.
8. Ellman R, Angeli N, Christians A, et al: Psychiatric morbidity associated with screening for breast cancer, *Br J Cancer* 60(5):781-784, 1989.
9. Fallenius AG, Skoog LK, Svane GE, Auer GU: Cytophotometrical and biochemical characterization of nonpalpable, mammographically detected mammary adenocarcinomas, *Cytometry* 5(4):426-429, 1984.
10. Fisher B, Anderson S, Fisher E, et al: Significance of ipsilateral breast tumour recurrence after lumpectomy, *Lancet* 338:327-331, 1991.
11. Fox CH: Innovation in medical diagnosis: the Scandinavian curiosity, *Lancet* 1:1387-1388, 1979.
12. Grant CS, Goellner JR, Welch JS, Martin JK: Fine-needle aspiration of the breast, *Mayo Clin Proc* 61:377-381, 1986.
13. Hakama M: Screening for cancer, *Scand J Soc Med* 37(suppl):17-25, 1986.
14. Heathfield HA, Kirkham N, Ellis IO, Winstanley G: Computer assisted diagnosis of fine needle aspirate of the breast, *J Clin Pathol* 43(2):168-170, 1990.
15. Lilleng R, Hagmar B, Marton PF: Aspiration cytology in palpable breast changes of the breast: too many specimens without cell material to examine, *Tidsskr Nor Laegeforen* 109(23):2287-2288, 1989.
16. Magarey CJ: Detection and diagnosis of early breast cancer, *Med J Aust* 2(22):834-837, 1976.
17. Mann LC, Bednar EJ, Ghods M, et al: Utilization of screening mammography: a comparison of different physician specialties, *Radiology* 164(1):121-123, 1987.
18. Mushlin AI: Diagnostic tests in breast cancer: clinical strategies based on diagnostic probabilities, *Ann Intern Med* 103(1):79-85, 1985.
19. Pamilo M, Anttinen I, Soiva M, et al: Mammography screening: reasons for recall and the influence of experience on recall in the Finnish system, *Clin Radiol* 41(6):384-387, 1990.
20. Peeters PH, Verbeek AL, Straatman H, et al: Evaluation of overdiagnosis of breast cancer in screening with mammography: results of the Nijmegen programme, *Int J Epidemiol* 18(2):295-299, 1989.
21. Plotkin D, Blankenberg F: Breast cancer: biology and malpractice, *Am J Clin Oncol* 14(3)254-266, 1991.
22. Salter DR, Bassett AA: Role of needle aspiration in reducing the number of unnecessary breast biopsies, *Can J Surg* 24(3):311-313, 1981.
23. Shapiro S: Evidence on screening for breast cancer from a randomized trial, *Cancer* 39:2772-2782, 1977.
24. Smeets HJ, Saltzstein SL, Meurer WT, Pilch YH: Needle biopsies in breast cancer diagnosis: techniques in search of an audience, *J Surg Oncol* 32(1):11-15, 1986.
25. Standertskjold-Nordenstam CG, Svinhufvud U: Mammography of symptomatic breasts: a report on 1119 consecutive patients, *Ann Chir Gynaecol* 69(2):48-53, 1980.
26. Stomper PC, Connolly JL, Meyer JE, Harris JR: Clinically occult ductal carcinoma in situ detected with mammography: analysis of 100 cases with radiologic-pathologic correlation, *Radiology* 172(1):235-241, 1989.
27. Thompson RS: Approaches to prevention in an HMO setting, *J Fam Pract* 9(1):71-82, 1979.
28. Young JO, Sadowsky NL, Young JW, Herman L: Mammography of women with suspicious breast lumps, *Arch Surg* 121(7):807-809, 1986.

Chapter 2

PROBLEMS IN BREAST CANCER DETECTION

The problem of non-palpable breast cancer is more extensive than breast cancer itself.

PHILIP STRAX

Breast cancer occurs in many women. When we attempt to diagnose presymptomatic breast cancer in "healthy" women, all women may become involved. If the system developed for cancer detection causes "dis-ease" through induced uncertainties and anxieties, it may be possible to cause more harm than good. Thus we must be ever vigilant to ensure that the diagnostic system we advocate does not cause more harm than good.

Many questions remain unanswered regarding screening mammography. Why use screening mammography? Which system works best? Will earlier detection lead to increased breast cancer cure? What do we mean by cure? What can be done to minimize the negative aspects of the diagnostic system? We will address the magnitude of the problem and the data that support the contention that mammographic detection of nonpalpable breast cancer is beneficial. An appreciation of the problem in breast cancer detection may reveal ways to further decrease deaths from this disease. We can do better than we are doing.

It is estimated that, in 1990, 150,000 new invasive breast cancer cases were identified in the United States.[280] In the same year some 44,000 women died from breast cancer. The age-adjusted death rate per 100,000 in 1984 to 1986 in the United States was 27.4; in England, it was 36; whereas in Sweden it was 22.2 (Fig. 2-1). The data from any locality may differ from a national aggregate. Reliable statistics from local regions have been more difficult to obtain. We are fortunate that the epidemiologic features of breast cancer were studied over a 40-year period from 1935 to 1974 in Rochester, Minnesota.[44] This community

is the home of a major medical center, which may account for its ability to gather the statistics and the improved survival. During this period the age-adjusted mortality from breast cancer declined slightly from 24.9 to 23.3 per 100,000 person years. This occurred while the age-adjusted incidence rate increased by 25% to 82.7 per 100,000 person years. Most of this increase occurred among women 45 to 64 years of age. The study found a prevalence of breast cancer of 9 per 1000 on January 1, 1975. The prevalence may be different in other communities.

This type of information could lead to the development of local breast cancer control programs targeted at women at most risk for breast cancer in any community, hospital, or screening program. If every breast cancer screening program developed an equivalent information system, each program could be better designed to meet the needs of the patients they are trying to serve. The quality of any medical decision depends on the quality of the information on which the decision is based. Better local information may be a way to improve decisions about breast cancer control.

In screening mammography it is important to define the risk for women who have radiologically negative findings and in whom malignancy might develop later in life. If we know the risk of each woman in a screening program, we should be able to keep those women at higher risk under appropriate observation, thereby detecting malignancy at the earliest sign and optimizing the chances of survival.[303] To do so we need to be well informed.

Death Rates

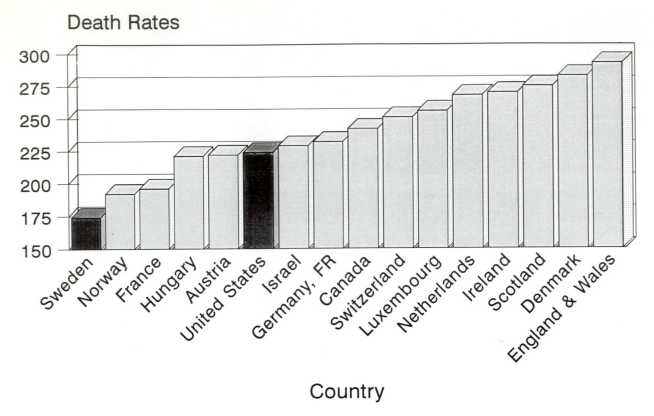

Country

Fig. 2-1. Breast cancer, 1986-1988 (death rate per million). (From Boring CC et al: *CA* 45:19-38, 1992.)

RISK AND INCIDENCE IN BREAST CANCER SCREENING

When we attempt to understand the role of screening mammography in detecting nonpalpable breast cancer, the risk profile of the patient assumes great importance. Which women should be screened? How often should a woman be screened? Is the clinical history relevant or useful in evaluating the indeterminate mammogram? Can a thorough understanding of the risk profiles assist us in understanding the etiologic factors of breast cancer? What information should we know about the patient to make the best diagnostic decision? What feature on the mammogram would we expect to correlate with breast cancer in this patient? What cytologic evidence do we expect to see with this mammographic pattern in a patient with this clinical history?

Answers to these questions may be difficult to obtain. However, clearly a thorough understanding of risk profiles is more important in performing screening mammography than in most other areas of radiologic practice. There are at least five important reasons why the understanding of risk factors is essential to the diagnosis of nonpalpable breast cancer.

First, every feature on a screening mammogram can be looked on as a risk factor for breast cancer. Mammograms contain positive risk factors, negative risk factors, and neutral risk factors. The absence of a mass is a negative risk factor. Any feature can be studied by correlating its incidence with that of breast cancer. That is how we determine which features of a mammogram are likely to indicate nonpalpable breast cancer. A history of having had a benign breast biopsy increases the risks for subsequent breast cancer. Many of these biopsies are indicated by the presence of "suspicious," although "benign," calcifications. One could reasonably ask if the presence of "benign-appearing" calcifications increases the risk for breast carcinoma at a later date. Are auxiliary nodes seen on a mammogram associated with an increased risk for breast cancer in otherwise asymptomatic women? This latter question has been addressed. Using a case control study, at Guy's Hospital in London, Hunter et al. demonstrated that the relative risk of breast cancer in an asymptomatic woman with mammographically demonstrable auxiliary lymph nodes was only 1.08 times that of asymptomatic women without auxiliary lymph nodes.[148] This difference was not significant. This example demonstrates the wide range of risk factors that may be important for the early detection of breast cancer in asymptomatic women. These can be assessed in any large screening program with an appropriate information system and knowledge of proper data analysis.

Observations on a mammogram itself should be considered as risk factors. High-quality diagnostic decisions depend on appropriately weighing all the risk factors, whether they emanate from the film, the patient's history, the clinical examination, or the community background.

Second, we must have an appreciation of which patients to select for screening and how often they are to be screened. This depends on risk factors. The dominant risk factor used in approaching this problem has been the age of the patient. Indeed, age is the criterion for the present American Cancer Society's recommendations for annual screening mammography in women over 50 years of age.

Even if some risk profiles were not used to identify women who should have mammograms, they may be used to target otherwise normal women for other interventions. For example, daughters of breast cancer patients may be specifically selected for education about breast cancer and breast self-examination. A knowledge of risk factors is essential to provide informed counseling of patients at increased risk.[106,219]

Third, a knowledge of risk factors is necessary if we are to use the clinical history to assist in evaluating the indeterminate mammogram. There is some controversy about the relative roles of clinical history in diagnostic decision making. However, it seems reasonable to maximize information when one is analyzing an indeterminate mammogram. In screening mammography 3% to 9% of cases will be indeterminate, requiring follow-up for further evaluation.[18,52] In these cases the decision about what to do for the patient should be based on the probability of the suspected mammographic abnormality representing cancer. The probabilities of cancer relate to risk factors. For example, if a woman under the age of 20 years has a history of radiation treatment for Hodgkin's disease, the probability that she will ultimately have cancer is more than 30 times that of other women.[121] She has a relative risk (RR) of 30 because of this risk factor. A relative risk can be thought of as a multiplier of a disease incidence. Knowledge of this is extremely important in interpreting a subtle abnormality on a dense mammogram. One is more likely to recommend further diagnostic studies based on slightly suspicious diagnostic criteria on the mammogram in patients with this increased risk than in patients less likely to have breast cancer.

Fourth, a knowledge of risk is important when we attempt to select patients, not only for diagnosis, but for potential chemoprevention of breast cancer. The recent tamoxifen trial to prevent breast cancer selected patients on the basis of the risks.[100] The risk factors used for prospective chemoprevention trials are equally important in the diagnosis of this disease. Whereas some may argue that all breast cancers are hormonally dependent, others suggest that chemoprevention trials such as tamoxifen would be appropriately limited to those patients with risk factors known to be hormonally dependent.

Fifth, a knowledge of risk factors may shed some light on what can cause breast cancer. Although we do not know what causes breast cancer, we do know some factors that influence whether or not it occurs. In analyzing the risk factors, we may develop a model to better understand which patient is likely to get breast cancer and why. We must have this insight if we are to develop strategies to prevent breast cancer and not merely diagnose it earlier.

The risks involved with the mammographic detection of breast cancer are more than merely the risk of cancer itself. They relate to the risk of noncompliance by the patient or referring physician with recommended screening protocols. They also relate to the risk of missing a cancer present on the mammogram. All of these risks should be understood as one attempts to appreciate the role of screening mammography in the early detection of nonpalpable cancer.

This discussion of breast cancer risk first assesses the ability to identify populations at risk for screening recommendations. Next, the specific risk factors important in understanding early breast cancer and the role of screening mammography are considered.

Risk profile

A major problem in the early detection of breast cancer concerns our ability to select accurately a subpopulation of women likely to develop the disease. It is often said that only 25% of breast cancers are related to some known risk factor.[267]

Carter et al. used the experience of the Group Health Cooperative of Puget Sound, based in Seattle, Washington, to develop a risk factor profile that concentrated 80% of breast cancer cases in some 60% to 65% of women.[56] They attained a 1.33 relative risk in the high-risk group versus 0.5 in the low-risk group. These groups were separated based on four levels of risk: high, moderate, borderline, and no measurable risk. They chose risk levels rather than a continuum of probabilities to prescribe specific screening recommendations for levels of prespecified risk. Their risk levels were calculated from chronologic age and accumulation of variable risk factors as seen in Table 2-1. The calculations were based on information available in 1983. They have an enrollment of 110,000 women in whom they suspect there are 150 new breast cancers per year. They calculate the relative risk for the four groups based on the incidence of breast cancer in all women they studied who were over 20 years of age. These figures are based on their experience rather than an estimated norm. They use these risk factors to selectively screen the women enrolled in this large health-maintenance organization

Table 2-1. Designation of breast cancer risk levels

Risk group	Relative risk	Group criteria	Variable risk factors (VRF)
High risk	6	Previous breast cancer, breast cancer in mother, or age 50+ yr *plus* any two VRF	Previous other cancer Other close relative with breast cancer Menarche at age 10 yr or earlier Nulliparity
Moderate risk	2	Under age 50 yr *plus* any two VRF or age 50+ yr *plus* any one VRF	First live birth at age 30+ years
Borderline risk	1.5	Under age 50 yr *plus* any one VRF	Menopause at age 50+ years
No measurable risk	1.2	No VRF, any age	Previous benign breast disease (other than in connection with lactation)

From Carter et al: *Prevent Med* 16:19-34, 1987.

(HMO). According to their initial screening protocol, only 57% of women over 40 years of age were eligible for screening mammography. By observing a large number of women over time, they can change their risk estimate based on their experience with this population of concern. Using these experiential data, this HMO revised their risk-based breast cancer screening program in 1990.[297] The revised program increased the number of women who were eligible for regular mammography to 83% of women over 40 years of age, rather than the initial 57%. They accomplished this by varying the screening intervals and therefore did not substantially increase the total number of mammograms (Table 2-2).

This example demonstrates the range of possible screening protocols that can be accomplished without adversely affecting the capacity of screening mammography to decrease death from breast cancer.

Schechter et al. identified a population of 40% of the women who had 85% of breast cancer cases.[260] They attained a relative risk level of 2 in the high-risk group and 0.25 in the low-risk group. They attempted to determine patient selection based on simple risk factors. Their method initially allocated risk by counting the number of risk factors present in an individual woman. They found this less satisfactory than the ultimate model used, which gave weighted risks in a logistic model. These weighted risks were developed using coefficients for discriminant scores obtained from the data in the Canadian National Breast Screening Study. The coefficients equal the natural logarithm of the odds ratio associated with a given risk

Table 2-2. Revised risk algorithm

Mammography frequency	Risk level	Risk-level criteria	Relative risk*		Percentage women†	
			Original	Revised	Original	Revised
Annual	1	Previous breast cancer or atypia on biopsy results; at least two first-degree relatives with breast cancer‡	1.2-44§	4-14	16	1
Every 2 years	2	One first-degree relative with breast cancer; age ≥50 yr and ≥2 MRFs	1.5-11§	1.9-3.5	27	15
Every 3 years	3	Age <50 yr and ≥1 MRF; age ≥50 yr and ≤1 MRF	1.2-2.0	1.2-1.9	12	66
Not recommended	4	Age <50 yr and no MRF	1.0-1.9	1.0	43	17
	TOTAL				100	100

From Taplin et al: *Cancer* 66:812-818, 1990.
*See Table 2-1.
†Among Group Health Cooperative women >40 years of age who completed the risk factor questionnaire by 1987 (*n* = 55,875) but excluding women with a history of breast cancer (*n* = 1460) or for whom information was missing (*n* = 1704).
‡*First-degree relative*, mother, sister, or daughter; *second-degree relative*, grandmother or aunt.
§At the time the original risking system was established, the risk of two first-degree relatives or atypical hyperplasia was not recognized. Women with these risk factors account for the upper limit of the "relative risk" in these risk levels.
MFR, Minor risk factors. Second-degree relative with breast cancer; menarche age ≤10 yr or menopause ≤30 yr; previous negative breast biopsy.

Table 2-3. Coefficients for discriminant scores

Variable	Premenopausal	Postmenopausal
Constant*	−6.50	−7.50
Age	0.133	0.182
Parity	−0.157	−0.288
Age at first childbirth	0.060	−0.025
Age at menarche	−0.074	
Smoking	0.0011	
Age at menopause		−0.017
Benign disease		0.396
Family history		0.234
Surgical menopause		−0.834
Lump (in past 6 mo)	2.720	2.560
Pain (in past 6 mo)	0.598	0.898
Discharge (in past 6 mo)	0.126	1.328

From Schechter MT et al: *J Chronic Dis* 39:253-260, 1986.
*Constant terms have been adjusted so that critical values for pre- and postmenopausal models coincide close to 0.

factor. Table 2-3 shows the coefficients they calculated.

These researchers markedly improved their discriminating ability by including the clinical variables of breast lump, pain, or discharge. Such clinical observations are not possible if one is analyzing only asymptomatic, nonpalpable breast cancers.

These risk factors were selected because no real improvement occurred when they added additional variables. This model was selected from alternatives using ROC analyses. They included seven major variables:

1. Age greater than 50 years
2. Age at first childbirth of greater than 27 years
3. Nulliparity
4. Positive family history
5. History of benign disease
6. Age at menarche under 12 years
7. Ever having been a smoker, for premenopausal women; or age at menopause and whether or not the menopause was natural for postmenopausal women

When the clinical symptoms of lumps, pain, or discharge in the preceding 6 months were added to these variables, the most efficient discriminating risks were obtained. This type of analysis allows for the calculation of relative risk using multiple factors. Experimentally based models such as this may be used to assist in diagnostic decisions involved in screening mammography.

Because Schechter's study population is composed of volunteers, there are questions about the ability to generalize from these results.[33] However, Schechter et al. believe that no index of discrimination thus far developed is sufficiently accurate to implement a risk-based screening program. Whatever discriminants are used, a large number of women with early breast cancer would not be detected by merely assessing their risk factors.

Previous investigators used discriminant functions to provide an indication of breast cancer risk for other purposes.[303] Their discriminant variables were primarily based on a systematic analysis of the various aspects of breast cancer detection. Their technique allowed for quantitative distinction of the merits in knowing any of the various symptoms associated with breast cancer. Toti et al. used a linear discriminant approach to define the merits in knowing any specific risk factor.[303]

Can a knowledge of risk factors be used to project the probability that a woman will ultimately develop breast cancer? The group from the epidemiology and biostatistics branches of the National Cancer Institute have sought to answer that question.[106] They consider this important data for counseling women who plan to be examined annually. They use the Breast Cancer Detection Demonstration Project (BCDDP) data base. Because of self-selection, these BCDDP data may not be uniformly applicable.[238] The technique used by Gail et al. differs from others; they used a proportional hazards model that has significant advantages over previous life table methods.[106] They were able to model relative risk for various combinations of factors and individualized breast cancer probabilities. This technique may be applicable in other populations, especially if a breast cancer screening program has an adequate number of examinations and an adequate data base of high-quality information that could be used to attach a probability of cancer to any woman being screened.

Gail et al. estimate that the calculation of an absolute rate of future breast cancer will require a long-term follow-up of thousands of individuals. This is exactly what should be happening when widespread screening programs are implemented. Collection of these data through proper encounter forms suggests that it may be feasible in major screening programs to develop an index of breast cancer risk specific for the women being screened. If high-risk women were better identified, more frequent examinations and recommendations for more radical approaches such as prophylactic mastectomy or less radical modifications such as chemoprevention could be based on an individual's profile. Only through better understanding of the risk profiles of individual patients will we be able to appreciate the merits of the various recommendations we provide these women. Models such as this should facilitate research in breast cancer prevention. And as Pickle and Johnson assert, the study of high-risk women is more likely to lead to the timely demonstration of desirable interventions.[238]

The work of Toti, Carter, Taplin, Schechter, and Gail suggests that there is enough potential of defining a population of patients at risk to warrant modification of the standardized screening protocols. Other investigators conclude that risk profiles other than age are not useful to select women who should be screened for breast cancer.[5,82,99] These authors conclude that knowledge of risk is

not of much use in designing a screening project.

Even if risk factors are not useful to define an appropriate screening population, a knowledge of risk factors is needed to properly use many mammographic observations. Therefore, we devote considerable attention to known and suspected risk factors useful in breast cancer detection. We consider risk factors when deciding which subtle mammographic abnormality warrants further attention. Risk factors form the basis for making any recommendation to a patient. Each mammographic observation affects the total risk profile. A risk profile is relevant to select those patients with minimally suspicious mammograms who require further studies.

Risk factors. Each patient is an amalgam of many risk factors. These risk factors are interdependent. Some attributes of a woman diminish her risk for breast cancer, others increase the risk. Because of this interdependence and the presence of both positive and negative cofactors in any one woman, a single factor may be difficult to isolate in a clinical context. However, an appreciation of the individual factors is needed to develop clinically relevant risk profiles used in diagnostic decisions. Risks are calculated from prospective cohort studies, case control studies, or differential incidence in populations of interest. Whatever the method, adjustments for other known risk factors are desirable to isolate as much of the risk factor of interest as possible. Risks are usually expressed as relative risks (RR), which relate the observed incidence to the expected incidence seen in the control population (O/E).

Hormonal burden. The probability that a woman will get breast cancer depends to some extent on the type and duration of estrogen exposure and the nature of her host response. It has also been found that the hormone level plays a role in male breast cancer. A prior history of mumps orchitis increases the risk of male breast cancer.[190] Curiously, bachelors and butchers are at a greater risk for male breast cancer.[177] The amount and duration of endogenous estrogen exposure is related to many of the risk factors discussed in this chapter. We must appreciate the interdependence of these risk factors when we try to isolate the relative risk contribution from any one factor. Table 2-4 displays the interrelation between the age of a woman at the birth of her first live child and family history. Risk factors are related to menstrual history, parity, marital status, benign breast disease, body build, obesity, and history of prior breast, ovary, or endometrial cancer.

Endogenous estrogen and progesterone. Endogenous estrogens and progesterone are factors involved in whether or not a woman will eventually get breast cancer. Numerous attributes of endogenous hormone levels have been used to identify high-risk patients. These attributes range from the age of menarche and menopause to the regularity of menses and age of the woman at the birth of her first live child.[167] The later the age at the first full-term pregnancy, the higher the cancer risk. This late age at first full-term pregnancy is a risk for estrogen receptor (ER)-rich breast cancer, but not for ER-poor breast cancer. This observation supports the hypothesis that early first birth protects against breast cancer by reducing the level of estrogen receptors in the breast epithelial cells from which carcinoma develops.[203] High parity is associated with a reduction in risk, independent of the age at first childbirth. Bruzzi et al. found a short-term increase of breast cancer after a full-term pregnancy.[51] They compared women who had given birth within the last 3 years to women who had given birth 10 years or more previously. After adjustment for age, age at first childbirth, and parity, this case control study found a relative risk for breast cancer of 2.66 in the women who were more recently pregnant. For a short time, this transient increase in breast cancer risk overcomes the long-term beneficial effect of pregnancy at a young age. A history of lactation may have an independent protective effect against breast cancer.[202]

The earlier the age at menarche and the later the age at menopause, the higher the risk. A late age at menarche is associated with a lower risk for premenopausal cancer, but not postmenopausal cancer.[127] Some hormonal risks for breast cancer have a substantially different effect on premenopausal versus postmenopausal breast cancer. Table 2-5 displays the hormonally dependent relative risks for pre- and postmenopausal breast cancer, as determined by McTiernan and Thomas.

Menstrual history has received a great deal of attention by those trying to identify which woman is more likely to get breast cancer. There is an increase in breast cancer risk if menarche begins under the age of 12 years. In addition, the risk increases if menopause begins after the age of 55

Table 2-4. Correlating risks relating age at first live childbirth to family history

Age at first live birth (yr)	First-degree relative with breast cancer	Relative risk
<20	0	1.00
	1	2.61
	≥2	6.80
20-24	0	1.24
	1	2.68
	≥2	5.78
25-29 or nulliparous	0	1.55
	1	2.76
	≥2	4.91
≥30	0	1.93
	1	2.83
	≥2	4.17

From Gail et al: *J Natl Cancer Inst* 81:1879-1886, 1989.

Table 2-5. Hormonally dependent risk factors for premenopausal and postmenopausal breast cancer

Risk factor	Premenopausal cancer RR (95% CI)	Postmenopausal cancer RR (95% CI)
Late age (yr) at menarche[a] (13+ yr vs. ≤13 yr)	1.6 (1.0-2.4)	1.3 (0.79-2.1)
Ever married[b]	0.29 (0.11-0.76)	2.3 (0.41-12.8)
No. of full-term pregnancies[c]		
3+	1.0	1.0
1-2	1.4 (0.79-2.4)	1.6 (0.91-2.9)
0	0.86 (0.38-1.4)	1.6 (0.53-5.0)
Age (yr) at first full-term pregnancy (parous only)[d]		
13-19	1.0	1.0
20-24	0.46 (0.24-0.89)	0.95 (0.47-1.9)
25-29	1.2 (0.59-2.6)	1.6 (0.70-3.6)
30+	1.3 (0.50-3.4)	1.9 (00.44-8.2)
History of benign breast disease[e]	2.7 (1.5-4.9)	1.1 (0.61-2.1)
Ever lactated (parous and nulliparous)[f]	0.49 (0.30-0.82)	1.0 (0.58-1.7)
Total lifetime duration of lactation (mo) (parous only)[f]		
Never	1.0	1.0
1-3	0.66 (0.35-1.2)	1.2 (0.62-2.2)
4-12	0.45 (0.24-0.87)	0.98 (0.46-2.1)
13+	0.45 (0.21-0.96)	0.38 (0.12-1.2)
Duration of nursing after first live birth (mo) (parous only)[f]		
Never	1.0	1.0
1-2	0.67 (0.36-1.2)	1.3 (0.72-2.5)
3-5	0.56 (0.27-1.1)	1.8 (0.74-4.4)
6+	0.54 (0.27-1.1)	0.66 (0.26-1.7)

From McTiernan A et al: *Am J Epidemiol* 124:353-358, 1986.
[a]Adjusted for age and age at first full-term pregnancy.
[b]Adjusted for age and education.
[c]Adjusted for age, age at first full-term pregnancy, and total lifetime duration of lactation.
[d]Adjusted for age, number of full-term pregnancies, and total lifetime duration of lactation.
[e]Adjusted for age.
[f]Adjusted for age, number of full-term pregnancies, and age at first full-term pregnancy.

years or if the individual has had more than 40 menstrual years (RR 1.5 to 2).[128] The regularity of menstrual cycles may increase breast cancer risk. If menses are more regular and frequent, there is thought to be more estrogen exposure and thus a greater breast cancer risk.

The timing of pregnancy is a risk factor. What does this add to the ultimate risk for breast cancer? An elderly primipara is more likely to develop breast cancer than a woman who has a child before the age of 30 years. A woman who has her first pregnancy after 30 years of age has a relative risk of 1.37 to 2.2.[46,50,318] If a woman never has a child, she has a relative risk of 1.5 to 1.6, as compared with women who have given birth.[85,202,318] The implications of menstrual history and pregnancy apparently relate to the total hormonal burden to which a woman's breast is exposed. This endogenous hormonal burden is considered by some to be the most important cause of breast cancer.

Ghys compared 200 patients with breast lesions (27 of whom had breast cancer) with 102 controls who had a family history of breast cancer but no breast pathologic

factors.[108] The frequency of hysterectomy in the control population was 62.5% and only 38.1% in those who had cancers. Others have shown that oophorectomies and hysterectomies to some degree protect against breast cancer in some susceptible patients.[161] The lower the age of premenopausal oophorectomy, the lower the risk for breast cancer. A bilateral oophorectomy reduces the risk more than hysterectomy alone.

Athletic activity at a young age that is sufficiently substantial to change menstrual activity is associated with a decrease in breast cancer. This suggests that regular participation in moderate physical activity may provide an opportunity for the primary prevention of breast cancer by reducing the ovulatory cycles in adolescence.[35] Former college athletes have a decreased risk for breast cancer.[105] Nonathletes had an RR of 2.53 (CI of 1.17 to 5.74) when matched against women who had been college athletes.

Kampert et al. used data obtained from the San Francisco hospitals to compare 1884 women with breast cancer to 3432 matched controls.[159] They developed incident rate functions that fit the observed data. This analysis reaffirmed many of the relationships between menses, parity, and body weight. They found that "(1) the protective effects of late menarche and of early first full-term pregnancy are greater in premenopausal than in postmenopausal women; (2) first full-term pregnancy initially boosts the level of risk, but incidence rates increase with age more slowly thereafter; (3) among the parous, multiparity is protective both in premenopausal and postmenopausal women, regardless of age at first full-term pregnancy; (4) both nulliparous and lean women are more protected by early menopause than are parous and overweight women; (5) increased body mass index is protective before, but detrimental after, menopause; and (6) postmenopausal incidence rates increase with age more rapidly among overweight than among lean women." Kvale and Heuch used 1565 cases of breast cancer in a prospective study of 63,090 Norwegian women, to calculate an average increase in breast cancer risk of 4% for each year of decreased age at menarche.[170] They observed a 3.6% increase in risk for each year of increased age at menopause. They found the protective effect of early menopause was strongest for breast cancer diagnosed in patients 80 years of age or older.

Exogenous estrogen and progesterone. Exogenous hormones, on the other hand, have not been shown to cause an increase in breast cancer. An Australian population-based case control study showed there was no evidence that oral contraceptives had a relationship to the risk of breast cancer. This confirmed many previous similar studies.[248] This study evaluated the age at first use and the total duration of contraceptive hormone use. Earlier concerns for possible breast cancer induction from exogenous estrogens and progesterone may have been related to dose. The more recent studies lend strong credence to the fact that there is no adverse risk effect caused by the use of oral contraceptive agents.

The recent World Health Organization (WHO) report on the study of neoplasia and steroid contraceptives provided reassurance that the use of injectable long-acting depot-medroxyprogesterone was not associated with an increased risk for breast cancer.[300]

Similarly, hormone replacement therapy in older women has been the subject of considerable investigation in relationship to breast cancer. Hulka reviewed five recent U.S. studies and four European studies to conclude that, although there may be a small increase in the risk of breast cancer after many years of estrogen use, "even this tentative conclusion is debatable since many rigorous studies show no association between estrogen use and breast cancer."[146] She notes that European studies exhibited a higher risk after a shorter duration of hormone use than those in the United States, and this may relate to the type of estrogen use and whether or not progesterones are added to the hormone replacement therapy. At best, current evidence strongly suggests that exogenous hormones at the doses currently prescribed do not lead to an increased risk for breast cancer.

Indeed, Dupont et al. observed an absolute decrease in the relative risk of developing breast cancer for women who took exogenous estrogens.[86] However, their observation was limited to women who had benign breast biopsy results. They obtained follow-up information on 3003 women with a median duration of estrogen therapy of 17 years. Of their total patient population originally selected for follow-up, 84% was observed. In women who took exogenous estrogens the risk of developing breast cancer over these 17 years was .98 versus 1.8 for women who did not take estrogens. This lowering of the observed breast cancer risk was seen in people with various types of benign breast disease. In atypical hyperplasia the risk for breast cancer was 3 for women taking estrogens versus 4.5 for those who did not. In women with proliferative disease without atypia, the relative risk was .92 versus 1.9 for women who did not take estrogens. In women without proliferative disease the relative risk was 0.69 for women taking estrogens versus 0.91 for women who did not take estrogens. Consistent with the other studies, the authors noted that more recent estrogen usage is less risky than the estrogens in use in earlier years. The women who took estrogens before 1956 had a 2.3 times greater risk of developing breast cancer than other estrogen users. Presumably, this was due to a dose effect. These authors conclude that exogenous estrogens are not associated with an increased risk of breast cancer in patients with benign breast disease, and suggest that exogenous estrogens may be somewhat protective against breast cancer in this patient population at risk.

Age. The most important single risk factor is patient age (Fig. 2-2). The incidence rates in Fig. 2-2 indicate the number of cancers that would be present in 1000 annual screening mammograms done in the specified age groups. The average risk that a woman will be diagnosed with breast cancer in the coming 10 years is about 13 per 1000 for a 40-year-old woman, 23 per 1000 for a 55-year-old woman, and 28 per 1000 for a 65-year-old woman.[87] Most recommendations for screening mammography depend on age. In women over 50 years of age, mammography can identify early cancers and thereby decrease breast cancer deaths. In premenopausal mammograms the denser breast may decrease the sensitivity of mammography in the detection of cancer. This increased masking of cancer in younger women increases the number of false-positive interpretations. Ghys observed that, in patients undergoing breast biopsies for suspected breast cancer, women with benign biopsy findings averaged 32.7 years of age and those with cancer averaged 52 years.[108] The combination of less sensitive mammography with less frequent disease is the major basis for the argument over the use of mam-

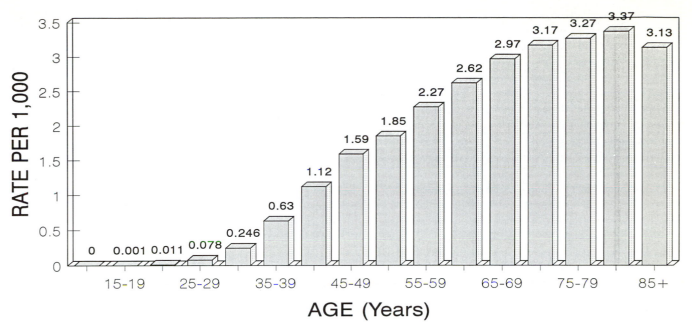

Fig. 2-2. Annual age-specific incidence of breast cancer per 1000 women. (From Eddy DM: *Ann Intern Med* 111:389-399, 1989.)

mography in women under 50 years of age. In women under 30 years of age there is no evidence that mammography is of benefit.[322]

Any recommendation to expand the mammographic screening pool to a younger age group must consider the potential risk from radiation to younger patients. The human breast exhibits an age-dependent sensitivity to radiation carcinogenesis.[38,94,171,302] The intense concern for mammographic-induced breast cancer of the 1970s has substantially diminished with the widespread use of low-dose mammography systems. However, there is a recent renewed concern, at least for relatives of patients with ataxia telangiectasia. These issues are discussed in greater detail later in this chapter. We do not have a strong opinion about the most appropriate age to initiate mammography because all opposing views have some merit.

Moskowitz[214,215] has been an important advocate of al-

tering the American Cancer Society's screening recommendation so that breast cancer may be detected in younger women.[322] The concern for the increased error rate in mammographic detection of premenopausal breast cancer is amply demonstrated in Paci's data.[228] There, screening examinations detected only 34% of the cancers in women between 40 and 49 years of age versus 82% of the cancers in women 50 to 59 years of age. The rest of the cancers were detected in the interval between screens. The average interval between these screening mammograms was 30 months (Table 2-6). The rationale for the theory that more frequent screening mammograms are needed in younger women (40 to 50 years of age) is that the disease in younger women usually grows more rapidly. At 40 to 50 years of age the preclinical interval appears to be less than after 50 years of age.[87]

The American Cancer Society's criteria promote a base-

Table 2-6. Effect of age on breast cancer prevalence and detection

Age	Women screened	Total cancers	Prevalence per thousand	Screen detected per thousand	Interval cancers per thousand[a]	Percentage detected on screen
40-49	12,604	47	3.7	16 (1.27)	31 (2.46)	34
50-59	5,932	36	6.1	27 (4.58)	9 (1.52)	75
60-69	4,444	44	9.9	39 (8.78)	5 (1.13)	88

From Paci et al: *Int J Cancer* 46(2):198-202, 1990. Reprinted by permission of Wiley-Liss, A Division of John Wiley & Sons, Copyright © 1990.
[a]Interval cancers are those cancers that presented between screening mammograms. The average interval between screens was 30 months.

line mammogram between 35 and 40 years of age, a mammogram every 2 years after 40 years of age in those women at risk, and an annual mammogram in all women after 50 years of age. This tends to find the more slowly growing tumors in older postmenopausal women and miss the more rapidly growing tumors of the premenopausal women. Moskowitz advocates annual or semiannual mammography in women 40 to 49 years of age and biannual mammography after 50 years of age. Fig. 2-3 describes a schema that forms the rationale for more frequent mammographic screening examinations in younger women. Rates I, II, and III represent three different growth rates in breast cancer. A is a threshold for mammographic detection. B is a threshold for palpable tumor or symptoms. C is the theoretic threshold for metastasis. Theoretically, in some women this threshold may be below threshold B or even threshold A. It is when the threshold for dissemination is between threshold A and B that screening mammography makes its unique contribution to the cure of breast cancer.

The tumor growing at rate I would be visible at year 1 on mammogram and would appear clinically in the interval between year 1 and 2. In a patient with a tumor growing at that rate, an annual mammogram would be necessary to detect the tumor before it metastasized. The interval between the mammographic threshold and the clinical threshold is the period when the mammogram may lead to the detection of an early lesion, thereby providing an opportunity to prevent a death from breast cancer. This is the purpose of mammographic screening.

A breast cancer at growth rate II could be detected at year 2 only on mammography. By year 3 it would be evident clinically. It would not metastasize until the interval between year 3 and year 4. If, however, a patient with this tumor was relegated to biannual screening, the lesion may well have metastasized before its detection.

On the other hand, a breast cancer growing at rate III could be detected on mammograms at years 4, 5, and 6. In such a case a 2-year interval between screenings would not diminish the chance of mammographic detection before the tumor reached its metastatic threshold. Growth rates represented by lines I and II are more characteristic in

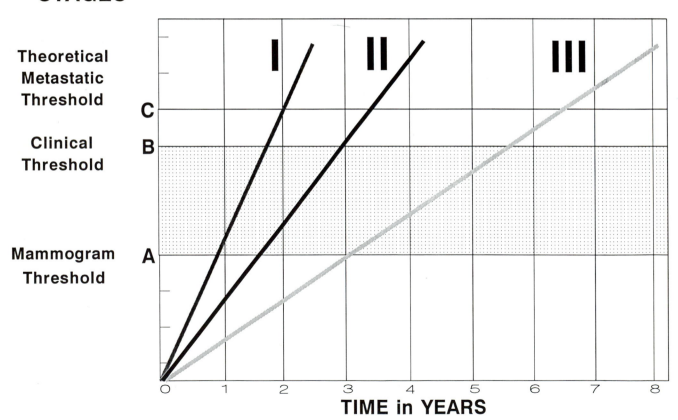

Fig. 2-3. Effect of different breast cancer growth on detection at a nonpalpable stage.

younger patients. Growth rate III is more typically seen in postmenopausal women.

The relative frequency of different time intervals is determined by the natural history of breast cancer—that is, the interval between initial detectability and the development of obvious signs and symptoms of breast cancer. The longer this "preclinical interval," the greater the chance for effective lengthening of the screening interval.

The actual effect of screening frequency varies considerably depending on the woman's age. At age 40 to 50 years, the preclinical interval appears to be short (less than 2 years). The 2-year screening interval used in Sweden has shown no beneficial effect on mortality in women 40 to 50 years of age after 6 years. If screening is to be done for those under 50 years of age, it should be done annually.

In women over 50 years of age the preclinical interval appears longer, so that the degree of effectiveness retained would be considerably better than the worst case in younger women. A 2-year interval between screens may not diminish screening effectiveness in this age group.[87]

Moskowitz advocates that younger patients receive more frequent mammographic screenings and that patients over 50 years of age receive less frequent mammographic screening. Biannual mammography in patients over 50 years of age is the present Karolinska approach. They do not perform screening mammographies in patients younger than 50 years of age. The probable yield is not considered sufficiently high to warrant earlier mammograms, although it is well recognized that earlier detection in younger patients will also aid in curing this disease.

Race. One problem in evaluating race as a risk factor for breast cancer is that race so often correlates with geography, diet, and social class. These related factors may interact in a complex way to affect the risk of breast cancer.[206] The issues of social class, geography, and dietary factors have been evaluated in many studies designed to assess the contribution of race to the risk for breast cancer. An interesting anecdote relates to finding that male breast cancer occurs more often in Jewish males. Mabuchi et al. studied 52 histologically diagnosed cases of male breast cancer and matched 52 controls for age, race, marital status, and hospital.[190] Their observations suggested a racial (Jewish) predisposition for testicular carcinoma and male breast cancer. The racial differences in breast cancer are generally felt to be on the genetic or familial basis. Indeed, the racial differences in population genetics are well recognized.[180]

Bondy et al. studied the ethnic differences in familial breast cancer and noted that there is relatively little data on the familial patterns of breast cancer in minority populations.[41] They did a case control study of first-degree relatives of black, white, and Hispanic breast cancer patients. They observed no overall increased cancer risk for the relatives of black women with breast cancer when compared

to relatives of white women with breast cancer. Both races had a similar standardized risk factor. However, the familial risk factor for Hispanics was somewhat less—that is, having a relative with breast cancer did not yield the same degree of risk for Hispanic women as it did both black and white women. They found a standardized incidence ratio of 12 for both black and white patients who had a first-degree relative with breast cancer. In blacks the risk was markedly increased if the diagnosis was made when the family member was less than 45 years of age. In those patients the standardized incidence ratio increased to 61.7 (CI of 12.4 to 180.4). That means that black patients who have a family member under 45 years of age with breast cancer have a higher risk of breast cancer than either whites or hispanics in a similar situation. This may be related to the unexplained racial crossover in cancer incidence rates between white and black women. Incidence crossover means that, in women over 40 years of age, the breast cancer incidence is higher in white Americans than in black Americans; under 40 years of age, the breast cancer incidence is higher in black Americans.

As can be seen in Fig. 2-4, the incidence of breast cancer is higher in premenopausal blacks and in postmenopausal whites. This relative incidence crosses over between 40 and 45 years. Thus, in this instance, breast cancer seems to be a different disease in black than in white women. Perhaps this is related to Clemmensen's hook, which is discussed later in this chapter.

Krieger relates this crossover to differences in social class.[168] Using the San Francisco Cancer Control Registry, Krieger demonstrated that the risk of breast cancer in younger black women was correlated with social class (Table 2-7). Why do younger black women get more breast cancer? Perhaps it is not entirely based on genetic predisposition. The crossover phenomenon is important to the understanding of the role of risk factors in breast cancer diagnosis and breast cancer etiologic factors. Risk factors other than race contribute to these findings. Krieger speculates that induced abortion and oral contraceptive use before the first full-term pregnancy are possible factors.

Age-related crossover in the incidence of breast cancer has also been observed in the factors of marital status, sex

Table 2-7. Racial crossover and social class

	Black/white incidence ratio	
	<40 yr	**>40 yr**
Working class	1.08 (.74-1.56)*	0.78 (0.68-0.89)
Nonworking class	1.96 (1.17-3.26)	0.98 (0.78-1.23)

From Krieger N. *Am J Epidemiol* 131:804-814, 1990.
* = 95% CI.

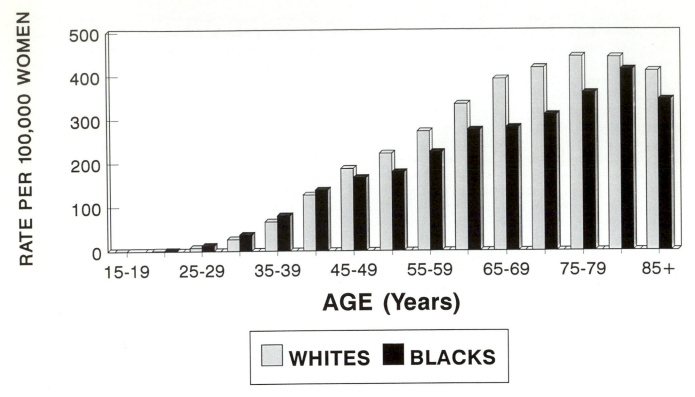

Fig. 2-4. Average annual breast cancer incidence rates per 100,000 women. (Based on data from the National Cancer Institute's Surveillance, Epidemiology and End Results (SEER) Program, 1983-1987.)

of the first child, and race. Janerich and Hoff used incidence data to show the presence of an excessive number of married women among the breast cancer cases, compared to other cancers, until approximately 40 years of age.[153] Their study revealed that, after 40 years of age, single women exhibited a higher incidence of breast cancer. They also noted an additional crossover risk factor. The sex of the first offspring had an effect on the survival of breast cancer patients. Breast cancer patients who were less than 45 years of age and whose first child was a female had a longer survival. Breast cancer patients who were over 45 years of age had a longer survival if their first child was a male. These preliminary observations need to be substantiated by a larger series. Multiple types of crossovers that are age dependent and, in part, race dependent may, in fact, be related to cultural or social differences. The crossover effect may be the result of premenopausal breast cancer being a different disease than postmenopausal breast cancer. If breast cancer is really two separate diseases, each disease may have different risk factors, biology, prognosis, diagnostic criteria, and therapeutic responses. Perhaps the only things in common between these two diseases are a common pathology and a common name— *breast cancer*. Further refinement in descriptive breast

cancer taxonomy may reveal a number of different diseases defined by attributes not limited to histology.

Schwartz et al. have shown a remarkable racial difference in patients with multiple primary cancers in a study of black and white residents of metropolitan Detroit.[265] In women with a history of breast cancer, black women experienced a higher risk of subsequent breast cancer than white women. The standard incidence ratio in blacks was 5.3, whereas in whites it was 3.6. The incidence ratio was considerably higher again in black women diagnosed before the age of 40 years; the standard incidence rate for blacks was 26.15, whereas for whites it was 10.87. These incidences of subsequent cancer occurred within 5 years of the initial diagnosis. This supports a contention that young black women are especially prone to develop a second primary breast cancer once an initial cancer is defined. In South Africa, blacks with breast cancer are seen at a younger age than whites.[218] These younger blacks in South Africa who developed breast cancer are more likely to have advanced disease. The opposite was seen in a study of breast cancer epidemiology in New York City. Black women in New York were twice as likely to develop minimal, as compared with clinical, breast cancer.[84] There is no doubt that some family-related breast cancers do occur in blacks, although there have been relatively few family histories of breast cancer published among minorities. Siraganian et al. did report on two black families with excesses of breast cancer.[282]

As far back as 1979, Austin et al. attempted to study the breast cancer risk in black Americans.[17] They noted that the incidence rate for breast cancer in younger blacks increased from 1947 to 1979. They state that, in 1979, it was similar to that of younger whites. This may be due to some cultural differences and may, in part, relate to the crossover evidence discussed above. The authors sought to explain the distinction between the incidence of breast cancer in younger and older blacks, suggesting it was related to common exposure to potential carcinogens between black and white patients born since about 1925. The possibility that the etiologic agents are either dietary or environmental factors poses interesting questions about racial predispositions for breast cancer.

A fascinating and intensely investigated racial variation for breast cancer was found in Hawaiian studies. Goodman et al. studied the breast cancer incidence in this multiethnic population.[109] The Hawaiian perspective provides an excellent opportunity to study the implications of racially dependent breast cancer incidences (Table 2-8).

Goodman notes that the Japanese in Hawaii have less postmenopausal breast cancer than Caucasians. Indeed, in Hawaii a woman of Japanese descent has a 50% less chance of developing breast cancer as compared with a white woman. Japanese women have fewer axillary lymph node metastases and their cancers are less invasive. Once the diagnosis is made, the risk of death in Chinese, Japanese, and white women is similar for the same stage of disease. However, Filipino and ethnic Hawaiian women have a considerably higher risk of death—1.5 to 1.7 times that of whites. In Hawaii, only 14% of the population studied was foreign born.

Other studies have attempted to assess the impact of dietary changes on the geographic increase in breast cancer incidence. This has been especially noted in Japanese women who immigrated to the United States. Nomura et al. studied the effect of dietary fat on breast cancer in Caucasian and Japanese women in Hawaii.[224] They used case control methods in breast cancer patients. Obese patients and those with a high fat intake had an increased risk of

dying from breast cancer once breast cancer was detected. This did not differ between the Japanese and white patients. Le Marchand observed that the better survival of Japanese patients with breast cancer in part may be due to the lower mean body weight and less dietary fat.[175]

Asians of lower body weight have a lower incidence of breast cancer; this lower incidence has also been seen in studies of other races. Barker observed that persons born in India, Pakistan, and Bangladesh had a lower incidence of breast cancer; however, this incidence increased toward the non-Asian level because of exposure to some risk factors. Perhaps these, too, were dietary in origin. Using the American College of Surgeons' Breast Cancer Survey, Natarajan et al. observed that Oriental patients with breast cancer were significantly younger than white women.[220] They had more localized breast cancer and a higher percentage of negative nodes compared with white patients. Nomura et al. studied breast cancer patients in Hawaii and observed that the standard risk factors, such as family history and late menopause, did not account for the difference in risk between Japanese and white women.[223] They emphasized the needs to focus attention on other environmental causes. Specifically, most attention has been given to the differences between the Japanese and standard U.S. diet. Rose studied migrating populations in an effort to assess the impact of diet on breast cancer.[249] He notes that, in Japanese women, each succeeding generation in the United States assumes an increased risk for breast cancer, and eventually they approach the breast cancer risk of white women. A contribution to this growth in breast cancer risk as progressive generations of Japanese women become integrated into American society seems related to fat consumption and the progression of obesity. Hill et al. emphasized the role of the dietary factors as possible etiologic agents in the increased risk of breast cancer as Asian women become westernized.[134] They conclude that such dietary factors may alter hormone metabolism and thereby alter breast cancer risks. Thus the link between racial risk for breast cancer and hormonal and dietary influences must be considered together as one attempts to appreciate the implications of these various risk factors. Although race may be an important risk factor, it appears that it is considerably more important when associated with the social situation and dietary habits of various races. That is not to

Table 2-8. Breast cancer in the multiethnic Hawaiian population

	White	Hawaiian	Chinese	Japanese	Filipino
Incidence	1.056	1.043	.641	.513	.292
Relative risk (RR)	1.00	0.99	0.61	0.49	0.48

From Goodman MJ: *Breast Cancer Res Treat* 18(suppl 1):S5-9, 1991.

say there is no genetic linkage in racial-based breast cancer incidence, but dietary and other factors may have an important effect on risk rates.

These epidemiologic studies have added to our understanding of breast cancer carcinogenesis. Croghan used a case control study to test the role of family history of breast cancer and high fat intake as co-risks.[72] She matched breast cancer cases from Roswell Park Memorial Institute to randomly selected females. There was no interaction for fat intake and family history of breast cancer. In this study both factors independently increased the risk of breast cancer. Hirohata et al., using a case control study between Japanese and white women in Hawaii, found no statistical difference between cases and controls in relation to total fat, saturated fat, linoleic acid, animal protein, and cholesterol.[136] Their case control study was consistent with others that did not support the hypothesis that a high-fat diet alone is a risk factor for breast cancer. Obviously, the influence of a fatty diet, social status, obesity, and race on the incidence of breast cancer is not yet clear.

Family history. A family history of breast cancer is a major risk factor for this disease. This risk depends on how many first-degree relatives have breast cancer and the age at which they were affected. It also depends on whether the disease was unilateral or bilateral.

Of women with breast cancer, 13.6% have at least one first-degree relative with the disease, whereas only 7.8% of women who do not have breast cancer have first-degree relatives with the disease. First-degree relatives are defined as the mother, sister, or daughter of the patient. A second-degree relative is an aunt or grandmother of the patient. The incidence in other relatives is usually not included as a risk factor for breast cancer in analyses of family history. In studying family histories as they affect breast cancer incidence rates, it appears that, in 5% of breast cancer cases, a true genetic syndrome of the disease can be demonstrated.[311]

Helmrich et al. used a hospital-based case control study involving 1185 women with breast cancer and 3227 controls to reveal a 2.9 relative risk (CI of 2.2 to 3.9) for breast cancer in women with a family history of breast cancer in a first-degree relative.[127] They did not segment the analysis by the age of either the patient or her relative when the cancer was diagnosed.

Sattin et al. studied the effect of family history on the risk for breast cancer in patients and controls involved in

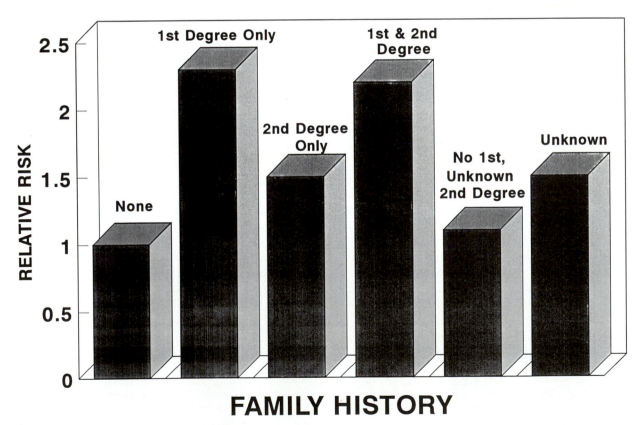

Fig. 2-5. Risk of breast cancer by family history of breast cancer. (From Sattin et al: *JAMA* 253:1908-1913, 1985.)

the cancer and steroid hormone study coordinated by the Division of Reproductive Health of the Centers for Disease Control.[257] This was done in collaboration with the surveillance, epidemiology, and end-results (SEER) centers of the National Cancer Institute.

Fig. 2-5 displays the risk of breast cancer in relationship to family history, as determined in this population of patients and controls. In this study 4735 patients with cancer were matched to 4688 controls. Of the cancer patients, 456 had first-degree relatives with breast cancer, whereas first-degree relatives with cancer were evident in only 231 of the controls. This amounts to a relative risk of 2.3 (95% CI of 1.9 to 2.7). Of the breast cancer patients, 741 had second-degree relatives with breast cancer (versus 569 second-degree relatives in the controls) for a relative risk of 1.5 (CI of 1.4 to 1.8). Having both a first- and second-degree relative with breast cancer occurred in 79 of the breast cancer patients (only 42 of the control cases) for a relative risk of 2.2 (CI of 1.5 to 3.3). The addition of a second-degree relative and a first-degree relative with cancer did not increase the relative risk above that which was seen when only a first-degree relative had breast cancer. In this study it did not make much difference whether the first-degree relative was a mother or a sister. Of the breast cancer patients, 364 had a mother with breast cancer, whereas only 196 of the controls had a mother with breast

cancer. This amounts to a relative risk of 2.1 (CI of 1.7 to 2.6). There were fewer sisters with breast cancer than there were mothers; 74 of the breast cancer patients had sisters with breast cancer, and 36 of the control patients had sisters with breast cancer, giving a relative risk of 2.1 (CI 1.5 to 2.8). However, if both the mother and the sister had breast cancer, the relative risk jumped substantially. In 35 instances breast cancer patients had both a mother and a sister who had breast cancer. This was seen in only 3 of 4688 control patients. The relative risk from having both a mother and a sister with breast cancer was 13.6 (4.1 to 44.8). Thus, if both a mother and a sister have breast cancer, the probability of getting breast cancer is 6.5 times greater and significantly different ($P < .005$) than if only a mother or a sister had breast cancer. Relative risks calculated in all of the instances were adjusted for age, area of residence, age at first full-term pregnancy, menopausal status, and a history of benign breast disease.

Sattin et al. and others have observed a substantial age-dependent effect on the family history risk for breast cancer.[257] Fig. 2-6 shows the estimated annual incidence rate per 100,000 women in relation to the age at which breast cancer will be found in a first- or second-degree relative with breast cancer. The annual incidence at ages 20 to 39 years is 17.3 (CI of 16.2 to 18.5) if there is no family history of breast cancer. However, the incidence increases to

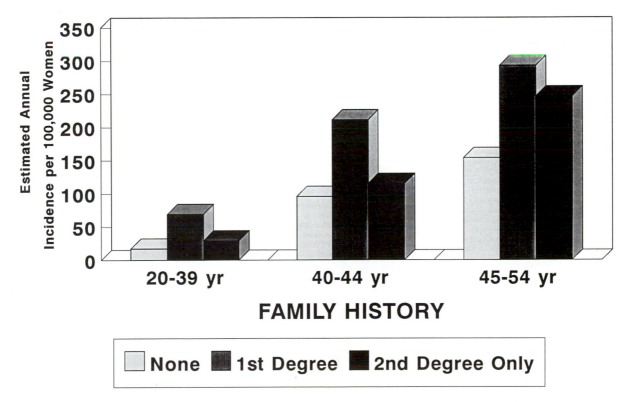

Fig. 2-6. Family history and breast cancer risk incidence estimates. (From Sattin et al: *JAMA* 253:1908-1913, 1985; and Neutra RR, Drolette ME: *Am J Epidemiol* 108:214-222, 1978.)

69.2 (CI of 45.7 to 104.7) with a first-degree relative with breast cancer and to 29.4 (CI 24.3 to 35.6) with a second-degree relative having breast cancer. At age 40 to 44 years the contribution of a family history of cancer to risk for breast cancer is somewhat less. Even though the relative risk contribution from such a family history is less, the annual incidence substantially increases with age. If there is no family history of breast cancer by ages 40 to 44 years, the authors found a 95.9 annual incidence per 100,000 women (CI of 87.7 to 104.9), whereas when a first-degree relative had cancer, they found an incidence of 211.0 (CI of 151.0 to 294.7), and when a second-degree relative had cancer, they found an incidence of 115.1 (CI of 92 to 144). Similarly, in the group between 45 and 54 years of age, the contribution of risk from a family history of breast cancer is less relatively, but the annual incidence of breast cancer per 100,000 women is more. If there is no family history of breast cancer by age 45 to 54 years, the incidence is 154 (CI of 145.7 to 162.8). However, when a first-degree relative has cancer, this incidence increases to 292.6 (CI of 246.2 to 347.7), and when a second-degree relative has cancer, it goes to 246.4 (CI of 214.3 to 283.3).

Compare Fig. 2-7, which displays the relative risks, with Fig. 2-6, which displays the absolute incidences. At 20 to 39 years of age the relative risk is 4 when a first-degree relative has cancer and 1.7 when a second-degree relative has cancer. For women 40 to 44 years of age who have a first-degree relative with breast cancer, the breast cancer risk increases by only 2.2, and in those who have a second-degree relative with cancer, it increases by only 1.1. For women 45 to 54 years of age who have a first-degree relative with breast cancer the risk of cancer increases by only 1.9 and with a second-degree relative with cancer the risk increase is 1.6. Patients are more likely to have breast cancer at a younger age than they would without a family history of breast cancer. Sattin et al. point out that the effect of having a second-degree relative with cancer should be interpreted cautiously because it is possible that patients do not accurately remember cancer treatment for grandmothers or aunts as well as they would have in their mother or sister.[257] However, there is no reason to suggest that the failure to remember in this study was any more or less than in routine history taking at the time of mammography. The calculated relative risks should be similar to those expected in clinical practice.

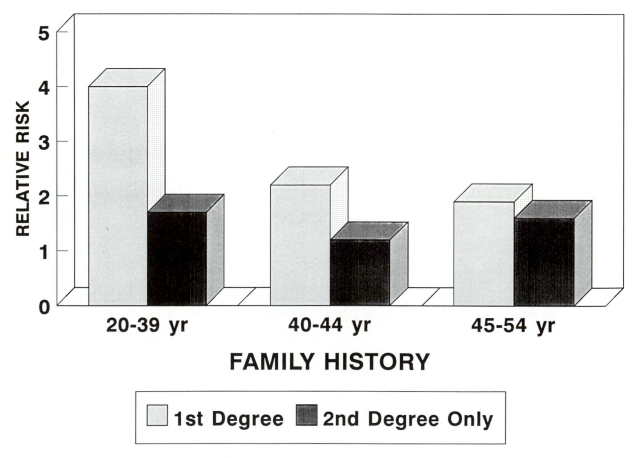

Fig. 2-7. Family history and breast cancer risk. (From Sattin et al: *JAMA* 253:1908-1913, 1985; and Neutra RR, Drolette ME: *Am J Epidemiol* 108:214-222, 1978.)

Obviously, this study strongly supports the notion that women with both a mother and a sister with breast cancer should be especially closely monitored by their physician. They estimate that in the 20 to 54 years of age group, the incidence of breast cancer in a woman with a mother and sister with breast cancer increases to a high of 8.28 cases (CL of 2.49 to 27.17) per 100,000 women from a low of 60.9 cases (CL of 58.6 to 63.3) in women without a family history of breast cancer.

Anderson observed a marked increase in the risk of breast cancer for women if a first-degree relative had bilateral rather than unilateral disease.[8] Sattin et al.'s study was unable to confirm this observation. Sattin et al. found an increased risk of breast cancer in women with either unilateral or bilateral disease.

Fig. 2-7 reveals that a woman is more likely to get breast cancer at a younger age if she has a first- or second-degree relative with breast cancer. The risk for breast cancer is, in part, related to the age when the relative's breast cancer was diagnosed. The risk for breast cancer is significantly less if a relative was diagnosed with breast cancer in a perimenopausal age group.

As seen in Fig. 2-8, the effect of a first-degree family history of breast cancer on the risk of developing breast cancer is less in the perimenopausal than in the premeno-pausal or postmenopausal woman. The risk associated with having a second-degree relative with breast cancer was not significantly influenced by the menopausal status. The basis for this perimenopausal decrease in family risk from breast cancer is not well understood. Sattin et al. conclude that the basis for this perimenopausal effect is unclear and may be due to chance, but it obviously warrants further research.[257] Other perimenopausal effects on the incidence of breast cancer have long been recognized. The incidence of breast cancer increases with age until menopause when the age effect on incidence diminishes, only to reappear after menopause. This "Clemmensen's hook" in age-dependent increases in the incidence of breast cancer is further discussed later in this chapter.

Genetic basis for breast cancer. It is not known how a family history of breast disease affects the risk of a woman developing breast cancer. However, in some families it is transmitted recessively and in others there may be an autosomal dominant trait. In 5% of breast cancer cases a true genetic syndrome of the breast cancer transmission can be demonstrated. Some genetically based breast cancer has been related to a locus involving two genes on chromosome 17p. Although racial and family history variations in the breast cancer incidence may have some environmental basis, they are primarily genetic in origin.

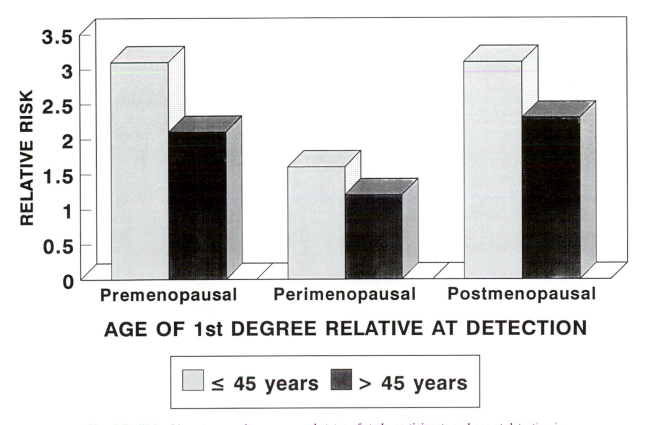

Fig. 2-8. Risk of breast cancer by menopausal status of study participants and age at detection in first-degree relatives. (From Sattin et al: *JAMA* 253:1908-1913, 1985.)

Goldstein et al. used segregation analyses in white patients from a cancer and steroid hormone study and found heterogeneity in the transmission of breast cancer.[111] They were unable to find evidence for a multifactorial component, such as a genetic and cultural basis for breast cancer incidence. Rather, their analysis revealed that, when cancer involved the entire ductal system, the transmission was consistent with an autosomal recessive trait. In this subanalysis, a recessive gene was sufficient to explain the breast cancer distribution when the patient had postmenopausal breast cancer. In contrast, however, when the patient had premenopausal breast cancer, the model was consistent with the dominant major gene and occasional sporadic cases of the disease.

In some families, breast cancer seems to be inherited by simple autosomal dominant transmission.[189,221] Studies on these high-risk families are important because genetic analysis of cancer susceptibility has made it possible to map genes for other selected neoplasms (e.g., retroblastoma). In some high-risk families, the probability of a woman having breast cancer by the age of 65 years approaches 50%. Newman used complex segregation analysis in a population-based study series of families to reveal that susceptibility was present in only 4% of the families.[221] He advocates using these high-risk families as models for studying breast cancer as a whole, which could potentially leading to a mapping of the responsible genes, at least in this subset of breast cancers. The analysis suggests that the etiologic factors of breast cancer in these patients may be analogous to the dual chromosome status evident in the retinoblastomas and Wilms' tumor.

Recently, there has been a virtual explosion of insight into the potential of genetic aspects for risk and analysis of families with breast carcinoma. Studies with human tumor cells revealed that the gene encoding p53, a 53-kilodalton cellular protein, was frequently mutated in human tumor cells. This suggested a role for this gene in human oncogenesis. Chen et al. demonstrated that mutation of two alleles of the p53 gene were essential for its role in oncogenesis.[59] They used exogenous p53 genes to suppress the neoplastic expression of a human osteosarcoma cell line.

Malkin et al. demonstrated that the p53 gene was mutated in a familial syndrome that is associated with breast cancer, sarcomas, and other neoplasms.[194] This Li-Fraumeni syndrome was discovered in 1969 by Li and Fraumeni in a review of 648 childhood rhabdomyosarcoma patients. They identified four families in which siblings or cousins had a childhood sarcoma. Malkin reported breast carcinoma in three of five families with this syndrome. The frequency of invasive carcinoma in individuals with the syndrome reaches almost 50% by 30 years of age when only 1% of the general population have cancer. It is estimated that over 90% of the gene carriers will develop cancer by 70 years of age. These cancers cannot be distinguished from cancers that are not associated with the gene. It is unknown how many of the general population carry the p53 mutations. Clearly the Li-Fraumeni syndrome is a rare lesion. It does, however, provide insight that some breast cancers are due to a genetic defect. Coles et al. used blood leukocyte samples in a larger series of breast cancer patients to map regions that lost heterozygosity on chromosome 17.[70] The structural gene p53 is located on this chromosome. They demonstrated distinct regions of the loss of heterozygosity in bands p13-3 and p13-1. Coles et al. conclude that lesions of this regulatory gene seemed to be involved in the majority of breast cancers.[70] Whereas the Li-Fraumeni syndrome is rare, some genetic basis enhancing the susceptibility to breast carcinoma seems to be rather common. Some breast cancers may be the result of a genetic alteration of somatic cells of the breast. These may involve the p53 locus.

Hall et al. linked early-onset familial breast cancer to chromosome 17q21.[120] This gene seems to be related to the inherited susceptibility to breast cancer in some families with early-onset disease. They based their analysis on 23 extended families with 146 cases of breast cancer, which was diagnosed early in both breasts or in male family members. A genetic analysis of 329 people in these families showed that the region of chromosome 17, which is ordinarily genetically variable, was similar among the family members associated with the breast cancers.

Claus et al. used segregation analysis of the patients and the controls involved in a cancer and steroid study.[65] They found evidence of a rare autosomal dominant allele (q = .0033) that led to an increased susceptibility to breast cancer. This susceptibility appeared to be a function of a woman's age. Although carriers of this gene are at greater risk at all ages, the risk is greatest during youth, and declines steadily thereafter. They estimate that among breast cancer patients aged 20 to 29 years, 36% carry this allele. This decreases to approximately 1% among breast cancer patients 80 years of age and older. Claus et al. have estimated that the cumulative lifetime risk for breast cancer approaches 92% in individuals with this allele, in contradistinction to the cumulative lifetime risk for noncarriers of approximately 10%.[65]

Skolnick et al. went further in analyzing the inheritance of the disease.[286] They used four-quadrant fine-needle aspiration cytology in women who have at least two first-degree relatives with breast cancer. These women had normal mammograms and normal clinical examinations. Of these clinically normal, female first-degree relatives of breast cancer patients, 35% had cytologic analysis that revealed proliferative breast disease, a well-recognized risk factor for breast cancer (see the section on p. 37). Although the finding of a genetically correlated prospective precursor of breast cancer is important, it is not yet possible to clearly define the genetic basis of this relationship, inasmuch as many of these patients will not get breast cancer. This research, however, does suggest that it may be possible to identify women at high risk for breast cancer either by analyzing peripheral blood cells for abnormalities of chromosome 17[70] or by sampling with fine-needle aspiration the breasts of patients who are known to have a strong family history for breast cancer.[70] These encouraging observations have led Vogel to suggest that it may be possible to provide a useful clinical assay for women at risk.[310] The ethical and other issues related to this have caused some problems. Vogel is so optimistic as to suggest that "deaths from breast cancer are, at least in theory, totally preventable. The trick is to identify the patients at risk."[328] This level of optimism, although encouraging, requires considerable further research and development to become a reasonable prospect.

Prior breast cancer. In an early study comparing cancerous versus noncancerous breasts Foote and Stewart asserted that "the most frequent antecedent of cancer in one breast is a history of having that cancer in the opposite breast."[103] The earliest demonstrations of mammographic use in diagnosing a second primary cancer were published by Byrne et al. who studied 102 postmastectomy patients every 6 months for 14 years.[53] They noted eight carcinomas in the remaining breasts, six of which were not palpable at the time of mammographic detection.

It is well established that a woman who has a history of cancer in one breast is at increased risk for cancer in the other breast. Many studies have sought to identify the exact risk of a second primary cancer in the opposite breast. Synchronous or simultaneous second primary cancers have been defined variously as a tumor diagnosed within a specified time of the first primary cancer or during the treatment of the first primary cancer. Most authors define a synchronous primary cancer in the contralateral breast as any tumor in the contralateral breast that is diagnosed within 6 months of the first primary cancer. Therefore asynchronous primary cancers are other tumors diagnosed at some later time. The advent of mammography has increased the proportion of second synchronous tumors (versus asynchronous). Obviously, this change in distribution is due to mammography's ability to detect the second primary cancer, sometimes long before it would have become clinically apparent. The frequency of a second primary cancer identified in the opposite breast, usually by mammography in recent studies, is demonstrated on Table 2-9.

In addition to the frequency of a simultaneous second primary cancer varying with the diagnostic method used, the interval between the first and second asynchronous primary cancer varies with the diagnostic method. In an interesting study from Holland, a group in Nijmengen used mammography to screen the remaining breast in patients following mastectomy, whereas a group in Eindhoven observed a similar number of patients without mammography. The interval between the first and second cancers, when they did occur in the opposite breast, had a mean of 34 months for the Nijmengen series (CI of 11 to 106) and a mean of 39 months for the series in (CI of 7 to 108) in Eindhoven.[204] Similarly, Senofsky et al., using a retrospective study from the University of Virginia Hospital, attempted to appraise the effect of mammography by separating patients into a group of contralateral breast cancers diagnosed before effective mammographic monitoring and a group diagnosed after effective mammographic monitoring.[269] Those diagnosed before effective mammographic monitoring had an average interval of 56 months from the original cancer until the second primary cancer, whereas those diagnosed after mammographic monitoring came into vogue had an average interval of 30 months.

Senofsky et al. sought to discover whether monitoring of the contralateral breast improved the prognosis for patients with primary breast cancer.[269] They had a similar number of patients in each group. The 33 patients before routine mammography (1969 to 1975) were compared with the 38 patients diagnosed after routine mammography was instituted (1977 to 1984). This study showed that 6.65% of the patients with primary cancer in the premammography era developed contralateral breast cancer, compared

Table 2-9. Incidence of second primary cancer and frequency of simultaneity

Reference	Incidence of second primary cancer (per 1000 women yr)	Frequency of "simultaneous" second primary cancer (%)
Prior and Waterhouse (1978)	4.4	0.4
Mueller and Ames (1978)	8-10 (to at least 15 yr)	0.9
Haagensen (1971)	5.8	0.6
Robbins and Berg (1964)	7.1 (to at least 20 yr)	0.3
Fukami et al. (1977)	3.4 (to at least 18 yr)	0.7
Schottenfeld and Berg (1971)	6.1	0.6
McCredie et al. (1975)	Approximately 10 (to at least 15 yr)	0.3
Hislop (1984)	3.8 (to at least 15 yr)	0.7

From Hislop TG et al: *Br J Cancer* 49:79-85, 1984.

Table 2-10. Stage of second breast cancer

Stage	Premammography monitoring (33 patients)	With mammography monitoring (32 patients)
0	6.1%	40.6%
I	51.5%	28.1%
II	6.1%	18.7%
III	21.2%	9.4%
IV	15.1%	3.2%

From Senofsky GM et al: *Cancer* 57:597-692, 1986.

with 6.79% of the patients after mammography was being used. The frequency of second primary cancers was similar in both eras. The proportion of synchronous tumors increased substantially with the use of mammography. In the premammography group only 15.2% of the contralateral breast cancers were diagnosed in a time closely related to the primary breast tumor. With the use of mammography, this increased to 28.1%. They also studied the use of a blind contralateral biopsy, which increased the frequency with which the second tumor was diagnosed at the time of the primary tumor to 39.5% (Table 2-10). The stage at which the second primary cancer was diagnosed was markedly affected by use of mammography. This use of mammography substantially increased the earlier detection of nonpalpable breast cancer.

The sensitivity of mammography in detecting second primary tumors in the contralateral breast is slightly less than the sensitivity of mammographic detection of the initial carcinoma in a screening population. In the series of Senofsky et al., 26% of the second breast cancers were missed on mammography. This is not dissimilar to the number of Mellink et al.; they found that 29% were missed on mammography and identified at clinical examination.[204] In screening series the frequency of false-negative mammograms in women with palpable cancers ranges from 11% to 17%. Thus, in seeking to diagnose cancer in the contralateral breast, mammography must be complemented by clinical examination. The routine use of blind contralateral biopsies is not recommended. When "cancer" is found, it usually is lobular carcinoma in situ (LCIS). These should not be included in calculation of clinical or mammographic diagnostic sensitivity. The clinical use of this diagnosis clearly differs from the diagnosis of invasive carcinoma or even ductal carcinoma in situ (DCIS) (see the section on The Cost and Benefit of Screening Mammography).

The risk of developing a second primary tumor is clearly related to other risk factors that influence the incidence of breast cancer. Horn et al. used the Connecticut Tumor Registry to study 338 cases of contralateral breast cancer diagnosed between 1979 and 1982.[141] Using a matched, randomly selected control study, they observed a significantly increased risk in women whose initial cancer was lobular carcinoma and during the first year following the diagnosis of the primary cancer. This increased incidence during the first year is related in part to combining the synchronous and asynchronous cancer in this group. Risk of second primary breast cancers primarily depends on the age at which the initial breast cancer diagnosis was made, the family history, and the histologic assessment (i.e., lobular carcinoma). Prior and Waterhouse defined the relative risk of a second primary breast tumor in relation to age at the first primary tumor (Fig. 2-9).[241] If the initial primary tumor was premenopausal, there is a greater probability of developing a second primary tumor. This probability decreases sharply as postmenopausal breast cancers develop. Thus *contralateral breast cancer is a disease that occurs primarily in patients with premenopausal breast cancer and a family history of breast cancer.*

Adami et al. calculated a cumulative risk of 13.3% for women whose primary breast cancer was diagnosed before 50 years of age and 3.5% for women whose cancer was diagnosed after 50 years of age.[2] They suggest that the occurrence of bilateral disease reflects a "multicentric neoplastic transformation of the breast epithelium, which is characteristic of early-occurring (premenopausal) disease." The risk for a second primary tumor is primarily related to the age of the patient at the diagnosis of the first primary. There is an effect of race on the risk for a second primary tumor.[265] Black women are more likely to develop a second primary tumor than are white women (RR = 1.47). This racial preponderance is even greater in women diagnosed before the age of 40 years (RR = 2.41).

The rate at which second primary cancers occur decreases in a linear fashion from the onset of the initial primary tumor, with a mean time of some 30 months and using mammography as the diagnostic criterion. There is a second high-risk group that appears at a later time and that has been related to radiation treatment of the primary tumor. Although the evidence is not yet convincing, there is a slight suggestion that radiation-induced second primary tumors occur in 10 to 14 years following the initial treatment. The study of Horn et al., using the Connecticut Tumor Registry, found a second peak of contralateral primary increase at 10 to 14 years following the initial treatment of premenopausal breast cancer, after which it declined.[141] Prior and Waterhouse observed a small peak of second primary tumors at 16 years after the initial breast cancer in women treated for premenopausal cancer.[241] The peak fell within a very narrow age range (55 to 59 years of age). They contrasted this with treated postmenopausal cancer, for which there is a much lower risk of a second primary tumor. The overall risk of a second primary tumor in their series was 2 times the risk of a first primary in the general population. When primary tumors are diagnosed

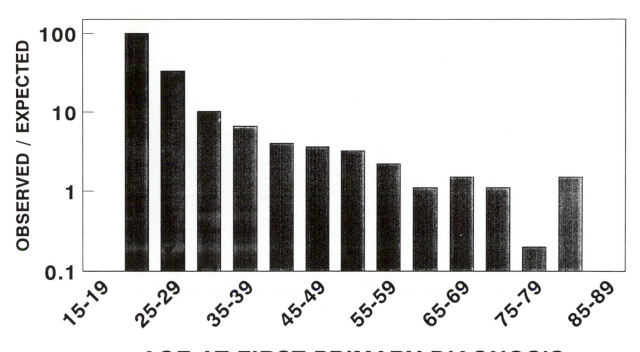

Fig. 2-9. Relative risk of a second primary tumor in breast in relation to age at primary diagnosis. (From Prior, Waterhouse: *Br J Cancer* 34:620, 1978.)

between the ages of 15 and 44 years, the risk is 5.6 times that for the general population; when the initial cancer is diagnosed from 45 to 59 years of age, the risk decreases to 3.76 times; and when the initial cancer is diagnosed after 60 years of age, the risk of a second primary tumor decreases to 1.8 times that seen in the general population.

Late second primary tumors may be related to the treatment of the initial cancer, although this has not been established. Prior and Waterhouse were unable to test this hypothesis.[241] However, radiation therapy for postpartum mastitis has been shown to cause breast cancer.[205]

Benign breast disease. It has long been recognized that a history of a prior benign breast biopsy findings increases the risk for breast cancer. Why is this so? Was the cancer there when the "benign biopsy" specimen was obtained and simply missed? Is benign disease a precursor of cancer in some patients? A problem in obtaining answers to these questions has been a lack of specificity in what has been termed *benign breast disease. Fibrocystic disease* is a common term used in most of the earlier studies intended to address these questions. In their study of risk factors for benign breast disease, Hislop et al. defined the benign breast disease as "comprising fibrocystic disease (such pathologic diagnosis as mammary dysplasia, lobular hyperplasia with evidence of cyst formation, apocrine metaplasia or atypia, collagenosis, fibrosclerosis, interstitial fibrosis, papillomatosis, sclerosing adenosis, and fi-

brosing adenosis), fibroadenoma and intraductal papilloma, but not such conditions as breast abscesses, eczema, or lipoma."[137] In 1988 Grady et al. classified the pathologic types of benign breast disease for the relative risk for cancer and included three categories of fibrocystic disease.[113] One category of fibrocystic disease had no increased risk for breast cancer. In this category they included adenosis, apocrine metaplasia, cyst(s), duct ectasia, fibrosis hyperplasia (mild), and squamous metaplasia. The second category of fibrocystic disease had a slight increased risk for breast cancer; this included the diagnoses of hyperplasia (moderate or florid) and papilloma. Finally, they classified atypical lobular hyperplasia and atypical ductal hyperplasia as fibrocystic disease with a moderate increased risk for breast cancer. These overall pathologic correlates are consistent with the Consensus Conference of the American College of Pathologists.[149,85] The diagnosis of "fibrocystic disease" alone has little merit when attempting to correlate it with a risk for breast cancer. Historically there has been a basis for stating that fibrocystic disease increases the risk for breast cancer, but it depends entirely on whether the pathologic state is proliferative, on whether that proliferation is atypia, and on whether that atypia is associated with a family history of breast cancer.

London et al. used the U.S. Registered Nurses' Prospective Study to assess the relationship of benign breast disease to the risk for breast cancer.[185] They nested a case control study within a prospective cohort, comparing women who had a benign breast biopsy and did not develop cancer with those who had a benign breast and did subsequently develop cancer. The median follow-up after the breast biopsy was 8 years. The relative risk for women who had a benign breast biopsy that revealed proliferative disease without atypia was 1.6 (CI of 1.0 to 2.5). If the woman had atypical hyperplasia, the relative risk increased to 3.7 (CI of 2.1 to 6.8). When the breast cancer was associated with atypical hyperplasia in premenopausal women, the relative risk increased to 5.9 (95% CI of 2.9 to 13.2). In postmenopausal women, however, the relative risk decreased from 5.9 to 2.3 (95% CI of 0.9 to 5.9). This pre- and postmenopausal variation in relative risk was limited to those women who had proliferative disease with atypical hyperplasia. In women who had proliferative disease without atypia there was no relationship to menopausal state in the risk for breast cancer. London et al. question Dupont and Page's correlation of family history with proliferative hyperplasia as risk factors. London et al. note that Dupont and Page's data were obtained retrospectively from the next of kin. This source may have been more completely reported by relatives of women who developed breast cancer than from relatives who did not. Carter et al. attempted to correlate the relationship between atypia and family history.[57] They obtained family history data from questionnaires from all the subjects before the biopsy. Carter et al. studied more patients than did Dupont and Page and did not observe an interaction between the atypia and family history. The difference between the data obtained by DuPont and Page and that obtained by Carter et al. points out some of the difficulties in ascribing risk to a specific condition when multiple conditions may be interacting. The way the data are obtained becomes very important in such risk assessments. Prospective cohort studies failed to demonstrate a synergistic association between family history of breast cancer and the presence of benign breast disease. As risk factors, these are perhaps totally isolated cofactors in the risk for breast cancer.

Some variations of what has been termed *fibrocystic disease,* particularly those that are at a low risk for breast cancer, may be entirely normal. Love et al. ask, "Is it reasonable to define as a disease any process that occurs clinically in 50% of patients and histologically in 90% of women?"[187] Hutter observed, "It is unfortunate that nodularity has been called a 'disease,' rather than a physiology process that may obscure disease" and "Breasts become nodular through cyclic hormonally modulated proliferative activity with incomplete resolution, due to either excess hormonal stimulation, or an exaggerated proliferative response by a hypersensitive breast epithelia."[149] The major

risk for cancer in these "normal" patients is the difficulty of distinguishing multiple benign nodules from a cancerous mass.

As can be seen from the foregoing, the incidence of benign breast disease is difficult to measure. Is the multinodular breast a pathologic condition, or does it represent a normal variant? Goodson et al. observed that routine breast examinations frequently find a difference in palpable densities and palpable nodularity of the breast.[110] They attempted to correlate these observations with high-risk histopathologic states. They found no correlation. Many of these patients had been diagnosed as having fibrocystic disease. These authors, using rigorous criteria for defining palpable nodularity, found no consistent pathologic conditions in excised breasts. Most "fibrocystic conditions" are benign and may indeed be considered a normal variant. Goodson found that 37% of patients with a "fibrocystic condition" had histologic conditions, which indicated an above average risk for cancer. The Consensus Conference of the American College of Pathologists concurs in the histologic risk factor used by Dupont and Page. The presence or absence of Dupont-Page high-risk group does not correlate with palpable nodularity that had been considered evidence of fibrocystic disease.

Ory et al. attempted to define the incidence of benign breast disease in their research, seeking to assess the role of oral contraceptives in reducing the risk of benign disease.[227] Their data and those of others have been based on the frequency with which people had surgery for potential breast cancer that was subsequently shown to be benign. This frequency depends heavily on the local criteria used to select women for surgical breast biopsy (see Chapter 5). A surgical biopsy revealing benign breast disease has formed the basis of the pathologic state called "fibrocystic disease." Vogel used the data of Ory et al. to formulate a theory about the incidence of benign breast disease.[310] He used these data as an indicator to the risk profile in the tamoxifen studies. The data were used in conjunction with Dupont and Page's data on how many patients were found at surgery to have histologic conditions that increased the risk for subsequent breast cancer.

Obviously, Dupont and Page's work formed the basis for much of our understanding today about high-risk histopathologic states, an understanding used to predict which patients will develop breast cancer. All subsequent studies correlating the histopathologic condition of prior breast disease to the incidence of subsequent breast cancer have been based on Dupont and Page's major contribution to our understanding of this field. They studied 10,366 consecutive breast biopsies performed in Nashville, Tennessee. They followed up 3003 of these patients for a 17-year period and correlated the histologic results of the breast biopsies with the ultimate outcome in the course of the pa-

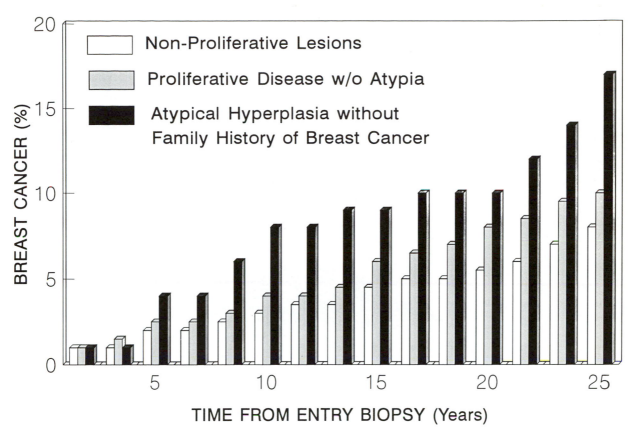

Fig. 2-10. Incidence of invasive breast cancer since time from entry biopsy. (Adapted from Dupont, Page: *N Engl J Med* 312:146-151, 1985.)

tient's disease. *This long-term follow-up provided an unusual insight into the implications of "benign" histology on prognosis* (Fig. 2-10).

In this study population of 3003 women, breast cancer ultimately developed in 134 patients. They found no evidence of an increased risk for breast cancer in women whose biopsy specimens did not reveal proliferative disease. Women who did have a histologic record of proliferative disease had 1.9 times the risk of breast cancer, as compared with the general population. The reference group of the study was a data base obtained from Atlanta, Georgia. The authors extensively studied the various combinations associated with proliferative disease in an effort to assess whether there were conjoint risks involved (e.g., whether calcification was found within the lesion). The relative risk increased from 1.8 to 2.4 in women with proliferative disease, but there was no effect in women who did not have proliferative disease. They found that, in women over 55 years of age who did not have proliferative disease, there was a marked reduction in the relative risk, as compared with women in this age group with proliferative disease. The risk was reduced to 0.3, as compared

with the 2.2 increase found in women over 55 years of age whose breast biopsies revealed proliferative disease. The major finding was that women with both atypia and a family history of breast cancer had an increased risk for developing breast cancer, as compared with women of a similar age without proliferative disease; this increase was only 5.3 for the entire population. In this study, there was a substantial impact on the ultimate incidence of breast cancer when both a family history and atypia were present. Table 2-11 summarizes the effects of age, hyperplasia, family history, and calcification on the risk for breast cancer in patients with known histologic conditions.

Dupont and Page's work provided a unique opportunity to look at the long-term implications, and Figure 2-11 demonstrates that the presence of atypical hyperplasia with a family history of breast cancer substantially increases the risk for breast cancer as long as 20 years from the time of biopsy.

Currently, if one is attempting to appraise the implications of benign breast disease on the risk of breast cancer, the work of Dupont and Page stands as the cornerstone of our knowledge. Their data have formed the basis for the

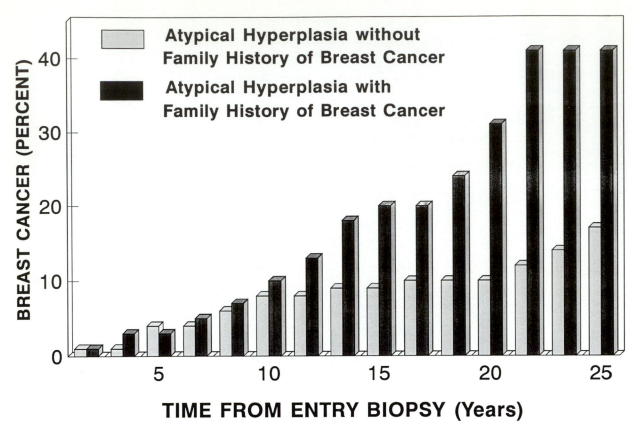

Fig. 2-11. Incidence of invasive breast cancer since time from entry biopsy. (Adapted from Dupont, Page: *N Engl J Med* 312:146-151, 1985.)

Table 2-11. Significant effect of hyperplasia, age, family history, and calcification on the risk for breast cancer

Numerator of relative risk	Denominator of relative risk	Relative risk	95% confidence interval	P value
PDWA	Non-PD	1.9	1.2-2.9	0.003
AH	Non-PD	5.3	3.1-8.8	<0.0001
CAL	No CAL	1.3	0.87-2.0	0.19
PDWA without FH	Non-PD without FH	1.9	1.2-3.0	0.007
PDWA with FH	Non-PD with FH	2.0	0.63-6.1	0.25
PDWA with FH	Non-PD without FH	2.7	1.4-5.3	0.004
AH without FH	Non-PD without FH	4.3	2.4-7.8	<0.0001
AH with FH	Non-PD with FH	8.4	2.6-28.0	0.0003
AH with FH	Non-PD without FH	11	5.5-24.0	<0.0001
PDWA, age 20-45 yr	Non-PD, age 20-45 yr	1.9	1.2-3.2	0.012
PDWA, age 46-55 yr	Non-PD, age 46-55 yr	1.4	0.57-3.3	0.49
PDWA, age >55 yr	Non-PD, age >55 yr	5.6	0.69-46.0	0.11
PDWA with CAL	Non-PD without CAL	2.3	1.2-4.3	0.008
AH with CAl	Non-PD with CAL	8.6	2.5-29.0	0.0006
AH with CAL	Non-PD without CAL	8.3	3.5-19.0	<0.0001

PDWA denotes proliferative disease without atypia; *AH*, atypical hyperplasia; *CAL*, calcification; and *FH*, family history of breast cancer (mother, sister, or daughter). Age refers to the age at the time of the entry biopsy.
Adapted from Dupont WD, Page DL: *New Engl J Med* 312:146-151, 1985.

Consensus Conference of the American College of Pathologists and others who have sought to define more clearly the risk for breast cancer. As of yet, no one has supplanted this research with more current insights into the implications of benign breast disease on the risk for breast cancer.

Mammographic pattern. Obviously, it would be an important advance if variations in the "normal" mammogram could be used to predict the possibility of developing future breast cancer. Wolfe has been the primary proponent of a system in which certain mammographic breast patterns are sought to define those patients at greater risk for breast cancer.[324] Wolfe defined breast parenchymal patterns as follows:

N1—The breast is composed primarily of fat, often with a fine trabeculated appearance.
P1—"Prominent" ducts occupy 25% or less of the breast volume.
P2—"Prominent" ducts occupy more than 25% of the breast volume.
DY—Mammary dysplasia (fibrocystic change) containing sheetlike areas of increased density.

Wolfe reported that the development of subsequent carcinoma over a 3-year period increased 30 fold for patients with DY patterns compared to patients with N1 patterns—that is, the incident increased from 1.45 cases per 1000 women with a N1 pattern to 44.6 cases per 1000 women with a DY pattern. The P1 and P2 patterns were intermediate. P1 had a 3.85 incidence, and P2 had a 17.45 incidence. Wolfe went on to assert that "the radiographic appearance of breast parenchyma provides a method of predicting who will develop breast cancer." This claim has become a highly controversial assertion. Many subsequent studies have sought to ascertain the use of mammographic patterns as a breast cancer risk factor. In our review of the available literature on the subject we reached a conclusion similar to that of Kalisher and McLelland who state that "parenchymal patterns of the breast may be a marker to identify patients at an increased risk for having carcinoma of the breast develop, but this has not been established, nor has it been established to what extent it is useful."[158] A major concern with Wolfe's claim has been his recommendation that these patterns be used to exclude certain women from standard screening. If one limits the screening criteria to certain breast parenchymal patterns, without further supporting data, many cancers that could have been diagnosed earlier may be missed.

However, we do not mean to claim that there is no use for breast parenchymal patterns as a risk factor in breast cancer. There is simply too much literature available supporting a contention that the volume of breast density is related to a risk for breast cancer in some patients.

Is the mammographic parenchymal pattern an independent risk factor for the subsequent development of breast cancer, or is it merely a reflection of another well-defined and more fundamental risk factor (e.g., hormonal status, menstrual history, or even family history)? Do mammographic patterns run in families? One approach to an evaluation of Wolfe's hypothesis is to identify the morphologic factors of this increased breast density and to correlate them to the subsequent development of breast cancer. Attempts to correlate the morphologic increase in breast density with the frequency of atypical ductal or lobular hyperplasia have not been successful.[29] Most authors agree that the radiographic densities of the breast correlate with increased fibrous tissue in the breast. These studies have relied on biopsy materials obtained from women with benign disease or from noncancerous areas of mastectomy specimens removed for carcinoma. Bartow et al. used breast samples obtained from forensic autopsies of otherwise "normal women" to study the prevalence of P2 and DY patterns in relation to the histologic risk factors of breast cancer.[29] They observed that the P2 and DY pattern is strongly affected by age and, to a lesser degree, by race, obesity, breast size, and total parity. They show a correlation between the P2 and DY pattern and the presence of intraductal and epithelial hyperplasia and microcalcification of terminal duct lobular unit epithelium in women over 50 years of age. However, they conclude that "because carcinoma of the breast is so common, a significant number of early cancers may be missed if further screening were suggested solely according to the radiologic characteristics."

Fisher et al. observed that mammographically dense breasts were most likely to contain dense supporting connective tissue without relation to epithelial alterations.[101] However, Wellings and Wolfe found a relationship between epithelial hyperplasia and mammographic patten.[315] They did not consider this relationship strong, however. Urbanski demonstrated a significant association between epithelial atypia, carcinoma in situ, and mammographic "dysplasia."[307] However, this association was weak and could not be reproduced on independent review by other radiologists. Arthur et al. studied the population from the Nottingham Breast Self-Examination Study, part of the U.K. trial for the early detection of breast cancer, which correlated mammographic patterns and histologic risk factors in breast cancer.[15] They concluded that radiographic densities, which are characteristic of Wolfe's four mammographic patterns, are simply the results of variation in fibrous tissue and the intralobular stroma and do not correlate with the proportion of epithelial parenchymal structure. Indeed, the epithelial parenchymal structures were highly variable between women, with no apparent relationship to the mammographic background pattern or histologic fibrous tissue and adipose tissue distribution. Their results demonstrate that any increased risk associated with P2 and DY patterns cannot be attributed to the greater por-

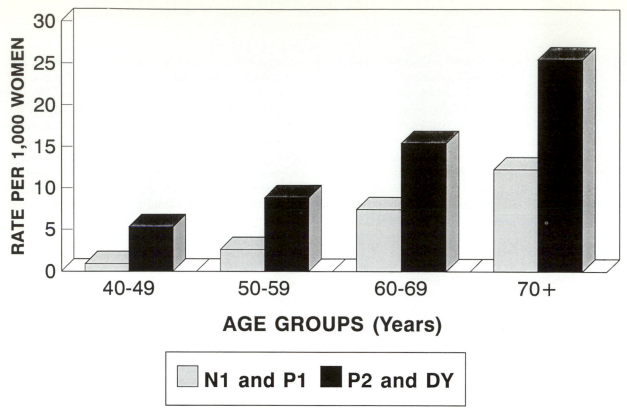

Fig. 2-12. Cancer prevalence based on mammographic parenchymal patterns. (From Tabar et al: *JAMA* 247:185-189, 1982.)

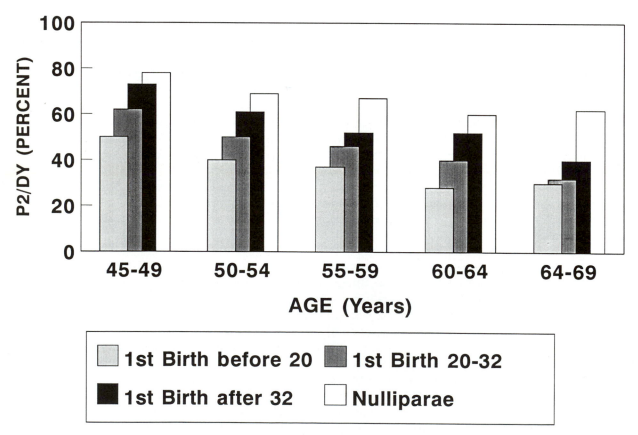

Fig. 2-13. Parenchymal patterns vs age at first birth. (From Andersson et al: *Radiology* 138:59-62, 1981.)

tion of high-risk epithelial abnormalities in the breast. The variations in Wolfe's pattern were due to the ratio of fibrous to adipose tissue in the breast with no apparent relationship to epithelial parenchymal content. These observations, however, do not necessarily dispel the claims of risk associated with P2 and DY patterns. This risk may be independent of the epithelial hyperplasia risk for breast cancer.

Andersson et al. studied the Malmo series of 15,110 women who were randomly selected from those 45- to 59-year-old women living in Malmo.[11] Their observations suggest that the P2 and DY patterns do produce a greater risk for cancer. The percentage of women with P2 and DY patterns correlated with the age of the patient and the age of the woman's first childbirth (Fig. 2-12).

Breast parenchymal patterns may be a correlated risk index of the time of a woman's first childbirth. MacMahon et al. previously estimated that the risk of breast cancer in women whose first childbirth occurred before age 20 years was about 40% of that found in women whose first childbirth occurred at 35 years of age or older and 50% of that found in women who have never had children.[193] Shapiro et al. and Adami et al. were unable to confirm this association.[3,271] Andersson et al. observed decreased P1 and DY patterns with age. This runs contrary to the growing risk of cancer with increasing age.[11] Tabar and Dean found that, when P2 and DY patterns are seen in postmenopausal women, the risk for breast cancer was greater than for premenopausal P2 and DY patterns.[293] Tabar and Dean correlated the mammographic parenchymal patterns with age, age at first pregnancy, and breast cancer detected on the first round of screening (Fig. 2-13).[293] They observed an increased frequency of P2 and DY patterns with advancing age at first pregnancy. They also observed that the incidence of cancer associated with P2 and DY patterns was 5.9 times greater than the incidence associated with N1 and P1 patterns in women 40 to 49 years of age. This incidence increased for older women. The relationship of the P2 and DY patterns to the N1 and P1 patterns for older versus younger women suggests an approximate 15-year displacement to the right. They consider that "this can be interpreted as approximately a 15 year delay in the risk of breast cancer in the N1/P1 group relative to the P2/DY group."

Recently, in an effort to enhance reproducibility in classifying mammographic parenchymal patterns, Saftlas et al. conducted a semiquantitative assessment of parenchymal patterns.[254] They used planimetry to measure the percentage of parenchymal density in relation to the total breast volume. They studied patients from the BCDDP whose mammograms were taken a minimum of 4 years before the development of breast cancer. The initial mammogram was measured using a planimetric assessment of density volume. The densities were classed according to percent-

age of total breast volume. Those with a density between 5% and 29% had breast cancer odds of 1.7. These odds increased to 2.5 with densities of 25% to 44.9% and 3.8 for 44% to 64%. Patients with densities of more than 65% had breast cancer odds of 4.3. The referent population for these assessments was those who had densities of less than 5%. This measurement isolated calcification, biopsy scars, and Cooper's ligaments. Breast masses were not considered in the measurement. The percentage of density was calculated by simply dividing the area with the densities by the total breast area using a planimeter. Table 2-12 reveals the age-adjusted odds ratio against the percentage of densities. The authors were unable to correlate the percentage of densities to other recognized breast cancer risk factors, such as family history and age at first live childbirth. They conclude that the measurement of density percentages provides a better definition of risk and is a positively associated risk factor for the subsequent development of breast cancer. Perhaps one important observation is that a first-degree family history of breast cancer was not a significant risk for postmenopausal women with densities of less than 5%. This essentially means that, if a mammogram reveals a density of less than 5%, a history of breast cancer in a first-degree relative is a less significant risk factor for the development of breast cancer.

They also note that increased body weight was associated with a reduction in the mammographic density percentages and concentrations. A higher body weight leads to a true reduction in the absolute number of mammographic densities. These authors suggest that longitudinal studies are needed to understand more fully the relationship between weight and the percentage of mammographic densities. In their series among control women, mammographic densities decrease with increasing patient age and body weight and the number of live-born children. Tall

Table 2-12. Adjusted breast cancer odds ratios associated with percentage of breast area containing mammographic densities seen in the Breast Cancer Detection and Demonstration Project*(BCDDP)

Densities (%)	Adjusted odds ratio†	95% confidence interval
<5	1.0	Referent
5-24.9	1.7	(1.0-3.1)
25-44.9	2.5	(1.4-4.6)
45-64.9	3.8	(2.0-7.1)
65+	4.3	(2.1-8.8)

From Saftlas AF et al: *Cancer* 67:2833-2838, 1991.
*Unknowns excluded from analysis.
†Simultaneously adjusted for age at entry (continuous variable), weight at entry (<55, 55-59, 60-64, 55-74, and 75+ kg), and number of live childbirths (0, 1, 2, 3, and 4+).

women were more likely than short women to have a high-density breast. Body weight and patient age, however, were the strongest associations with density percentages. The decrease in breast density patterns in obese women, which is associated with a decrease in breast cancer risk, runs counter to the well-recognized role of obesity as a positive risk factor for breast cancer.

The exact role of mammographic parenchymal patterns as risk factors for the subsequent development of breast cancer is uncertain. Clearly, it cannot yet be used to define patient populations at risk sufficiently to warrant changing screening practices. However, further studies, perhaps with more quantitative assessment, may yield greater insight into an additional risk factor for the subsequent development of breast cancer. This work remains to be done.

Obesity. Obesity is a risk factor for breast cancer. This risk may be more closely correlated with breast cancer mortality than with breast cancer incidence. The relative risk for breast cancer reported in obese women is between 2 to 4 times the control population. In many incidents, obesity may act as a co-risk factor. Obesity varies with age, hormonal influence, race, social situation, nutrition, family history, and mammographic patterns. Oken et al. presented a detailed analysis of the relationship that exists between social economic status and obesity changes in women.[225]

The relationship of obesity to the incidence of breast cancer has long been recognized.[75,290] The Statistical Research Division of the American Cancer Society has thoroughly reviewed the variations in mortality by weight.[179] Women who have less than a normal body weight for their age have less than a normal risk for breast cancer. There is a dose-dependent relationship as weight increases above the normal. The more the weight is above a standard, the greater is the risk for breast cancer. Lew and Garfinkel used a weight index that is calculated by dividing the actual weight by the corresponding normative weight for sex, inches of height, and 5-year age group multiplied by 100.[179] This is similar to the Quetelet index, which associates body weight with height and is the predominant measure in epidemiologic studies of body build. Fig. 2-14 reveals the mortality ratios for breast cancer for all ages in the 90% to 109% of average weight groups. Those who are over 140% of their average weight have a mortality ratio for breast cancer 1.53 times above those whose weight is normal. Thus breast cancer mortality is 1.53 times greater than the normal in women whose body weight of more than 140%.

Cohort data from the Framingham Heart Study have been used to study the relation of central to peripheral body fat as an index of breast cancer risk.[26] They calculated a central adiposity ratio from the sum of truncal skinfolds (chest, scapular, and abdomen) divided by the sum of extremity skinfolds (triceps and thigh). In following a

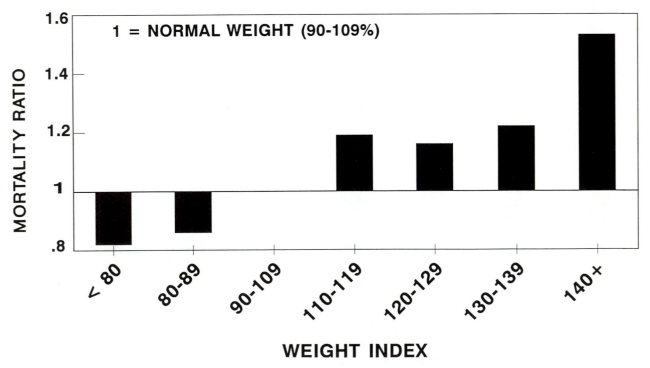

Fig. 2-14. Mortality ratios for breast cancer in relation to female patients 90% to 109% of average weight. (From Lew EA, Garfinkel L: *J Chron Dis* 32:563-576, 1979.)

cohort for up to 28 years, they found 106 cases of breast cancer. Women in the higher quintile of central to peripheral body fat distribution demonstrated an increased risk for breast cancer. This central adiposity ratio was independent of total body weight.

The mechanisms of this relationship between obesity and the incidence of breast cancer are not known. Initially, it was thought that the worldwide incidence differences were (in part) related to dietary differences and specifically dietary fat. The dietary fat hypothesis has been refuted by the work of Willett et al., who studied the nutrition of 89,000 U.S. nurses and observed that there was no relationship between dietary fat and the risk of breast cancer.[320] Mills et al. reached a similar conclusion in a study of the breast cancer incidence in Seventh-Day Adventists.[210] Others have formulated alternative hypotheses. Cole and Crammer observed a moderate relationship between obesity and breast cancer risk in postmenopausal women.[69] They suggest that this may be related to the conversion of androstenedione to estrone. Estrone is an estrogen that was found to be carcinogenic in animals. The greater the amount of adipose tissue, the greater the degree of conversion.[261] In postmenopausal women, obesity is an increased risk factor, possibly because of the greater rate of androstenedione conversion to estrone in adipose tissue and the lower levels of sex hormone–binding globulin in obese (as compared with nonobese) women. Sex hormone–binding globulin in obese postmenopausal women is about 50% of the value observed in lean controls. These changes are reversible and tend toward normality with weight reduction.[89] In breast cancer patients, sex hormone–binding globulin correlates negatively with cytosolic andione concentrations ($P < 0.01$). In susceptible postmenopausal women, obesity implies a double risk for breast cancer by inducing a decrease in sex hormone–binding globulin and a concomitant increase in the supply of free andione in the absence of cyclic endogenous progesterone. The increased risk of breast cancer caused by obesity is not related to an incremental increase in dietary fat.

Although many authors have found an increase in the incidence of breast cancer with an increase in postmenopausal body weight, a similar correlation has not been found for premenopausal women.[81,182,211,242] In a study comparing the Netherlands with Japan, De Waard et al. further observed that the incidence of breast cancer in thin women does not rise with age after menopause such as it does in women of normal body weight.[81] These authors thought that perhaps half the variation in incidence rates between the Netherlands and Japan could be explained by differences in body build. Le Marchand et al. further studied body sizes at different periods of life in association with breast cancer risks.[176] This work from the Cancer Research Center of Hawaii included data on cohorts of women born from 1918 to 1943. Body weights were available from 1942, 1943, and 1972. The Quetelet index,

which was more clearly associated with breast cancer risk than was mere body weight, takes into account the relationship of weight and height. Weight alone was not an equivalent correlate for breast cancer risk. The authors observed a breast cancer risk associated with postmenopausal obesity. They did not observe this risk to increase once a threshold was reached in the Quetelet index.

These investigators reported a protective role of adolescent obesity against premenopausal breast cancer. In the women who had an increase in body size between the ages of 10 to 14 years in 1942, the risk of breast cancer was substantially less ($P = 0.004$) than in individuals who were of normal body weight or slim in their adolescent years. This observation was present in all ethnic groups and persisted in overweight adolescents who remained overweight into adulthood. Both prepubertal and peripubertal obesity seem to have a protective affect against the subsequent development of premenopausal and postmenopausal breast cancer. Miller concludes that obesity in premenopausal women is protective against breast cancer.[208] London et al. found that the risk of premenopausal breast cancer decreased significantly with increasing relative weight.[183] At the highest weight category, this decrease reached an RR of 0.6.

Height and obesity appear to be independent risk factors for breast cancer among postmenopausal, but not premenopausal, women. Hsieh et al. found that postmenopausal women who were 10 cm taller than average height of 158 cm had a 12% (CI of 11 to 22) higher risk of breast cancer.[145] Postmenopausal women of average height had an 11% (CI of 7 to 16) higher risk of breast cancer when they were 10 kg heavier than the norm.

Obesity is also associated with early menarche, which is another hormonally dependent risk factor for breast cancer. Is early menarche a greater risk factor for breast cancer than peripubertal obesity is a protection against breast cancer? If obesity persists into the second decade, the effect of obesity seems to dominate. Curiously, Hsieh et al. imply that the protective effect of late menarche may not apply to women with postmenopausal obesity.[145] Late menarche may not apply to women with postmenopausal obesity and may be detrimental in obese women. Henderson et al. considered that it is not merely the age of menarche that accounts for the increased risk of breast cancer, but the cumulative number of regular ovulatory cycles.[128] This number may be altered by adolescent obesity.

In summary, obesity in postmenopausal women is a factor causing an increased risk for postmenopausal breast cancer. Adult women with less than normal body weight have a decreased risk for postmenopausal breast cancer. Obesity in prepubertal, peripubertal, or premenopausal women appears to decrease the risk for breast cancer. The mechanisms of obesity-dependent breast cancer risks may be related to endocrine factors within the adipose tissue.

Radiation. It is well known that radiation exposure to the breast can increase the incidence of breast cancer. The breast is one of the organs most susceptible to radiation carcinogenesis.[140] Follow-up studies of the Japanese survivors of the atomic bomb revealed a substantial increase in breast carcinoma.[199] The risk is especially high in women who are exposed at 10 to 19 years of age. The adolescent breast is remarkably sensitive to radiation, and this is especially true for the time just around menarche.[38] Long-term follow-up data have revealed that the incidence of breast cancer occurs even in women exposed before 10 years of age. Perhaps even more important, it has been observed in long-term follow-up that the risk of radiogenic breast cancer decreases with increasing age at exposure. This occurs whether the incidence is expressed in relative or absolute terms.[132,302] There is a substantial decrease in breast cancer risk from radiation after the age of 30 years, with virtually no evidence of increased breast cancer risk from radiation in postmenopausal women. Mettler et al. studied breast cancers in women treated for acute postpartum mastitis by radiation.[205] This radiation treatment was associated with an increase in the risk of breast cancer. Many of the patients studied were over the age of 30 years. It is not known whether lactation affects the radiation risk of breast cancer, but this study suggests that some radiation-induced breast cancer risks can occur at a later age than has been seen in other high-dose radiation studies. Perhaps the difference is that these researchers studied lactating breasts.

In addition to high-dose radiation effects, low-dose radiation has also been shown to increase the risk for breast cancer. The most compelling evidence comes from the studies of fluoroscopic examinations in patients being treated for scoliosis or tuberculosis.[39,209] Land observed that studies of different exposed populations yield remarkably consistent results despite wide differences in underlying breast cancer rates and conditions of exposure.[172] He states "that the excess risk is approximately proportional to dose and is independent of the ionizing density and fractualization. It is, however, heavily dependent on age at exposure but relatively independent of population difference in normal risks. It appears that multiple exposures of low doses have a cumulative effect and these effects appear to be permanent, as they are still apparent for as long as the exposed women have been followed (up to 40 years)."[39]

The effect of radiation on breast cancer risk is obviously of considerable concern in screening mammography for the detection of breast cancer. Bailar strongly believed that the radiation hazard from mammography exceeded the potential gains.[20] This argument has been refuted by Shapiro.[270] Much of the concern resulted because controls for radiation doses in mammography were not as good as current controls. When using low-dose film screen techniques, the radiation risks from mammography are considerably lower than was previously available. The overwhelming evidence supports the contention that diagnostic radiology has only a small, if any, influence on the incidence of breast cancer.[90]

Recently, however, renewed concern about the radiation from mammography was raised in a report on families who are affected by the ataxia telangiectasia gene and who have an increased risk for radiation-induced carcinogenesis (see the sections on Family History and The Hazard of Ionizing Radiation). This gene occurs in approximately 1.4% of the population. Perhaps blood relatives of individuals who have ataxia telangiectasia should not receive the same frequency of screening mammography as other women. However, the effect of radiation occurs predominantly in younger age groups, so that, if one restricts radiation exposure according to the American Cancer Society's recommendations (i.e., examinations given only in women over the age of 40 years and only annual examinations given to women over the age of 50 years), one would anticipate a minimal to absent increase in the incidence of breast cancer caused by the radiation from the mammogram, even in women who are heterozygous for the ataxia telangiectasia gene. The futility of mammography in women under the age of 30 years is well recognized. Williams et al. reviewed mammograms of 76 patients who were 18 to 29 years of age.[322] In 74% of the patients referred for the study of a palpable mass, no mass was evident on the mammogram. Mammography in younger women, when the breast is more sensitive to radiation, has relatively little to no clinical use. As long as screening mammograms are performed in individuals who are at higher risk for breast cancer and at lower risk for radiation-induced breast carcinogenesis, it seems prudent to advocate screening mammogram.

Alcohol. Is the drinking of alcoholic beverages associated with an increased risk for breast cancer? Ever since the case control study of Williams and Horn in 1977, there have been repeated efforts to answer that question. They demonstrated an increase in risk of 1.6 (CI of 1.1 to 2.3) in women who drank alcoholic beverages versus those who abstained.[323] They compared the drinking history of 1127 patients with breast cancer with 2380 matched controls, but they did not adjust for the classic risk factors. The dose of alcohol ingested was not clearly defined. This article stimulated a large number of subsequent studies, which attested to the difficulty of identifying weak correlations between a risk factor and breast cancer. The reason why alcohol may be an important risk factor is that it is one of the few risks that could be avoided. However, many authors have pointed out that the benefit of low doses of alcohol in decreasing the risk for cardiovascular disease may overcome the relative risk for whatever breast cancer is caused by alcohol. However, if alcohol were a significant risk factor, patients who are already at high risk for breast cancer from other risk factors may choose not to consume alcohol. For that to become a viable contention, the issue of whether alcohol is a risk factor for breast cancer must be resolved. Expending considerable effort to clarify risk factors that are potentially reversible is worthwhile.

Harris et al. attempted to analyze the weak associations between breast cancer and alcohol consumption.[122] They presented 10 case control studies and 3 prospective (cohort follow-up) studies. They pointed out that there are substantial socioeconomic factors correlated with alcohol consumption that may produce an elevated unadjusted odds ratio relating breast cancer to alcohol. Educational level correlates with people who drink. Some say there is approximately a 5% increase in alcohol consumption per year of education. Career-oriented women drink 10% to 20% more alcohol than women in other occupations. In addition, any study on a weak association is especially subject to biases in risk factors that are difficult to measure. Rosner et al. notes that the error in risk factor measurement substantially affects biases in risk factor calculation.[250] The amount of alcohol previously consumed is difficult to measure. The authors sought to correct reported alcohol consumption by validating the questionnaire used to determine the reported measurement. In this study they observed that the age-adjusted relative risk for 25 g of alcohol was 1.33 (CI of 1.14 to 1.55). After correcting for the measurement, the relative risk increased to 1.62 (CI of 1.23 to 2.12). Thus validation of the questionnaire used to obtain the data resulted in an increased risk factor calculation.

Harris and Wynder noted several factors that influence alcohol consumption.[123] These include age, religion, education, occupation, marital status, body mass, and cigarette smoking. These confounding variables mitigated against evidence that alcohol, in and of itself, is a risk factor for breast cancer. They point out that an important question relates to biologic plausibility—that is, the mechanism by which alcohol affects the breast epithelium either directly or through hormones must be identified. In addition, if alcohol consumption were a risk factor for breast cancer, one would expect the relationship to be stronger in heavier drinkers. Both of these issues have been subsequently addressed. Rohan and Cook studied the association between alcohol and the presence of benign proliferative epithelial disorders of the breast in breast biopsies.[247] They found no correlation. Their unadjusted relative risk for proliferative epithelial disorders in drinkers versus nondrinkers was 0.9 (CI of 0.6 to 1.3). The relative risk derived after comparing breast cancer cases with benign disorder cases (as controls) was 1 (CI of 0.6 to 1.4). Dupont et al. conducted a 17-year follow-up of 10,366 women with benign biopsy specimens and found no effect of alcohol in those patients who subsequently developed breast cancer.[86] Thus there is no evidence that alcohol consumption is related to benign proliferative disorders of the breast that develop into breast cancers. Thus far the only research on this subject has failed to confirm a correlation. However, alcohol may have another mechanism by which it influences the incidence of breast cancer, independent of benign proliferative disorders.

Longnecker et al. used a metaanalysis to study the effect of alcohol dose on breast cancer risk.[186] They studied the results obtained in four cohort follow-up studies and twelve case control studies. Their analysis employed rigorous assessment of the quality of the data reported in the

Table 2-13. Studies on alcohol as a risk factor for breast cancer

Cohort studies	Year	Cases (n)	Controls	Risk	95% CI	Dose	Location	Comments
Willett	1987	601	89,538	1.3	(1.1-1.7)	5-14 g/wk,	Massachusetts	
				1.6	(1.3-2.0)	3-9 drinks/wk		
						15 g+		
Schatzkin	1987	121	7188	1.5	(1.1-2.2)	Drinking vs.	Massachusetts	
				1.4	(0.9-2.3)	no drinking		
				1.5	(0.9-2.6)	Low drinking		
				1.6	(1.0-2.7)	Moderate drinking		
						Heavy drinking		
Hiatt	1988	303	69,000	1.5	(1.0-2.3)	1-2 drinks/day	California	Adjusted
				1.5	(0.8-2.8)	3-5 drinks/day		
				3.3	(1.2-9.3)	6+/day		
Schatzkin (Framingham Heart Study)	1989	143	2636	0.8	(0.5-1.1)	Multiple risk factor adjustment	Massachusetts	
				1.0	(0.6-1.5)			
				0.7	(0.4-1.1)	0.1-1.4 g/day		
				0.6	(0.4-1.0)	1.5-4.9 g/day		
						5+/day		
Dupont	1989	17-yr follow-up of 10,366 women with benign biopsy specimens				No effect of alcohol	Tennessee	

Table 2-14. Comparative analysis of studies on alcohol as a risk factor for breast cancer

Case control studies	Year	Cases (n)	Controls	Risk	99% CI	Dose	Country	Comments
Williams and Horn	1977	1127	2380	1.6	(1.1-2.3)			1st case control study
Rosenberg et al.	1982	1152	2702	1.9	(1.5-2.1)			Population control
			519	1.5	(1.1-2.1)	<7 g/day ovarian and endo-metrial		
				2.0	(1.4-2.9)	>7 g/day cancer control		
Byers and Funch	1982	1314	770	1.1	(0.9-1.4)	Studied only small amounts of alcohol ingestion; did not adjust		
Paganini-Hill	1983	239	239	1.0	(0.7-1.4)	Adjusted for risk factors but mostly upper class and postmenopausal females		
Webster et al.	1983	1226	1279	1.0	(0.8-1.2)	Adjusted for important risk factors; no dose effect		
Begg et al.	1983	997	730	1.4	(0.9-2.0)			
Le et al.	1986	1010	1050	1.5	(1.3-1.7)			
O'Connell	1987	276	1591	1.5	(1.0-2.1)	≥2 g/day		
Harvey et al.	1987	1524	1896	1.7	(1.2-2.4)	N/A	Australia	
Rohan	1988	451	451	1.5	(1.0-2.1)	9.3 g/day	USA (New York)	
Harris and Wynder	1988	1467	10178	0.87-1.4	(not significant)			
Adami	1988	422	527	0.6	(0.4-0.9)	5+ g/day	Sweden	
Young	1989	277	372	2.2	(1.34-3.5)	10 vs. 0 drinks/wk	USA (Wisconsin)	Young drinkers
				1.8	(1.2-2.6)			Older drinkers
			433	2.0	(1.3-3.1)			Young drinkers
				1.6	(1.2-2.2)			Older drinkers
Richardson et al.	1989	349	459	1.8	(1.2-2.8)	1-2 drinks/wk	France	
				3.5	(2.0-6.1)	>17 drinks/wk		
Toniolo	1989	250	499	1.0		<40 g/day	Italy	
Meara et al.	1989	998	998	1		No effect	United Kingdom (Oxford)	Clinical cases detected by screening mammog-raphy
vant Veer et al.	1989	120	164	8.5	(1.1-65.1)	30 g vs. 1-4 g/day	Netherlands	Premenopausal only
				4.0	(1.0-15.6)	15+ vs. 1-14 g/day		
				2.8	(0.8-9.8)	>3 X/wk vs. <3 X/wk		

Study	Year			RR	(95% CI)	Measure	Location	Comments
Kato et al.	1989	1740	8920	1.36	(1.04-1.78)	Daily alcohol intake vs. nondrinker	Japan	
Chu et al.	1989	3498	3157	1.0	(0.9-1.2)	Any alcohol vs. nondrinkers	USA (Georgia)	
				1.1	N/A	8-14 drinks/wk		
				1.0	N/A	15-21 drinks/wk		
				1.2	N/A	22+ drinks/wk		
Cusimano et al.	1989	N/A	N/A	1.97	(1.2-3.2)	N/A	Italy (Palermo)	
LaVecchia et al.	1989	2402	2220	1.4	(1.2-1.6)	Nondrinkers vs. drinkers	Italy (Milan)	
				1.3	N/A	<1 g drink/day (10 g of ethanol)		
				1.3	N/A	<2 drinks/day		
				1.4	N/A	2.03 drinks/day		
				2.2	N/A	>3 drinks/day		
Rosenberg et al.	1990	607	1214	0.9	(0.6-1.2)	1 drink/day vs. <1 drink/mo	Canada (Toronto)	
				1.7	N/A	1 beer/day		
				0.7	N/A	1 glass wine/day		
Rosner et al.	1990	N/A	N/A	1.33	(1.14-1.55)		USA (Massachusetts)	
				1.62	(1.23-2.12)	After correction for measurement error		
Nasca et al.	1990	1617	1617	1.37	(1.07-1.75)	15+ g/day	USA (New York)	
Unger et al.	1991	992	492	1.59	$P < 0.001$		Switzerland (Zurich)	
Howe et al.	1991	1575	1974	1.0		Up to 40 g/day	Canada (Toronto)	
				1.69	(1.19-2.4)	40+ g/day		
Zaridze et al.	1991	139	139	3.39	(1.37-8.38)	Alcohol use	Russia (Moscow)	
Sneyd et al.	1991	891	1864	1.0	(0.64-1.7)	Current drinkers vs. never drink	New Zealand	Risk may be increased in females who began drinking at a later age
				1.3	(0.74-2.5)	Ex-drinkers		Ages 25-54
				1.0				
				1.8				
Francesci et al.	1991	132	499	1.0	N/A	Up to 14 drinks/wk	Italy (Aviano)	
				1.8	(0.87-3.8)	>14 drinks/wk		
				1.5	(0.8-2.6)	Drinkers vs. nondrinkers		
				1.2		<1 drink/day		
				1.4		2 drinks/day		
				1.9		3 drinks/day		
				1.6		>3 drinks/day		

literature. At the time of their study, these authors concluded that the world data strongly support an association between the consumption of 1 oz of alcohol per day and an increased risk for breast cancer. At less than 1 oz, there seems to be a weaker association. They assert that "the evidence in favor of a dose response relationship between alcohol consumption, and the risk of breast cancer is compelling." They and others caution that the apparent risk from alcohol should not be considered separately from the protective effect of alcohol against cardiovascular disease when recommending social policy.

Table 2-13 presents an outline of the various studies on alcohol as a risk factor for breast cancer. The studies of Willett et al., Schatzkin et al., Hiatt, and Dupont et al. are all cohort-type studies.[86,130,259,321] They found an increased risk of 1.6 (CI 1.3 to 2.0) with 15 g or greater of alcohol consumption. The first report by Schatzkin et al. presented data from the epidemiologic follow-up of the first National Health and Nutrition Examination Survey.[259] The second report of Schatzkin et al. used the results from the Framingham Heart Study and reached a different conclusion.[258] They pointed out in the latter article that there is no readily apparent source of bias to explain the discrepancy of findings between the Framingham Study and the previous National Health and Nutrition Examination Survey on the effects of at least one drink per day or less. These types of discrepancies have lead to uncertainty about the relationship of alcohol consumption to breast cancer risk.

The first nine case control studies were used in the metaanalysis of Longnecker et al. (Table 2-14).[186] Subsequent case studies have been reported since that time. Currently, 20 additional case control studies can be added to the metaanalysis review. These case control studies vary in quality, as can be observed from the comments. Many showed a dose-related effect, others did not. There are now studies from many countries, including the United States, France, Italy, Switzerland, Canada, Russia, Sweden, England, the Netherlands, Japan, New Zealand, and Australia. The worldwide interest in this subject reflects the importance of this issue.

Although we have not subjected all these studies to the rigorous metaanalysis of Longnecker et al., the additional evidence continues to show a trend toward a substantial relationship between alcohol consumption and breast cancer.[186] The risk is commonly reported as 1.6 versus a control of 1. This is a relatively weak association, but overall the evidence is compelling and seems to be greatest for the highest doses. Could this be related to the hepatic effect of alcohol and the liver's function in estrogen metabolism? This review of alcohol consumption as a risk factor for breast cancer provides an opportunity to better understand the methodologies and difficulties in appraising risk factors that have weak relationships to breast cancer. A summation of many weak risk factors may be important if we are attempting to develop techniques to prevent breast cancer or better understand the implications of risk factors in the diagnosis of nonpalpable breast carcinoma.

Other risk factors. There are many different variables that have been studied as potential risk factors for breast cancer. Most relative risk estimates are fairly modest. In most women there are undoubtedly many variables acting together to determine the total risk for breast cancer. Quite possibly, many known risk factors are related to some common underlying mechanism, such as hormonal profile. There may be other risk factors that do not lend themselves to epidemiologic assessment to determine their exact nature. However, others have been suggested in the literature and may or may not play a role in the probability of developing breast cancer in any specific woman. Here, we briefly discuss some of the other suggested risk factors in an effort to portray some of the difficulties encountered when one is attempting to assess weak relationships in which multiple possible factors interact.

Paternal age. Does the age of a woman's mother or father at the time she was born affect her chances for breast cancer? The evidence for prenatal influences on the subsequent incidence of breast cancer during adulthood has been studied by many investigators. Thompson and Janerich used a case control study involving 5000 women (both breast cancer patients and controls) to determine that a 15-year increase in maternal age was associated with an estimated 25% (CI of 8 to 46) increase in breast cancer risk.[318] Janerich et al. from Yale University studied 5489 cancer patients compared with 2647 controls.[152] They observed that an increase of 10 years in maternal age was associated with a 24% increase in the risk for breast cancer (odds ratio 1.24; CI of 1.09 to 1.41). They also found a relationship with paternal age. A 10-year increase in the father's age at the time a woman was born was associated with a 19% increased incidence of breast cancer (odds ratio 1.19; CI of 1.07 to 1.33). The authors observed that each parent's age may have an independent contribution to the risk of breast cancer. However, they found no statistically significant effects of birth order on adult breast cancer. They concluded that factors affecting the parents in the prenatal period may have a stronger influence on adult cancers than were previously recognized. Panagiotopoulou et al. observed that the risk of breast cancer increases monotonically with maternal age at birth.[234] They hypothesized a relation linking the levels of prenatal estrogen to the risk of breast cancer in the offspring. However, Colditz et al. from Harvard University Medical School examined the risk of breast cancer among daughters in a population of over 100,000 women 30 to 55 years of age in 1976.[68] These women had no prior diagnosis of cancer. Over 1,000,000 person-years of follow-up was reported, and 1799 cases of cancer were documented. The authors observed only a weak and nonsignificant trend of increased risk of cancer with increasing maternal age at birth. Daughters born to mothers between 30 and 34 years of age had an age-adjusted relative risk of breast cancer of 1.11 (CI of 0.89 to 1.37) when compared with daughters born to mothers less than 20 years of age. They were unable to find any relationship whatsoever between paternal age and the risk of breast cancer in a daughter. The authors suggest that there is either a weak or no association between parental age and the risk of breast cancer.

Obviously, there is some discrepancy between these various epidemiologic studies. This type of discrepancy is typical for the weak factors that may or may not be risk factors for breast cancer. If they were better understood, some of them might indicate the cause of cancers in some patients. Perhaps some breast cancers are associated with a genetically based prenatal problem. The fact that there are so many stronger factors in the incidence of breast cancer makes it difficult to uncover the subtle or weak associations. Perhaps it will take a metaanalysis of all of the available literature (when more literature is available) in an effort to ascertain the validity of the various assertions that parental age is or is not a risk factor for breast cancer.

Lactation. Breast-feeding was once thought to decrease the risk for breast cancer. As early as 1931 Wainwright observed an association between a history of lactation and breast cancer.[312] Women with a history of lactation had fewer breast cancers. Since that study, many authors have sought to define the factors that relate breast cancer risk to lactation. Salber el al. considered that lactation had no effect on the incidence of breast cancer when parity was taken into account.[255] More recently this controversy has been revisited. Petrakis et al. attempted to assess the relationship between parity and lactation as separate or co-risk factors for breast cancer by studying the breast-fluid estrogen levels, which were positively correlated with months since last birth or breast-feeding.[238] The prolonged low levels of breast-fluid estrogens following a full-term birth and lactation may in part provide a mechanism by which parity reduces the risk of breast cancer. Yuan et al. observed a clear effect of lactation on breast cancer risk in a Chinese population studied in Shanghai.[329] The majority of the women were characterized by a long cumulative duration of nursing. A substantial beneficial effect of nursing on the risk of breast cancer was observed in this population. Similar data were noted by McTiernan and Thomas, who studied the female residents of King County, Washington.[202] They found that premenopausal women who had lactated had a 0.49 relative risk of developing breast cancer when compared with premenopausal women who have never lactated (CI of 0.30 to 0.82). They noted that the risk of breast cancer decreased with an increasing duration of lifetime lactation experienced in both pre- and postmenopausal women. The effect was consistently stronger for premenopausal than postmenopausal women. This protective effect persisted even after adjustment for age, parity, and age at first full-term pregnancy. In a study of Japanese women, Tashiro et al. showed that those women who had never lactated had an increased risk of breast cancer (odds ratio 2.67; $P = 0.02$) when compared with women who had lactated.[298] This, however, was apparently not corrected for parity or age at first childbirth.

On the other hand, London et al. studied a cohort of almost 90,000 registered nurses between the ages of 30 and 55 years and observed 1262 cases of breast cancer between 1976 and 1986.[184] They found no independent association between lactation and the risk for breast cancer after adjustment for age and parity when compared with women who had never lactated. They found a relative risk of 0.95 (CI of 0.84 to 1.08). Similar relative risks were observed for women who had lactated for various periods of time. Siskind et al., in an Australian case control study, found no significant relationship between any lactation versus no lactation (odds ratio of 0.85; CI of 0.55 to 1.30).[283] They did, however, find a statistically significant nonlinear association with breast-feeding of the first live-born child; a slightly elevated odds ratio existed for lactations of less than 1 month. Perhaps the effect of lactation is more subtle and requires a more detailed analysis than other risk factors in breast cancer research. The findings of Siskind suggest that the lactation occurring after the first infant's birth may have a different effect than subsequent lactations or comparison of lactation versus no lactation at all. Based on a case control study of 50,000 women (of whom 1136 had breast cancer), Kvale and Heuch concluded that they found a very weak association between the mean duration of lactation per birth and the duration for each of the first three births. They suggested there may be a nonlinear relation between lactation and breast cancer.[170] They were left with the overall impression that breast-feeding is not strongly related to the risk for breast cancer.

Smoking. The role of cigarette smoking as a cause of breast cancer is small, if it is at all present. The efforts to define the relationship between smoking and breast cancer have produced inconsistent results. Schlemmer et al., using a case control study, found that there was a decreased risk of endometrial and breast cancer associated with cigarette smoking.[262] They concluded this may be mediated by androgenic protection. Palmer et al. used two case control studies—the Canadian study, in which 670 women with breast cancer were matched with 1214 controls, and the United States study, in which 1955 breast cancer patients were matched with 805 controls.[232] In both of these studies, they concluded that the risk of breast cancer was more strongly associated with the commencement of smoking at a young age. Their findings suggest the hypothesis that exposure to cigarette smoking during adolescence increases a woman's risk of breast cancer. Chu et al. used the cancer and steroid hormone study data to conclude that the risk of breast cancer in women who smoke is the same as or perhaps slightly higher than women who have never smoked.[62] Vatten and Kvinnsland used a prospective study of 24,329 Norwegian women and found no overall association between cigarette smoking and breast cancer risk.[309] However, they did find an interaction between cigarette smoking, body mass index, and age at diagnosis—$P = 0.01$. Ewertz found no association between smoking and the risk for breast cancer in Danish women.[91] Overall, the data suggest that, if there is a relationship between smoking and breast cancer, it is related more to other things smokers do than to smoking per se.

Previous cancer in other organs. A previous history of ovarian cancer and endometrial cancer has been well documented as risk factors for the subsequent development of breast cancer. The range of risk factors for ovarian cancer is 1.4 to 4.0.[243,264] Endometrial cancer has a relative risk factor ranging from 1.2 to 2.[22,192] The incidence of endometrial cancer is most evident in women who are over 60 years age and within 10 years of the presence of the endometrial cancer. Other cancers have also been related to an increased risk for breast cancer. Salivary gland cancer and meningiomas are most often associated with breast cancer.[34,263]

Other factors. A number of other factors appear to be associated with a risk for breast cancer. For example, women who live in North America and Northern Europe have a greater probability of breast cancer than women who live in Asia and Africa. Women of a higher social economic class who have never married and who live in urban rather than rural areas and in the northern part of the United States are more likely to develop breast cancer.[160] A relationship between education and breast cancer has been suggested by many authors.[58,127] Carter et al. observed that a high level of education (compared with less than a high school education) was associated with a relative risk of 2.1 (CI of 0.95 to 5.1).[127] Helmrich also noted an association between the Jewish religion and 12 or more years of education, which was independently associated with an increased risk for breast cancer.[127] Hsieh and Trichopoulos found a relationship between handedness and breast cancer laterality.[144] Left-handed or ambidextrous women more often had a left-sided breast cancer with a relative risk of 1.22 (CI of 0.96 to 1.56). These authors also found a relationship between the size of the breast and the probabilities of breast cancer. This was only found in postmenopausal women and, in part, may have been accounted for by obesity. Jasmin et al. attempted to relate psychologic factors with the risk for breast cancer. These authors attempted to correlate excessive self-esteem, hysterical disposition, and unresolved recent grief to a significant increased risk for breast cancer.[154] Obviously, there are many things that make up different women. Any one of these may or may not be correlated, depending on (in part) the statistical validity and the design of the research project. Many of these relationships may have some basis in fact. However, it is extremely difficult to isolate a specific risk factor when so many weak risk factors may interplay.

Incidence and the detection of breast cancer

Risk factors define the relative incidence between two compared populations. A study of incidence tells us the absolute number of cases we can expect in a population. For example, in screening mammography, how many mammograms can we expect to yield positive findings? If a radiologist found that 5% of annual mammograms of 50-year-old women were sufficiently suspicious to warrant a surgical biopsy, then (barring other risks) there would be 27 biopsies per cancer. The incidence of breast cancer in 50-year-old women is 1.85 per 1000 women. If these were baseline rather than annual mammograms, using the same hypothetical there would be only nine biopsies per cancer found. The prevalence of breast cancer in 50-year-old women is approximately 5.5 per 1000 women.[228] The ratio of prevalence to incidence is 2.72 at age 40 to 49 years, 2.96 at age 50 to 59 years, and 3.54 at ages 60 to 69 years. The ratio of prevalence to incidence increases with age. This is due to slower growing tumors in older women. To responsibly interpret mammograms, the radiologist must understand the probability of cancer being present on any examination. This necessitates knowledge of prevalence and incidence.

The prevalence of breast cancer is defined as the number of cases present in a population. This is usually reported by age group. The number of breast cancers in the population differs from the incidence of breast cancer. Incidence refers to how many new cases occur per year. The distinction between prevalent breast cancers and incident breast cancers is well exemplified in screening mammography. A cancer discovered on a baseline mammogram would be defined as a prevalent breast cancer. A cancer newly identified on a subsequent mammogram would be defined as an incident cancer. A "true" interval cancer occurs in the interval between the two mammographic examinations. Screening mammography has provided an opportunity to appreciate the implications of breast cancer incidence and breast cancer prevalence.

It may be possible to perform geographic targeting if we know geographic prevalences. Such targeting would be most useful where between-area-variability in a prevalence is large and within-area-variability is small.[162] The knowledge of the local prevalence rate is useful for other purposes. If one knows the expected prevalence of breast cancer in a screening population, the ability of screening mammography to detect early cancer can be better evaluated. The true prevalence rate in Rochester was 9 per 1000. Patchefsky et al. reported a prevalence rate of 8.9

per 1000 on mammographic screens in 17,526 asymptomatic women 45 to 64 years of age.[235] This may suggest that the screening system used in these women was sufficiently sensitive to detect almost all of the cancers anticipated.

However, these 17,526 women were not randomly selected from the population at large, although they were asymptomatic. Common intuition suggests that this may have led to a self-selection bias where women at higher risk chose to have the screening mammogram. The opposite may well be true. There is both epidemiologic and survey evidence to suggest that women who are at a higher risk for breast cancer do not tend to self-select screening mammograms as readily as do women at a lower risk.[178] A heightened anxiety about cancer and the consequences of screening may dissuade some women at higher risk from entering a screening program. Gregorio et al. found a fear of finding cancer as the reason for not being screened in 9% of women surveyed by telephone.[115] In a recent assessment of breast cancer screening data, Wald et al. suggest an explanation for some of the observed differences between the self-selected and randomized screening studies.[313] "It would seem that in nonrandomized studies a self-selection bias occurred, in which women who attended for screening were in any case at lower risk of dying of breast cancer than were women who did not attend."[313] This "detection rate" may not represent the "prevalence rate" in the population at large. In the BCDDP, the asymptomatic women self-selected themselves to participate. Some of the women had a definite concern that they had breast cancer.[266]

A better estimate of the actual ability of screening mammography to detect the presence of breast cancer can be found by noting the detection rate of prevalence mammograms in a randomly selected population. It is, however, difficult to obtain a truly random population for mammography. No program has had a 100% response to invitations for screening mammograms. A 70% response is considered very good.[12] It is not possible to determine whether those women who do not respond to the invitation have the same prevalence rate as those who

do respond. If we assume a similar prevalence rate in responders and nonresponders, the detection rate of prevalence mammograms may be a surrogate for mammographic deductibility of breast cancer in lieu of accurate false-negative data.

We have reviewed six reported series in which screening mammograms were used to detect breast cancer (Table 2-15). In these series the women were invited to participate from a population at large rather than from a preselected or self-selected risk group. The observed detection rate of breast cancer on these prevalence screens ranged from 2.7 to 7.6 per 1000 women screened.

It is difficult to compare reliably one series with another. There are many variables that may influence the detection of breast cancer. These variables range from the quality of mammographic technique and interpretation to the marketing methods used to enhance the participation of the invited. In a truly random series, as the detection rate approaches a known prevalence rate, it is reasonable to assume that a screening system is accurate in detecting breast cancer. As the detection rate approaches a known prevalence rate, there are proportionately fewer false-negative results. Very few cancers would be missed by a system in which the detection rate on prevalence mammograms equals the expected prevalence. Though the quality of a mammographic screening program may be difficult to evaluate, Day et al.[77] point out that the data from the Swedish two-county randomized trial provide targets that can be achieved.[295]

The single most important risk factor in selecting patients to be screened for breast cancer is the patient's age. It is important to adjust the data for age, if one is to use it on detection rates to evaluate a screening system. There is considerable controversy about the appropriate age to initiate screening mammography.

The current American Cancer Society guidelines recommend a baseline mammogram at age 35 to 40 years, biannual mammograms at 40 to 49 years of age, and annual mammograms after age 50 years. These guidelines have been endorsed by many organizations (Table 2-16).[87,278]

The Canadian Association of Radiologists recommends

Table 2-15. Reported breast cancer detection rates at prevalence screens in population-based invited screening programs

	Detection rate per thousand				
Author	**45-64**	**50-64**	**50-69**	**Attendance (%)**	**Location**
Shapiro (1971)	2.7	—	—	66	New York, USA
Andersson (1979)	7.4	7.6	—	73	Malmo, Sweden
Anderson (1986)	5.7	—	—	NA	Edinburgh, Scotland
Cirelli (1989)	—	7.3	—	69.2	Brescia, Italy
Paci (1990)	4.1	4.8	6.4		Florence, Italy
Azavedo (1991)			7.7	68.6	Stockholm, Sweden

Table 2-16. Recommendations of organizations for screening mammography

	Women under 50 yr of age	Women over 50 yr of age
American Cancer Society	A baseline mammogram for women between the ages of 35 and 40 yr, annual breast physical examinations from 40 to 50 yr of age, and a mammogram every 1 to 2 yr from 40 to 50 yr of age.	Annual breast physical examinations and annual mammograms
The National Cancer Institute	Breast physical examinations at every periodic examination; encourages mammography every 1 to 2 yr starting at age 40 yr; and encourages annual mammograms for women with a personal history of breast cancer.	Breast physical examinations at every periodic examination and mammography annually
The American College of Obstetricians and Gynecologists	A baseline mammogram for women between the ages of 35 and 50 yr, and a breast physical examination in the same age group. At any age, mammograms are recommended if there are strong indications, such as a family or personal history of breast cancer, breast augmentation implants, or first pregnancy after age 30 yr.	Mammograms and breast physical examinations at a frequency determined by the woman's physician
The American College of Radiology	A baseline mammogram before the age of 40 yr and subsequent mammograms every 1 to 2 yr or more frequently based on the physician's assessment.	Annual mammograms and breast physical examinations
The American College of Physicians	Does not recommend mammography for women below 50 yr of age.	Mammograms for women between the ages of 50 and 59 yr "on a routine basis"; mammograms are recommended for women 60 yr of age and over, with the screening interval chosen by the physician and patient
The U.S. Preventive Services Task Force	Annual clinical breast examinations for women 40 to 49 yr of age, but does not recommend mammograms for this age group.	Annual mammograms and clinical breast examinations for women over 50 yr of age

Reproduced with permission from Eddy DM: *Ann Intern Med* 111:389-399, 1989.

mammography after 25 years of age for any woman with breast symptoms, with metastasis from cancer of an unknown primary site, and before any breast surgery. They advise women with a strong family history of breast cancer and those women with large breasts, which may confound efforts to palpate a cancer, to have a mammogram between the ages of 25 and 35 years. Baseline mammograms for asymptomatic women should be obtained between the ages of 35 and 39 years. After 39 years of age and up to 50 years of age, women should consult their physicians annually for a clinical palpation examination and to determine when and how frequently mammography should be performed. After 50 years of age, annual mammography and physical examination is recommended. The practice of breast self-examination is advocated by both the American and Canadian groups.

Others advocate variations on these programs. Moskowitz uses epidemiologic evidence to argue for annual mammography screens for women from ages 40 to 50 years and biannual screens over 50 years of age.[215] Andersson et al. observed a reduction in breast cancer mortality resulting from an invitation to breast cancer screening only in women over 55 years of age.[13] Indeed,

Andersson et al. noted a slight increase in breast cancer mortality in women less than 55 years of age in the screened group, as compared to a control group.[13] They calculated a relative risk of dying from breast cancer in women who were screened under the age of 55 years to be 1.29 (0.74 to 2.25). Similar results in women in the under 50-years-of-age group have apparently been noted in unpublished reports from the Canadian study. Thus far there has been no satisfactory explanation about why mammography performed at an earlier age may be associated with a greater likelihood of death from breast cancer. This association could not be due to an alleged radiation effect. There is insufficient lag time for a radiation effect to be observed. No explanation for these observations yet given seems reasonable. The observations themselves are in doubt. Both the Malmo and the Canadian data have been subjected to attack in the literature.[166]

Others have shown a reduction in mortality in women who were screened prior to 50 years of age. As they followed the women under 50 years of age at the time of entry in the HIP study group for 18 years, Shapiro et al. have shown a similar reduction in mortality, as compared with women who were over 50 years of age at the time of entry into the program.[272] Tabar et al. have observed a reduction in mortality in those women who were 40 to 50 years of age at the time of their screening mammography.[295] They proved a reduction in mortality for the whole group and for women above 50 years of age. There is an ongoing study to evaluate the group between 40 and 50 years of age. The final results are not yet available. Preliminary results did not show a reduced mortality for younger women. Seidman et al. compared the survival experience of the women who participated in the BCDDP project with the survival of breast cancer patients in the SEER database to affirm a beneficial effect of breast cancer screening.[266] The 8-year case fatality rate of women screened in the BCDDP was 19%, whereas those unscreened women in the SEER group had a case fatality rate of 35%. Seidman et al. state that this connotes that 46% fewer women in the BCDDP group died of their breast cancer.[266]

Using these survival experience data, Seidman et al. concluded "Some authorities are of the opinion that the benefits of mammography after age 50 are well documented, but at younger ages the evidence is still inconclusive. The findings in this study show there is no doubt of the very successful results of screening for breast cancer with mammography in younger as well as older women."[266] The controversy of screening younger women continues. An editorial in *Lancet* analyzes the arguments and carefully points out the need to keep an open mind on both sides of the debate.[43] Age, no doubt, has a substantial effect on the efficacy of a screening program (Fig. 2-15).

A knowledge of breast cancer incidence serves many purposes. The incidence of breast cancer is most important in appreciating the ambient frequency of the disease when one seeks to diagnose it in a screened population. By knowing the ambient frequency, one can modify a diagnostic opinion in relationship to the probability that a pathologic disorder exists. However, that is not the only reason why incidence is important in diagnosing nonpalpable breast cancer. A study of incidence trends can suggest a change in probability, which is used to anticipate a diagnosis of breast cancer. All risk factors are merely assays of relative incidence in relationship to some diagnostic attribute held by the patient. These risk factors may change over time. What is the natural frequency of breast cancer, and is it changing over time or in the population under study? Are there cohorts of populations more susceptible to breast cancer as the result of something that happened in their past? Is the pathologic diagnosis of breast cancer one disease or multiple diseases? If these are multiple diseases, should they be diagnosed or managed differently? Some of these problems can be clarified by analyzing incidence rates.

de Waard used the cancer incidence in five continents to study and evaluate the time trends of cancer incidence.[80] In 1978 he noted that the age-standardized incidence of breast cancer had increased in almost all countries. This

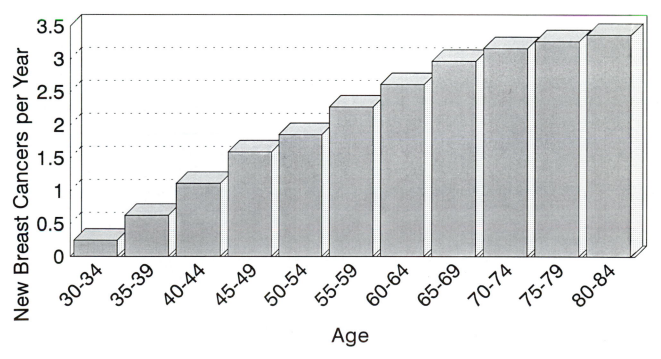

Fig. 2-15. Effect of age on breast cancer incidence (incidence rate per 1000 women, 1983-1985). (From Eddy DM: *Ann Intern Med* 111:389-399, 1989.)

rising incidence was not apparent before 1960. He observed some populations with an especially steep rise in breast cancer incidence. These were women in Iceland, Israel's Sabras, and Hawaiian Japanese. In some populations (e.g., the Japanese in Hawaii), the increase involved cohorts born after 1905. He concludes that these were the Japanese immigrants who grew up in an American environment. He suggests that the regional variations in incidence may be related to regional differences in height, weight, or both and that this may also be the basis for the overall international increase. An improvement in nutrition may account for both the increase in height and weight. Women are taller because of better early nutrition, and postmenopausal obesity occurs because of more total caloric intake. The change in both of these phenomena tracks the rising breast cancer incidence in various countries. The relative magnitude of their change resembles the regional variation in changing breast cancer incidence. de Waard's observations may be used to understand some factors that may predispose specific populations to breast cancer.

This overall rise in breast cancer incidence has been replicated by the SEER program analysis of 1973 to 1988 in the United States (Fig. 2-16). Note that there are some fluctuating incidence rates between 1973 and 1984. Since 1985 the total incidence of breast cancer has increased dra-

matically. Remember, breast cancer incidence is defined as the number of new breast cancer cases *diagnosed* in a population. Without a diagnosis being made, we do not know a disease is present. Undoubtedly, there are many patients with cancer that is at an earlier stage than can be diagnosed by any present modality. As an improved diagnostic method becomes available, some of these cases will now be diagnosed and temporarily increase the disease incidence. Thus, an increased incidence may not mean that more breast cancer exists in the population, it may only mean that previously obsure cases are now being uncovered. If these are cases that would have developed into more advanced cancer (and thus would be diagnosed by older methods), the apparent increase in incidence will eventually decline. However, if these "new cancers," seen by an improved diagnostic modality, are not of biologic significance, the increased incidence will be maintained at the higher level brought on by the new diagnostic modality. Finally, these may actually represent an increase in the frequency of breast cancer not related to improved diagnosis. If there was an absolute increase in breast cancer occurrence, it may be due to any one of the factors causally related to breast cancer, ranging from a new environmental toxin to an increase in predisposition caused by a change in the genetic pool.

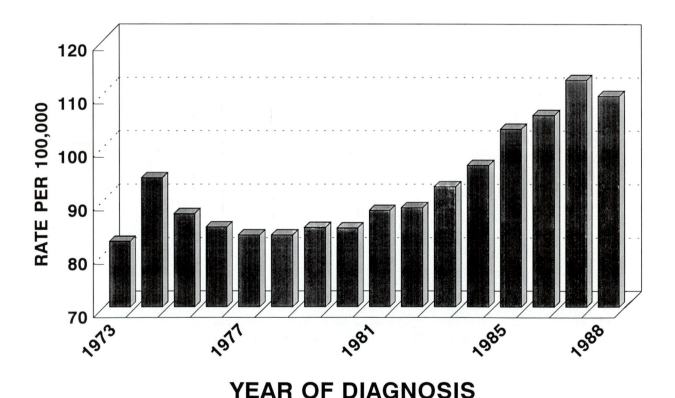

Fig. 2-16. Age-adjusted incidence rates for female breast cancer, all races. (Based on data from the National Cancer Institute's Surveillance, Epidemiology and End Results [SEER] Program, 1973-1988.)

There is some question about whether observed increases in incidence are due to an earlier diagnosis of nonpalpable lesions through the advent of the more frequent use of mammography. Some of the increase is undoubtedly the result of earlier diagnosis. Some of these cases would have appeared at a later time, in an advanced stage, and would thereby be diagnosed in other years. We envision that the future will hold a continued decreasing incidence of breast cancer as this cohort of early cancers, uncovered through the advent of widespread screening mammography, passes through the system. The decline in 1988 is somewhat encouraging. Some evidence suggests that the current increases are the result of the major impact of early breast cancer diagnosis. However, not all of this increase is likely the result of earlier diagnosis alone. Fig. 2-17 demonstrates the age-adjusted change in breast cancer incidence in pre- and postmenopausal women. In women under 50 years of age, there has been relatively little change in the incidence of breast cancer from 1973 to 1988. However, there has been dramatic increase in the incidence of breast cancer women over 50 years of age. Almost all of the age-adjusted incidence rate increases evident in Fig. 2-16 can be accounted for by a

change in breast cancer incidence in postmenopausal women. The earlier diagnosis of nonpalpable breast cancer through screening mammography has largely occurred in postmenopausal women. Thus this observation is consistent with a hypothesis that earlier diagnosis is a major factor in the increased incidence seen in the period from 1985 through 1990.

Another way to look at this changing incidence rate is to look at the effect that the overall age-adjusted incidence has on the racial population being studied. Does the incidence of breast cancer increase in black as much as in white women? Are they separable cohorts? Is there a racial cohort with a similar probability of the disease advancing through the population? Is some of the apparent change in the incidence of breast cancer caused by population shifts in women who are being diagnosed?

In Fig. 2-18 one can see that the age-adjusted incidence rates for breast cancer from 1973 to 1988 reveal no significant trends of racial differences. On the average, black women are less frequently diagnosed with breast cancer than are white women, as was discussed earlier. Although the recent increased incidence is more evident in white women, the increase is not significant.

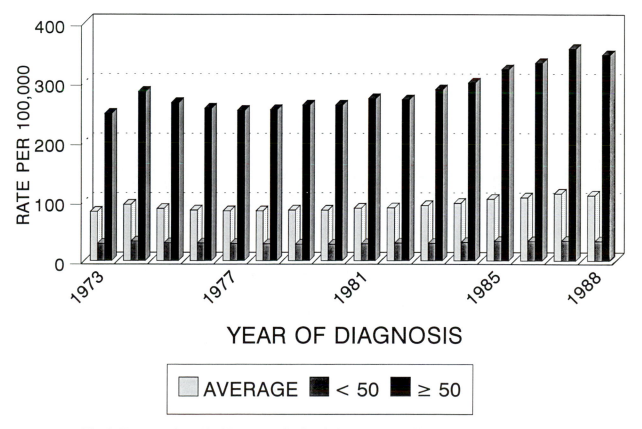

Fig. 2-17. Age-adjusted incidence rates for female breast cancer, all races. (Based on data from the National Cancer Institute's Surveillance, Epidemiology and End Results [SEER] Program, 1973-1988.)

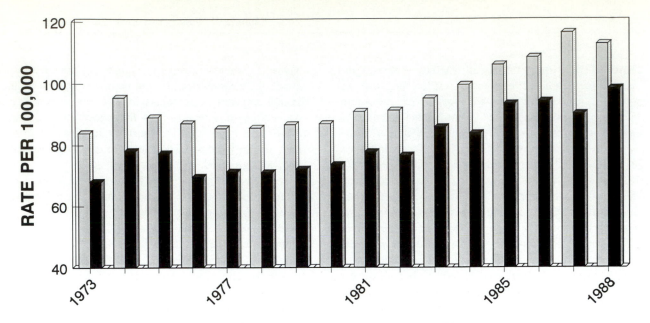

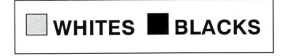

Fig. 2-18. Age-adjusted incidence rates for female breast cancer. (Based on data from the National Cancer Institute's Surveillance, Epidemiology and End Results [SEER] Program, 1973-1988.)

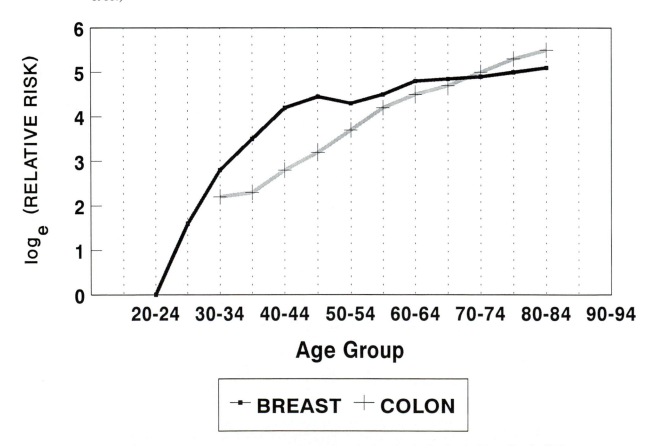

Fig. 2-19. Breast cancer and colon cancer incidence in females in Scotland. (From Boyle, Robertson: *J Natl Cancer Inst* 79:1175-1179, 1987.)

Incidence models can also be used to look at time trends in incidence according to age groups in an effort to observe a change in the probability for a specific cancer versus cancer as a whole. Boyle and Robertson studied the incidence of breast and colon cancer in females in Scotland (Fig. 2-19).[42] They observed a linear relative increase in colon cancer with aging, from 30 to 84 years of age. Breast cancer had a different pattern. There was a relative peak at 45 years of age and a relative decrease at 54 years of age with a subsequent resurgence of incidence with increasing age. This plateau of changing age-specific breast cancer incidence at or around the time of menopause had been well studied. This bimodal age-specific incidence curve for cancer of the breast has been termed *Clemmensen's hook,* after the work of Clemmensen in the late 1940s.[66,67]

Clemmensen's hook is not seen in male breast carcinoma.[147] However, it was observed in the age-dependent incidence of sinonasal cancer.[252] Hill et al. observed a Clemmensen's hook inflection at menopause in their studies of the incidence rates of female breast cancer in Alberta, Canada, from 1953 to 1977.[133] Clemmensen's hook

may reflect that the pathologic diagnosis of breast cancer is really two separate diseases, or it may mean that there are two separate temporal cohorts of patients.[42] Some recent data suggest a temporal cohort hypothesis because there is a decline in the appearance of Clemmensen's hook in many western countries. Boyle and Robertson suggest that the declining incidence of breast cancer in younger cohorts suggests the possible existence of a factor that protects against breast cancer, at least at younger ages.[42] This factor remains yet to be identified.

The bimodal incidence of breast cancer was studied by de Waard et al.[81] They separated their populations into those with obesity, hypertension, glucose intolerance, or a combination of these and those with none of these features. Obesity and hypertension were related to increased breast cancer in older postmenopausal breast cancer patients, whereas there was no such relation in the younger breast cancer patients.

This bimodal distribution in some patient populations is well demonstrated in the work of Hakama.[119] Figs. 2-20 and 2-21 show a plateau breast cancer incidence increase at about 40 to 45 years of age in four Scandinavian coun-

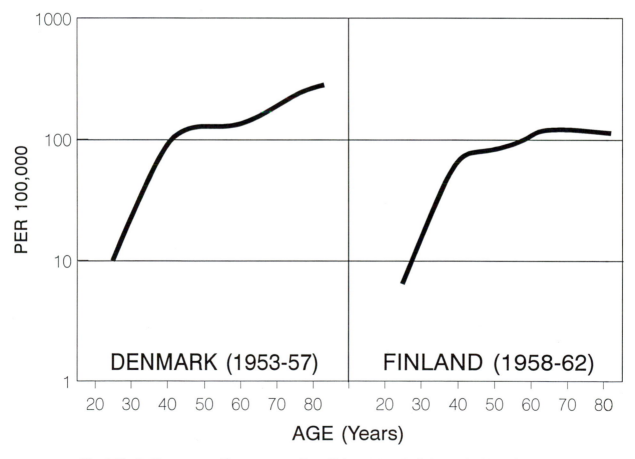

Fig. 2-20. Incidence rates of breast cancer. (From Hakama: *Acta Pathol Microbiol Scand* 75:340-374, 1969.)

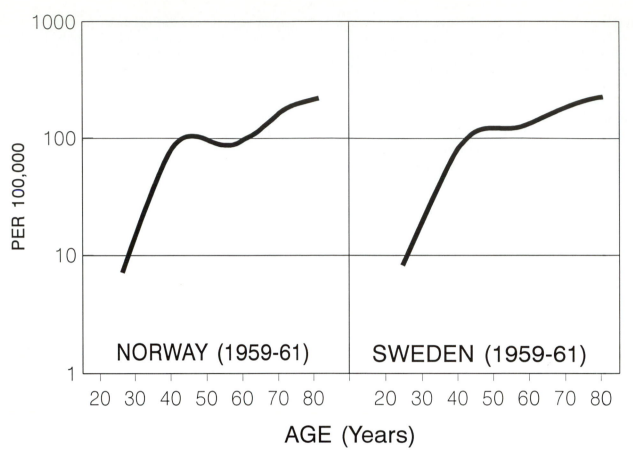

Fig. 2-21. Incidence rates of breast cancer. (From Hakama: *Acta Pathol Microbiol Scand* 75:340-374, 1969.)

tries. Lilienfeld and Johnson considered that the age-specific incidence rate for breast cancer can be resolved into two linear components.[181] One component occurred in the younger group (20 to 40 years of age) and the second began at about 40 years of age and persisted into old age. Hakama observed that the hypothesis of two forms of mammary cancer is supported by the fact that Clemmensen's hook diminishes when mortality data, rather than incidence data, are considered. He concludes that there is "some evidence in favor of the conclusion that Clemmensen's hook is caused by two complements of a disease both of which are called breast cancer."[119] These patterns can be seen in Figs. 2-22 and 2-23.

A bimodal population of breast cancer patients can be clearly discerned from the data obtained from these Scandinavian countries. There are a number of features that distinguish the typical case of premenopausal breast cancer from the typical case of postmenopausal breast cancer. It is possible that these are two separate disease entities having only histopathologic states in common. One conclusion of the clinical distinction may be that screening mammography is a more effective diagnostic strategy in post-

menopausal women. A recognition of multiple diseases grouped into one histologic nomenclature would be useful as we look for alternative diagnostic strategies or even alternative treatments. It is important to keep in mind that there may be multiple diseases that have common histopathologic characteristics called breast cancer. These diseases may be etiologically, biologically, and clinically distinct. That clinical distinction can include a distinction in appropriate diagnostic strategy.

Previously, we discuss the experience of Carter et al. in the Group Health Cooperative of Puget Sound.[56] They studied a clinically effective breast cancer screening program, which was modified on the basis of risk factors in an effort to diminish the cost of screening and still not substantially decrease the ability to detect early breast cancer. They were concerned that the early detection rate was at 55% for 20 years and that the addition of the American Cancer Society's recommendations would have increased it to only 70%. This 15% increase in their experience would amount to only 23 women and would have required the screening of an additional 50,000 women. Thus the marginal costs of detecting breast cancer (above that which

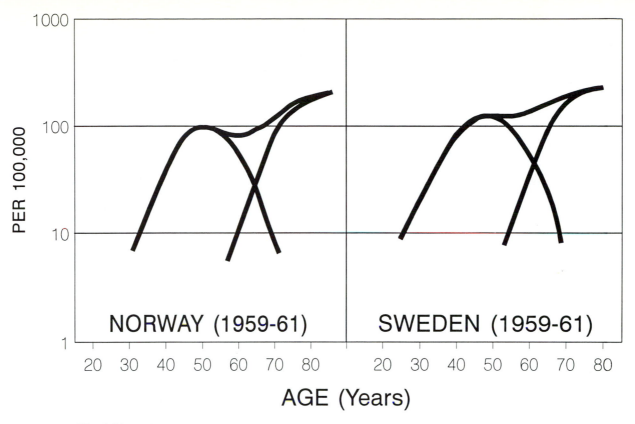

Fig. 2-22. Incidence rates of breast cancer of Clemmensen's hook. (From Hakama: *Acta Pathol Microbiol Scand* 75:340-374, 1969.)

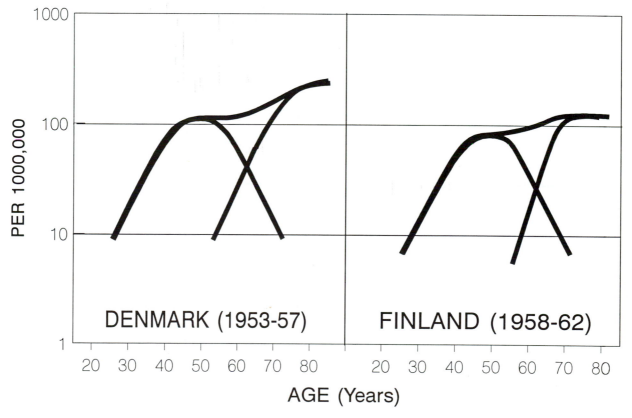

Fig. 2-23. Incidence rates of breast cancer of Clemmensen's hook. (From Hakama: *Acta Pathol Microbiol Scand* 75:340-374, 1969.)

was already extant before the implementation of the American Cancer Society's recommendations) were such that an effort was made to assess the merits of alternative strategies in screening for breast cancer. They analyzed the implications of seven different program options in recommending screening profiles. The option that detected the most cancers at the lowest costs for implementation used nurse practitioners for physical examination and breast self-examination instruction, with mammography performed only for reported risk. Thus in this study only 25% to 30% of women over the age of 40 years would be asked to undergo a mammography each year. The risk profile used by this group has been revised based on their own experience (see the section on Age). Using a cost-effective model, screening criteria based on relative incidence data may be a reasonable alternative to the standard recommendation and warrants further attention.

Recently, Paci et al. used age-related prevalence and incidence data as early indicators to evaluate the efficacy of breast cancer screening programs.[228] They observed a prevalence rate in a case controlled study in Florence, Italy. They obtained data on all breast cancer cases occurring within 5 years in any women who had been screened in their program. Thus they observed their false-negative cases. Using their data one can readily appreciate the difficulty of mammographic detection of breast cancer in the 40- to 50-year-old age group, as compared to the group of women over 50 years of age.

The dense glandular premenopausal breast may mask a cancer that may be more readily observed in an older woman's breast (see Table 2-6).

Further analysis reveals a significant difference between cancers detected in women over and under 45 years of age. The percentage of breast cancers detected on the first screen increased from 23% in the 40- to 45-year-old age group to 53% in women 45 to 49 years of age. In women under 50 years of age only 34% of the breast cancers were detected on the screening examination, whereas 82% of the cancers ultimately found in women age 50 to 69 years of age were detected on the mammographic screening examination. The authors detected 1.27 cancers per 1000 women between 40 and 49 years of age and 6.36 cancers per 1000 women between 50 and 69 years of age. The reason for this difference in detection is not evident from the statistical data alone.

Does increased breast density in premenopausal women mask breast cancer that is more readily detected in older women? Is the biology of premenopausal breast cancer not as mammographically obvious as postmenopausal breast cancer? Are these two separate diseases, or was there a length-time bias in the cancers detected on the prevalence screen in older women? To address these concerns, it is necessary to review some basic theories of cancer screening.

EARLY CANCER AND THE UNCERTAIN MAMMOGRAM
Interval cancer problem

If most cancers were diagnosed as interval cancers, a screening program would have little efficacy. Nonpalpable or asymptomatic breast cancer does not occur as interval cancer unless a mammogram is performed between the two screens. Martin et al. define interval cancers as "those whose signs or symptoms were first detected by the woman or her personal physician subsequent to a screening examination in which she had both a negative mammogram and a negative physical examination."[196] Thus interval cancers are symptomatic by definition. Some symptoms must have occurred between the screens to warrant a diagnostic procedure. Interval breast cancer usually is diagnosed after the patient identifies a breast lump that was not detected at the prior screen. Of the 48 interval cancer patients reported by Martin et al., two had crusting of the nipple, two had bleeding from the nipple, one had pain in the breast, and 43 had palpable masses.[196]

In a breast cancer screening program, interval cancer is defined as breast cancer diagnosed during the interval between two mammography screening periods. This cancer is distinguished from breast cancers found by the screening program. Cancers found by the screening program are either prevalence cancers or incident cancers. A change in a mammogram between two screening studies may reveal a cancer that occurred in the interval between the two screens. A "true" interval cancer is diagnosed in the interval between screens. The discovery of a breast cancer on any screening examination, other than the initial baseline study, is an incident cancer. Incident cancer is any cancer that occurs during the interval between two screens and that is detected by the screen. Any cancer found on an initial baseline screening mammogram is considered to be representative of breast cancer prevalence in the community being screened. A cancer apparent in retrospect is a false-negative screening examination. It could be representative of breast cancer prevalence or incidence, depending on when it is found. A "true" interval cancer is not present at the initial screen, but develops and becomes sufficiently symptomatic to be detected during the interval between two screens. "True" interval cancer represents a new cancer that has developed since the previous screen. This distinction between prevalence, incident, and interval cancer has been used to evaluate the natural history of early breast cancer. The way a breast cancer is diagnosed (i.e., prevalence screen, incidence screen, or interval symptoms) has an effect on a number of issues ranging from lead-time and length-time bias to the efficacy of the screening program.

Whitehead et al. sought to distinguish the features between breast cancer cases diagnosed at screening and interval cancers.[319] He studied 409 breast cancer patients in a case control study. He found no distinction between interval and screen detected cancers in relation to method of detection (mammography or palpation), age at menarche, first live childbirth, time of menopause, contraceptive use, or history of maternal cancer. He did, however, observe a relative increase in interval cancers over screen-detected cancers around the time of menopause.

When an interval cancer is found, it always raises questions concerning the efficacy of the screening program. Breast cancer screening is performed to find and treat the earliest cancers before they become symptomatic. When interval cancer occurs, was the cancer missed on the screen or was it not present?

Fig. 2-24 depicts the chances of finding a cancer that was diagnosed during an average of 30 months on a prevalence screen rather than during the interval. Some of the cancers found in this 30-month period would have been present at the time of the screen and missed. The fact that an interval cancer is more likely to be found in younger women is important to the design of screening programs. Fewer cancers will be detected on prevalence screens in women under 45 years old. This is not only because fewer cancers exist at this age, but also because the cancers that are subsequently shown to have existed are less likely to be diagnosed on the prevalence screen. This effect of age

on interval cancer has also been shown in a review of BCDDP data by Martin et al. in which one half of the 48 interval cancers occurred in women 50 years of age or younger.[196]

A similar but less dramatic age effect on the interval cancer occurrence is seen on screens subsequent to the prevalence screen (Fig. 2-25). In the 2953 tests of women from 40 to 44 years of age 11 cancers were found on repeated screens. Of these 11 cancers, 2 were interval cancer and the rest were diagnosed by screening. The follow-up period was only 3 years for this age group, whereas it is up to 11 years in the other groups. Even with repeated screens, a cancer that is eventually diagnosed will more often be found on a screen in older women. Is this because younger women have more rapidly growing cancers or because existing cancer is more often missed in the denser breasts seen in premenopausal women? Both of these are likely explanations.

Forty-eight cases of interval cancer were found in 630 biopsies performed in the interval between screening examinations in the BCDDP project.[196] This represents 13.1 biopsies per cancer found in the interval between screening examinations, as compared with 5.9 biopsies per cancer (2641:451) in the cases detected by screening. These in-

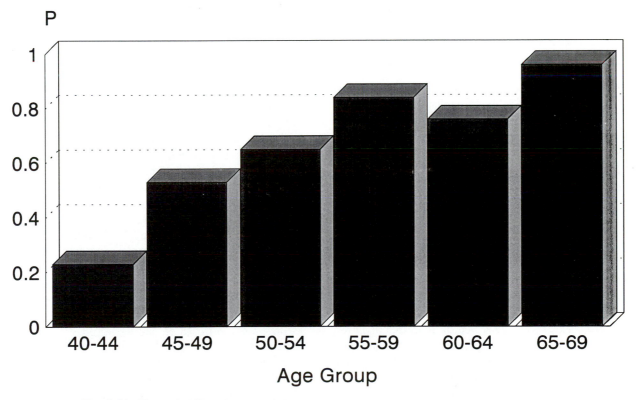

Fig. 2-24. The probability of a cancer being found on the first screen rather than during the interval between the first and second screen (average interval of 30 months). (Calculated from Paci et al: *Int J Cancer* 46:198, 1990. Reprinted by permission of Wiley-Liss, A Division of John Wiley & Sons, © 1990.)

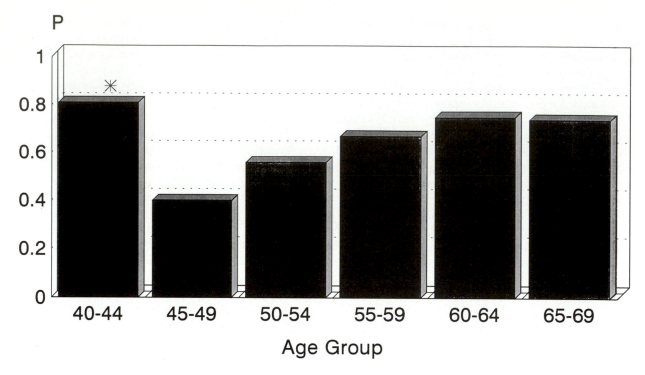

✳ only 3 year followup

Fig. 2-25. The probability that a cancer will be found on a screen rather than during the interval between screens 2 to 7 (average interval of 30 months). (Calculated from Paci et al: *Int J Cancer* 46:198, 1990. Reprinted by permission of Wiley-Liss, A Division of John Wiley & Sons., Inc. © 1990.)

terval biopsies were conducted because of the presence of new symptoms since the last screen. The false-positive indicators for biopsy were greater in the interval cases than on the screen. This suggests that mammograms suspicious for cancer caused fewer "unnecessary" biopsies than did clinical examinations that were sufficiently suspicious to warrant a biopsy. Of the 43 palpable masses that led to interval biopsy and in which cancer was found, 10 of the masses were cysts and the cancers were found incidentally. Five of these were intraductal carcinoma, and five were lobular carcinoma in situ. Martin et al.[196] consider that this observation may lend support to the hypothesis that some breast cancers cause excitation of surrounding tissues with increased collagen or even excitation of fibrocystic disease.[107] Similar results were observed in the HIP study,[97] in which cancers suspected by mammography resulted in only 4.6 biopsies per cancer (203:44) and those indicated on clinical grounds required 6.6 biopsies to find a cancer (392:59). In the HIP study, when the biopsy was based on both mammographic and clinical indicators, only 1.8 biopsies per cancer were found (54:29).

Interval cancers occur because the cancer was not diagnosed at the screening examination. Either it was missed by the screen or it became detectable only since the screen. If it was missed by the screen, can something be done to improve the screening process to recognize more of the detectable cancers? If it became detectable since the screen, should the screening interval be shortened? Can we detect more of these cancers earlier, or does interval cancer represent a tumor with an unusually rapid growth and poor prognosis? Kirch and Klein observed that interval cancers have a poorer prognosis than those found by screening.[165] They considered a low interval cancer rate in a screening series as a weak measure of programmatic success because interval cancers are usually due to cancers that are more rapidly growing than prevalence cancers. Calculations show that a large reduction in interval cancer cases does not imply an equivalent reduction in positive axillary node cases. Kirch and Klein found interval counts to be useful because they reveal programs that are less dependent on efficient patient self-examination.

Interval or incidence cancers have a poorer prognosis than do cancers detected on a prevalence screen.[165] The Edinburgh Breast Screening Project results agree with the theory that incidence screens find faster growing, more aggressive tumors. Tumors found at prevalence screens have a more favorable prognosis.[9] This is thought to be due to the lengthy presence of prevalence cancers before they were diagnosed. Does some subset of prevalence cancers have a sufficiently benign course, so that recognizing them in the preclinical state constitutes overdiagnosis? In their analysis of the BCDDP, Seidman et al. suggest that this is not the case.[266]

Some interval cancers are undoubtedly the result of the presence of rapidly growing, aggressive cancers. Undoubtedly, many interval cancers could have or should have been detected by screening. The mortality observed in any screening program will be adversely affected by these interval cancers. The 48 interval cancers reported by Martin et al.[196] were due to three major reasons: (1) poor radiographic technique; (2) absence of radiographic criteria of cancer; and (3) obvious oversight by the radiologist or failure to recognize subtle radiologic signs. Observer or technical error accounted for 36% of the 64 interval cancers reported by Holland.[139] Thirty-three percent were present but masked and not detectable on the screening mammogram; 31% of the cancers diagnosed in the interval between two mammographic screens were "true" interval cancers. These "true" interval cancers were those that occurred between scans and were not present as detectable breast cancer at the time of the screen. Holland distinguishes "masked" interval cancers from "true" interval cancers by calculating tumor doubling times and estimating that 20 of the 41 cases not due to technical or observer error were probably too small to be detected at the last screening. The "masked" cancers tended to be found in women with dense breasts or were caused by histologic features, in situ intraductal, or diffuse infiltrative lobular carcinoma.

Peeters et al. reviewed 158 breast cancers diagnosed in the 2-year interval between screens.[236] Over a period of six screening rounds, they did not observe a significant trend in the incidence of interval cancers (which ranged from 0.9 to 1.3 per 1000 women years after each screening round). Twenty-six percent of these cases were due to technical or observer error and an additional 16% were radiographically occult but detectable on the mammogram in retrospect. They regard "true" interval cancers as those that could not have been seen on previous mammograms. Of all the interval cancers, 58% were of this type.

These interval cancers occurred more commonly in younger women, perhaps because the "masked" cancers, as described by Holland, are especially prone to occur in dense breasts. Peeters noted that even with annual screening in women under 50 years of age, 66% of all interval cancers were undetectable on a previous mammogram. Holland suggests that women with dense breasts be more frequently screened, using more views and broader criteria for recommending a surgical biopsy for these women. Others suggest that this is one of the reasons for not advo-

cating the use of screening mammography in younger women.

Holland et al. reported a greater proportion of interval cancers than that seen in more recent publications.[139] This study included 209 cancers in a regular screening program and 66 interval cancers. Of every 4.2 cancers diagnosed at the screen, one was found in the interval (66:275, or 24%). In an American case control study, Whitehead et al. observed 78 interval cancers in a total of 409 cancers diagnosed (1 of 5.2, or 17%).[319] In the Canadian study, 34 breast cancers were diagnosed within 1 year after the first screen, in which 238 breast cancers were detected (1 of 8, or 12.5%).[23]

Survival, cure, and minimal cancer

Cancer is the leading cause of death in women 35 to 74 years of age. Breast cancer accounts for 29% of the total cancers in women and 18% of cancer deaths. In 1986 breast cancer was the most common death-causing cancer in women 35 to 54 years of age, and the second most common death-causing cancer in women 55 years of age and older. Smaller nonpalpable lesions have a much better prognosis than larger palpable lesions because larger lesions are more likely to have auxiliary node and distant metastases at the time of diagnosis. Mammographic screening enhances the capacity to diagnose nonpalpable breast cancer. Because of this aspect of screening mammography, it is considered to decrease the proportion of women who will die from breast cancer. In two large series the screened population had fewer breast cancer deaths than did the controlled population.[270,295] The diminished mortality from breast cancer, related to diagnoses at an earlier stage, has been responsible for the enthusiastic dissemination of screening mammography as an appropriate public health policy. These results conflict with other studies that found no evidence of change in the breast cancer mortality, despite the social policy attempted. Studies based on large registries using relative survival rates and age-adjusted mortality tables have inferred that there is as yet no demonstrable effect of modern breast cancer diagnosis and therapy. The age-adjusted mortality from breast cancer has changed very little over the past 50 years (Fig. 2-26).

The differences seen in mortality table analyses versus those seen in individual patient studies and control cohort studies have been difficult to reconcile. This contrast between population-based mortality data and the merits of earlier diagnosis represents an important conundrum in breast cancer control. This disparity has caused major controversies regarding the role of screening mammography in the diagnosis of nonpalpable breast cancer. In view of the important competing opinions, it is worthwhile to clarify both sides of the argument to appreciate their implications. First, we must understand the outcome measures used by

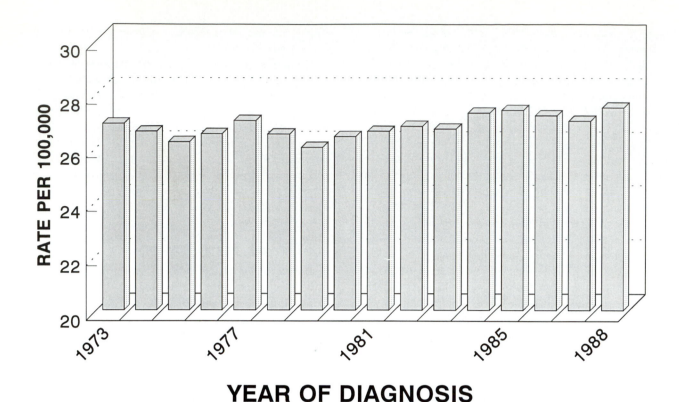

YEAR OF DIAGNOSIS

Fig. 2-26. Age-adjusted mortality rates for female breast cancer, all races. (Based on data from the National Cancer Institute's Surveillance, Epidemiology and End Results [SEER] Program, 1973-1988.)

the various proponents. We then must evaluate the effect of earlier diagnosis.

Measures of outcome. The impact of any medical intervention on the natural history of disease can be analyzed in many ways. What differences does it make to the patient if a different diagnostic strategy or course of treatment is used to modify the disease? The effect on populations of patients can be monitored using population death rates. Relative survival rates compare those who do with those who do not have breast cancer.

There are many possible factors that can change when a different diagnostic strategy or therapeutic approach is used. Population studies may reveal a change in total mortality from the disease. Paired control studies may demonstrate an effect on survival, disease-free survival, symptom-free interval, metastasis-free survival, proportion of patients with metastasis at the time of diagnosis, hazard rate, or even cure.

Mortality is defined in terms of deaths per 100,000 women and is usually adjusted for the age of the population. Survival is variously described as being alive at a specified time after the disease was diagnosed. These times are usually 5 years, 10 years, 15 years, or longer. A symptom-free interval is the duration between the diagno-

sis of the disease and the time when ultimate symptoms occur. Similarly, a metastasis-free interval is the duration between the diagnosis and when metastases are first recognized. In comparing diagnostic approaches, we determine the proportion of patients who are at an earlier stage of the disease at the time of diagnosis. The staging of breast cancer is used to compare patients diagnosed by one modality with those diagnosed using an alternative diagnostic strategy. Stage 0 and stage 1 cancers are more likely to result in longer term survival than are stage 3 or 4 cancers. Hazard rates are measures of the probability that a woman will manifest a clinical cancer. Once breast cancer is diagnosed, the subsequent hazard rate is approximately 4% per year.[60]

Finally, breast cancer "cure" is a different concept than other cures seen in medicine. A patient cured of pneumonia means that there is no residual disease. A patient "cured" of breast cancer means that the patient's probability of dying from the disease is no different from other women who have not had a previous diagnosis of breast cancer. If the woman has an unusually high-risk profile for breast cancer, she may not be "cured" because her chances of developing subsequent primary breast cancer are greater than women who have never had the disease. Thus, the issue of second primary in the other breast takes on a special significance when attempting to define which patients, if any, are "cured" of breast cancer. Perhaps a preferred definition of breast cancer "cure" is: A breast cancer can be considered as cured when the probability of dying from the residuum of the initial breast cancer is no greater than the probability of breast cancer death in other women who have never had the disease. Thus cured breast cancer could be defined as a return to a healthy state, as regards the chances of dying from any residuum of the primary disease.

Haybittle has defined three concepts for cure: a statistical cure, a clinical cure, and a personal cure.[125] The statistical cure is defined as the fraction of the original group of patients, showing an annual death-rate from all causes similar to that of a normal population of the same age distribution. Most long-term studies of breast cancer patients followed for 20 years or more have failed to show convincingly that a statistically cured fraction exists. The death rate of long-term survivors approaches, but does not reach, that of the similarly aged matched population. This approach compares relative survival. Relative survival is defined as crude survival rate divided by the expected survival rate multiplied by 100. If the relative survival rate equals the survival rate of persons without the disease, the relative survival rate becomes horizontal. One can con-

clude that the remainder of the individuals who originally had breast cancer have a risk for death from breast cancer precisely the same as the overall population (Fig. 2-27).

In most breast cancer studies there is a persistent negative slope of the relative survival cure. There have been a few very long-term studies. In these studies, although death approaches that of the control group at 20 to 30 years, there is a persistent excess mortality. Excess breast cancer mortality has been seen as long as 40 years after the diagnosis of breast cancer.[253]

In a study from Cambridge University, Brinkley and Haybittle have shown that the death rate from breast cancer at 20 to 30 years after its diagnosis remains 15 times greater than the rate from breast cancer deaths seen in the general population.[45] Le et al. had similar results.[174] These two long-term studies demonstrate the difficulty in eliminating breast cancer as a cause of death in women who have been diagnosed once with the disease. Brinkley and Haybittle studied 696 breast cancer patients and were able to follow-up 693 for at least 31 years.[45] Of these, 183 women died. Of these, 16 (26%) died from causes other than breast cancer. Eight deaths from breast cancer, however, occurred 25 years after the initial breast cancer, which was 15 times the number expected in a normal population. There was a constant decrease in the deaths from breast cancer from the years of diagnosis to approximately

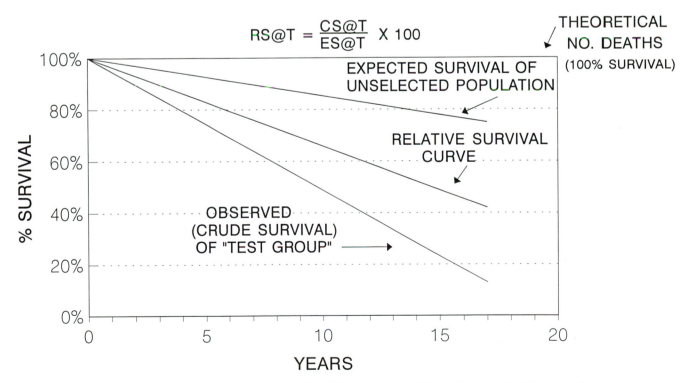

Fig. 2-27. Idealized relative survival. *RS,* Relative survival; *CS,* crude survival; *ES,* expected survival; *T,* time. (From Plotkin, Blankenberg: *Am J Clin Oncol* 14[3]:254-266, 1991.)

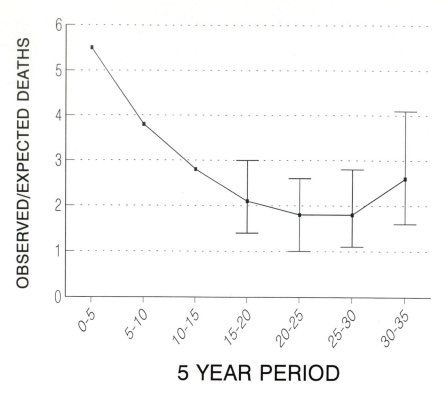

Error bars on last four points are 95% confidence limits.

Fig. 2-28. Breast cancer death rates: ratios of observed to expected. (From Brinkley et al: *Lancet* 1:1118, 1984.)

25 years. After 25 years there was an unexpected increase in deaths from breast cancer in this patient population (Fig. 2-28).

Similarly, Le et al. reported on the long-term survival of 2151 breast cancer patients treated at the Institute Gustave-Roussy from 1954 to 1967.[174] These patients were followed for at least 22 years. There appeared to be a statistical cure at approximately 22 years, when the number of patients dying from breast cancer equaled the expected number of deaths in the population who had never had the disease. However, after approximately 28 years, there was a resurgence of deaths from breast cancer (Fig. 2-29).

This late appearance of breast cancer deaths following initial breast cancer has led to considerable debate about the prospect for ultimate breast cancer cure. Some have considered that the late increase in mortality may be due to inadequate local treatment or the adverse effect of radiotherapy. Le et al. have effectively established that the late increase in mortality from breast cancer is not due to radiation therapy or other conservative approaches to the initial breast cancer treatment. A possible explanation for the late resurgence of breast cancer mortality after 25 years is the occurrence of a second primary tumor in women who are at demonstrable increased risk (as evidenced by the initial breast cancer). Perhaps this late mortality population

are those women who had some specific risk factors related to the initial breast cancer development. Thus far no one has done a comparative risk profile of women with and without late recurrent breast cancers. Obviously, these long-term studies do not include women with nonpalpable breast cancer diagnosed by screening mammography. Very few patients who were seen 25 years ago had their tumors diagnosed before the development of a palpable mass. Hopefully, earlier diagnosis will improve long-term survival. Large registry-based studies suggest that, once a woman has been diagnosed as having breast cancer, there is approximately a 75% chance that her death will ultimately be from this disease. These long-term studies are limited to patients whose disease was diagnosed at a more advanced stage then is usually accomplished by screening mammography. Mueller et al. observed an age-dependent relationship in the probability of ultimate death from breast cancer once the disease has been diagnosed.[217] They observed that breast cancer occurring at a younger age will more likely lead to ultimate death from the disease than would be the case for breast cancers occurring at an older age. This difference is not necessarily due to more virulent cancer in younger women because, in younger women, death from other causes is less probable. Mueller noted that breast cancer was ultimately a cause of death in 96.5% of women who had their breast cancers diagnosed

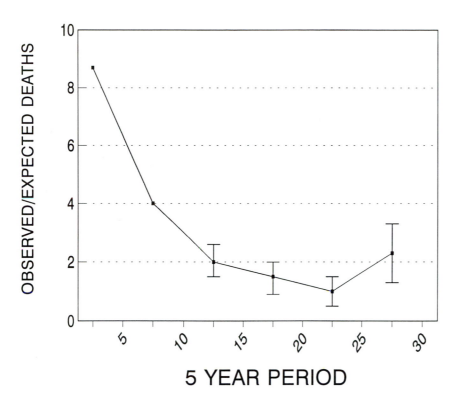

Error bars on last four points are 95% confidence limits.

Fig. 2-29. Breast cancer death rates: ratios of observed to expected. (From Le et al: *Lancet* 2:922, 1984.)

between the ages of 21 and 50.[217] In the 50 to 71 years of age group, 90% of the women ultimately died from breast cancer. Among women older than 70 years of age at the time of diagnosis, only 77.5% died from breast cancer. Younger women with breast cancer have a greater chance of ultimately dying from the disease because these younger women have fewer other lethal disease prospects, whereas many more causes of death could ensue in older women during the duration of observation. Plotkin and Blankenberg assert that, after the diagnosis of breast cancer at a relative young age, a survival of 30 to 40 years is so rarely seen that its occurrence warrants the reexamination of the original tissue for accuracy.[239] They concluded that "surviving breast cancer by dying of something else is more an expression of a pyrrhic victory than therapeutic efficacy." Needless to say, the same view holds true for diagnostic efficacy. Again, it must be appreciated that any woman whose breast cancer was diagnosed 30 to 40 years ago had a more advanced disease than can be found with modern mammographic screening.

In the United States, the constant age-adjusted mortality for breast cancer from 1973 to 1988 (Fig. 2-26) has been attributed in part to the increase in breast cancer mortality among blacks despite "improved" earlier diagnosis and "more effective" treatment. Fig. 2-30 shows the age-adjusted mortality by race. This reveals an increase in breast cancer mortality among blacks that is disproportionate to the relatively stable breast cancer mortality seen in whites. Before 1977 the mortality among whites was considerably higher than that among blacks. From 1977 to 1981 the mortality was roughly equivalent between the races. Only after 1981 has there been a dramatic increase in the absolute mortality among blacks or the mortality as compared to whites. This increased breast cancer mortality among black women may be due to a number of causes. No single explanation readily accounts for the total increase in breast cancer mortality among black U.S. women. This higher relative mortality is seen even though black women have a lower incidence of breast cancer than do white women. Is this difference between black women and white women biologic or sociologic? For example, the relative increase in longevity exposes more black women to breast cancer than was evident in prior years. Is this mortality difference the result of an increased virulence of the disease in black women, or is it due to socioeconomic conditions in which black women do not have equivalent access to modern diagnosis and therapeutic approaches to breast cancer control? If the latter is true, it suggests that diagnosis, treatment, or both have the effect of decreasing mortality in white women, although aggregate age-adjusted death rates do not appear to improve.

Over the past 50 years there has been a persistent small

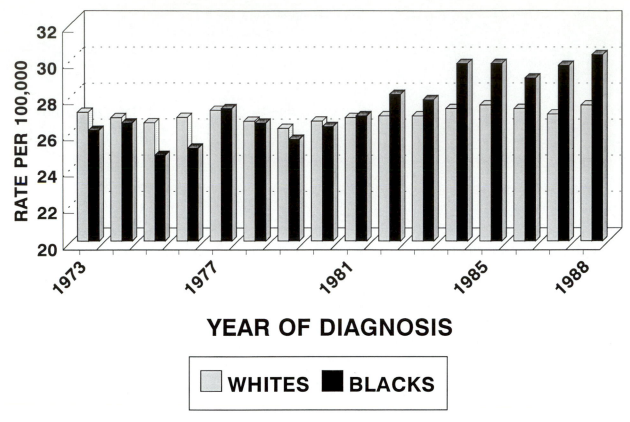

YEAR OF DIAGNOSIS

☐ WHITES ■ BLACKS

Fig. 2-30. Age-adjusted mortality rates for female breast cancer. (Based on data from the National Cancer Institute's Surveillance, Epidemiology and End Results [SEER] Program, 1973-1988.)

increase in age-adjusted mortality from breast cancer, despite advances in medicine and surgery and overall improvement in the practice of medicine. This breast cancer mortality is associated with the steady increase in the incidence of breast cancer over the past 50 years. The increasing incidence of breast cancer may be responsible for a constant mortality despite improvements in breast cancer control. Plotkin and Blankenberg argue that, if this is true, it is remarkable that the advances in breast cancer control have succeeded "in numerically nearly perfectly off-setting the potential increase in deaths so that the mortality rate remains stable."[239] They pose an alternative view, which they find more plausible. They suggest that the "extra cancers" may not have the biologic significance of cancers seen in previous years. The additional breast cancer incidence may be due to better diagnosis—in particular, mammography. Hayward et al. observed that an increase in the diagnosis of less malignant cancers occurred at a steady rise of approximately 1% per year from the 1930s to the 1960s and that it has jumped to 2% per year since 1960.[126]

Haybittle, in defining statistical cures, clinical cures, and personal cures, observed that true clinical cures infrequently occur, if they do at all.[125] The calculated risk of a second breast cancer over a follow-up period in the Cambridge series was 12%, as compared with the normal of 7% for the overall risk in England and Wales. Adair et al. observed a 16% increase,[1] whereas Le et al. observed an increase of 14%.[174] All of these population-based studies suggest that there is continued risk for breast cancer mortality long after apparent clinical cure in women with palpable (clinically evident) lesions that were diagnosed many years ago.

Personal cure is defined as an individual who has no further symptoms from the disease for the remainder of her lifetime and who dies from another cause. McBride et al., from the M.D. Anderson Hospital, reported a 12% personal cure rate for breast cancer.[197] Using the Cambridge series data, Brinkley and Haybittle observed that 26% of patients died from causes without overt signs of breast cancer present.[45]

Based on the experiences of the past 50 years, the proportion of personal cures, clinical cures, and statistical cures seems very low once a patient has received a diagnosis of breast cancer. Is the enthusiasm for early detection and alternative treatment unfounded, if the ultimate outcome of the disease may be modified very little by whatever approach is attempted? Have the results of widespread screening mammography in detecting nonpalpable breast cancer not yet had an impact on major population or controlled studies? The initial studies that demonstrated the ability of breast cancer screening to diminish deaths from breast cancer, done 20 years ago, have only recently achieved a widespread acceptance. Widespread screening mammography has only been established as a standard of care in most Western countries in the past 5 to 10 years. Will we see this effect of widespread earlier diagnosis in years to come? If we do not anticipate that this will have an effect on overall age-adjusted mortality, how can we justify our continued advocacy of breast cancer screening?

The effect of earlier diagnosis. The evidence from the HIP and the Swedish two-county study reveals that the proportion of women who die from breast cancer will be diminished if they are in the group that has been screened (Fig. 2-31). The HIP study and an 18-year follow-up study clearly showed a decline in mortality from breast cancer (Fig. 2-32). This was seen even in the 40- to 49-year old age group at entry. The differences between the groups who were 40 to 49 years of age at entry and those who were 50 to 64 years of age in part are due to the effects of

lag time on the ability to demonstrate an effect. The significant results were first observed 9 years after the HIP study for women 40 to 49 years of age at entry, and similar results were observed 4 years later in the women 50 to 64 years of age at entry. Chu et al. conclude that the benefit of screening in younger women was demonstrated.[61] However, the exact extent of mortality reduction attributable to mammography must await the evaluation of an extended follow-up. The impact of early breast cancer diagnosis by screening on women 40 to 49 years of age may not be demonstrable for a long time.

Some have argued that the effect of early screening is merely the identification of cancer at a preclinical stage, when identification would have occurred at a later time. This earlier diagnosis may have no effect on the ultimate "cure rate" despite an evident change in 5-year survival rate. The difference in survival rates may occur because the cancer is "clinically" observed for a longer period of time. Because the survival of the patient is measured from the time of the initial diagnosis, cancers found earlier by physical examination or mammography will, by their very nature, have a longer survival time. When survival is expressed as the percent of the original group alive 5 years after the diagnosis, any earlier sampling of the patient pop-

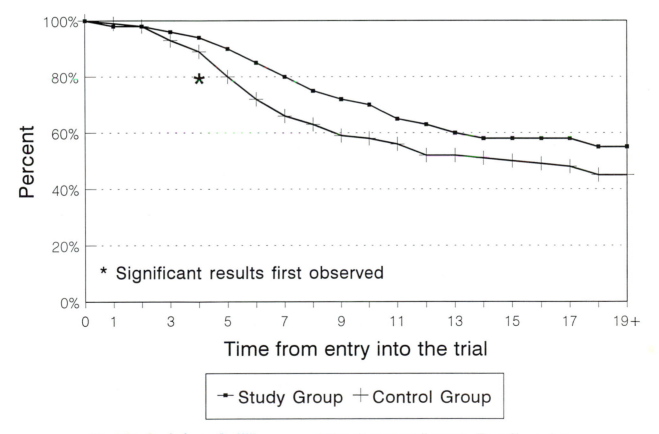

Fig. 2-31. Survival rates for HIP women aged 50 to 64 at entry (all stages). (From Chu et al: *J Natl Cancer Inst* 80:1125-1132, 1988.)

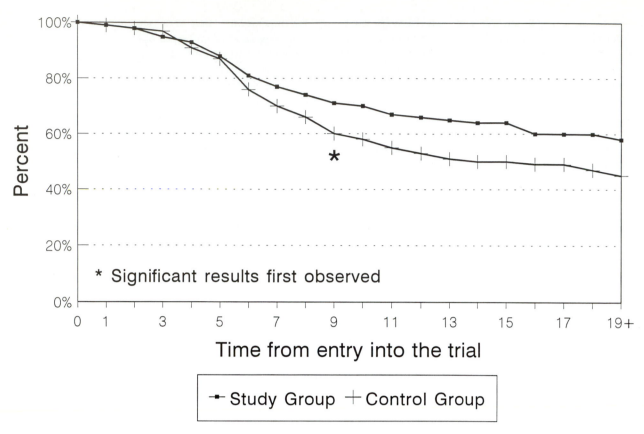

Fig. 2-32. Survival rates for HIP women aged 40 to 49 at entry (all stages). From Chu et al: *J Natl Cancer Inst* 80:1125-1132, 1988.)

ulation will result in an improved 5-year survival rate. This results in the classic "lead-time bias." Therefore merely following the 5-year survival rate of patients with breast cancer may be misleading if one wishes to find out if earlier diagnosis altered the natural course of the disease.

Adami et al. used data from Sweden to analyze the possible causes of an observed improvement in survival rates.[4] Changing diagnostic criteria (or even an increase in diagnostic activity) may result in a higher proportion of "biologically benign tumors." Increased diagnostic activity could also lead to earlier diagnosis, which would result in a lead-time bias or apparent "increased curability." Improved survival rates may be due to improved treatment. Finally, they suggest that the difference in the time trends of survival may be due to a changing natural history of the disease. Diagnostic or therapeutic interventions in breast cancer are intended to increase curability by whatever definition curability is assessed.

In addition to the effects on survival, earlier diagnosis may have an impact on treatment choice. Breast-conserving surgery may be possible with earlier diagnoses, independent of whether or not the patient ultimately dies from the disease. Thus earlier diagnosis may decrease morbidity of the disease. An improvement in morbidity can occur whether or not there is improvement in mortality. The opportunity to perform less radical surgery or to prolong the symptom-free interval may justify efforts to attain earlier diagnosis through mammographic screening.

The stage of breast cancer at diagnosis has a substantial impact on longevity. Thus the staging of breast cancer is useful to determine the effectiveness of alternative diagnostic systems. The diagnosis of earlier cancers by mammography screening necessitated modification of the standard TNM system of breast cancer staging. The revised system allows for recognition of smaller cancers.[31] *T1a* indicates cancers of 5 mm or less at the greatest diameter. *T1b* indicates primary cancers of between 5 mm and 1 cm in diameter. *T1c* indicates cancers between 1 and 2 cm in diameter. The median diameter of breast cancers currently diagnosed in the United States is less than 2 cm. It is important to have this subset staging available to develop more sophisticated analyses of the implications of alternative diagnostic and therapeutic strategies.[54] In addition to the newer staging criteria for the primary cancers, node metastases are separated into more precise categories. *N1a* are micrometastases of less than 0.2 mm in diameter. *N1b1* metastases are those with one to three lymph nodes of larger than 0.2 mm, but less than 2 cm. *N1b3* nodes have extensions through the capsule, but are less than 2 cm in overall diameter. This improved staging hopefully will allow for more reliable assessments of diagnostic strategies and therapeutic approaches to treat early nonpalpable breast cancer.

Joensuu and Toikkenen compared breast cancers diagnosed in the 1980s with those diagnosed in the 1940s to 1960s.[157] They did a retrospective cohort study of patients seen in Turku, Finland. They observed that breast cancers diagnosed in the 1980s had a smaller primary tumor size and fewer axillary metastases than those diagnosed in the 1940s to 1960s. The later cancers had more favorable histologic features and were associated with better prognosis than cancers diagnosed in earlier years. They concluded that the improved survival rate for breast cancer can partially be explained by the detection of more and smaller cancers with favorable histologic characteristics. There was no change in the histologic type or DNA ploidy. Rather, the more recent cancers had less nuclear pleomorphism and lower mitotic counts with less tumor necrosis and a better defined tumor margin. The patients from the 1980s had a much higher proportion of smaller tumors at the time of diagnosis, presumably the result, in part, of the impact of the mammographic detection of nonpalpable tumors. The proportion of the T0T1 cancers increased from 13% to 41% ($P < 0.0001$). The survival rate curves for

these two groups are readily distinguishable. Fig. 2-33 displays the survival rate corrected for intercurrent deaths in these two groups of patients. Patients diagnosed in the 1980s had a 21% better 5-year survival rate than those cases diagnosed from 1945 to 1965. This improved survival was correlated with a smaller primary tumor size and less advanced stage at diagnosis. The tumors were associated with fewer axillary nodes and distant metastasis ($P < 0.0001$). The improved 5-year survival rate in the 1980s was seen even in those patients with a poorer histologic grade of tumor ($P < 0.001$). Interestingly, the cancers seen in 1980 to 1984 occurred in older women than those diagnosed in 1945 to 1955. The mean age at diagnosis increased from 55.5 to 62.5 years of age (Table 2-17).

Does this improved survival rate mean that the patients in Turku are faring better in the 1980s than they were in prior years? Or is this apparent improvement the result of a "lead-time bias," with cancers merely detected earlier and observed for a longer period of time? The increased breast cancer incidence with a stable mortality suggests some possible contribution of a lead-time bias (Fig. 2-34). The age-adjusted incidence increased from 30.8 of 100,000 person years in 1953 through 1957 to 62.2 in 1983 through 1987. This occurred while the mortality was relatively stable, increasing only from 16.7 to 17.2 of 100,000 person years.

The staging of breast cancer had a substantial impact on 5-year survival rates in the SEER program. Data revealed that the 5-year program survival rate correlated closely to

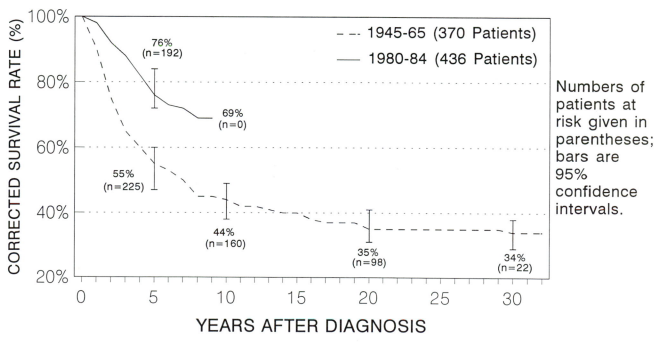

Fig. 2-33. Survival corrected for intercurrent deaths of patients diagnosed with breast cancer. (From Joensuu, Toikkanen: *Br Med J* 303:155-158, 1991.)

Table 2-17. Effect of year of diagnosis on breast cancer characteristics

| | No. survived for 5 years | | | | |
| | Diagnosis, 1945-1965 | | Diagnosis, 1980-1984 | | |
	N	%	N	%	P value
Primary tumor size*					
pT1 (≤2 cm)	56	52(93)	149	133(89)	0.43
pT2 (2-5 cm)	244	151(62)	160	114(71)	0.03
pT3 (>5 cm)	73	19(26)	19	9(47)	0.10
pT4	58	11(19)	35	18(51)	0.001
Stage†					
I	41	40(98)	96	94(98)	0.68
II	194	120(62)	168	128(76)	0.0
					0.0001
III	81	20(25)	41	20(49)	0.02
IV†	18	1(6)	13	8(62)	0.001
Histologic grade					
1	111	101(91)	126	122(97)	0.004
2	173	99(57)	142	101(71)	0.005
3	155	43(28)	102	58(57)	<0.0001

From Joensuu H, Toikkanen: *Br Med J* 303:155-158, 1991.

*Not known in two cases; intraductal cancer (eight in 1945-1965 and five in 1980-1984) not shown.

†Given only for patients who had axillary nodal evacuation.

‡Two-year survival figures; data missing in three cases.

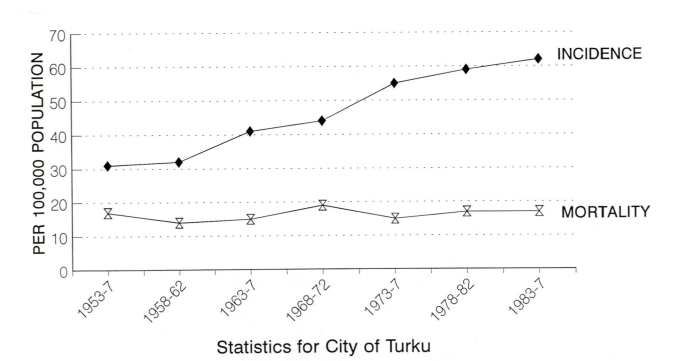

Fig. 2-34. Age-adjusted incidence of breast cancer and resulting mortality in Finland. (From Joensuu, Toikkanen: *Br Med J* 303:155-158, 1991.)

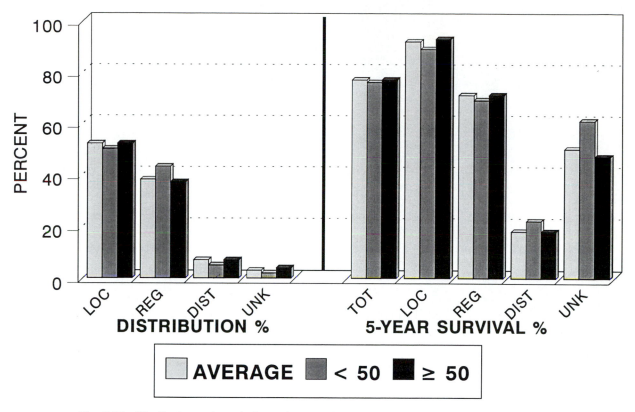

Fig. 2-35. Distribution and survival rates by stage for female breast cancer, all races (number of cases = 74,219). (Based on data from the National Cancer Institute's Surveillance, Epidemiology and End Results [SEER] Program, 1981-1987.)

the stage at diagnosis (Fig. 2-35). The SEER program data reveal that most breast cancers are diagnosed at a localized stage. More patients under 50 years of age have regional spread than do patients older than 50 years of age. The 5-year survival rate of patients under 50 years of age with distant metastases is statistically greater than the 5-year survival rate of the patients over 50 years of age. This distinction may (in part) be due to lead-time bias, but the exact basis for it is not clearly established. More than 50% of the cancers seen in the SEER program in the years 1981 to 1987 were localized at the time of diagnosis. This varied slightly with age and substantially with race (Figs. 2-36 and 2-37). The 5-year survival rate for breast cancer from 1974 to 1985 in white U.S. women was 75%. However, if the cancer was identified as a localized cancer, the survival rate increased to 91%. When the cancer had spread to regional lymph nodes, the survival rate dropped to 69%. Only 19% of patients with distant spread survived for 5 years. For black women the comparable figures were a 63% total 5-year survival rate, 86% if the cancer was localized, 55% if the cancer was regional, and 14% if distant metastases were present. The 5% difference in localized cancer may be due to biologic differences, but the differ-

ences seen once the cancer has spread may be due to differences in the care received.[291] Black women with breast cancer have a lower 5-year survival rate at all ages. This difference is even more pronounced in older black women (Fig. 2-37).

Between 1974 and 1985, 48% of breast cancers were localized, 41% were regional, and 7% had distant metastases when diagnosed. The 5-year survival trends for breast cancer in the United States have improved between the years 1960 and 1985 (Fig. 2-38).

In Rochester, Minnesota, even before the advent of screening mammography, they observed a slight improvement in the length of survival after breast cancer diagnosis in women who were less than 45 or more than 65 years of age at the time of diagnosis. Brian et al. studied the epidemiologic features of breast cancer in Rochester, Minnesota, over the 40-year period from 1935 to 1974.[44] The age-adjusted incidence rose 25%, to 82.7 per 100,000 person years. Similar to the Finnish experience the breast cancer incidence increased with advancing age, as did the prevalence. They observed a prevalence of 9 cases per 1000 women on January 1, 1975. The age-adjusted mortality declined from 24.9 to 23.3 per 100,000 person years

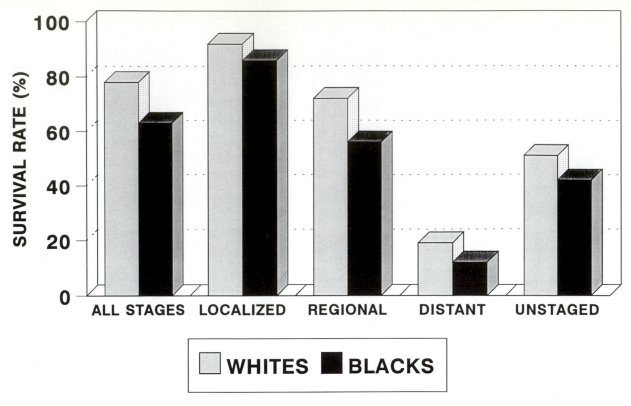

Fig. 2-36. Five-year survival rates for female breast cancer. (Based on data from the National Cancer Institute's Surveillance, Epidemiology and End Results [SEER] Program, 1981-1987.)

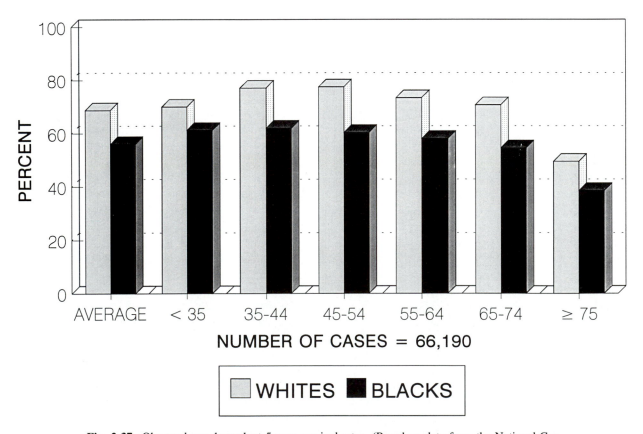

Fig. 2-37. Observed age-dependent 5-year survival rates. (Based on data from the National Cancer Institute's Surveillance, Epidemiology and End Results [SEER] Program, 1981-1987.)

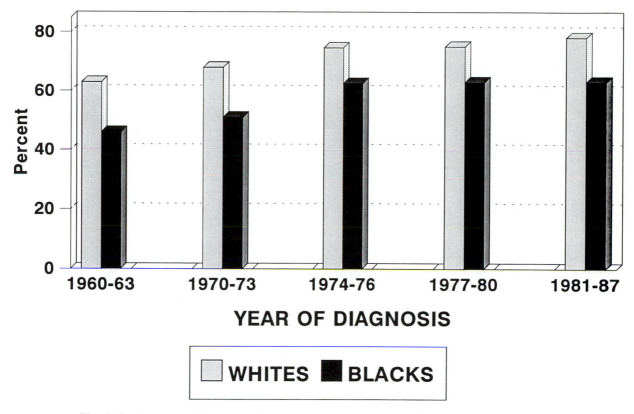

Fig. 2-38. Five-year relative survival rates for female breast cancer. (Based on data from the National Cancer Institute's Surveillance, Epidemiology and End Results [SEER] Program, 1960-1987.)

over a 40-year period. The increase in survival in the mammographic era is also associated with the decline in regional lymph node and distant metastases at the time of diagnosis. Perhaps this is related to more vigilant early clinical diagnosis by palpation. Ballard-Barbash et al. compared the incidence and survival rates of breast cancer patients in Rochester, Minnesota, from 1935 to 1982.[25] The age-adjusted incidence rate was determined after excluding patients with carcinoma in situ. The incidence rates rose 14% when comparing patients from 1965 to 1974 with those from 1975 to 1982. The incidence increased from 87.2 to 99.5 per 100,000 person years. Similar to the Finnish study findings, the Minnesota study found that the frequency of axillary node and distant metastases at the time of initial diagnosis decreased significantly. Thus the increased incidence was related to the diagnosis of patients with less advanced disease. In this study the authors noted no increase in overall survival rates, and they relate this to the lack of sufficient time to observe the effects of the improved earlier diagnosis. The only patients in whom they observed a statistical improvement in survival were those patients with distant metastatic disease at the time of diagnosis ($P < 0.01$). Their survival

increased from a median of 21 months to a median of 28 months when comparing the period of 1955 to 1974 versus the period of 1975 to 1982. The authors relate this increased survival rate to advances in therapy—inasmuch as it is improbable that advances in earlier diagnosis were the causes because these lesions were all metastatic at the time of diagnosis. As long ago as the 1940s Haagensen reported a doubling of the 5-year cure rate in women operated on at Presbyterian Hospital.[118] When he compared patients from 1940 to 1942 with those operated on from 1915 to 1919, the 5-year "clinical cure rates" increased from 26.6% in the 1915 to 1919 period to 52.5% in the 1940 to 1942 period. Similarly, Cutler et al. described long-term breast cancer treatment results in 53,330 women with breast cancer treated from 1940 to 1964.[73] They observed a steady improvement in 5-year survival rates from 1940 to 1969. They noted a 53% survival in the period from 1940 to 1949, a 60% survival in the period from 1950 to 1959, a 62% survival in the period from 1960 to 1964, and a 64% survival in the period from 1965 to 1969. Chism et al. studied 530 women from Brookside Hospital in San Pablo, California, from 1968 to 1983.[60] During this time, mammography became available in 1970 and fine-needle aspiration became widely used by 1982. They noted a slight improvement in 5-, 10-, and 15-year survival rates in the intervals of 1972 to 1975, 1975 to 1979, and 1980 to 1983 when compared to the earliest interval of 1968 to 1971. These differences, however, were not statistically significant. The frequency of stage I disease increased from 16% to 31%. They concluded that, although progress has been made in diagnosis and breast conservation with palliation of symptoms, the end results for the total breast cancer population remain stable during a time when the treatment evolved markedly. In the United States, 5-year survival rates in white women have increased from 63% in the period from 1960 to 1963 to 76% in the period from 1980 to 1985. In the 1974 to 1976 period to the 1980 to 1985 period, the rate increased from 75% to 76%. This 1% increase was statistically significant ($P < 0.05$).[279]

Minimal cancer. Breast cancer screening involves other conceptual problems. What is the smallest cancer we can expect to find by mammography? Is it small enough to remove before it is too late? Is breast cancer ever cured? Martin and Gallager established a concept of minimal cancer.[195] They defined it to be a noninvasive intraductal carcinoma, a lobular carcinoma in situ, or an invasive carcinoma forming a mass with a volume no greater than a sphere of 0.5 cm in diameter. The National Cancer Institute guidelines state that "a lesion no more than 1 cm in diameter" is the criterion for minimal cancer.[196] Obviously, it would be ideal if mammographic screens could be timed to coincide with the period when cancer is minimally detectable. This would maximize the probability of "curing the cancer" through early detection. However, the probability of mammographic detection increases over time. A mammographic examination is more likely to miss the earliest detectable cancer than a more obvious lesion. There is a continuum of increasing detectability occurring during the mammographically detectable phase of a breast cancer's life cycle. The earlier the detection, the greater the duration of time between detection and the last chance for "cure."

Some investigators have argued against the concept of "minimal cancer." Often, they take the position that there is no cured breast cancer.[239] This is based on the observation that even "minimal" breast cancer can be "satisfactorily treated" only to recur at some later time, perhaps in a remote site. However, in many treated breast cancer cases, the patient dies from other causes long after the cancer was treated and the patient had no evidence of residual or metastatic breast cancer. We consider those patients to have been cured of their cancer. The object of a breast cancer screening program is to maximize the number of such "cures." Because breast cancer screening programs have clearly demonstrated a possible reduction in the number and proportion of women who die from breast cancer, this

is a reasonable objective. This leads to a need to clearly define breast cancer and when it occurs.

What is the earliest time an abnormal can be termed *breast cancer?* In biopsies to detect minimal cancer, we often find breast variations, such as atypia or hyperplasia, which are considered by some to be precursors of cancer. Biologically significant breast cancer may never develop in these patients.[230] Dupont and Page distinguished between proliferative atypia and the nonproliferative variations.[85] They correlated subsequent cancer to atypical hyperplasia. Clinical cancer is much more likely to develop if atypical hyperplasia is found in a patient with a family history of breast cancer (see the section on p. 37). Atypical hyperplasia and family history have a highly synergistic effect on the risk for breast cancer.

One problem in trying to identify the earliest breast cancer has been the inclusion in many reports of carcinoma in situ. Carcinoma in situ probability does not represent clinically significant breast cancer. Carcinoma in situ is a marker of risk for subsequent invasive cancer. Will every carcinoma in situ develop into invasive cancer? Probably not.

Hyperplasia, cellular atypia, and even carcinoma in situ may belong to a continuum of precancer. The questions about preinvasive breast cancer have been studied extensively. In 1913 MacCarty recognized and reported on preinvasive breast carcinoma.[191] This was defined by Broders in 1932 as carcinoma in situ.[47] Broders observed that in situ carcinoma consists of malignant epithelial cells that move into positions previously occupied by normal cells. These cells do not migrate beyond the normal epithelial basement membrane. The work of Foote and Stewart clarified lobular carcinoma in situ.[102] Their work has been the basis for subsequent literature in this field. Most researchers consider that lobular carcinoma in situ is a preinvasive cancer. Normal epithelial elements are transformed into invasive neoplastic cells only after going through intermediate morphologic states. Ductal carcinoma in situ and lobular carcinoma in situ are considered intermediate states in the development of ultimate invasive and metastatic cancer. Not all ductal carcinomas in situ or lobular carcinomas in situ will eventually progress to clinical cancer. The passage of these cells through the various states may take many months or years. Breast carcinoma appears to grow in spurts. The various inducers and restrainers of growth activation are not constant, despite the use of doubling times as indices of cancer origin.

Lobular carcinoma in situ is a lesion occurring primarily in premenopausal women. It tends to be diffuse and bilateral and is most often an incidental finding at breast biopsy. Table 2-18, taken from Ketcham and Moffat, summarizes the distinctions between DCIS and LCIS.[163] *DCIS is a premalignant lesion, whereas LCIS is a marker of*

Table 2-18. Ductal carcinoma in situ versus lobular carcinoma in situ

	DCIS	LCIS
Age profile	Parallels that of invasive breast cancer	Younger, premenopausal
Presentation	Mass or mammographic abnormality	Often incidental
Mammographic appearance	Microcalcifications	Variable
Associated with infiltrating carcinoma	Up to 40%	Up to 35%
Multicentricity	50%-65%	60%-65%
Axillary metastases in the absence of demonstrable invasive cancer	Up to 7%	Approximately 1%
Subsequent invasive cancer		
Incidence	25%-55%	20%-30%
Laterality	Largely ipsilateral	Both breasts equally at risk
Mean time to diagnosis	Approximately 10 yr	Approximately 20 yr

From Ketcham AS, Moffat FL: *Cancer* 65:387-393, 1990.
DCIS indicates ductal carcinoma in situ; *LCIS,* lobular carcinoma in situ.

breast cancer risk. Ketcham and Moffat do not agree on the use of the term *minimal,* or *microinvasive, breast cancer.* They consider that, from a clinical point of view, "invasiveness is a binomial variable with definitive treatment implications in the context of breast cancer."

In situ lobular carcinoma is usually an incidental finding. There are no specific clinical or radiologic signs (see Chapter 4). Calcification may be associated with some in situ lobular carcinomas and this calcification can be seen on histologic examination. However, most often LCIS is not detectable by mammography and the association with calcifications is merely coincidental. The radiologic signs of DCIS are exceptional. They are infrequently associated with focal density and periductal fibrosis with localized ductasia.[107,240] Holland et al., in a study of mammographically occult breast cancer, found only one intraductal carcinoma in situ, discovered as a mammographic sign other than microcalcification.[138] This cancer was found as an incidental finding adjacent to a fibroadenoma. Holland et al. observed that the threshold size of a radiologically detected invasive breast cancer in a radiolucent breast is about 5 mm, whereas cancer in a dense breast may grow to 20 to 30 mm and still remain mammographically occult when imbedded in dense fibroglandular tissue. The authors distinguished the mammographic presence of intralobular carcinomas from intraductal carcinomas by the lack of a desmoplastic reaction with LCIS. Some cases of DCIS produce a desmoplastic reaction and can be detected by mammography. These DCISs are manifest by the presence of microcalcifications. Jensen et al. studied preneoplastic lesions of the human breast using a sampling technique, with histologic confirmation made by the presence of a pathologic disorder of whole human breasts.[155] They observed that, in animals, "atypical lobules" were seen more frequently in breasts associated with cancer than in other

breasts. They identified atypical lobules in human breasts that were associated with cancer. They found this to be similar to the cancer-associated hyperplastic alveolar nodules (HAN) observed in mice. When comparing cancerous and noncancerous human breasts, papillary hyperplasia and cytologic atypia were more frequently found in cancerous breasts. These lesions appeared to be histologically identical to the higher grade atypia, which they call atypical lobules (AL). They felt that the presence of atypical lobules in breast biopsy specimens should alert clinicians and pathologists to the tendency of such women to develop breast cancer.

Others have sought to identify a means of detecting clinically obscure proliferative breast disease. A major effort was conducted by Ward et al., who sought to detect proliferative breast disease in four-quadrant needle aspiration.[314] They examined women with a strong family history of breast cancer. Fourteen families were studied. The subjects were evaluated in a clinical research center with physical examinations, screening mammography, and fine-needle aspiration. They classified the cytologic findings into normal epithelium, benign ductal hyperplasia, or atypical ductal hyperplasia. Proliferative breast disease occurred in 39% of women who otherwise had no evidence of breast cancer on mammography. Were these preneoplastic lesions? Is fine-needle aspiration a reasonable adjunct to mammography and clinical diagnosis for screening people at extremely high risk for breast cancer? In women under 50 years of age, Ward et al. found that 43% of those with first-degree relatives with breast cancer had proliferative breast disease.[314] This decreased to 29% in women over 50 years of age, for a total of 39% in the entire population. This work has been criticized by Page and Dupont.[229] They think that the term *proliferative breast disease* should be limited to histologic diagnosis. They do not feel that cytology is effective in distinguishing proliferative breast disease. Skolnick et al.[284] responded to the concerns of Page and Dupont by reviewing a series of studies in which histologic and cytologic diagnosis were concordant for severe atypical hyperplasia. Cytologic analysis revealed a continuum of changes in proliferative lesions. They noted that histopathologists do not agree with each other about the diagnosis of proliferative breast disease any more than do cytologists. Skolnick et al. think that inherited proliferative breast disease will eventually be defined "genotypically by specific DNA sequences at specific loci, and phenotypically by molecular analysis of expression of specific oncogenies, the inactivation of specific tumor suppressor genes, and quantitative histologic and cytologic analysis." To some degree this summarizes the level of certainty in the diagnosis of the earliest of breast cancers.

The diagnosis of in situ carcinoma has changed over the past 10 years. The frequency with which the diagnosis is made is increasing. Simon et al. studied the trends in the diagnosis of in situ carcinoma in the Detroit Metropolitan area from 1973 to 1987.[281] They observed that the largest increase in the diagnosis of in situ carcinoma occurred in black women older than 70 years of age. Their data, obtained from the SEER, suggested that in situ carcinoma represented only 5% of all breast cancers. The Detroit study had a cohort of 1316 women with a mean age of 56 years of age. Of these, 957 had ductal carcinoma in situ, 313 had lobular carcinoma in situ, and 40 had both. Of these, 73 were DCIS and 24% were LCIS. *The increasing incidence of carcinoma in situ is largely due to increased number of biopsies detecting otherwise benign lesions at mammography.* The increasing diagnosis of LCIS may be merely an offshoot of the efforts to screen for early breast cancer.

Wertheimer et al. observed that mammography alone was responsible for a biopsy recommendation in 42% of the cancers detected, as compared with only 33% in the HIP study.[316] Less than 20% of all the women with cancer detected in the BCDD study had positive nodes at surgery, as compared with the previous standard of 50%. The increased number of biopsies performed because of mammography has resulted in a decreased number of axillary nodes at the time the diagnosis is made. As many as one third of all the breast cancers detected in the BCDD study were "minimal breast cancers. Only 2.5% of the breast cancers detected by physical examination in the San Diego study were "minimal."[256] The frequency with which minimal cancers are found on screening studies varies with the study. Bland et al., using the BCDD data from the University of Louisville, defined minimal cancers as in situ or invasive carcinomas of less than 1 cm in diameter.[37] They found that approximately 30% of the cancers in the screened population were minimal, as compared with less

than 5% in an unscreened population. Ketcham and Moffat reviewed the proportions of DCIS to LCIS in the in situ carcinomas.[163] Sixty-eight percent of the SEER cases were DCIS; 63% of the American Cancer Society cases were DCIS; and 80% of the BCDD cases were DCIS.

What is the significance of ductal carcinoma in situ? Ketcham and Moffat reviewed 83 patients from a series of articles on the diagnosis of carcinoma in situ.[163] In those patients, 42% subsequently developed invasive cancer. The incidence of multicentricity in the intraductal carcinomas observed on total mastectomy specimens was approximately 30%. Multicentricity was found more often in clinically palpable than in mammographically detected ductal carcinoma in situ. Ketcham and Moffat note that the therapeutic problem presented by multicentricity is not limited to lobular carcinoma in situ. Gump compared grossly palpable with mammographically detected ductal carcinoma in situ.[116] They found that palpable ductal carcinoma in situ had a much higher instance of occult invasion and residual disease in the breast after incisional biopsy. DCIS has been classified into subtypes that correlate with a specific biologic behavior. In situ comedocarcinoma has a much greater long-term risk for infiltrating cancer and is more apt to be invasive than either the papillary or cribriform DCIS.[163]

Page et al. studied 28 patients with ductal carcinoma in situ who underwent biopsy.[230] These patients were observed from the years 1950 to 1968. In 25 women followed for more than 3 years, 7 developed invasive breast carcinoma. These were all in the same breast. Four of these seven patients with invasive carcinoma developed distant metastasis after mastectomy. This study suggests that 28% of women who are treated with biopsy only and in whom DCIS is an incidental histologic finding will develop invasive carcinoma in a follow-up period of approximately 15 years.

Subsequent invasive carcinoma in patients with ductal carcinoma in situ ranges from the 25% found by Farrow[93] to the 75% found by Dean and Geschickter.[78] In patients with DCIS most of the subsequent invasive cancers are found in the same quadrant of the affected breast—that is, at the original in situ lesion. However, despite meticulous follow-up, 20% to 30% of the new lesions have already metastasized to the axillary nodes at the time they are discovered. In view of this, it has been suggested that patients with ductal carcinoma in situ may wish to undergo a total mastectomy. Ketcham and Moffat reviewed some 510 patients from the published literature who underwent total mastectomy for ductal carcinoma in situ.[163] In this series 29 patients (or 5.7%) had recurrences, and 7 (or 1.4%) died from breast cancer despite undergoing total mastectomy. The recurrence rate ranged from 0.9% to 10.4%.[16,251] LCIS and DCIS are incidental findings in up to 10% of benign breast biopsy specimens. They occur in approximately 30% to 40% of patients who have other invasive carcinoma. Clearly, there seems to be some relationship between the presence of ductal carcinoma in situs and the ultimate development of invasive carcinoma.

The outcome for lobular carcinoma in situ is clearly different than that for ductal carcinoma in situ. Because lobular carcinoma in situ is a premenopausal disease and is not as evident in postmenopausal women, one wonders what happens to it. Does it become invasive cancer with age, or does it disappear? Is it merely a marker for subsequent breast cancer in some patients but not in all and therefore remains in older women? Because breast specimens from postmenopausal women do not have the incidence of LCIS seen in premenopausal patients, perhaps LCIS regresses with age. The ultimate outcome of patients with LCIS has been reported on by Ketcham and Moffat from a series of 346 patients they found in the literature.[163] Of these, 19.9% developed cancer during surveillance. Of these, 13% were ipsilateral cancers, 9% were contralateral cancers, and 3% were bilateral cancers. Of the total 346 patients with LCIS, 16 ultimately died from breast cancer, yielding a 4.6% mortality. The patients in these series were followed for a period of 4 to 27 years with an average of approximately 15 years. The deaths from breast cancer ranged from 2.9% to 11.5%.[7,117]

Haagensen et al. found 211 examples of LCIS, which they prefer to call lobular proliferation rather than carcinoma in situ.[117] The designation of carcinoma for a lesion that will probably not become malignant has ominous overtones that can influence therapy and patient anxiety. They note that this pathologic disorder should be recognized as a risk factor that is cumulative with gross cystic disease and a family history of breast cancer in a first-degree relative. When all three risk factors were present (i.e., LCIS, gross cystic disease, and first-degree family history), the ratio of observed to expected risk of breast cancer was only 13:8. Wheeler et al. observed even a lower risk for LCIS.[317] They found only 25 out of 98 women with LCIS who did not undergo mastectomy. The follow-up of these 25 women averaged 17 years. Only 1 of the 25 women developed ipsilateral breast cancer (4%). Of the 98 women, 32 had a contralateral breast at risk, and in this group only 3 developed infiltrating carcinoma (9.7%). The authors recommended only careful follow-up for LCIS because most patients will not develop infiltrating breast cancer. LCIS can most reasonably be viewed as a marker for subsequent cancer in 20% of patients. This cancer can occur in either breast, and therefore unilateral mastectomy is not a reasonable approach.

In discussing minimal breast cancers one asks the question, when does cancer begin? Is early cancer cytologic evidence of atypia, or is there the continuum? Many attempts to identify the earliest cancer used tumor doubling times to appreciate when the cancer began. A tumor dou-

bling time is observed, and the time since the origin of the tumor is extrapolated back to zero. This method of determining when a cancer began assumes a constant log doubling of the tumor. This assumption is probably incorrect. Tumor doubling times have been used in the medicolegal arena to identify when during the normal biology of the tumor intervention may have made a difference to the outcome of the patient.

Plotkin and Blankenberg argue for doubling-time analysis to assess the screening mammography.[239] They are of the opinion that doubling time remains constant throughout the course of the tumor biology. Growth rate is visually assumed to be exponential. This growth rate is substantially dampened as the tumor becomes large.[48] There is a significant slowing of doubling time at the time the tumor mass becomes clinically visible.[287] Breast cancer grows in spurts. These spurts depend on various promoters or inhibitors that affect the tumor growth rate. Tamoxifen can slow or stop the growth of some breast tumors and thereby markedly affect doubling time. Similarly endogenous estrogen and other promoters can effect a variance in doubling time.

Plotkin and Blankenberg state that it will take approximately 20 doubling times to develop the 1 million cells that make up 1 mg and measure 1 mm in diameter.[239] An additional 10 doubling times are required before the tumor would be diagnosed by palpation (i.e., measure 10 mm in diameter). They state that mammography can detect a tumor 6 to 7 doubling times before palpation—that is, 20% earlier in the life of a cancer. They point out that the earliest breast cancer diagnosis, even by mammography, is by no means early in the biologic sense. They state that no matter when the early diagnosis is made, the biologic life of a cancer is approximately 75% concluded when a diagnosis can be made. Fournier et al. observed that the distribution of primary breast cancer doubling time had a wide variability.[104] They found a range of doubling time from 2 months to 11 years. All of their doubling times showed exponential growth, but they had no evidence that there was constant doubling time throughout the course of the cancer. Plotkin and Blankenberg point out that "noninvasive cancer, which is destined to become invasive, is probably eliminated as a cause of death by mammographic detection that leads to treatment.[239] It may well be that in addition, a very small subset of patients, those often referred to as having 'minimal breast cancer' are amenable to surgical cure because of truly localized state. It is even more clear, however, that in the BCDDP, in which selection bias occurred, the proportion of such patients is only around 20%." They opine that screening studies showing a decreased mortality for the test group should also demonstrate no compensatory increase in deaths from other causes in the control population.

These observations have substantial legal implications.

In malpractice litigation for failure to diagnose breast cancer, expert witnesses must testify that the damage resulted from the delay in diagnosis. They usually base their opinion on the fact that there is an improved 5-year survival rate with earlier diagnosis. They may fail to consider the issues of lead-time bias, which affects the 5-year survival percentage without having an impact on the ultimate outcome of the disease. An Aetna Life and Casualty malpractice study observed that a failure to diagnose was the claim for malpractice in 75% of 67 cases. Breast cancer was involved in 20% of their series. For a failure to diagnosis to be legal negligence, the failure to diagnose must be the proximate cause of some substantial injury. This proximate cause heavily depends on the time at which a change in the outcome of the patient's illness would have been affected by the earlier diagnosis. Thus the use of doubling time, or minimal cancer detection, as an index of opportunity to "save lives" is a common legal basis for the finding of medical malpractice in failing to diagnose breast cancer. The temporal delay in diagnosis often becomes an issue in breast cancer litigation. How long does such a delay have to be before the delay in diagnosis is responsible for substantial injury? The substantial injury is usually considered to be cancer that can no longer be successfully treated because of delay. That assumes, of course, that the cancer could have been successfully treated. A delay in diagnosis has not been demonstrated to have an effect on the ultimate outcome of the woman's illness, except for those relatively infrequent rapidly growing cancers. However, the other point of view asserts that there must be some moment in time when a breast cancer grew beyond a threshold where it can be successfully eliminated by treatment before dissemination.

Sometimes even invasive cancer may have an indolent course. Breast cancer is notorious for its wide variation in rate of progression. A 6- to 12-month delay in diagnosis may make very little difference in some cases, whereas in others such a delay may be devastating. In some reported series, normal cytologic variants, precancer, and nonvirulent invasive cancer are lumped with invasive cancer when establishing the prevalence of "minimal" cancer. This confounds efforts to estimate the impact of baseline (prevalence) detection of early breast cancer. This problem is not as evident in those cancers that become detectable in the interval between two screening mammograms.

The problem of what is breast cancer on a prevalence screening mammogram is related to the issue of multifocal cancers. Which of the many suspect areas on an initial mammogram is the one that will become sufficiently virulent to be lethal? If a patient has multifocal cancer and only one is sufficiently obvious to detect and remove by excision, earlier diagnosis may make little difference to what will ultimately happen to the patient. A failure to diagnose only one of many breast cancers in a patient will

not be the proximate cause of the patient's death from breast cancer. Should we have a different attitude to a near normal variant on a baseline mammogram in which there is evidence of probable cancer elsewhere in the breast or even in the other breast? The degree of vigilance directed toward a suspected abnormality relates to the risk profile of an individual patient.

Masked and missed cancers and malpractice in breast cancer diagnosis

Screening mammography is somewhat unique in radiologic diagnosis because, even when a mammogram is read as normal, a subsequent mammogram will be done if the recommendations of the American Cancer Society are followed. Thus the radiologist interpreting the screening mammogram is aware that another radiologist will observe that film at a subsequent time, even if the diagnosis is "normal mammogram." With abnormal studies in other areas of radiology subsequent examinations are anticipated. The possibility of having a missed lesion recognized on subsequent examinations is higher for screening mammograms than for other radiologic procedures. The primary concern of most radiologists appears to be that of missing subtle breast cancer. This results in a substantial false-positive interpretation of screening mammograms in the United States. This is evidenced by the number of surgical biopsies performed per cancer (as compared with that in other countries). In the United States, some of the increase in false-positive findings and in surgical biopsies per cancer is the result of a defensive position assumed by radiologists when interpreting screening mammograms.

This defensive practice is further augmented by U.S. radiologists reading considerably fewer examinations per year than in other countries in which mammography is performed by mammographic specialists. The American College of Radiology accreditation requires that only 480 mammograms be read per year. This number was apparently selected arbitrarily—it amounts to 10 examinations per week. Although there is little scientific evidence that such low volume influences the number of false-negative interpretations, the evidence strongly suggests that low-volume mammography will increase false-positive interpretations. Ciatto et al. studied the preclinical cancer diagnostic rate by reporting radiologists from 1978 to 1985 in Florence, Italy.[63] They observed that there was a relationship between false-positive interpretations and lower volume mammography interpretation (Fig. 2-39). No such relationship was observed in the true-positive diagnoses. Thus low volumes of mammography interpretations further accentuate the false-positive findings rate in U.S. radiologic practice. It has been suggested that the number of radiologic centers in the United States that perform mammography exceeds the number necessary if high-volume

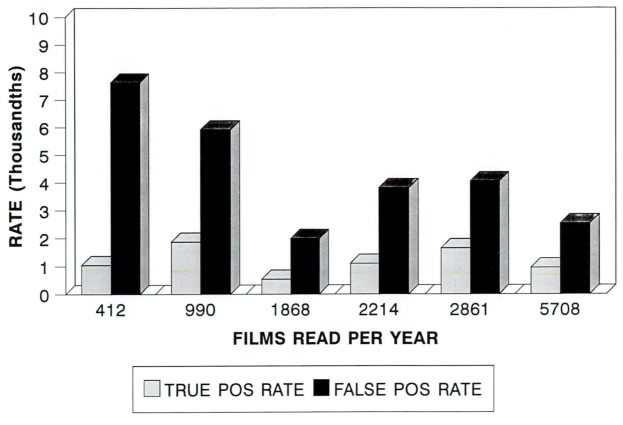

Fig. 2-39. Effect of reading volume on ROC. (From Ciatto S, Cataliotti L, Distante V: *Radiology* 165:99-102, 1987.)

mammography was concentrated in centers where there are dedicated specialists performing the procedures.[49]

The excessive false-positive mammogram findings leading to surgical biopsy are, in part, engendered by the defensive practice of U.S. radiologists, combined with the low volume of interpretations made by many radiologists. This has an adverse effect on the system of screening mammography. Excessive false-positive findings decrease patient compliance with screening mammography and significantly increase the cost of the system of breast cancer diagnoses. We must do what we can to decrease the false-positive finding rate without adversely affecting the true-positive rate in breast cancer diagnosis.

To better understand some of the problems, it is worthwhile to review quality-control issues in systems of screening mammography. The American College of Radiology has established the major quality-control system in the United States. This system concentrates on the quality of the image obtained. It credits the machine and system for obtaining the image based on the physics and engineering of image quality. Although there are requirements for the volume of use, they have no quality assurance on issues such as interpretations (observer performance), communi-

cation, recommendations, or outcome. Outcome measures such as decreased deaths from breast cancer may be the most reliable but are difficult to assess. Process outcomes are important. For example, we should monitor the observer false-positive and false-negative findings rate (ROC), the communication of information, and the results of surgery. A lack of observer performance monitoring is a major deficiency of quality control in breast cancer diagnosis. Once an abnormality or variation in normal is recognized, we must also monitor how it is interpreted. To be comprehensive, a quality-control system should also monitor the reporting of the interpretation and the implications of the report on the outcome of the patient. *By putting a major emphasis on the generation of the image, we may be missing opportunities to improve quality-control systems in screening mammography.* A comprehensive system should include observer performance studies, interpretive studies, and communication studies related to the report. These additions to the generation of the image are important if one wishes to demonstrate quality-control standards that can replace the current quality-control measures imposed by medical malpractice litigation.

Medical malpractice litigation has been thought of by

some as a means for the public to have quality control. However, this system causes defensive medicine and results in false-positive interpretations.

Diagnostic delay. Many radiologists believe that the major problem in medical malpractice is the false-negative finding, or missed cancer. What factors do influence a delay in breast cancer diagnosis?

Finley studied the factors that influence diagnostic delay in symptomatic breast cancers.[98] Diagnostic delay was considered to have occurred when the time between first physician visit for the symptoms and the diagnosis of breast cancers was made exceeded 30 days. Such a delay occurred in 30% of the cases. Patients who experienced delay were more often younger and employed and their initial symptoms did not include a lump. Patients who were seeing their regular physicians or obstetrician-gynecologists or physicians in smaller practice settings were more likely to experience delay. Patients in these settings were more likely to be told to watch and wait or have their cases dismissed after the initial evaluation. When delay occurred, patients in HMOs experienced a shorter delay (31 to 90 days) as compared with patients in other practice settings. The delay in the HMO setting was largely caused by scheduling. Board certification, medical school affiliations, or sex of the physician was not related to diagnostic delay.

In 1990 the Physicians' Insurers Association of America (PIAA) presented 269 cases in which the alleged delay in diagnosis was cited in malpractice claims.[289] More than one reason per case may have been provided. As is evident in Table 2-19, in over 50% of the cases a referring physician was not impressed with the physical findings. In only 35% of cases was a negative mammogram reported. Most of the negative mammogram reports occur in cases in which there is a palpable lesion and the referring physician

relied on a normal mammogram and did not do a further examination. Indeed, in 16% of these cases, no mammogram was ordered. Only 8.9% of malpractice litigation included a misread mammogram as one of the causes for action. Thus misread mammograms are relatively infrequent causes for medical malpractice litigation. It appears that radiologists' defensive behavior, as seen in false-positive interpretations, may exceed the rational basis for such defensive behavior.

Misread mammograms. A misread mammogram is less frequently a cause of delay in breast cancer diagnosis leading to malpractice litigation than are other causes. Despite this fact, however, misread mammograms remain the radiologist's major concern for malpractice litigation. This concern alters the behavior of radiologists and is becoming an increasing source of prospective litigation. Why does this occur? Some of the increased concern about malpractice litigation in screening mammography is because subsequent serial mammograms may often reveal a lesion that was either missed or not readily apparent on the prior mammogram. Some of the concern is due to the enhanced anxiety of patients when they are referred for a biopsy and the biopsy is deemed unnecessary. In those cases, two different radiologists disagree in the mammographic interpretation. Meyer et al. studied 603 patients scheduled for biopsy.[207] Of these, 58 (8.8%) were canceled on the day of the procedure. In 22 cases (38%) the reasons given for cancellation included the statement that no mass was present—that is, the initial mammographic interpretation suggested that a mass warranted surgical biopsy and the patient was prepared for biopsy. However, subsequent mammographic interpretation was unable to confirm the presence of a mass. In 13 of the 658 cases (22%), aspiration of the mass revealed that it was benign and therefore no surgical biopsy was necessary. The remaining cases (Table 2-20) were due to inappropriately overreading mammograms from benign calcifications or artifacts.

These disagreements concerning the appearance of an

Table 2-19. Most common reasons for delay in breast cancer diagnosis

Suspected reason	Frequency	% of cases
Not impressed with physical findings	147	54.7
Negative mammogram report	96	35.7
No appropriate biopsy	72	26.8
Repeat examinations did not arouse suspicion	66	24.5
Delay or failure to confer	49	18.2
Mass history ignored	44	16.4
No mammogram ordered	44	16.4
Lack of physician-to-physician communication	37	13.8
Other health problems	33	12.2
Misread mammogram	24	8.9

From Stephenson G et al: *Diagn Imag* July:31-35, 1990.

Table 2-20. Cancellation of preoperation breast localization procedure*

n	Reasons given for cancellation
22 (38%)	No mass present
13 (22%)	Aspiration of a mass
9 (16%)	Skin calcifications
4 (7%)	Random calcifications
3 (5%)	Skin artifacts
2 (3%)	Other

From Meyer JE et al: *Radiology* 169(3):629-630, 1988.
*Of 603 patients scheduled for biopsy, 58 (8.8%) cancelled on the day of the procedure. N = 58.

abnormal mammogram are cause for alarm in some patients. However, most often they can readily be clarified through adequate physician-to-patient rapport. The greatest potential for malpractice litigation arises in the distinguishing of missed breast cancer from a lesion that is masked although present on a prior screening mammogram. The lesion is subsequently revealed on subsequent mammograms as it enlarges.

Martin et al. reported 48 cases of interval cancer that they were able to separate into true interval cancers, observer errors, and masked cancers.[196] The true interval cancer was the cancer in which there was no radiographic sign of the cancer, even in retrospect. This was found in 16 (33%) of 48 patients. There was obvious observer error in 14 (29%) of the patients. Perhaps even more important were the masked cancers. These are cancers that would not be expected to be interpreted on the initial mammogram because of the difficulty of interpretation. Martin et al. advocate more vigilance for the subtle radiologic clues of masked cancer in their series.[196] They specifically emphasize the need to pay attention to degrees of asymmetry or a developing density or to calcifications that are interpreted as benign. Although the developing density sign in misinterpreted calcifications resulted in only 10% of their interval cancer, most of their interval cancers were cases in which there was breast asymmetry that was missed by failure to compare the two breasts. They noted the indirect signs of masked cancers to be the following:

1. Solitary ducts under the areola or complex of dilated ducts extending 3 cm or more within the breast
2. Intraductal and intralobular calcifications
3. Progressive density in a specific area
4. Asymmetry of breast tissue, especially if there is a palpable lesion
5. Benign-appearing mass in the perimenopausal or postmenopausal woman

They specifically note that in the involuting breast, a new mass should not develop. This is evident on serial mammograms, and it is the most important cause of missed cancer. Of their 48 interval cancers, 66% were either masked or missed because of observer error.

Similar data were obtained by Holland et al. who reported on 64 cases of interval cancer.[139] Of the interval cancers not seen in retrospect, they considered 20 (31%) to be true interval cancers. They define these cancers as too small to have been detected at a prior screening. Masked cancers, they concluded, were large enough but masked from radiologic detection usually because of a dense breast, a poorly outlined tumor mass of the diffuse infiltrative type, a mainly lobular carcinoma, or an intraductal localization. In their series of interval cancers, they noted that 30% of the missed cases were due to observer error in which direct or indirect signs of the tumors were seen in

retrospect. In addition, they noted that 6% of the missed cases were due to technical error because the tumor lay outside the imaging field on the initial mammogram and was evident only on the subsequent study. The observer error rate of 30% of the interval cancers compares with the 29% observer error reported by Martin et al. The criteria of Holland et al. for masked cancer depended in part on the concept of tumor doubling time, in which the lesion would be too small to be identified on the initial examination.[139] They make the important point that dense breasts often obscure underlying cancer. This type of masking is the most common situation in which it would not be a breach of the standard of care to not have identified the lesion on the initial study. The obvious observer errors or technical errors are more likely to lead to malpractice litigation.

Peeters et al. reported on 153 cases of interval cancers in 1989. In this series, there were 89 (58%) true interval cancers.[236] A true interval cancer was defined as a cancer that showed a clear lesion on a diagnostic mammogram but no suspected signs at the preceding screening examination. This type of case is not likely to lead to medical malpractice litigation. One should not be accused of missing a breast cancer that is not seen even in retrospect. Peeters et al. found that 26% of interval cancers were missed on a prior mammogram.[236] Nine percent were due to technical error, which compared with the 6% technical error of Holland. Another 17% were observer error, which they broke down into obvious errors in 11%. They define the masked cancers as those that, although seen in retrospect, may have been too subtle to warrant suspicion on a screening mammogram. They class 10 of the 18 masked cancers as observer error and 8 as radiographically occult. Perhaps this distinction should be used to separate the missed breast cancer from one that is masked. One would not be expected to recognize a masked cancer. In this study, Peeters et al. missed cancers were 26% of interval cancers.[236] They were present on a prior screening mammogram and due to either technical error (9%) or observer error (17%). These missed cancers will most likely lead to malpractice litigation because missing a cancer seen in retrospect may be interpreted as practice outside the standard of care.

It becomes important to distinguish whether breast cancer identified in the second of two serial mammograms represents a missed cancer, for which the lack of proper interpretation constitutes practice outside the standard of care, from those lesions seen on subsequent mammograms, which are recognized only as subtle lesion on the initial mammogram after analysis. To find all the lesions on an initial mammogram would markedly increase the false-positive mammographic interpretations. This would be unacceptably costly and has the possibility of causing more "dis-ease" than could be potentially eliminated by advocating a program of screening mammography. Some reasonable boundaries short of perfect detection of all cancers is necessary for screening mammography to be made widely available to the U.S. public.

One approach to the distinction between a missed breast cancer and a masked lesion is the conspicuity of the lesion on the mammogram. Conspicuity is a concept developed by Kundel and Revesz[169] to identify those lesions that can be seen on a chest x-ray examinations. They define conspicuity as the lesion contrast divided by the surrounding complexity, using contrast or edge enhancement. If the surrounding complexity increases faster than the contrast, the conspicuity decreases. In mammographic diagnosis, conspicuity is a reasonable concept to allow for the distinction between the conspicuous lesion (i.e., when failure to identify it could be considered a breach of the standard of care) and the inconspicuous or masked lesion (i.e., one would not anticipate being able to identify). This conspicuity concept is directly influenced by the surrounding complexity (Figs. 2-40 and 2-41).

In summary, interval breast cancer increases the prospects for identifying missed and masked breast cancers. This may be the basis for medical malpractice litigation.

This concern can lead to excessive false-positive mammographic interpretations, which can adversely affect the system of screening mammography in breast cancer control. By limiting the breach of the standard of care in screening mammographic interpretation to those obvious lesions readily identifiable on the initial and subsequent mammograms it may be possible to decrease unnecessary or nuisance litigation. The distinction between a masked lesion that is inconspicuous and a missed lesion that is readily conspicuous provides more scientific grounds for attesting as to whether the radiologist who did not observe the cancer on the initial two serial studies was guilty of a breach of the standard of care.

COMPLIANCE AND SCREENING RECOMMENDATIONS

Never trouble trouble until trouble troubles you.

A WOMAN ON WHY SHE WOULDN'T GET A MAMMOGRAM[260]

Many women have screening mammograms. Others do not comply with the recommendations for periodic screen-

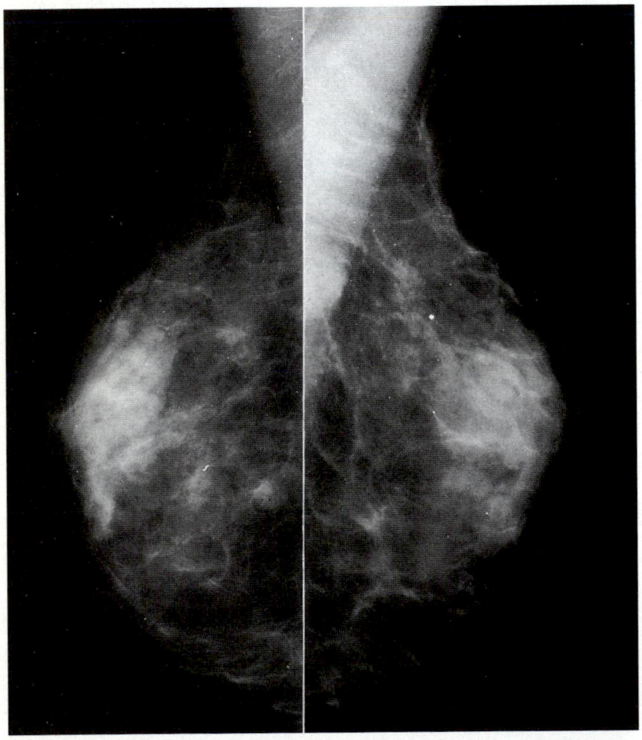

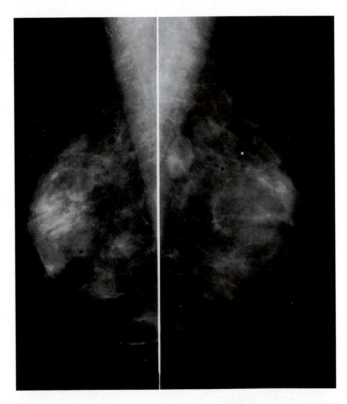

Fig. 2-40. Serial mammograms taken in 1990 do not separate the abnormality from the pectoralis muscle, so the lesion was not sufficiently conspicuous and was not identified. This would represent an error caused by the interference of the pectoralis muscle with the conspicuity of the abnormality. Failure to observe this lesion would be considered within the standard of care.

Fig. 2-41. Mammograms taken 1 year after the study in Fig. 2-40, clearly show the lesion. The greater obliquity of this view clearly delineates a lesion separate from the pectoralis muscle. In retrospect, this lesion was apparent 1 year before and the film was not adequate to detect the lesion. Failure to identify the lesion on this set of films would be an observer error and outside the standard of care.

ing. Why do some women participate, whereas others do not? What can be done to improve compliance?

Recent trends in mammography in the United States have shown a dramatic increase in usage from 1980 to 1989. Lantz studied mammography trends in Wisconsin.[173] He found an 18-fold increase from 1980 to 1989. In 1980, 31,000 mammograms were performed in Wisconsin, whereas in 1989 the number approached 573,000. In 1984 the mammography rate began to show an accelerated increase, which continued through 1988, when a dramatic doubling in the number of mammograms occurred between 1988 and 1989. Lantz observed an increase from 278,000 in 1988 to 573,000 in 1989. Even with this dramatic change in the number of mammograms performed, only 66% of the women in the recommended age groups had mammograms. Thirty-three percent or 289,000 Wisconsin women who met the recommended ACS guidelines for screening mammograms in 1989 did not have a mammogram.

In the State of Michigan, it is relatively easy to estimate compliance rates. State law requires that all mammographic machines be registered and their annual volume is a required component of accreditation of the device. The annual volume for a standard of mammography can be readily assessed in any standard metropolitan area.

We have made an effort to assess the use of mammography within Michigan. The regional distribution of use has been assessed in 10 regions of the state (Fig. 2-42).

In Michigan on January 1, 1992, there were 482 registered mammographic machines. The 1990 census revealed

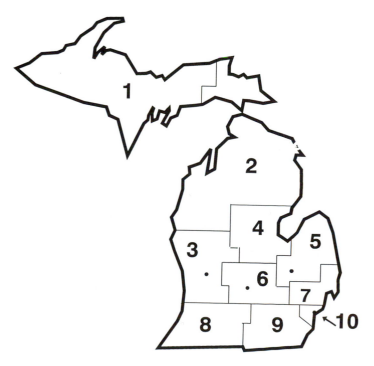

Fig. 2-42. Michigan mammography study zones.

a population of 1,467,210 women over the age of 45 years. The use rate per machine was estimated at the time of accreditation. Based on this use rate in 1991 there were 935,580 mammograms performed. Thus there are .64 mammograms per women over 45 years of age. This is a rough estimate of compliance because many of these mammograms may have been done on the same women. This would be especially true for those women in whom there was some perceived difficulty with the mammogram. In any event, there is no more than a 64% compliance in Michigan, which compares with the 68% seen in the Wisconsin study. Admittedly, many of these mammograms may have been done on women under 45 years of age. Experience shows that the dominant mammographic usage is in the younger age groups of the recommended population. The standard in Michigan has been annual mammography after 50 years of age and baseline mammograms sometime between 35 and 50 years of age. From 35 to 50 years of age, the average woman has approximately one mammogram every 3 years. Relatively few women over 70 years of age obtain mammograms in Michigan. These estimates suggest that there is a persistent deficiency in compliance with the American Cancer Society's recommendations.

The regional variation in mammography use in Michigan is quite remarkable. The 10 population regions indicated in Fig. 2-42 are reasonably reflective of metropolitan areas that have a homogeneity in medical care. The number of machines per women over 45 years of age ranges from 4.46 to 2.41 for an average of 3.29. The annual examinations per women over 45 years of age range from a high of 90% in one region in the state to a low of 36% in another region, with a statewide average of 64%. This means that in Michigan in 1991, 6.4 women obtained mammograms for every 10 women in the population who were 45 years of age or older. (Fig. 2-43).

Fig. 2-44 shows the relationship between women per machine and examinations per women over 45 years of age. There is some relation of the number of examinations to the number of available machines in any specific area. Part of the variations in mammography use seems to depend on the accessibility of mammographic machines. This evidence suggests that Brown's[49] contention of an excessive number of mammographic machines throughout the United States does not take into account their regional distribution. There are areas in Michigan where there are over 4000 women to be screened per available machine. In no place in the state are the examinations per machine that high. Indeed, the average number of examinations per machine in Michigan is 1941 (with a range of 2800 to 1500). Similarly, however, there are other places in Michigan with an adequate number of machines and still relatively low compliance. This may, in part, be related to population density. The most sparsely populated region of the state is in the Upper Peninsula. This zone has 16 machines for 47,577 eligible women. They achieve a compliance

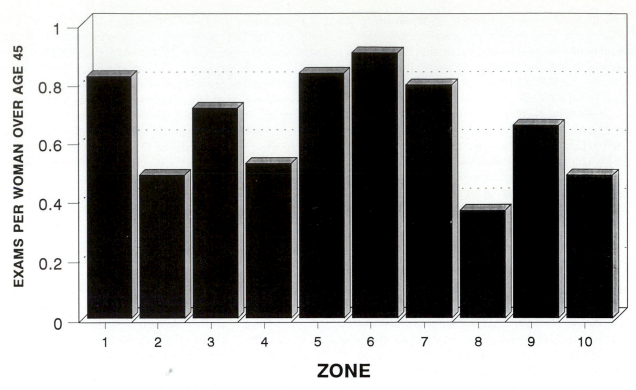

Fig. 2-43. Mammography examinations per woman over 45 years of age.

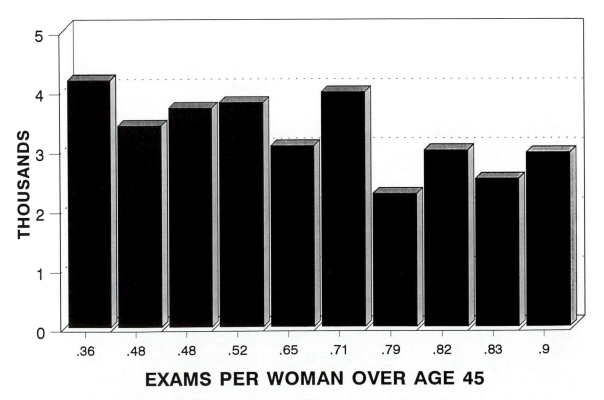

Fig. 2-44. Women over 45 years old per mammography machine.

rate of 82%. However, the most densely populated region of the state, zone 10, has 101 machines for a population of 342,000 and achieves a compliance rate of 48%. Factors other than the population density and regional accessibility to mammography are obviously important in establishing how many mammograms are done per year per eligible woman. The rates may well be changing. Currently, every mammographic machine is required to report the volume of mammographies performed each year to the State; thus it will be possible to monitor these compliance rates and direct efforts toward enhancing mammographic use in areas where the greatest results could be obtained (Table 2-21).

The change in mammography use in the past few years makes it difficult to compare various published series on compliance. The year when the study was done becomes critical. Hayward et al. found a 42% compliance rate in a national survey.[126] Houts et al. sought to increase compliance rates in sisters and daughters of breast cancer patients.[142] They found a 52% compliance in their control group. The most recent comprehensive survey in the United States was done in February 1990.[308] The Mammography Attitudes and Usage Study (MAUS) entailed a random multistage cluster sample of households with telephones. They interviewed 980 women over 39 years of age. They obtained a 64% response rate. They compared their results with those observed in the National Health Interview Survey (NHIS) of 1987. The percentage of white women over 39 years of age who reported ever having a mammogram increased from 39% (between 38% and 40%, 95% CI) in 1987 to 65% (between 62% and 68%, 95% CI) in 1990. For black women a similar increase was observed (i.e., 30% [between 28% and 32%] to 58% [between 47% and 69%]. They note that mammography use increased during the period of increased publicity encouraging women to have mammograms. Perhaps some of this increase is the result of the July 1990 requirement by 29 states that insurance carriers provide some level of coverage for mammography.

The 65% rate in the MAUS study is strikingly similar to the 66% rate observed in the Wisconsin data and the estimate of 64% in our Michigan study. In the MAUS survey, 35% of the study population had had more than one mammogram. Only 31% followed the guidelines for screening mammography established by the American Cancer Society and the National Cancer Institute. The failure to obtain follow-up mammograms is similar to the observation of DeNeef in his study of the indeterminate mammogram.[79] In that study, only 26% of the women with indeterminate mammograms who were advised to return in 6 months for follow-up mammograms complied with the recommendation. A failure to comply with a recommendation for a 6-month follow-up mammogram is more serious than a failure to return for an annual screen following a normal mammogram. The probability of finding cancer on a 6-month follow-up of an indeterminate mammogram was 2% (between 0.2% and 5.9%; 95% CI) or more than twice what would be expected on an annual screening mammogram following a prior normal mammogram (i.e., an incidence screen versus a screen in a patient at higher risk because of questionable findings on a prior examination).

The relationship between the risk for breast cancer and the participation in mammographic screening is especially important. Taylor and Billingham studied the relationship between the recognition of risk and the use of breast self-examination in daughters with a maternal history of breast cancer.[299] They matched women with a maternal history with control subjects for race, age, and education. They observed that one third of the experimental group did not report being susceptible to breast cancer, although their mothers were treated for the disease. This rate was not different between the experimental and the control group.

Vogel et al. studied a community-based, low-cost mammography program to determine whether the attitudes, be-

Table 2-21. Mammography use data, State of Michigan, January 1, 1992

Zone	Machines	Exams/machine	Exams/year	Exams/woman >45	Population woman >45	Woman >45/machine	Machines/1000 women
1	16	2439	39024	0.82	47577	2974	3.36
2	26	1770	46032	0.48	95817	3685	2.71
3	42	2817	118332	0.71	165968	3952	2.53
4	24	1954	46884	0.52	90631	3776	2.65
5	40	2080	83184	0.83	99775	2494	4.01
6	31	2633	81612	0.90	90888	2932	3.41
7	141	1766	249024	0.79	316490	2245	4.46
8	29	1493	43308	0.36	120492	4155	2.41
9	32	1990	63684	0.65	97506	3047	3.28
10	101	1629	154496	0.48	342065	3387	2.95
Total/average	482	1941	935580	0.64	1467210	3044	3.29

liefs, and practices of women at an increased risk for breast cancer because of family history differed from those without that risk factor.[311] They compared age-matched controls of women without family histories of breast cancer with women with family histories of breast cancer. The reasons for mammography were most often related to the physician's order. Both cases and controls ranked lack of a physician's order as a "very important" reason for not undergoing a prior mammogram. In this study women were reported as having a family history of breast cancer if any relative had breast cancer. Of these women with a family history of breast cancer, some 79% perceived their risk to be moderate or greater compared with controls (54%, $P <$ 0.0001). The mammographic histories were not different when these investigators controlled for poorly perceived risk. The authors conclude that, although these women are aware of their increased risk for breast cancer because of family history, they are not undergoing regular mammographic screening.

Taplin et al. studied breast cancer risk in relation to participation in mammographic screening.[296] They observed that participation was decreased among women with late menopause and was increased among women with either increased age, a family history of breast cancer, or a previous breast biopsy. The effect of increased risk was highest among women 50 to 59 years of age, as compared with women 60 to 79 years of age. These results suggest that individuals at a higher risk for breast cancer are more likely to participate in voluntary breast cancer screening.

Ethnicity, socioeconomic status, and psychologic barriers affect the use of screening mammography.[288] Hispanic women were more often affected by socioeconomic status in failing to get a mammogram than were either white or black U.S. patients. In all ethnic and socioeconomic groups a concern about cost was the principal perceived barrier to the use of screening mammography. Gram and Slenker reported on attitudes toward screening mammography among Norwegian women.[114] Although 33% of the population sample expressed anxiety about breast cancer, only 18% of nonattendees expressed this concern. Of the women who attended screening mammography, 99% had a positive attitude toward mammography. This was not adversely affected by the screening experience. In this Norwegian study the most frequent reason for not getting a screening mammogram was the lack of an opportunity to have the examination.

Most compliance studies use large population surveys or statistics from geographic regions. There are some subsets of the population in which compliance with screening recommendations is even worse. For example, Coll et al. studied screening mammography compliance in a nursing home setting.[71] In 139 subjects studied in 1986, 93% had a chest x-ray during their nursing home stay, whereas only 1 of the 139 women had a mammogram. The mean stay was 6.5 years and the mean age of the subjects was 78 years of age. They found no association between functional status and the use of the mammogram. This study revealed a less than 1% compliance rate, despite the evidence that screening mammograms may benefit this age population. Is being an elderly nursing home resident reason not to comply with screening recommendations?

Physician behavior

The recommendations of physicians play a dominant role in a woman's choice of whether or not to have a mammogram. The 1989 survey of physicians' attitudes and practices in early cancer detection revealed substantial changes in physician attitudes concerning screening mammography over the prior 5 years. The percentage of physicians who recommended mammograms for asymptomatic patients increased from 49% in 1984 to 96% in 1989. The percentage of physicians who acknowledged giving more attention to screening mammography increased from 14% in 1984 to 44% in 1989. Despite this improved compliance of physicians, only 37% of physicians follow or exceed ACS guidelines for their patients. This increased from 11% in 1984.

The 1989 physicians' survey continued to reveal a discrepancy between physicians' agreement with the ACS guidelines and their application of these guidelines to their patients. In 1989, 72% of physicians agreed completely with the guidelines, yet only 37% followed the guidelines for all their patients. This difference is due to other factors that influence a physician's decision to recommend a screening mammogram. In this survey, 53% of the physicians say their decision is influenced by whether or not a patient can afford the mammogram, and 47% are influenced by the cost of the mammogram to the patient. The usual cost for screening mammogram and interpretation was $93. Of all physicians, 71% knew what the usual cost was. Of physicians 42% report they are influenced by the reliability of a mammogram; 29% by the availability of a qualified radiologist; and 16% by the availability of a breast x-ray machine, despite the oversupply of mammographic machines in the United States.[49]

Less rational influences acknowledged by physicians may be easier to address because physician education alone may overcome some of the hesitancy to perform a mammogram in an asymptomatic patient. The low chance of finding a breast abnormality was a concern of 26% of physicians; and concerns about radiation exposure were expressed by 17% of physicians.

Even with all these concerns, 81% of physicians report they are more inclined to order a screening mammogram on an asymptomatic patient than they were 5 years ago. Of the 9% of physicians who disagree with the guidelines (288 in the survey), most have understandable reasons for their disagreement. Of these physicians, 35% think a baseline mammogram at 35 years of age is too early; 29% consider annual testing after 50 years of age to be too frequent; and 18% assert that the recommendations are too costly. Other reasons given seem less rational and may be addressed by physician education.

Of those physicians who disagree with the ACS guidelines, 16% believe that mammography is not needed if there are no symptoms. Why do they not know better? This belief is contrary to the true role of mammography in detecting nonpalpable breast cancer. Some 12% of those physicians who disagree with the guidelines claim that screening mammography is not needed if there is no family history. Clearly, these physicians do not realize that selecting a screening population on the basis of risk factors is not possible. Of physicians who disagree with the guidelines, 9% do not advocate screening mammography because of its low yield.[6]

Women's views

A practice audit is one way to evaluate the use of screening mammography by primary care physicians. Selinger el al. reported on the Department of Family Medicine at Jefferson Medical College in Philadelphia.[268] They studied a random sample of 88 women over 55 years of age who were patients for at least 5 years. Within this sample, 56% had received no recorded mammograms over the 5-year period, and only 19% had a mammogram in the most recent year. The average interval between mammograms in the patients who had one or more mammograms was 3.5 years. In addition, for 18% of all mammograms ordered, the results could not be located within the chart. Thus it would seem reasonable to increase an emphasis on auditing the practices of primary care physicians for their use of screening mammography as one index of quality of care. If more practices were audited, perhaps there would be an increased vigilance of physicians in performing and requesting mammograms for their appropriate patient populations and in ensuring that the results are available to influence the patient's management. Selinger et al. conclude that family physicians need to improve adherence to recommended guidelines for mammography and to improve the documentation of screening activities in the medical records.[268]

Although physician recommendations are important, there are other reasons why women do not comply with the recommendations for screening mammography. The sociology of screening mammography has been extensively analyzed. Theories such as Health Belief Model[55] and Fishbein's Theory of Reasoned Action[212] have been applied to assess the relationship between behavior and beliefs that are presumably based on knowledge (to some extent).[156] Montano used Fishbein's theory of reasoned action to study women's behavior in having a mammogram.[212] This analysis found attitude, affect, subject

norm, and facilitating conditions to be significantly associated with participation in a breast screening program. One of the problems with this study and many others is that the data are gathered from respondents to questionnaires who were more likely to participate in screening than were nonrespondents (65% versus 20%). We do not know what factors influence a nonrespondent's participation or lack of participation in a breast cancer screening program. Indeed, a major problem in attempting to market the idea of screening mammography to asymptomatic women has been the failure to understand the woman's view. Opinions, sociologic studies, and survey instruments have all been used to shed light on why some women do not choose to obtain screening mammograms. The validity of surveys has been questioned because they often tried to reach the unreachable (nonrespondent) women. The validity of telephone surveys was tested by King et al.[164] They telephoned HMO patients whose medical history was recorded to test the validity of self-reported mammography experience. All of the patients who said they did not have a prior mammogram had not had one. For 96% of those who said they had had a mammogram, one was recorded. This gives reason for optimism about the use of telephone surveys to gather data on mammography usage.

The attitudes of the involved women are essential to an understanding of why some women do not obtain screening mammograms. If we seek to improve compliance, we should know why some women choose not to comply. Women's views are usually studied by open-ended questions or survey instruments. Both methods have their advantages and disadvantages. These can be reviewed in the context of known factors that affect mammography use. These factors include knowledge, education, age, fear, and risk.

Knowledge. McCance et al. found that a woman's knowledge of breast cancer screening was associated with the use of screening mammograms and clinical breast examination, but not with breast self-examination.[198] Fallowfield surveyed women's knowledge of breast cancer on the premise that knowledge will influence the decision to have a screening mammogram.[92] He found that most women were poorly informed about what would increase their chances of having breast cancer. Only 49% knew that having relatives with breast cancer could affect their likelihood of having the disease. Although a substantial number of women thought that actions under their control would increase the chance of eventually having breast cancer, some of these perceptions are erroneous. Of the women surveyed, 13% thought that having children increased the chance of breast cancer, whereas 6% thought that being married and not having children increased the risk. Forty percent of the women were convinced that regular use of the contraceptive pill increased breast cancer risk and 35% considered prior breast trauma (hit in the breast) to be associated with an increased cancer risk. These beliefs about breast cancer risks may influence a woman's choice to have a screening mammogram. The 1987 National Health Interview Survey revealed that 20.5% of white women and 30.8% of black women agreed or strongly agreed that breast cancer death was not preventable.[156] This racial difference was largely due to differences in education.[308]

Education. The effect of education on the participation in screening mammography differs in relation to the culture being studied. In the United States the percentage of women who reported ever having a mammogram increased with the level of education in every large series studied. The MAUS survey found a gradual increase in mammogram usage between women who had less than a high school education (58% [50% to 66%; 95% CI]), high school education (65% [60% to 70%]), some college (72% [66% to 78%]), and a college degree or more (74% [68% to 80%]). There is a clear increase in mammogram compliance with increasing level of education. The opposite effect was observed in Italy.[83] In the Brescia study they reported on the percentage of women who attended a breast screening clinic after once being invited to do so. Of women with less than 12 years of school 61% (818:1346) attended the screening program. Of women with 12 to 15 years of education, 51% (164:298) attended, whereas only 47% (42:90) of those women with a university education obtained screening mammograms. The difference between the U.S. survey and the Italian attendance study may be a cultural distinction regarding who is likely to comply with a suggestion to be screened.

Age. The effect of age on breast screening compliance is similar in all reported studies. Younger women are more likely to comply with mammography screening. Donato et al. reported a 57% (933:1625) attendance rate for women 50 to 59 years of age, whereas they observed a 49% (99:201) attendance rate for women over 60 years of age.[83] The 1990 MAUS survey of U.S. women who reported ever having had a mammogram revealed an age-dependent effect of 71% for those 50 to 59 years of age, 65% for those 60 to 69 years of age, and only 56% for those over 70 years of age. This relative lack of compliance was also noted in the 1987 NHIS survey in which the figures were 44%, 38%, and 28%, respectively. Each of these earlier figures was 27% to 28% lower than the respective data obtained in 1990. The increase in mammography compliance seen between these two studies did not appear to be affected by the woman's age.

Fear and risk. Why do some studies show that women with a greater risk of breast cancer are even less likely to comply with the screening guidelines? Some 10% of the women in the Brescia study reported that the reason they did not attend the screening program was that they were afraid that breast cancer may be detected. In a New

Zealand study, Richardson reported on the principal reason given for not participating in screening.[245] The main reasons were fear (42%) and embarrassment (31%).

One way to shed light on the concerns of women who do not participate in screening is to quote directly from open-ended responses. Schechter et al. evaluated women's attitudes and perceptions to develop mammography promotion messages.[260] They used small-group discussions as focus groups in Philadelphia and Kansas City. They quote a number of women, and these vignettes may serve as a background when considering what may be done to improve compliance. Schechter quotes participants as saying, "I never think about getting one . . . I mean I'm not opposed to it, I just never think about it." "People think it's not going to happen to them. It happens to everyone else but it won't affect me. I think a lot of people have that attitude." "Never trouble trouble 'til trouble troubles you." "If it ain't broke don't fix it." "Why spend the money?" "You just don't know what they're going to find." "Fear of the results—not the test itself." "I worry about too many x-rays . . . because I've had a lot . . . and I'm concerned about having too much radiation." "I'm scared of the results." "It's fear on the back burner whether we want to admit it or not." "If a doctor told me to get one, I probably would. But until somebody tells me, I'm not going to call up and say I want one." These statements place in vivid perspective the type of issues that we must deal with as we seek to increase compliance.

Irwig et al. recently completed a telephone survey in Sydney, Australia.[151] They sought to study women's perceptions of screening mammography. Prior research on compliance demonstrated that women who attended screening services felt more personally vulnerable to breast cancer than nonattendees. Irwig et al. observed that compliance with screening mammography depends on knowledge, attitudes, and perception of personal susceptibility.[151] They argue that compliance is more affected by attitudes about perceived benefits and barriers than by knowledge. The best correlate with knowledge of screening mammography was occupational status and whether or not a language other than English was spoken at home. Women in professional households more often had heard of mammography, whether or not a language other than English was spoken at home. In Australian homes where languages other than English were spoken, women were much less likely to have knowledge of the benefits of screening mammography.

They found that 79% of women had a favorable attitude to screening mammography. Attitude was associated with the level of education and knowledge of mammography. Women with more education had a more favorable attitude than those who had less education. Women who had previously heard of screening mammography had a more favorable attitude toward screening mammography than those women for whom screening mammography was explained at the time of the encounter.

In this study the most important predictors of perceived personal susceptibility were whether women had had a previous breast lump. Women with a previous breast lump considered themselves considerably more susceptible than if they had not had a lump. The second major factor associated with perceived personal susceptibility was an erroneous perception. Compared with those 65 to 70 years of age, 17% more women 40 to 49 years of age regarded themselves as susceptible to having breast cancer. The younger women considered themselves more susceptible to breast cancer although their risk was lower. Perhaps older women considered themselves less susceptible because they have outlived women they know who have died from breast cancer. Is this why younger women are more likely to comply with the recommendations for screening mammography even though they are less likely to have the disease?

How to improve compliance

Compliance with the American Cancer Society's recommendations for breast cancer screening varies with different populations. If we target nonwhite older patients with no college education, the results may be more effective. Perhaps compliance efforts should target populations at a higher risk for breast cancer or at a higher risk for noncompliance. Most efforts have been made to target people on the basis of risk for breast cancer rather than on risk for failing to comply. Both issues should be addressed when attempting to improve compliance.

Many investigators have designed techniques to increase the number of women who seek and use screening mammography. Most consist of reminders or encouragement through educational programs either to physicians or to the public at large. Wolosin studied the effect of appointment scheduling and reminders.[325] In their control group the women were examined and told about mammography and instructed to make an appointment themselves. They compared this group with another for whom an appointment was made on the spot and followed up with a reminding postcard. These investigators studied nine different sites and sought to determine whether a change in the price of the mammogram would affect the compliance. This reminder increased adherence at every site studied. Do lower cost mammograms increase the number of women who seek and use mammography? In this study the average cost per mammogram was $54.66 and five of the nine were priced below $50. The range of prices was from $45 to $90. Despite this range, the use of a follow-up reminder and postcard increased adherence, independent of the cost of the mammogram.

Turnbull et al. used a randomized trial of women invited to attend screening mammography.[304] They observed

that the invitation to a screening from either a personal physician or a source not personally known to the woman achieved comparable compliance. Nielson studied the effect of the availability of information and a realistic perception of risk on women's use of screening mammography.[222] They found that these alone were not sufficient motivators to obtain a mammogram. They, like others, observed that higher education and income increased mammogram use independent of mammogram cost. In this study, in which there was an attempt to motivate women to use mammography, they found that 71% of the women found the recommendation of the health professional to be the single most important motivating factor in obtaining a mammogram. Thus there must be widespread physician compliance if one is to improve patient compliance in obtaining screening mammography. Harris et al. studied ways of prompting physicians for preventive procedures in North Carolina.[124] They compared manual and computer reminders versus no reminders at all. The manual reminders were nurse initiated. They found they could increase mammography use by computer prompting on case records. With no prompt or with nurse prompting alone, the percentage increase was 4% and 7%, respectively, whereas with computer prompting the percentage increase in mammographic use versus the controls was 33%.

Compliance requires an ability to address the specific barriers of women to acceptance of mammography.[244] Gregorio et al. used mass media campaigning to encourage screening mammography in the Connecticut Breast Cancer Awareness campaign.[115] Women's reasons for obtaining more mammograms in this study were enhanced awareness that the baseline examination was due and the availability of low-cost service, at least for the initial mammogram. This study suggests that low cost may initially increase the use of mammography and subsequent mammograms may well be obtained by follow-up reminders. *The price sensitivity does not seem to be as great for subsequent mammograms as it is for the baseline mammogram.* Once a woman's initial barrier to the acceptance of mammography is found, it seems that reminders alone may be more effective. Initial mammography depends more on knowledge, education, and attitude. Subsequent mammograms in the screening series seem to depend more on constant reminders and the patient's awareness that the mammogram is due.

Thus efforts to increase mammography should include:
1. Widespread public awareness (e.g., advertising campaigns and mass media via communication to the public at large)
2. Increased physician recognition that mammography is useful, a barrier that has (for the most part) been overcome in the United States and may account for the remarkable recent increase in screening mammography

3. Direct reminders to patients that it is time to have either a baseline or an initial mammogram, often by direct invitation for screening (In the United States, initial screening at lower cost decreases one of the potential barriers to the acceptance of mammography. Cost in later mammograms does not seem to be as substantial an inhibitor of mammographic use.)
4. Asking women who have had mammograms to bring along a friend at their next examination (This is especially useful on reminder examinations when women already accept mammography as useful. The direct word of mouth to friends seems to be an effective way to widely encourage the use of mammography to the public at large.)

THE COST AND BENEFIT OF SCREENING MAMMOGRAPHY
Adverse effects of screening mammography

The basic principle of medical care—"First do no harm"—is an important consideration in advocating screening mammography. If we are to responsibly advocate and use screening mammography, we must be aware of the potential negative consequences of our actions. We must be aware of the criticisms of screening mammography. Even if an objective improvement in health is achieved, this may not be accompanied by a subjective one.[28]

The advocacy of screening mammography may have a negative effect on society. Skrabanek[286] is one of the most vehement spokesmen against screening mammography.[246] He argues that screening is presented to women using emotive language (e.g., "saving lives") without any attempt to inform them about the risks associated with screening. Because any screening program can be justified only if the potential benefit outweighs the harm, both the benefit and the harm must be quantified. Skrabanek[286] notes the following potential harms of screening mammography:

1. False-negative mammogram findings resulting in false reassurance and a delay in treatment
2. False-positive mammogram findings, resulting in unnecessary diagnostic tests and surgical interventions
3. Mammograms that detect premalignant lesions, of which only some would progress to invasive carcinoma in a lifetime, resulting in unnecessary mastectomies in a proportion of women
4. Mammograms that detect true cancers earlier than accidental discovery, but do not change their natural history by early treatment
5. Psychologic effects of increased anxiety and fear through constant reminders that a woman is at risk for breast cancer and should keep her appointments for screening[286]

Skrabanek emphasizes that the ethics of screening differ from the ethics of ordinary medical care. A doctor offering screening to a healthy woman must have much better evidence that the benefit outweighs the harm than when dealing with an ill patient—for whom "something must be done." Skrabanek warns "When a symptomatic patient asks for help, the doctor does the best he or she can, without promising a benefit, and with informed consent. In screening, a healthy person is solicited by a screener with a promise of a benefit, without any form of consent and without any guarantee that the potential benefits of screening outweigh the potential harms, i.e., without any information on the number of women who have to be screened for one death postponed and on the number of unnecessary surgical procedures for each breast cancer death prevented."[286]

We will attempt to analyze some of these concerns. We do not seek to either magnify their importance or diminish their significance. We believe that responsible advocacy of screening mammography requires an appreciation of its limitations and potential for untoward outcomes.

Iatrogenic induction of "dis-ease." Breast cancer is a disease that often strikes women at the prime of life and thereby decreases the total amount of contributing lives of a society. The breast cancer problem primarily affects the developed world. Other causes of death in developing countries overshadow the problems caused by carcinoma of the breast. In Europe and the United States, breast cancer is a frequent disease. Most adults know someone who has suffered from the disease. This knowledge instills an appropriate concern in most women when they are at their peak of productive life.

In advocating efforts to decrease the number of women who will die from breast cancer, it is important to appreciate that any system of diagnosis may induce "dis-ease." It can do so by increasing unnecessarily the anxiety and concern of women to a level at which concern for the disease may exceed the ramifications of having the disease itself. Earlier diagnosis of breast cancer can lead to the identification of cancers at a stage when cure is more probable; thus there has been great push for efforts to diagnose breast cancer earlier. Thus far mammography is the only reliable means by which nonpalpable breast cancers can be diagnosed. In our efforts to continually seek out earlier breast cancers, we encounter the ill-defined border between breast cancer and normal breasts. When we diagnose breast cancer at an earlier stage, are we possibly identifying cases that would never have developed into clinically significant breast cancer?

It is possible to analyze the cost and harm of screening mammography in relation to the benefit and to conclude that "mass screening for breast cancer should be abandoned and the procedure should be reserved for those women with high risk factors."[327] To reach that conclusion requires an analysis based on an estimate that 5% of screened women have a suspicious mammogram and are referred for further assessment. In established programs, this number is 2% to 5%.[7,19,64,233] The reduction in breast cancer mortality attributed to screening ranges from 0.049% to 0.144% in the screened population. More than 2000 women must be screened for each woman who will benefit. In addition to the direct financial cost of mammographic screening and the opportunity costs that entails, Wright considers that women who are subjected to surgery for benign disease are harmed by the screening program, resulting in a harm/benefit ratio of up to 62:1.[327]

Obviously, any responsible implementation of a screening program requires attention to the prospects for causing more harm than good in a population of "healthy" women, in addition to the direct financial implications of the program. Those who advocate screening mammography have a duty to minimize the financial cost of the system and the potential for harm to "healthy" women. This harm can come from uncertainties and anxieties induced by the system and from "unnecessary" surgical procedures. Because the psychologic aspects of screening are difficult to quantify, they are generally dismissed as unimportant.[95] As is seen later in this book, a major theme of the Karolinska system of breast cancer control is the reduction of "unnecessary" surgical biopsies through reasonable interpretation of screening mammograms and the liberal use of stereotactic fine-needle biopsy. In our experience, fine-needle biopsy substantially reduces patient anxiety and uncertainties and the number of surgical biopsies initiated by the screening program.

Inappropriate assurance of normality. The concern that mammography may induce inappropriate confidence in a woman, leading her to believe she has no breast cancer, has been exemplified in the writings of many investigators. Skrabanek asserts it is unclear whether this is a major problem.[286] He feels it is difficult to demonstrate any direct relationship between the length of delay in breast cancer diagnosis and the outcome of the disease (see the section on minimal cancer). Indeed, in most instances the damage incurred by delayed diagnosis of breast cancer is not readily apparent (see the section on minimal cancer). The delay must be sufficiently long for the tumor to advance to a stage at which the chances for cure are less than they would have been had the tumor been detected at the earlier time. No one has shown the exact effect of delay in various situations and sizes of tumors. This is partially because small tumors can metastasize and some larger tumors are readily curable. In any event, at some time in the stage of all lethal breast cancers, a moment is reached when cure is less likely to occur. It is reasonable to presume that, as time elapses from the opportunity to detect a nonpalpable breast cancer until it is ultimately detected, there is an increased risk that the cancer will not be cured. As the tumor becomes larger, there is an increased

chance for metastases. Thus the false-negative mammogram finding may give the patient and her physician inappropriate reassurance, so that a cancer occurring in the interval between two screening mammographic examinations is ignored (see the section on diagnostic delay). For the purposes of this discussion, it does not make much difference whether the mammogram was abnormal and interpreted as normal or whether the lesion did not exist on the screening mammogram. In either case the detection of a palpable lesion in the interval between two screening mammograms warrants attention. In breast cancer diagnosis the most common malpractice claim in the United States has been inappropriate reliance on a normal mammogram in the face of a palpable mass. Physicians and patients should be informed that a mammogram is not intended to (nor does it) find every malignancy. The purpose of mammography is to find cancers before they become symptomatic (i.e., the nonpalpable breast cancer). Screening mammography will have an adverse effect if patients and physicians ignore interval cancer until the next screen and then rely on the mammogram, even in the face of a palpable mass. The way to address this problem is to increase the education and understanding of the proper role of mammography among referring physicians and patients.

A second issue related to the reliance on a normal mammogram concerns the analysis of researchers seeking to explain the apparent increase in mortality among younger screened patients compared to their control population in the studies recently completed in Canada. The initial publicity accompanying the release of the unpublished Canadian data was troublesome. They alleged more cancer deaths in the screened population than in the controls. The authors have since retracted this proclamation. They acknowledge that the data were biased by the selection of patients who had mammograms. Some of the patients were symptomatic with a breast mass and therefore much more likely to have cancer than would a group of asymptomatic women, like the controls. The Canadian breast project was initially designed to observe a phenomenon. They sought to observe how mammographic screening was being performed in Canada. There was no effort to control the quality of either the mammogram or its interpretation. Image quality control was essentially nonexistent. Others have discussed problems of the Canadian research project.[24] In some patients there is a natural tendency to rely on a normal mammogram finding. In younger patients, who may experience a more rapidly growing tumor, this reliance may have an especially adverse affect. In young patients in whom the tumor may be difficult to detect on screening mammography, it is even more important to emphasize that any change in breast symptoms on breast self-examination warrants attention, regardless of what was demonstrated on the past mammogram. It is not reasonable to wait until the next screening mammogram to do something about a newly palpable mass.

The current recommendation of 2-year intervals between mammograms for women 40 to 50 years of age increases the chance for false reliance on a prior screening mammogram. A subsequent observation would not be made for 2 years. Here again, the obvious approach is to better educate patients about the use and implications of mammography. We must diminish the number of patients who will falsely rely on a normal mammogram finding. False reliance on a prior mammogram can and will occur, despite whether the mammogram was falsely interpreted as normal. A true interval cancer can occur even with a completely normal screening mammogram finding. Findings from the screening mammogram may be normal even in retrospect, and an interval cancer can grow so fast that it is beyond cure by the time of the next screening mammogram.

Hazard of ionizing radiation. Young breast tissue has long been known to be more radiosensitive than most other soft tissues. The breast, thyroid, and bone marrow are the organs most susceptible to radiation carcinogenesis.[140] In 1970 there was a major international scare about the potential for mammography to cause breast cancer. Indeed, Bailar was of the opinion that mammography could potentially cause as much breast cancer as the early detection of cancer might cure.[21] He based this opinion partially on the fact that, at that time, 15% of those undergoing mammography were exposed to radiation doses that exceeded reasonable dose limits. Since the advent of low-dose screening mammography, there has been the widely held view that the dose is simply too low to warrant concern about radiation carcinogenesis in the human breast. This is especially true in view of the age in which mammography is being done. In women over 40 years of age the breast is less radiosensitive than at a younger age. In addition, the long lag time between the exposure and the incidence of radiation carcinogenesis suggests that women may die from other causes before radiation breast carcinogenesis occurs. Recently, however, there has been renewed concern about radiation carcinogenesis in a small population with a genetic trait that apparently predisposes them to increased breast sensitivity to radiation, leading to breast cancer.[292] It is well known that xeroderma pigmentosa and ataxia-telangiectasia predispose patients to radiation carcinogenesis, probably as the result of an abnormal DNA repair system inhibited by the gene causing the primary disease. Swift recently showed that, in individuals who are heterozygous for the ataxia telangiectasia gene, the incidence of breast carcinoma following diagnostic radiology examinations exceeds that of normal controls. They studied women who underwent documented diagnostic x-ray procedures, including fluoroscopic examinations of the chest, back, and abdomen, or documented therapeutic radiation. The diagnostic examinations studied were limited to upper gastrointestinal series, cholecystography or cholangiography, cardiac catheterization, barium enema, lumbar myelography, or intravenous or retrograde pyelography. They did not study any patients who had undergone a previous mammography, probably because those who have undergone mammography are at an older age than individuals who received most of the diagnostic examinations used in this study. They used a 5-year latency period from the time of the diagnostic study. They counted only those exposures in both the patients and the controls that occurred five years or more before the year of the cancer diagnosis. Cancers were diagnosed in patients ranging from 20 to 79 years of age. Of the 23 breast cancers, 5 occurred in patients who were under 50 years of age at the time of diagnosis.

Table 2-22 presents the incidence of breast cancer in blood relatives compared with their spouses. Swift et al. concluded that there is a five- to sixfold greater risk for breast cancer among blood relatives of patients with ataxia telangiectasia who have had a single or multiple fluoroscopic examinations of the chest or abdomen.[292] They estimated the mean glandular dose to the breast to be on the order of 1 to 9 MGy in a single exposure. Because they have calculated that 1.4% of the general population are heterozygous for the ataxic telangiectasia gene, it may be possible for mammography to cause breast cancer in a population of patients heterozygous for the ataxia telangi-

Table 2-22. Incidence of female breast cancer in 854 blood relatives and 415 spouses in families affected by ataxia-telangiectasia who were studied prospectively

Age (yr)	No. of breast cancers	Blood relatives No. of person-years	Rate per 1000	No. of breast cancers	Spouses No. of person-years	Rate per 1000
20-39	2	1490	1.3	0	947	0
40-49	3	1034	2.9	0	654	0
50-59	8	1132	7.1	2	593	3.4
60-69	6	985	6.1	1	355	2.8
≥70	4	736	5.4	0	157	0
All	23	5377	—	3	2706	—

Adapted from information appearing in: Swift et al: *N Engl J Med* 325:1831-1836, 1991.

ectasia gene. Because it is not possible to distinguish those persons with the gene from those without, this may become an important adverse effect of mammography, at least in the population under study. Curiously, other than for the suspect Canadian data for women 40 to 50 years of age, there has been no evidence of an increase in breast cancer incidence related to mammography. One might expect a slight incremental increase in this incidence, if as many as 60% to 70% of the population between 50 and 70 years of age receive mammograms (i.e., the extent in many localities in the United States).

Because of this concern it is reasonable to review the evidence for radiation breast carcinogenesis. The early data on radiation breast sensitivity were derived from the atomic bomb experience. In studies on the mortality of atomic bomb survivors, there was a significant dose response observed for leukemia; cancers of the esophagus, the stomach, colon, breast, and ovary; and urinary bladder and multiple myeloma.[273] In subsequent studies, patients undergoing radiation therapy for the thymus in infancy,[131] postpartum mastitis,[274] and Hodgkin's disease[121] have been observed. It was shown that breast radiation sensitivity is less likely to be carcinogenic at high doses than at considerably lower doses. This difference may be the result of permanent DNA damage. Upton considered that permanent damage to DNA may depend as much on the effectiveness of repair mechanisms as on the nature of the primary chemical lesion itself.[306] This may explain the susceptibility of persons with ataxia-telangiectasia and xeroderma pigmentosa.

There is evidence that doses as low as those given during chest fluoroscopy may induce breast carcinoma.[39,40,143] These studies have all shown a remarkable age dependency in the breast's susceptibility to radiation carcinogenesis. This was initially seen in the A-bomb studies. Younger patients (even those under 10 years of age) are susceptible to radiation carcinogenesis of the breast. The immature breast is more susceptible than the older breast.[38] There is no evidence of breast radiation carcinogenesis in women who receive radiation therapy after 30 years of age.[121] Radiation carcinogenesis is nonexistent in the postmenopausal breast.[94] This difference between the pre-menopausal and postmenopausal breast may be due to the strong hormone-promotion action seen in radiogenic breast cancer.[76] Feig believes that the decrease with age may be due to a progressive decline in the amount of glandular and ductal tissue after 20 years of age.[94] Indeed, the premenopausal decrease in the age-dependent rate of breast cancer incidence may support the theory of two populations of patients (see the section on Clemmensen's hook). This populations can be defined as:

1. A younger population, which may well be more radiosensitive

2. An older population, which appears to be somewhat, if not strongly, radioresistant

An age-dependent change in radiation sensitivity may occur in patients heterozygous for the ataxia telangiectasia gene.

The available evidence suggests that the recent concern about radiation-induced breast cancer from mammograms is unwarranted. As long as one adheres to the American Cancer Society's recommendations and performs most screening mammography in patients over 40 years of age, one would be performing the examinations at a time when the breasts were relatively radioresistant. This new "radiation scare" may be inappropriate if one considers its social impact—that is, it will decrease compliance with recommendations for mammography screening to detect early breast cancer. Further studies are necessary to ascertain the exact magnitude of the ataxia telangiectasia effect on induction of potential carcinogenesis from radiation. Until further evidence is in, it seems reasonable to conclude that this effect has been documented only for fluoroscopy performed in premenopausal women. It has not been documented at radiation doses as low as those used in the film screen mammography or in patients at the age when mammography is recommended.

Economics of screening mammography

The cost of screening mammography can be approached from many viewpoints. There are the "costs" of harming the patient by causing "unnecessary" anxieties and inducing "dis-ease." There are opportunity costs of advocating screening mammography to reduce morbidity and mortality from breast cancer. However, there may be other ways this money could be spent that would result in even more reduction in mortality and morbidity. There are social and political costs of advocating such a program and, more important, of not advocating breast cancer control as an important sociopolitical agenda. This has an impact on governmental priorities in resource allocation. Finally, there are the direct financial costs of a screening system and questions about what can be done to decrease these costs without compromising the quality of or accessibility to screening mammography.

These wide-ranging costs have been considered by Mooney et al. in a study of the long-run average screening cost for breast cancer detection by the British National Health Service.[213] They define cost widely, including not only screening and biopsy costs, but also anxiety costs for women biopsied and costs of such results as false-negative findings. When they defined costs this way, their analysis concluded that mammography with a single clinical examination is the "best buy." Similarly, the cost-benefit analysis of Kopans et al. concluded that mammography is the only imaging technique that has proved effective for screening.[166] They stated that "the cost for each curable cancer that is detected must be compared with the psychological, social and personal losses that accrue, as well as the numerous medical expenses incurred in a frequently protracted death from breast cancer."

Moskowitz includes these medical and philosophic considerations in his cost equation.[214] He states that "a reduction in cancer deaths is not easy to come by." When a method is available to achieve this result, every effort should be made to see that it is used "until it can be satisfactorily replaced by a less expensive, equally effective modality." He quotes Bierman, who said that "ultimately, when the scent is of flesh rather than figures, even the economist concedes that it will be important to insulate the individual practitioner (from cost-benefit/cost-effectiveness analysis) on a day-to-day basis because of potential conflict with the commitment to do what is best for each patient. Here is the crux. The economist's reference to the 'nation's health' is at best ambiguous and more likely meaningless. The physician's commitment to the patient's health is neither of these; it is clear, undeniable, and profoundly meaningful."

Carter et al. evaluated the breast cancer cohort at the Group Health Cooperative of Puget Sound.[56] They compared the service's utilization and cost for various stages of cancer at diagnosis. Their data clearly support the contention that diagnosis at an earlier stage substantially diminishes the total use of health care services in the management of breast cancer patients.

Table 2-23 demonstrates that patients diagnosed at a more advanced stage have 1.87 times as many clinic visits, 1.4 times as many diagnostic radiology examinations, and 4.8 times as much hospitalization over the 10 years studied than those diagnosed at an earlier stage. This type of data provides insight into the relative cost effectiveness of early detection of breast cancer through mammographic screening programs.

Tabar and Dean's analysis asserts that decision makers will have to realize that screening mammography can lead to a reduction in health care costs in the long run.[294] They caution that the cost of screening may outweigh the savings until the number of advanced cancers decreases. However, once this number is attained, the expense of screening will be far less than the savings. Savings will come from the smaller number of advanced—that is, more costly—cases. After reviewing this evidence, the "Swedish government has recommended screening mammography for all women aged 40-74." This recommendation emphasizes the need for high-quality examinations interpreted by well-trained radiologists. Similarly, Carter et al. showed how the start-up and maintenance costs of an organized program can be offset by future cost savings.[56] These cost savings occur from the reduced long-term disability in patients diagnosed at stage 0 and I, as opposed to those diagnosed at stages II or later. Carter asserts that a careful selection of the delivery model before implementation can make a breast cancer screening program both cost effective and "health effective." McLelland observed that "low cost, high-quality screening is feasible and can be expected to reduce the overall mortality from breast cancer."[200] He feels that a recognition of the need for and a desire to provide the service are the essential motivating factors. This involves a basic economic principle—the more it costs, the fewer the women who will undergo mammography. How to effectively reduce the cost without compromising the service remains a major worldwide problem in screening mammography and breast cancer control. Thus we review some basic economic principles of screening mammography as it applies in the United States.

The direct financial costs of breast cancer screening have been widely discussed and analyzed. In 1991 the U.S. Congress approved a payment of $55 per screening mammogram. This covers all women over 65 years of age. Previous charges for mammography in Michigan ranged from $60 to $180 per two-view examination of both breasts. A number of efforts have been made to reduce the charges and thereby increase the access to screening mammography. The number of mammograms read by a typical radiologist in mid-Michigan varies from 6 to 20 per day. Those who are considered dedicated mammographers may read as many as 80 examinations per day. The professional component of the fees paid for mammography ranges from 20% to 60% of the payments. Screening mammography is not a profit center in most radiologic practices and hospitals. As the payments for the procedure and its interpretation edge lower, it is often considered to be a loss leader. Thus this creates tension between the available social resources to pay for screening mammography and the capacity to perform them. In the early 1980s when many mammographic devices were sold, there was considerable enthusiasm about the potential profits to be attained from widespread screening. The needs of only a small proportion of the recommended population were being met. Only 15% to 30% of women who the American Cancer Society

Table 2-23. GHC 1972 breast cancer cohort: comparison of service utilization by stage at diagnosis

Mean units of service utilization per follow-up year	Stage at diagnosis		Increased utilization by stages II-III
	0-I	II-III	
Clinic visits	3.05	5.67	×1.87
Diagnostic radiology	1.60	2.27	×1.42
Hospital days	0.73	3.49	×4.78

From Carter et al: *Prevent Med* 16:19-34, 1987.

said should have annual screening mammograms were having them done. The number of mammography machines installed in the United States increased from 6500 to 10,000 between 1987 and 1990.[49] Some authorities feel that this number exceeds that needed if they were used at a reasonable rate. Indeed, Brown estimates that the projected demand for mammography would require only 2600 machines. In an effort to amortize this excessive capital, charges were either increased or maintained at a level too high to maximize market potential. The volume of patients being filmed with each machine is too low. In Michigan the average mammography machine does 1941 examinations per year with a range of 100 to 8700 per year. There probably are too many mammographic machines installed in the United States. This is especially true in view of the wide range in the number of examinations done per machine. Many radiologists interpret too few examinations to maintain their clinical skills. Low-volume mammography is beset with problems of both economics and quality. There simply are too few women, at the present cost of mammography, to recoup the capital investment in mammographic machines. Typically, U.S. medicine pricing policy has been to increase charges when it appears that there are insufficient patients and a prospect of economic loss. In more rational economic systems, profits are increased by market pricing rather than marginal pricing. The distinction is this— *marginal pricing* is done by calculating costs (e.g., equipment, operations, and film) and adding on a marginal profit, which is needed to sustain the enterprise. *Market pricing* applies the laws of market supply and demand. It asks at what price are profits maximized. If the use of invested capital is a substantial component of the cost and if that use is not saturated, profits may be increased by lowering charges to increase volume. This presupposes an elastic market, which is a market in which the demand (volume of use) increases as prices are lowered. (Similarly, as prices are increased, fewer people will demand the product.) In U.S. medical practice, it has not been customary to lower prices to increase volume. It was thought that the public will demand as much medical care as they need, regardless of costs. That may still be true for the individual consumer. However, access to and cost of screening mammography has become a social and political issue in the United States and elsewhere.[23,30,96,129,294] There are still serious questions about whether the cost of the procedure is a substantial barrier to demand for more mammograms. If it is such a barrier, perhaps lowering prices will increase the volume of screening mammography, thus permitting a more efficient use of the capital invested in equipment. Brown et al. assert that "the price of $100 is above the $50 usually associated with low-cost screening mammography programs and may impede the desirable public health trend to increase use of mammography screening."[49] If there were

fewer mammographic machines doing a higher volume of mammographies, more radiologists could devote themselves to mammography.[201] Unlike those seeing 6 to 12 cases per day, the radiologist seeing 80 to 100 mammograms should be more proficient and better able to monitor his or her false-negative and false-positive findings. The feedback from practice audit and continued ROC analysis should markedly improve the quality of mammographic services.

The price of mammography is an issue. Because the value of screening mammography to society partially depends on how much it costs, what else could be done with those monies to more effectively and efficiently decrease that component of human misery caused by breast cancer?

Moskowitz et al. analyzed the cost of screening mammography in terms of cost per person year gained.[216] For 1979 he estimated the cost per cancer found at $9000 and for each highly curable cancer at $26,961. Each death averted cost $61,100. He estimates that 60 person years are to be gained by each 1000 women screened by mammography and clinical examination. Mammography alone gains 40 person years per 1000 women screened. Therefore he calculates the gain of combined screening to be $3866 per person year, whereas the cost of screening by clinical examination alone is $4550. This difference is due to the fact that clinical examination alone would miss many of the more "curable" cancers.

Cyrlak obtained hard data by a telephone follow-up of a low-cost screening mammography project in Orange County, California.[74] The charges per mammogram were set at $50. Of the 2261 women screened, 18% required additional evaluation. This additional evaluation ranged from additional mammographic views to surgical biopsy. The average cost of additional evaluation was $607. The cost of screening mammograms accounted for less than one third of the total cost, with surgical consultation and biopsies for benign disease representing the major induced costs of screening. In this series five cancers were detected per 1000 women screened, and 17% of the cancers involved axillary lymph nodes. The actual cost for cancer detected was $25,500. This could obviously be reduced if we could decrease the false-positive mammogram findings or reduce the number of surgical biopsies. In large established programs, 3% to 5% is atypical for additional studies. This is a reasonable objective.[12,19,64,233] A lower rate of additional evaluations—from 18% to 3%—would substantially reduce the total cost. The surgical biopsy rate is the most important determinant of cost added by the finding of a suspicious mammogram. Azavedo and Svane have reduced this number to 1.14 biopsies per cancer found, compared with the 6 to 8 biopsies per cancer in the United States. They decreased the surgical biopsy rate to three biopsies per cancer by adding stereotactic fine-needle biopsy. The savings of 1.86 biopsies per cancer is beneficial from a purely financial standpoint because this 50% savings in total cost is accomplished by a procedure that costs 25% that of a surgical biopsy.

The rate of cancer detected also markedly affects these calculations. Prevalence screens in older women detect many more cancers than incident screens in younger women. In the face of limited resources should we perform only prevalence screens? Should we begin screening at an older age to improve the yield and thereby make screening more cost effective? Should we lengthen the time between screens to increase the number of detectable incident cancers per 1000 women screened? These issues were considered when the Karolinska screening program was established. Although the Swedish Board of Health and Welfare recommended screening mammography for all women 40 to 74 years of age, the Karolinska program screens all women between 50 and 69 years of age in an effort to maximize the benefit/cost ratio per cancer detected. The Swedish policy also screens at 2-year intervals (not the annual screen recommended by the American Cancer Society). The Swedish approach increases the number of incident cancers per screen. Whether there will be a related decrease in the proportion of "curable" cancers detected remains in doubt. The best available evidence suggests that the 2-year interval attains a better cost/benefit ratio.

Eddy et al. have carefully analyzed the cost implications of screening at a younger age.[88] They calculated that women between 40 and 50 years of age have a 128 in 10,000 chance of having breast cancer in 10 years. Of these 10,000, 82 will die from such a cancer. The addition of mammography to annual physical examination reduces the probability of death from 82 to about 60 per 10,000 women. They used a 25% compliance rate to estimate a decrease in total deaths by the year 2000 of 373 women and a surgical biopsy-to-cancer ratio of 9 to 1 to calculate a cost of some $1 million per death avoided by the year 2000 (1989 dollars). Although this represents an interesting and useful analysis, some of the assumptions are not valid. A surgical rate of nine biopsies per cancer would be found currently only if the mammographic interpretation were inept. Using mammograms alone one should be able to attain a biopsy-to-cancer ratio of three (or five) to one for early (nonpalpable) cancers. With the addition of fine-needle biopsy, this number can be reduced even further and approach a limit of one to one.[19] In addition to increasing the accuracy of mammographic interpretation and using aspiration cytology to decrease the cost of 'unnecessary" surgery, there are a number of other strategies that may lead to a reduction in the cost of screening mammography. Anything that can reduce the cost without decreasing the benefit will improve the cost/benefit ratio. Anything that could be done to increase the risk profile of patients being screened would improve the cost benefit.[88] The initiation of population screens probably should be

limited to women over 50 years of age. Perhaps women under 50 years of age should be screened only if they have a high-risk profile. These thoughts are embodied in the policies developed by the American Cancer Society and others.

Eddy's analysis suggests that screening in women under 50 years of age be limited to annual physical examination and breast self-examination. O'Malley et al. point out that no controlled prospective trial links breast self-examination to lives saved from breast cancer.[226] They state that the psychologic effects of teaching and performing breast self-examination are not yet clear. The cost of screening by breast self-examination is unknown, but it depends on the accuracy of the test and the training method used. The sensitivity of breast self-examination is low and reliance on it may decrease the potential benefits of screening in detecting early (nonpalpable) breast cancers. O'Malley feels that breast self-examination has potential as a screening test, but "many questions require additional scientific examination before it can be advocated as a screening test for breast cancer." The National Cancer Institute recently funded major projects to evaluate the effect of breast self-examination and physical examination on the control of breast cancer. This may be rather late because self-examination is already advocated as an educational policy of the American Cancer Society.

Other efforts to decrease the cost of screening mammography have been attempted. Reducing the number of films on follow-up (incident) screens has been investigated by Sickles et al., Gozzi et al., and Ikeda et al.[112,150,277] Sickles' group compared one-view with two-view screening mammograms in 22,500 consecutive asymptomatic women undergoing baseline mammography. They made two separate interpretations, one using only the oblique projection image and the other using both the oblique and the craniocaudal view. Two-view interpretations identified more cancers (27 versus 25). Perhaps even more important in terms of cost analysis was the observation that a one-view interpretation resulted in a need for many more additional mammograms to evaluate potential abnormalities. The "callback" rate for additional evaluation was 26% for one-view and only 7% for two-view interpretation. As we discussed, call-back rate is an important component of cost, in terms of both increased subsequent care and induced anxiety. Sickles' evidence suggests that a reduction of the number of views on prevalence screens may actually increase the cost. He, however, did not study the effect of one-view screens on incident examinations after a baseline had been established on a prevalence screen. Gozzi et al. advocate a two-film baseline examination followed by a one-view oblique projection on follow-up mammograms.[112] They claim a decreased cost of screening without decreased sensitivity using this approach. They were able to increase the number of women examined by 20% without increasing the total cost.

In a study of 1000 consecutive asymptomatic women who had prior normal baseline mammograms, Ikeda et al. observed that the density of the breast on the initial mammogram may be useful in selecting women who will require a two-view versus a one-view follow-up examination.[150] In women with dense breasts, the single oblique view resulted in an abnormal interpretation four times as often as the two-view reading (5.3% versus 1.3%). In these patients "the induced cost from these abnormal interpretations would have more than effected the small savings and operating expense associated with one-view screening." This difference was not seen in women with primarily fatty breasts on the baseline mammogram. The authors concluded that, "in these women, considering the cost, it may be reasonable to obtain a single oblique projection for follow-up mammograms."

Hillman et al. used another approach to provide low-cost high-quality mammography.[135] They trained physician's assistants (PAs) to interpret screening mammograms. The PAs' interpretations were more sensitive and as specific as those made by six radiologists who interpreted the same mammograms. Both groups were as effective as radiologists described in the literature. The ROC curves for PAs were larger than those of the radiologists. The PA interpretations took less time and cost less, and the dispositions recommended by the PAs were similar to those recommended by the radiologists. Hillman concluded that properly trained, evaluated, and supervised PAs can interpret screening mammograms at less cost and as well as radiologists. He feels that this should be attempted only under the direction of radiologists who are well trained in mammography.

Sickles et al. demonstrated how operational efficiency in screening mammographic practice can markedly reduce cost without sacrificing quality.[277] Screening mammography requires a different approach than is necessary for solving the more complex problems seen in symptomatic patients. In screening practice "operational procedures can be streamlined to maximize patient throughput" and achieve a substantial cost savings through the economies of scale. They recommend computerized record keeping and interpretation reporting to lower the cost of screening examinations. "With only 15 patients per day" operation is feasible at a charge of $50 per patient. They are very sensitive to the implications this lower charge may have on the practice of mammography.[276] Low-cost screening attracts a very different group of women than the population seen in traditional mammographic practices. They estimate that lower charges resulted in 93% of the patients being new rather than established mammographic patients seeking examination at a lower price. "Although low-cost screening does divert women away from more expensive nearby practices, it also generates an approximately equal number of breast imaging cases for these neighboring practices, including problem-solving examinations to further evaluate screening detected abnormalities." A survey of a nearby practice revealed that "the introduction of low-cost screening had no measurable impact on the steadily increasing mammography case load observed during the study period." They reached the conclusion that low-cost screening is not much of an economic threat to existing mammography practice.

We must do whatever we can reasonably do to reduce the financial costs of screening mammography programs. Cost reduction is necessary for improved access to the benefits. Each additional cost of screening mammography may tip the balance, so that society does nothing rather than embraces life-saving preventive health measures. Therefore we must do whatever we can do to reduce the cost of this system as perceived by society if we believe the benefits to be gained warrant our efforts. The most effective way to lower the cost to society—in the face of fixed benefit—is to remove the negatives. Efforts directed toward improved reliability of mammography and reduction of "unnecessary" surgical biopsy should be the most efficient way to diminish the costs of breast cancer screening to society.

Effect of screening mammography

Can we develop a system for early breast cancer detection? If this could be done, what are the costs and implications of such a system? If fewer women died from breast cancer, what would they eventually die from?

Screening mammography has a major effect on the stage in which breast cancer is diagnosed. Detection at an earlier stage of the disease has an impact on survival. The hallmark of success in the HIP study was the decreased mortality of patients who underwent screening mammography in relation to those who did not have such an opportunity.[272]

Ansell et al. reported on a nurse-run breast cancer detection program.[14] Of those cancers diagnosed by mammographic screen in the preclinical state, 16% (44 of 72) had localized disease, whereas only 33% (7 of 213) of women whose cancer was diagnosed outside of the screening program had localized breast cancer.

Tabar and Dean noted that women who participate in screening have half the risk of dying from breast cancer they would have had if they had not been screened.[294] Lung et al. analyzed the impact of breast cancer screening in 166 women whose tumors were detected by screening a population of 10,000 women.[188] In this series the mammogram was abnormal in only 55 women. An abnormal physical examination was present with or without an abnormal mammogram in 111 women. Recurrent tumor occurred in only 14.5% of those patients diagnosed by mammography alone and in 24.5% of patients who had abnormal physical findings with or without an abnormal mammogram. This shows that mammography is able to detect nonpalpable disease, which has a considerably lower recurrence rate than palpable lesions. In the Breast Cancer Detection and Demonstration Program, 33% of the tumors were less than 1 cm in diameter and considered minimal.[32]

In the first year of the Brescia screening project, Cirelli et al. found breast cancer in 39 patients.[64] Of these, 69.2% were stage I, 17.9% were stage II, none were stage III, and 2.6% were stage IV. This is a considerably higher number of stage I tumors than would traditionally be found in a symptomatic population.

In the Malmo screening project, Andersson et al. found 53 of 97 cancers (55%) to be either in situ or invasive, with a diameter of less than 1 cm.[12] They observed axillary metastases in 19.6% of the breast cancer cases detected on a population-based randomized screening trial. They observed a higher number of tubular carcinomas among the cancers detected by mammographic screening, suggesting a more benign course. Andersson et al. subsequently reported on the Malmo screening trial with controls.[13] They found stage II to IV cancer in 33% (190/588) of the study group and 52% (231/447) of their control group. In this series, screening mammography clearly led to the detection of breast cancer at an earlier stage.

Bird found 31% of the cancers detected at a low-cost screening center to be minimal (i.e., in situ or less than 1 cm in diameter with no positive nodes).[36] Sickles et al. reported on 170 patients with breast cancer detected on a screening practice; 94% were asymptomatic.[276] Their median size cancers were 12 mm and axillary metastases occurred in only 11%, with systemic metastases in 1.2%. Of the cancers detected in this program, 76.5% were either stage 0 or stage I. These studies establish that screening mammography can lead to the detection of breast cancer at an earlier stage. What about the reduction in fatalities?

In addition to marked improvement in the stage of the cancers detected in screening programs, screening programs have also been demonstrated to lead to a decrease in mortality from breast cancer. Shapiro et al. studied the HIP follow-up for 16 years.[272] He demonstrated again that the mortality from breast cancer continues to be lower among the study women, as compared with their controls. He estimated a 30% reduction of breast cancer mortality if screening had been maintained. Shapiro compared the survival rate curves for 14 years after diagnosis and showed a change in the contour of the trend lines resulting from the screening. The study group had a concave survival curve in contrast to the convex survival curve usually seen and seen in the controls. Those cases detected through mammography had an even more decided change in the contour of the survival curves. The relative survival rate remained the highest in the "mammography only" detected group. The Florence study observed that the chances of dying from breast cancer for patients who have been screened versus those never screened was 53%.[231] In women who had only one screen, the chances of dying were 57%, whereas those who had had two screens had a 32% chance of dying of breast cancer, as compared with the control population. Thus screening patients more than once yielded a significant improvement over a single screen in the reduction of mortality from breast cancer. Seidman et al. used the BCDDP data on 4240 women with breast cancer.[266] There is a remarkably high survival rate, with a 5-year survival rate of 88%, an 8-year rate of 83%, and a 10-year rate of 79%. The improved survival rates were as good for the women in their fourth decade of life as for the women in their fifth decade of life. More importantly, 46% fewer women died in the BCDDP group than in the comparable SEER group from 1977 to 1982. The authors concluded that this substantial gain in survival is due to cancers being diagnosed and treated at a more favorable stage as a result of screening. Only 19% of the BCDDP patients had died, whereas 35% of the SEER patients died.

In 1988, Seidman reviewed the cohort of HIP women whose breast cancer was diagnosed within 6 years of entry into the trial and followed for at least 18 years after the trial. Study group women and each age cohort had significantly lower breast cancer mortality than the control group. The Malmo mammographic screening trial yielded some interesting results on the impact of screening on survival.[13] The 1988 report from the Malmo mammographic screening trial warrants special attention. They screened women over 45 years old at intervals of 18 to 24 months. They invited 2188 women for screening, and 21,195 other women were placed in a control group and similarly followed for the appearance of breast cancer and for death from all causes. Five screening rounds were completed at the time of the report with a mean follow-up of 8.8 years. They treated all breast cancers according to the stage at diagnosis and the end-point of the study was mortality from breast cancer.

Breast cancer was diagnosed in 579 of the study group and in 443 of the control group. The rate of breast cancer diagnosis over the duration of the study was 27.9 cancers per 1000 women invited for screening and 22.5 breast cancers per 1000 women in the control group. The relative increase in cancers detected in the study group raises issues of lead-time and length bias, which should result in less mortality in the study versus the control group. That is not what was observed. In the study group, 63 women died from breast cancer, and in the control group, 66 died from breast cancer. There was no significant difference in the number of women dying from breast cancer between these two groups. The breast cancer death rate over this period of time was 2.99 per 1000 invited women in the study group and 3.11 per 1000 women in the control group.

However, the authors did observe an age-related effect of mammographic screening on breast cancer control. In the study group, 35 women over 55 years of age died from breast cancer, whereas 44 women over 55 years of age in the control group died. This represents a 20% reduction in mortality from breast cancer in women older than 55 years of age. Women under 55 years of age who entered the study had the opposite effect. In the study group 28 died versus 22 in the control group. This is difficult to explain because, on the average, the cancers in the study group were detected at an earlier stage than those in the control group. The authors concluded that an invitation to screening can lead to reduced mortality from breast cancer, at least in women over 55 years of age.

Lopez reported on 136 breast cancer patients who were found among 10,087 symptom-free patients in a screening program.[186a] In 76 patients, mammography was the sole diagnostic modality. If the diagnosis was made by mammography alone the breast cancer–related fatality rate was 2.6% (2 of 76). Breast cancer–related mortality in patients whose tumors were palpable at the time of detection was 30% (8 out of 60). The difference between those patients whose tumors were diagnosed only by mammography and those patients whose tumors were palpable is statistically significant with a P of 0.00001.

The 1990 statistics from the American Cancer Society indicate conclusive evidence on the 18-year follow-up of the HIP data, showing that the detection of the disease at an earlier than usual stage leads to a substantial savings of lives. Past screening procedures reduced the death rate from the disease up to 30%.

SUMMARY OF PROBLEMS

The problems in the diagnosis and management of breast cancer concern (1) the number of women who will die from the disease and what can be done to decrease that number; (2) the implications of a scheme for control, including the diagnosis of the disease by screening techniques; (3) the definition of what is early breast cancer and the implications of assessing data on diseases that may be related to, but are not, breast cancer; (4) and the risk factors that could be used to identify a population more likely to have breast cancer, thereby limiting the screening protocols to individuals at greater risk. These problems are partially compounded by a final problem: Why are more patients not cured once the diagnosis is established? In part, this is due to the limitations of early breast cancer treatment. Initially, radical mastectomy was the most common approach to the management of breast cancer. Efforts to change the surgical treatment of the disease over a period of almost 50 years did not greatly improve on the number of mastectomies or decrease the number of women who eventually would die from the disease. Surgical management at times did lengthen the symptom-free interval—that is, the time from the onset of breast cancer symptoms until the final symptoms of life's termi-

nus occur. It did not, however, have a substantial impact on the number of patients who die from the disease. The variations in treatments—ranging from the Halstead radical mastectomy to more recent breast-conserving treatments—have yielded little improvement in ultimate cure rates from the disease.

The model of the disease has changed dramatically. Breast cancer is not merely considered to be a local disease with axillary lymph node invasion but rather is a local disease that may or may not have early systemic complications. Which patient is more likely to have early systemic disease is still difficult to assess before surgery. Breast-conserving surgery, therefore, is in vogue and seems most appropriate. Breast conservation has as effective a cure rate as any alternative strategy in most cases of nonpalpable breast cancer. When the lesion is small, the breast can be preserved. This has great implications on the acceptance of breast cancer screening. Women are more likely to obtain diagnostic procedures that will not lead to radical, deforming breast surgery. The combination of radiation treatment, breast-conserving surgery, and appropriate chemotherapy has become a standard of care that maximizes benefit. The cure rate most heavily depends on the stage at which the cancer is diagnosed. Thus at our present stage of knowledge, any efforts that can establish an earlier diagnosis of breast cancer are more likely to lead to improvements in the cure of breast cancer than efforts to improve treatment.

The definition of breast cancer cure itself is controversial. Some investigators assert that no breast cancer is ever cured because it can possibly recur at much later times. A long, symptom-free interval can be followed by a reappearance of the disease in some patients. However, many authors perceive that a minimal breast cancer—fully excised and treated with appropriate radiation therapy—can result in a complete diminution of subsequent cancer in a patient's breasts. The probability of death from breast cancer in these patients is no greater than that in the general population with a similar risk profile. Women who undergo screening mammography are less likely to die from breast cancer than women who do not comply with the recommendations of the American Cancer Society.

REFERENCES

1. Adair F, Berg J, Lourdes J, Robbins GF: Long-term follow-up of breast cancer patients: the 30-year report, *Cancer* 33:1145, 1974.
2. Adami H, Bergstrom R, Hansen J: Age at first primary as a determinant of the incidence of bilateral breast cancer, *Cancer* 55:643-647, 1985.
3. Adami HO, Rimsten A, Stenkvist B, Vegelius J: Reproductive history and risk of breast cancer: a case-control study in an unselected Swedish population, *Cancer* 41:747-757, 1978.
4. Adami HO, Malker B, Rutqvist LE, et al: Temporal trends in breast cancer survival in Sweden: significant improvement in 20 years, *J Natl Cancer Inst* 76(4):653-659, 1986.
5. Alexander FE, Roberts MM, Huggins A, Muir BB: Use of risk fac-

tors to allocate schedules for breast cancer screening. *J Epidemiol Comm Health* 42(2):193-199, 1988.

6. American Cancer Society: Cost of screening mammography: issues, recommendations, and solutions, *Cancer* 60(7 suppl): 1694-1699, 1987.

7. Andersen JA: Lobular carcinoma *in situ:* a long term follow-up of 52 cases, *Acta Pathol Microbiol Scand* 82:A519-A533, 1974.

8. Anderson DE: Breast cancer in families, *Cancer* 40:1855, 1977.

9. Anderson TJ, Lamb J, Alexander F, et al: Comparative pathology of prevalent and incident cancers detected by breast screening: Edinburgh Breast Screening project, *Lancet* 1(8480):519-523, 1986.

10. Reference deleted in proof.

11. Andersson I: Radiographic patterns of the mammary parenchyma; variations with age at examination and age at first birth, *Radiology* 138:59-62, 1981.

12. Andersson I, Andren L, Hildell J, et al: Breast cancer screening with mammography: a population-based, randomized trial with mammography as the only screening mode, *Radiology* 132(2):273-276, 1979.

13. Andersson I, Aspergren K, Janzon L, et al: Mammographic screening and mortality from breast cancer: the Malmo mammographic screening trial, *Br Med J* 297(6654):943-948, 1988.

14. Ansell DA, Dillard J, Rothenberg M, et al: Breast cancer screening in an urban black population: a preliminary report, *Cancer* 62(2):425-428, 1988.

15. Arthur JE, Ellis IO, Flowers C, et al: The relationship of "high risk" mammographic patterns to histological risk factors for development of cancer in the human breast, *Br J Radiol* 63:845-849, 1990.

16. Ashikari R, Hajdu SI, Robbins GF: Intraductal carcinoma of the breast (1960-1969), *Cancer* 28:1182-1187, 1971.

17. Austin H, Cole P, Wynder E: Breast cancer in black American women, *Int J Cancer* 24(5):541-544, 1979.

18. Reference deleted in proof.

19. Azavedo E, Svane G: Radiologic aspects of breast cancers detected through a breast cancer screening program, *Eur J Radiol* 13:88-90, 1991.

20. Bailar JC III: Mammography: a contrary view, *Ann Intern Med* 84:77-84, 1976.

21. Bailar JC III: Mammographic screening: a reappraisal of benefits and risks, *Clin Obstet Gynecol* 21(1):1-14, 1978.

22. Bailar JC III: The incidence of independent tumors among uterine cancer patients, *Cancer* 16:842-853, 1963.

23. Baines CJ: Impediments to recruitment in the Canadian National Breast Screening Study: Response and resolution, *Controlled Clin Trials* 5(2):129-140, 1984.

24. Baines CJ, Miller AB, Kopans DB, et al: Canadian National Breast Screening Study: assessment of technical equality by external review, *AJR* 155(4):743-747, 1990.

25. Ballard-Barbash R, Griffin MR, Wold LE, O'Fallon WM: Breast cancer in residents of Rochester, Minnesota: incidence in survival, 1935 to 1982, *Mayo Clin Proc* 62:192-198, 1987.

26. Ballard-Barbash R, Schatzkin A, Kannel WB, et al: Body fat distribution and breast cancer in the Framingham Study, *J Natl Cancer Inst* 82:286-290, 1990.

27. Barker RM, Baker MR: Incidence of cancer in Bradford Asians, *J Epidemiol Comm Health* 44(2):125-129, 1990.

28. Barsky AJ: The paradox of health, *N Engl J Med* 318:414-418, 1988.

29. Bartow SA, Pathak DR, Mettler FA: Radiographic microcalcification and parenchyma pattern as indicators of histologic "high-risk" benign breast disease, *Cancer* 66:1721-1725, 1990.

30. Bassett LW, Bunnell DH, Cerny JA, Gold RH: Screening mammography: referral practices of Los Angeles physicians, *AJR* 147(4):689-692, 1986.

31. Beahrs O: *American Joint Committee on Cancer: Manual for staging of cancer,* ed 3, Philadelphia, 1988, Lippincott.

32. Beahrs OH, Smart CR: Diagnosis of minimal breast cancer in the BCDDP: the 66 questionable cases, *Cancer* 43(3):851-856, 1979.

33. Begg CB: Risk factor analysis of screening data, *J Chronic Dis* 40:989-991, 1987.

34. Berg J, Hutter RVP, Foote FW Jr: The unique association between salivary gland cancer and breast cancer, *JAMA* 204:771-774, 1968.

35. Bernstein L, Ross RK, Labo RA, et al: The effects of moderate physical activity on menstrual cycle patterns in adolescence: implication for breast cancer prevention, *Br J Cancer* 55:681-685, 1987.

36. Bird RE: Low cost screening mammography: report of finances and review of 21,716 consecutive cases, *Radiology* 171(1):87-90, 1989.

37. Bland KI, Buchanan JB, Mills DL, et al: Analysis of breast cancer screening in women younger than 50 years, *JAMA* 245:1037-1042, 1981.

38. Boice JD: Carcinogenesis: a synopsis of human experience with external exposure in medicine, *Health Phys* 55:621-630, 1988.

39. Boice JD, Monson RR: Breast cancer in women after repeated fluoroscopic examinations of the chest, *J Natl Cancer Inst* 59:823-832, 1977.

40. Boice JD Jr, Rosenstein M, Trout ED: Estimation of breast doses and breast cancer risk associated with repeated fluoroscopic chest examinations of women with tuberculosis, *Radiat Res* 73(2):373-390, 1978.

41. Bondy ML, Fueger JJ, Vogel VG, Spitz MH: Ethnic differences in familial breast cancer, *Am Assoc Cancer Res* 32:PA1316, 1991.

42. Boyle P, Robertson C: Breast cancer and colon cancer incidence in females in Scotland, 1960-84, *J Natl Cancer Inst* 79:1175-1179, 1987.

43. Breast cancer screening in women under fifty, *Lancet* 337:1575-1576, 1991 (editorial).

44. Brian DD, Melton LJ III, Goellner JR, et al: Breast cancer incidence, prevalence, mortality, and survivorship in Rochester, Minnesota— 1935 to 1974, *Mayo Clin Proc* 55(6):355-359, 1980.

45. Brinkley D, Haybittle JL: Long-term survival of women with breast cancer, *Lancet* I:1118 and II:353, 1984.

46. Brinton LA, William RR, Hoover RN, et al: Breast cancer risk factors among screening program participants, *J Natl Cancer Inst* 62(1):37-44, 1979.

47. Broders AC: Carcinoma *in situ* contrasted with benign penetrating epithelium, *JAMA* 99:1670-1674, 1932.

48. Brown BW, Atkinson EN, Bartoszynski, et al: Estimation of human tumor growth rate from distribution of tumor size at detection, *J Natl Cancer Inst* 72:31-38, 1984.

49. Brown ML, Kessler LG, Rueter FG: Is the supply of mammography machines outstripping need and demand? An economic analysis, *Ann Intern Med* 113(7):547-552, 1990.

50. Bruzzi P, Green SB, Byar DP, et al: Estimating the population attributable risk for multiple risk factors using case-control data, *Am J Epidemiol* 122:904-914, 1985.

51. Bruzzi P, Negri E, LaVecchia C, et al: Short term increase in the risk of breast cancer after full term pregnancy, *Br Med J* 297:1096-1098, 1988.

52. Burhenne LJW, Hislop TG, Burhenne HJ: The British Columbia Mammography Screening Program: evaluation of the first 15 months, *AJR* 158:45-49, 1992.

53. Byrne RN, Bringhurst LS, Gershon-Cohen J: Postoperative detection of cancer by periodic mammography of the remaining breast, *Surg Gynecol Obstet* 115:282-286, 1962.

54. Cady B: New diagnostic, staging, and therapeutic aspects of early breast cancer, *Cancer* 65:634-647, 1990.

55. Calnan M: The health belief model and participation in programmes for the early detection of breast cancer: a comparative analysis, *Soc Sci Med* 19(8):823-830, 1984.

56. Carter AP, Thompson RS, Bourdeau RV, et al: A clinically effective breast cancer screening program can be cost-effective, too, *Prevent Med* 16(1):19-34, 1987.

57. Carter CL, Corle DK, Micozzi MS, et al: A prospective study of the development of breast cancer in women with proliferative breast disease, *Am J Epidemiol* 128:467-477, 1988.

58. Carter CL, Jones DY, Schatzkin A, Brinton LA: A prospective study of reproductive, familial and socioeconomic risk factors for breast cancer using NHANES I data, *Pub Health Rep* 104:45-50, 1989.

59. Chen PL, Chen Y, Bookstein R, Lee WH: Genetic mechanisms of tumor suppression by the human p53 gene, *Science* 250:1576-1580, 1990.

60. Chism SE, Brown BS, Hoyle BA: Breast cancer treatment: evolving approaches, but stable results, *Int J Radiat Oncol Biol Phys* 12:2073-2078, 1986.

61. Chu KC, Smart CR, Tarone RE: Analysis of breast cancer mortality and stage distribution by age for the health insurance plan clinical trial, *J Natl Cancer Inst* 80:1125-1132, 1988.

62. Chu SY, Stroup NE, Wingo PA, et al: Cigarette smoking and the risk of breast cancer, *Am J Epidemiol* 131:244-253, 1990.

63. Ciatto S, Cataliotti L, Distante V: Nonpalpable lesions detected with mammography: review of 512 consecutive cases, *Radiology* 165:99-102, 1987.

64. Cirelli L, Donato F, Carafa M, Spiazzi R: Risultati del primo passaggio di uno screening mammografico nell'USSL 43, Leno della Lombardia (BS). [Results of the first round of mammographic screening at local health unit No. 43, Leno, Lombardy (Brescia)]. *Radiol Med (Torino)* 77(4):382-385, 1989.

65. Claus EB, Risch N, Thompson WD: Genetic analysis of breast cancer in the cancer and steroid hormone study, *Am J Hum Genet* 48:232-242, 1991.

66. Clemmensen J: Carcinoma of the breast, symposium: results from statistical research, *Br J Radiol* 21:583-590, 1948.

67. Clemmensen J: On the etiology of some human cancers, *J Natl Cancer Inst* 12:1-21, 1951.

68. Colditz GA, Willett WC, Stampfer MJ, et al: Parental age at birth and risk of breast cancer in daughters: a prospective study among US women, *Cancer, Causes, Control* 2(1):31-36, 1991.

69. Cole P, Crammer D: Diet and cancer of the endocrine target organs, *Cancer* 40:434-437, 1977.

70. Coles C, Thompson AM, Elder PA, et al: Evidence implicating at least two genes on chromosome 17p in breast carcinogenesis, *Lancet* 336:761-763, 1990.

71. Coll PP, O'Connor PJ, Crabtree BF, Besdine RW: Prevalence of mammography use in a nursing home population, *J Fam Pract* 30(6):682-685, 1990.

72. Croghan IT: A study to determine the effects of genetic and dietary factors on the etiology of breast cancer, *Dis Abstr Int (Sci)* 48(3):799, 1987.

73. Cutler SJ, Myers H, Green SB: Trends in survival rates of patients with cancer, *N Engl J Med* 293:122-124, 1975.

74. Cyrlak D: Induced costs of low-cost screening mammography, *Radiology* 168(3):661-663, 1988.

75. Damon A: Host factors in cancer of the breast and uterine cervix and corpus, *J Natl Cancer Inst* 24(2):483-516, 1960.

76. Day NE: Radiation and multistage carcinogenesis, *Prog Cancer Res Ther* 26:437-443, 1984.

77. Day NE, Williams DR, Khaw KT: Breast cancer screening programmes: the development of a monitoring and evaluation system, *Br J Cancer* 59(6):954-958, 1989.

78. Dean L, Geschickter CF: Comedocarcinoma of the breast, *Arch Surg* 36:225-234, 1938.

79. DeNeef P, Gandara J: Experience with indeterminate mammograms, *West J Med* 154(1):36-39, 1991.

80. de Waard F: Recent trends in breast cancer incidence, *Prevent Med* 7:160-167, 1978.

81. de Waard F, Baandersvan-Halewijnea EA, Huzinga J: The bimodal age distribution of patients with mammary cancer: evidence for the existence of two types of human breast cancer, *Cancer* 17:141-151, 1964.

82. de Waard F, Collette HJ, Rombach JJ, Collette C: Breast cancer screening, with particular reference to the concept of "high risk" groups, *Breast Cancer Res Treat* 11(2):125-132, 1988.

83. Donato F, Bollani A, Spiazzi R, et al: Factors associated with non-participation of women in a breast cancer screening programme in a town in northern Italy, *J Epidemiol Comm Health* 45(1):59-64, 1991.

84. Dublin N, Hutter RV, Strax P, et al: Epidemiology of minimal breast cancer among women screened in New York City, *J Natl Cancer Inst* 73:1273-1279, 1984.

85. Dupont WD, Page DL: Risk factors for breast cancer in women with proliferative breast disease, *N Engl J Med* 312:146-151, 1985.

86. Dupont WD, Page DL, Rogers LAW, Parl FF: Influence of exogenous estrogens, proliferative breast disease, and other variables on breast cancer risk, *Cancer* 63:948-957, 1989.

87. Eddy DM: Screening for breast cancer, *Ann Intern Med* 111:389-399, 1989.

88. Eddy DM, Hasselblad V, McGivney W, Hendee W: The value of mammography screening in women under age 50 years, *JAMA* 259(10):1512-1519, 1988.

89. Enriori CL, Orsini W, del Carmen-Cermona M, et al: Decrease of circulating level of SHBG in postmenopausal obese women as a risk factor in breast cancer, reversible effect of weight loss, *Gynecol Oncol* 23:77-86, 1986.

90. Evans JS, Wennberg JE, McNeil BJ: The influence of diagnostic radiology on the incidence of breast cancer and leukemia, *N Engl J Med* 315:810-815, 1986.

91. Ewertz M: Smoking and breast cancer risk in Denmark, *Cancer Causes Control* 1:31-37, 1990.

92. Fallowfield LJ, Rodway A, Baum M: What are the psychological factors influencing attendance, non-attendance and re-attendance at a breast screening centre? *J R Soc Med* 83(9):547-551, 1990.

93. Farrow JH: Current concepts in the detection and treatment of the earliest of the early breast cancer, *Cancer* 25:468-477, 1970.

94. Feig SA: Biologic determinants of radiation induced human breast cancer, *CRC Crit Rev Diagn Imaging* 13:229-248, 1980.

95. Fentiman S: Pensive women, painful vigils: consequences of delay in assessment of mammographic abnormalities, *Lancet* 1:1041-1042, 1988.

96. Fernandez L, Buch ML, Molina A, et al: Risk factors in mass screening for breast cancer, multivariate analysis of data from the Cuban diagnosis pilot study, *Neoplasma* 33(4):535-541, 1986.

97. Fink R: Delay behavior in breast cancer screening. In Cullen JW et al, editors: *Cancer: the behavioral dimensions,* New York, 1976, Raven Press.

98. Finley ML: Social and medical factors associated with diagnostic delay in breast cancer patients, *Dis Abstr Int* 46:[A]3864, 1986.

99. Fischedick O, Plum R: Reihenuntersuchungen bei Frauen mit einem erhohten Risiko fur eine Brustkrebserkrankung mit Hilfe der Mammographie. [Mass radiography via mammography in women with enhanced risk of cancer of the breast (author's transl).] *Rontgenblatter* 32(5):242-250, 1979.

100. Fisher ER, Redmond C, Fisher B, Bass G: Pathologic findings from the National Surgical Adjuvant Breast and Bowel Project (NSABP), *Cancer* 65:2121-2128, 1990.

101. Fisher ER, Palekar A, Kim WS, Redmond C: The histopathology of mammographic patterns, *Am J Clin Pathol* 69:241-246, 1978.

102. Foote FW, Stewart FW: Lobular carcinoma in situ: a rare form of mammary cancer, *Am J Pathol* 17:490-496, 1941.

103. Foote FW, Stewart FW: Comparative studies of cancerous vs. non-cancerous breasts, *Ann Surg* 131:197-222, 1945.

104. Fournier DV, Schiller U: Natural growth rate in 300 primary breast carcinomas and correlation to hormone factors, *Ann NY Acad Sci* 464:563-565, 1986.

105. Frisch RE. Wyshak G, Witschi J, et al: Lower lifetime occurrence of breast cancer and cancers of the reproductive system among former college athletes, *Int J Fertil* 32:217-225, 1987.

106. Gail MH, Brinton LA, Byar DP, et al: Projecting individualized probabilities of developing breast cancer for white females who are being examined annually, *J Natl Cancer Inst* 81:1879-1886, 1989.

107. Gallager HS, Martin JE: The study of mammary carcinoma by mammography in whole organ sectioning: early observations, *Cancer* 23:855-873, 1969.

108. Ghys R: Natural history of benign and malignant breast tumors seen in a screening center; 15-year retrospective study, *Cancer* 57(8):1618-1626, 1986.

109. Goodman MJ: Breast cancer in multi-ethnic populations: the Hawaii perspective, *Breast Cancer Res Treat* 18(Suppl 1):S5-9, 1991.

110. Goodson WH, Miller TR, Sickles EA, Upton RA: Lack of correlation of clinical breast examination with high-risk histopathology, *Am J Med* 89:752-756, 1990.

111. Goldstein AM, Amos CI: Segregation analysis of breast cancer from the cancer in steroid hormone study: histologic subtypes, *J Natl Cancer Inst* 82:911-917, 1990.

112. Gozzi G, Vidali C, Polonio G, et al: Mammographic diagnosis based on oblique projection: personal experience, *Radiol Med* 75(4):365-369, 1988.

113. Grady D, Hodgkins ML, Goodson WH: The lumpy breast, *West J Med* 149:226-229, 1988.

114. Gram IT, Slenker SE: Cancer anxiety and attitudes toward mammography among screening attenders, nonattenders and women never invited, *Am J Public Health* 82:249-251, 1992.

115. Gregorio DI, Kegeles S, Parker C, Benn S: Encouraging screening mammograms: results of the 1988 Connecticut Breast Cancer Detection Awareness Campaign, *Conn Med* 54(7):370-373, 1990.

116. Gump FE, Jicha DL, Ozello L: Ductal carcinoma *in situ* (DCIS): a revised concept, *Surgery* 102:790-795, 1987.

117. Haagensen CD, Lane N, Lattes R, Bodian C: Lobular neoplasia (so called lobular carcinoma *in situ*) of the breast, *Cancer* 42:737-769, 1978.

118. Haagensen CE: The treatment and results in cancers of the breast at Presbyterian Hospital, New York, *Am J Roentgenol* 62:328-334, 1949.

119. Hakama M: The peculiar age specific incidence curve for cancer of the breast—Clemmensen's hook, *Acta Pathol Microbiol Scand* 75:370-374, 1969.

120. Hall JM, Lee MK, Newman B, et al: Linkage of early-onset familial breast cancer to chromosome 17q21, *Science* 250:1684-1689, 1990.

121. Hancock, SLH: Personal communication, Stanford University, Department of Radiation Therapy, 1992.

122. Harris RE, Spritz N, Wynder EL: Studies of breast cancer and alcohol consumption, *Prevent Med* 17:676-682, 1988.

123. Harris RE, Wynder EL: Breast cancer and alcohol consumption: a study in weak associations, *JAMA* 259:2867-2871, 1988.

124. Harris RP, O'Malley MS, Fletcher SW, Knight BP: Prompting physicians for preventive procedures: a five-year study of manual and computer reminders, *Am J Prevent Med* 6(3):145-152, 1990.

125. Haybittle JL: Curability of breast cancer, *Breast Dis* 47:319-323, 1990.

126. Hayward RA, Shapiro MF, Freeman HE, Corey CR: Who gets screened for breast cancer? Results from a new national survey, *Arch Intern Med* 148:1177-1181, 1988.

127. Helmrich SP, Shapiro S, Rosenberg L, et al: Risk factors for breast cancer, *Am J Epidemiol* 117:35-45, 1983.

128. Henderson BE, Ross RK, Judd HL, et al: Do regular ovulatory cycles increase breast cancer risk? *Cancer* 56:1206-1208, 1985.

129. Hessler C: Screening for breast cancer, *Schweiz Med Wochenschr* 25(Suppl):72-75, 1988.

130. Hiatt RA: Alcohol consumption and breast cancer, *Med Oncol Tumor Pharmacother* 7:143-151, 1990.

131. Hildreth NG, Shore RE, Dvoretsky PM: The risk of breast cancer after irradiation of the thymus in infancy, *N Engl J Med* 321:1281-1284, 1989.

132. Hildreth NG, Shore RE, Hempelmann LH: Risk of extrathyroidal tumors following radiation treatment in infancy for thymic enlargement, *Radiation Res* 102:378-391, 1985.

133. Hill GB, Burns PE, Koch M, et al: Trends in the incidence of cancer of the female breast and reproductive tract in Alberta, 1953 to 1977, *Prevent Med* 12(2):296-303, 1983.

134. Hill P, Garbaczewski L, Helman P, et al: Environmental factors and breast and prostatic cancer, *Cancer Res* 41(9,pt 2):3817-3818, 1981.

135. Hillman BJ, Fajardo LL, Hunter TB, et al: Mammogram interpretation by physician assistants, *Am J Roentgenol* 149(5):907-912, 1987.

136. Hirohata T, Nomura AM, Hankin JH, et al: An epidemiologic study on the association between diet and breast cancer, *J Natl Cancer Inst* 78(4):595-600, 1987.

137. Hislop TG, Elwood JM: Risk factors for benign breast disease: a 30-year cohort study, *Can Med Assoc J* 124:283-291, 1981.

138. Holland R, Hendriks JHCL, Mravunac M: Mammographically occult breast cancer, *Cancer* 52:1810-1819, 1983.

139. Holland R, Mravunac M, Hendriks JH, Bekker BV: So-called interval cancers of the breast: pathologic and radiologic analysis of sixty-four cases, *Cancer* 49:(12)2527-2533, 1982.

140. Holm LE: Cancer occurring after radiotherapy and chemotherapy, *Int J Radiation Oncol Biol Physics* 99:1303-1308, 1990.

141. Horn PL, Thompson WD, Schwartz SM: Factors associated with the risk of second primary breast cancer: an analysis of data from the connective tumor registry, *J Chron Dis* 40:1003-1011, 1987.

142. Houts PS, Wojtkowiak SL, Simmonds MA, et al: Using a state cancer registry to increase screening behaviors of sisters and daughters of breast cancer patients, *Am J Public Health* 81(3):386-388, 1991.

143. Howe GR, Miller AB, Sherman GJ: Breast cancer mortality following fluoroscopic irradiation in a cohort of tuberculosis patients, *Cancer Detect Prevent* 5(2):175-178, 1982.

144. Hsieh CC, Trichopoulos D: Breast size, handedness and breast cancer risk, *Eur J Cancer* 27:131-135, 1991.

145. Hsieh CC, Trichopolos D, Katsouyanni K, Yuasa S: Age at menarche, age at menopause, height and obesity as risk factors for breast cancer: associations and interactions in an international case control study, *Int J Cancer* 46:796-800, 1990.

146. Hulka BS: Hormone-replacement therapy and the risk of breast cancer, *CA* 40(5):289-296, 1990.

147. Hultborn R, Friberg S, Hultborn KA: Male breast carcinoma. I. A study of the total material reported to the Swedish Cancer Registry 1958-1967 with respect to clinical and histopathologic parameters, *Acta Oncol* 26:241-256, 1987.

148. Hunter JV, Hunter GJ, Tucker AK: Patterns of axillary lymphadenopathy demonstrated by mammography: implications for the asymptomatic woman in a breast screening programme, *Clin Radiol* 38:515-517, 1987.

149. Hutter RVP: Goodbye to "fibrocystic disease," *N Engl J Med* 312:179-181, 1985.

150. Ikeda DM, Sickles EA: Second-screening mammography: one versus two views per breast, *Radiology* 168(3):651-656, 1988.

151. Irwig L, Cockburn J, Turnbull D, et al: Women's perception of screening mammography, *Aust J Pub Health* 15:24-32, 1991.

152. Janerich DT, Hayden CL, Thompson WD, et al: Epidemiologic evidence of perinatal influence in the etiology of adult cancers, *J Clin Epidemiol* 42:151-157, 1989.

153. Janerich DT, Hoff MB: Evidence for a cross over in breast cancer risk factors, *Am J Epidemiol* 116:737-742, 1982.

154. Jasmin C, Le MG, Marty P, Herzberg R: Evidence for a link between certain psychological factors and the risk of breast cancer in a case-control study, *Ann Oncol* 1:22-29, 1990.

155. Jensen HM, Rice JR, Wellings SR: Preneoplastic lesions in the human breast, *Science* 191:295-297, 1976.

156. Jepson C, Kessler LG, Portnoy B, Gibbs T: Black-white differences in cancer prevention knowledge and behavior, *Am J Public Health* 81(4):501-504, 1991.

157. Joensuu H, Toikkenen S: Comparison of breast carcinomas diagnosed in the 1980s and those diagnosed in the 1940s to 1960s, *Br Med J* 303:155-158, 1991.

158. Kalisher L, McLelland R: The role of mammographic parenchymal patterns in screening for carcinoma of the breast, *Surg Gynecol Obstet* 172:81-88, 1991.

159. Kampert JB, Whittemore AS, Paffenbarger RS: Combined effect of childbearing, menstrual events, and body size on age-specific breast cancer risk, *Am J Epidemiol* 128:962-979, 1988.

160. Kelsey JL: A review of the epidemiology of human breast cancer, *Epidemiol Rev* 1:74-109, 1979.

161. Kelsey JL, Berkowitz GS: Breast cancer epidemiology, *Cancer Res* 48:5615-5623, 1988.

162. Kerner JF, Andrews H, Zauber A, Struening E: Geographically-based cancer control: methods for targeting and evaluating the impact of screening interventions on defined populations, *J Clin Epidemiol* 41(6):543-553, 1988.

163. Ketcham AS, Moffat FL: Vexed surgeons, perplexed patients, and breast cancers which may not be cancer, *Cancer* 65:387-393, 1990.

164. King ES, Rimer BK, Trock B, et al: How valid are mammography self-reports? *Am J Public Health* 80(11):1386-1388, 1990.

165. Kirch RL, Klein M: Prospective evaluation of periodic breast examination programs: interval cases, *Cancer* 41(2):728-736, 1978.

166. Kopans DB, Meyer JE, Sadowsky N: Breast imaging (review), *N Engl J Med* 310(15):960-967, 1984.

167. Korenman SG: The endocrinology of breast cancer, *Cancer* 46:874-878, 1980.

168. Krieger N: Social class and the black/white crossover in the age specific incidence of breast cancer: a study linking census-derived data to population-based registry records, *Am J Epidemiol* 131:804-814, 1990.

169. Kundel HL, Revesz G: Lesion conspicuity, structured noise and film reader error, *AJR* 126:1233-1235, 1976.

170. Kvale G, Heuch I: Lactation and cancer risk: is there a relation specific to breast cancer? *J Epidemiol Commun Health* 42:30-37, 1988.

171. Land CE: Low dose radiation—a cause of breast cancer, *Cancer* 46:868-873, 1980.

172. Land CE: New understanding from epidemiology—the next 25 years, *Health Phys* 55:269-278, 1988.

173. Lantz P, Bunge M, Remington PL: Trends in mammography in Wisconsin, *Wisc Med J* 89:281-282, 1990.

174. Le MG, Hill C, Rezvani A, et al: Long-term survival of women with breast cancer, *Lancet* 11:922, 1984.

175. Le Marchand L: Ethnic variation in breast cancer survival: a review, *Breast Cancer Res Treat* 18(Suppl 1):S119-S126, 1991.

176. Le Marchand L, Kolonel LN, Earle ME, Mi MP: Body size at different periods of life in breast cancer risk, *Am J Epidemiol* 128:137-152, 1988.

177. Lenfant Pejovic MH, Mlika Cabanne N, Bouchardy C, Auquier A: Risk factors for male breast cancer: a Franco-Swiss case-control study, *Int J Cancer* 45:661-665, 1990.

178. Lerman C, Rimer B, Trock B, et al: Factors associated with repeat adherence to breast cancer screening, *Prevent Med* 19(3):279-290, 1990.

179. Lew EA, Garfinkel L: Variations in mortality by weight among 750,000 men and women, *J Chron Dis* 32:563-576, 1979.

180. Lewontin RC, Hartl DL: Population genetics in forensic DNA typing, *Science* 254:1745-1750, 1991.

181. Lilienfeld A, Johnson E: The age distribution in female breast and genital cancers, *Cancer* 8:875-882, 1955.

182. Lin TM, Chen KP, MacMahon B: Epidemiologic characteristics of cancer of the breast in Taiwan, *Cancer* 27:1497-1504, 1971.

183. London SJ, Colditz GA, Stampfer MJ, et al: Prospective study of relative weight, height and risk of breast cancer, *JAMA* 262:2853-2858, 1989.

184. London SJ, Colditz GA, Stampfer MJ, et al: Lactation and risk of breast cancer in a cohort of US women, *Am J Epidemiol* 132:17-26, 1990.

185. London SJ, Connolly JL, Schnitt SJ, Colditz GA: A prospective study of benign breast disease and the risk of breast cancer, *JAMA* 267:941-944, 1992.

186. Longnecker MP, Berlin JA, Arza MJ, Chalmers TC: A meta-analysis of alcohol consumption in relation to risk of breast cancer, *JAMA* 260:652-656, 1988.

186a. Lopez MJ, Blackwell CW: Breast cancer detected by screening: the importance of long-term follow-up, *Surgery* 106(4):590-594, 1989.

187. Love SM, Gelman RS, Silent W: Fibrocystic "disease" of the breast: a non-disease, *N Engl J Med* 307:1010-1014, 1982.

188. Lung JA, Hart NE, Woodbury R: An overview and critical analysis of breast cancer screening, *Arch Surg* 123(7):833-838, 1988.

189. Lynch HT, Krush AJ: Genetic predictability in breast cancer risk, *Arch Surg* 103:84-88, 1971.

190. Mabuchi K, Bross DS, Kessler II: Risk factors for male breast cancer, *J Natl Cancer Inst* 74:371-375, 1985.

191. MacCarty WC: The histogenesis of cancer of the breast and its clinical significance, *Surg Gynecol Obstet* 17:441-446, 1913.

192. MacMahon B, Austin JH: Association of carcinomas of the breast and corpus uteri, *Cancer* 23:275-280, 1969.

193. MacMahon B, Cole P, Lin TM, et al: Age at first birth and breast cancer risk, *Bull WHO* 43:209-221, 1970.

194. Malkin D, Li FD, Strong LC, et al: Germ line p53 mutations in a familial syndrome of breast cancer, sarcomas, and other neoplasms, *Science* 250:1233-1238, 1990.

195. Martin JE, Gallager HS: Mammographic diagnosis of minimal breast cancer, *Cancer* 28(6):1519-1526, 1971.

196. Martin JE, Moskowitz M, Milbrath JR: Breast cancer missed by mammography, *Am J Roentgenol* 132(5):737-739, 1979.

197. McBride CM, Brown BW, Thompson JR, et al: Can patients with breast cancer be cured of their disease? *Cancer* 51:938, 1983.

198. McCance KL, Mooney KH, Smith KR, Field R: Validity and reliability of a breast cancer knowledge test, *Am J Prevent Med* 6(2):93-98, 1990.

199. McGregor DH, Land CE, Choi K, et al: Breast cancer incidence among atomic bomb survivors, Hiroshima and Nagasaki, 1950-1969, *J Natl Cancer Inst* 59:799-811, 1977.

200. McLelland R: Low-cost mass screening with mammography as a means of reducing overall mortality from breast cancer (review), *Radiol Clin North Am* 25(5):1007-1013, 1987.

201. McLelland R: Screening mammography, *Cancer* 67:1129-1131, 1991.

202. McTiernan A, Thomas DB: Evidence for a protective effect of lac-

tation on risk of breast cancer in young women, *Am J Epidemiol* 124:353-358, 1986.

203. McTiernan A, Thomas DB, Johnson LK, Roseman D: Risk factors for estrogen-rich and receptor poor breast cancers, *J Natl Cancer Inst* 77:849-854, 1986.

204. Mellink WAM, Holland R, Hendriks JHCL, et al: The contribution of routine follow-up mammography to an early detection of asynchronous contralateral breast cancer, *Cancer* 67:1844-1848, 1991.

205. Mettler FA, Hempelmann LH, Dutton AM, et al: Breast neoplasms in women treated with x-rays for acute postpartum mastitis: a pilot study, *J Natl Cancer Inst* 43:803-811, 1969.

206. Mettlin C, Schoenfeld ER: The effect of race geography and social class, *Dev Oncol* 57:15-25, 1989.

207. Meyer JE, Sonnenfeld MR, Greenes RA, Stomper PC: Preoperative localization of clinically occult breast lesions: experience at a referral hospital, *Radiology* 169(3):629-630, 1988.

208. Miller AB: Diet and cancer: a review, *Acta Oncol* 29:87-95, 1990.

209. Miller AB, Howe GR, Sherman GJ, et al: Mortality from breast cancer after irradiation during fluoroscopic examinations in patients being treated for tuberculosis, *N Engl J Med* 321:1285-1289, 1989.

210. Mills PK, Beeson WL, Phillips RL, Fraser GE: Dietary habits and breast cancer incidence among Seventh Day Adventists, *Cancer* 64:582-590, 1989.

211. Mirra AP, Cole P, MacMahon B: Breast cancer in an area of high parity: Sao Paulo, Brazil, *Cancer Res* 31:77-83, 1971.

212. Montano DE, Taplin SH: A test of an expanded theory of reasoned action to predict mammography participation, *Soc Sci Med* 32(6):733-741, 1991.

213. Mooney G: Breast cancer screening: a study in cost-effectiveness analysis, *Soc Sci Med* 16(13):1277-1283, 1982.

214. Moskowitz M: Costs of screening for breast cancer, *Radiol Clin North Am* 25(5):1031-1037, 1987.

215. Moskowitz M: Cost-benefit determinations in screening mammography, *Cancer* 60(7 Suppl):1680-1683, 1989.

216. Moskowitz M, Fox SH: Cost analysis of aggressive breast cancer screening, *Radiology* 130(1):253-256, 1979.

217. Mueller CB, Ames F, Anderson GD: Breast cancer in 3,558 women: age as a significant determinant in the rate of dying and causes of death, *Surgery* 83:123-132, 1978.

218. Muller AB: Mammography: a critical evaluation of its role in breast cancer screening, especially in developing countries, *J Pub Health Policy* 10(4):486-498, 1989.

219. Mulvihill JJ, Safyer AW, Bening JK: Prevention in familial breast cancer: counseling and prophylactic mastectomy, *Prevent Med* 11:500-511, 1982.

220. Natarajan N, Nemoto D, Nemoto T, Mettlin C: Breast cancer survival among orientals and whites living in the United States, *J Surg Oncol* 39(3):206-209, 1988.

221. Newman B, Austin MA, Lee M, King MC: Inheritance of human breast cancer: evidence for autosomal dominant transmission in high risk families, *Proc Natl Acad Sci USA* 85:3044-3048, 1988.

222. Nielsen BB: The nurse's role in mammography screening, *Cancer Nursing* 12(5):271-275, 1989.

223. Nomura AM, Lee J, Kolonel LN, Hirohata T: Breast cancer in two populations with different levels of risk for the disease, *Am J Epidemiol* 19(4):496-502, 1984.

224. Nomura AM, Marchand LL, Kolonel LN, Hankin JH: The effect of dietary fat on breast cancer survival among Caucasian and Japanese women in Hawaii, *Breast Cancer Res Treat* 18(Suppl 1):S135-S141, 1991.

225. Oken B, Hartz A, Giefer E, Rimm AA: Relation between socioeconomic status and obesity changes in 9046 women, *Prevent Med* 6:447-453, 1977.

226. O'Malley MS, Fletcher SW, US Preventive Services Task Force: Screening for breast cancer with breast self-examination: a critical review, *JAMA* 257(16):2196-2203, 1987.

227. Ory H, Cole P, MacMahon B, Hoover R: Oral contraceptives and reduced risk of benign breast diseases, *N Engl J Med* 294:419-422, 1976.

228. Paci E, Ciatto S, Buiatti E, et al: Early indicators of efficacy of breast cancer screening programmes: results of the Florence District Programme, *Int J Cancer* 46(2):198-202, 1990.

229. Page DL, DuPont WD: Proliferative breast disease: diagnosis and implications, *Science* 253:915, 1991.

230. Page DL, Dupont WD, Rogers LW, Landenberger M: Intraductal carcinoma of the breast: follow up after biopsy only, *Cancer* 49:751-758, 1982.

231. Palli D, Del Turco MR, Buiatti E, et al: A case-control study of the efficacy of a non-randomized breast cancer screening program in Florence (Italy), *Int J Cancer* 38(4):501-504, 1986.

232. Palmer JR, Rosenberg L, Clarke EA, et al: Breast cancer and cigarette smoking: a hypothesis, *Am J Epidemiol* 134(1):1-13, 1991.

233. Pamilo M, Anttinen I, Roiha M, et al: Mammography screening for breast cancer: first year results from Helsinki and surroundings, *Ann Med* 21(4):277-279, 1989.

234. Panagiotopoulou K, Katsouyanni K, Petridou E, et al: Maternal age, parity, and pregnancy estrogens, *Cancer—Causes—Control* 1(2):119-124, 1990.

235. Patchefsky AS, Shaber GS, Schwartz GF, et al: The pathology of breast cancer detected by mass population screening, *Cancer* 40(4):1659-1670, 1977.

236. Peeters PH, Verbeek AL, Hendriks JH, van Bon MJ: Screening for breast cancer in Nijmegen: report of 6 screening rounds, 1975-1986, *Int J Cancer* 43(2):226-230, 1989.

237. Petrakis NL, Wrensch MR, Ernster VL, et al: Influence of pregnancy and lactation on serum and breast fluid estrogen levels: implications for breast cancer risk, *Int J Cancer* 40:587-591, 1987.

238. Pickle LW, Johnson KA: Estimating the long-term probability of developing breast cancer, *J Natl Cancer Inst* 81:1854-1855, 1989.

239. Plotkin D, Blankenberg F: Breast cancer—biology and malpractice, *Am J Clin Oncol* 14:254-266, 1991.

240. Price JL, Gibbs NM: The relationship between microcalcifications and in situ carcinoma of the breast, *Clin Radiol* 29:447-452, 1978.

241. Prior P, Waterhouse JA: Incidence of bilateral tumours in a population-based series of breast-cancer patients. I. Two approaches to an epidemiological analysis, *Br J Cancer* 37:620-634, 1978.

242. Ravnihar B, MacMahon B, Lindtner J: Epidemiologic features of breast cancer in Slovenia, 1965-1967, *Eur J Cancer* 7:295-306, 1971.

243. Reemer RR, Hoover R, Fraumeni JF Jr, et al: Second primary neoplasms following ovarian cancer, *J Natl Cancer Inst* 61:1195-1197, 1978.

244. Reynolds KD, West SG, Aiken LS: Increasing the use of mammography: a pilot program, *Health Ed Q* 17(4):429-441, 1990.

245. Richardson A: Factors likely to affect participation in mammographic screening, *N Z Med J* 103(887):155-156, 1990.

246. Rodgers A: The UK breast cancer screening program: an expensive mistake, *J Public Health Med* 12:197-204, 1990.

247. Rohan TE, Cook MG: Alcohol consumption and risk of benign proliferative epithelial disorders of the breast in women, *Int J Cancer* 43:631-636, 1989.

248. Rohan TE, McMichael AJ: Alcohol consumption and risk of breast cancer, *Int J Cancer* 41:695-699, 1988.

249. Rose DP: Diet, hormones and cancer, *Food Technol* 37(3):588-562,567, 1983.

250. Rosner B, Spiegelman D, Willett WC: Correction of logistic regressive relative risk estimates and confidence intervals for measurement error: the case of multiple covariates measured with error, *Am J Epidemiol* 132(4):734-745, 1990.

251. Rosner D, Bedwani RN, Vana J, et al: Noninvasive breast carcinoma: results of a national survey by the American College of Surgeons, *Ann Surg* 192:139-147, 1980.

252. Roush GC, Schymura MJ, Stevenson JM, Holford TR: Time and age trends for sinonasal cancer in Connecticut incidence and US mortality rates, *Cancer* 60:422-428, 1987.

253. Rutqvist LE, Wallgren A: Long term survival of 458 young breast cancer patients, *Cancer* 55:658-665, 1985.

254. Saftlas AF, Hoover RN, Brinton LA, et al: Mammographic densities and risk of breast cancer, *Cancer* 67:2833-2838, 1991.

255. Salber EJ, Trichopoulos D, MacMahon B: Lactation and reproductive histories of breast cancer patients in Boston 1965-1966, *J Natl Cancer Inst* 43:1013-1024, 1969.

256. Saltzstein Sl: Potential limits of physical examination and breast self-examination in detecting small cancers of the breast: an unselected population-based study of 1302 cases, *CA* 54:1443-1446, 1984.

257. Sattin RW, Rubin GL, Webster LA, et al and the Cancer and Steroid Hormone Study: Family history and the risk of breast cancer, *JAMA* 253:1908-1913, 1985.

258. Schatzkin A, Carter CL, Green SB, et al: Is alcohol consumption related to breast cancer? Results from the Framingham Heart Study, *J Natl Cancer Inst* 81:31-35, 1989.

259. Schatzkin A, Jones DY, Hoover RN, et al: Alcohol consumption and breast cancer in the epidemiologic follow-up study of the first national health and nutrition examination survey, *N Engl J Med* 316:1169-1173, 1987.

260. Schechter MT, Miller AB, Baines CJ, Howe GR: Selection of women at high risk of breast cancer for initial screening, *J Chron Dis* 39:253-260, 1986.

261. Schindler AE, Ebert A, Friedrich E: Conversion of androstenedione to estrone by human fat tissue, *J Clin Endocrinol Metab* 35:627-630, 1972.

262. Schlemmer A, Jensen J, Ris BJ, Christiansen: Smoking induces increased androgen levels in early post-menopausal women, *Maturitas* 12:99-104, 1990.

263. Schoenberg BS: Nervous system neoplasms and primary malignancies of other sites: the unique association between meningiomas and breast cancer, *Neurology* 25:705-712, 1975.

264. Schottenfeld D, Berg J: Incidence of multiple primary cancers. IV. Cancers of the female breast and genital organs, *J Natl Cancer Inst* 46:161-170, 1971.

265. Schwartz AG, Ragheb ME, Swanson GM, Satariano WA: Racial and age difference in multiple primary cancers after breast: a population based analysis, *Breast Cancer Res Treat* 42:126-131, 1989.

266. Seidman H, Gelb SK, Silverberg E, et al: Survival experience in the Breast Cancer Detection Demonstration Project, *Cancer* 37(5):258-290, 1987.

267. Seidman H, Stellman SD, Mushinski MH: A different perspective on breast cancer risk factors: some implications of the nonattributable risk, *CA* 32(5):301-313, 1982.

268. Selinger HA, Goldfarb NI, Perkel RL, Carlson BL: Physician compliance with mammography guidelines: a retrospective chart review, *Family Med* 21(1):56-58, 1989.

269. Senofsky GM, Wanebo HJ, Wilhelm MC, et al: Has monitoring of the contralateral breast improved the prognosis in patients treated for primary breast cancer? *Cancer* 57:597-602, 1986.

270. Shapiro S: Evidence on screening for breast cancer from a randomized trial, *Cancer* 39:2772-2782, 1977.

271. Shapiro S, Strax P, Venet L, Rink R: The search for risk factors in breast cancer, *Am J Public Health* 58:820-835, 1968.

272. Shapiro S, Venet W, Strax P, et al: Selection, follow-up, and analysis in the Health Insurance Plan Study: a randomized trial with breast cancer screening, *Natl Cancer Inst Monogr* 67:65-74, 1985.

273. Shimizu Y, Kato H, Schull WJ: Studies of the mortality of A bomb survivors. IX. Mortality. 1950-1985; part 2. Cancer mortality based on recently revised doses (ds86), *Radiation Res* 121:120-141, 1990.

274. Shore RE, Hempelmann LH, Kowaluk E, et al: Breast neoplasms in women treated with x-rays for acute postpartum mastitis, *J Natl Cancer Inst* 59:813-822, 1977.

275. Reference deleted in proof.

276. Sickles EA, Ominsky SH, Sollitto RA, et al: Medical audit of a rapid-throughput mammography screening practice: methodology and results of 27,114 examinations, *Radiology* 175(2):323-327, 1990.

277. Sickles EA, Weber WN, Galvin HB, et al: Baseline screening mammography: one vs two views per breast, *Am J Roentgenol* 147(6):1149-1153, 1986.

278. Sierra AE, Potchen EJ: Use of mammography in screening for breast cancer, *Obstet Gynecol Clin North Am* 17(4):927-938, 1991.

279. Silverberg E: Cancer statistics, 1985, *CA* 35(1):19-35, 1985.

280. Silverberg E, Boring CC, Squires TS: Cancer statistics, 1990, *CA* 40:9-26, 1990.

281. Simon MS, Schwartz AG, Martino S, Swanson GM: Trends in the diagnosis of in situ breast cancer in the Detroit metropolitan area, 1973 to 1987, *Cancer* 69:466-469, 1992.

282. Siraganian PA, Levine PH, Madigan P, Mulvihill JJ: Familial breast cancer in black Americans, *Cancer* 60(7):1657-1660, 1987.

283. Siskind B, Schofield F, Rice D, Bain C: Breast cancer and breast feeding: results from an Australian case-control study, *Am J Epidemiol* 130:229-236, 1989.

284. Skolnick M, Marshall CJ, McWhorter W, et al: Proliferative breast disease: diagnosis and implications, *Science* 253:915-916, 1991.

285. Skolnick MH, Cannon-Albright LA, Goldgar DE, et al: Inheritance of proliferative breast disease in breast cancer kindreds, *Science* 250:1715-1720, 1990.

286. Skrabanek P: Mass mammography, the time for reappraisal, *Int J Technol Assess Health Care* 5:423-430, 1989.

287. Spratt JS, Greenberg RA, Heuser LS: Geometry, growth rates and duration of cancer and carcinoma in situ of the breast before detection by screening, *Cancer Res* 46:970-974, 1986.

288. Stein JA, Fox SA, Murata PJ: The influence of ethnicity, socioeconomic status and psychologic barriers on the use of mammography, *J Health Soc Behav* 32:101-113, 1991.

289. Stephenson G, Freiherr G: Insurers pay dearly for breast cancer "misses," *Diagnostic Imaging* July 1990, pp 31-35.

290. Straszewski J: Breast cancer and body build, *Prevent Med* 6:410-415, 1977.

291. Swanson GM, Satariano ER, Satariano WA, Threatt BA: Racial differences in early detection of breast cancer in metropolitan Detroit, 1978-1987, *Cancer* 66:1297-1301, 1990.

292. Swift M, Morrell D, Massey RB, Chase CL: Incidence of cancer in 161 families affected by ataxia-telangiectasia, *N Engl J Med* 325:1831-1836, 1991.

293. Tabar L, Dean PB: Mammographic parenchymal patterns, *JAMA* 247:185-189, 1982.

294. Tabar L, Dean PB: The control of breast cancer through mammography screening. What is the evidence? (review), *Radiol Clin North Am* 25(5):993-1005, 1987.

295. Tabar L, Gad A, Holberg LH, et al: Reduction in mortality from breast cancer after mass screening with mammography, *Lancet* 1:829-832, 1985.

296. Taplin S, Anderman C, Grothaus L: Breast cancer risk and participation in mammographic screening, *Am J Public Health* 79:1494-1498, 1989.

297. Taplin SH, Thompson RS, Schnitzer F, et al: Revisions in the risk-based breast cancer screening program at Group Health Cooperative, *Cancer* 66:812-818, 1990.

298. Tashiro H, Nomura Y, Hisamatu K: A case-control study of risk

factors of breast cancer detected by mass screening, *Gan No Rinsho* 36:2127-2130, 1990.

299. Taylor B, Billingham KA: Failure to recognize risk and use breast self-examination in daughters with maternal history of breast cancer (meeting abstract), *Proc Annu Meet Am Soc Clin Oncol* 7:A306, 1988.

300. Thomas D, Noonan E: Breast cancer and depot-medroxyprogesterone acetate: a multinational study. WHO collaborative study of neoplasia and steroid contraceptives, *Lancet* 338:833-838, 1991.

301. Thompson WD, Janerich DT: Maternal age at birth and risk of breast cancer in daughters, *Epidemiology* 1(2):101-106, 1990.

302. Tokunaga M, Land CE, Yamonoto T, et al: Incidence of female breast cancer among atomic bomb survivors, Hiroshima and Nagasaki, 1950-1980, *Radiati Res* 112:243-272, 1987.

303. Toti A, Piffanelli A, Pavanelli T, et al: Possible indication of breast cancer risk through discriminant functions, *Cancer* 46:1280-1285, 1980.

304. Turnbull D, Irwig L, Adelson P: A randomized trial of invitations to attend for screening mammography, *Aust J Public Health* 15:33-36, 1991.

305. Reference deleted in proof.

306. Upton AC: The biologic effects of low-level ionizing radiation, *Sci Am* 246:41-49, 1982.

307. Urbanski S, Jensen HM, Cooke G, et al: The association of histological and radiological indicators of breast cancer risk, *Br J Cancer* 58:474-479, 1988.

308. Use of mammography—United States, 1990, *MMWR* 39(36):621, 627-630, 1990.

309. Vatten LJ, Kvinnsland S: Cigarette smoking and risk of breast cancer: a prospective study of 24,329 Norwegian women, *Eur J Cancer* 26:830-833, 1990.

310. Vogel VG: High risk populations as target for breast cancer prevention trials, *Prevent Med* 20:86-100, 1991.

311. Vogel VG, Schreiber Graves D, Vernon SW, et al: Mammographic screening of women with increased risk of breast cancer, *Cancer* 66:1613-1620, 1990.

312. Wainwright JM: A comparison of conditions associated with breast cancers in Great Britain and America, *Am J Cancer* 15:2610-2645, 1931.

313. Wald N, Frost C, Cuckle H: Breast cancer screening: the current position (letter), *Br Med J* 302(6780):845-846, 1991.

314. Ward JH, Marshall CJ, Schumann GB, et al: Detection of proliferative breast disease by four-quadrant, fine-needle aspiration, *J Natl Cancer Inst* 82:964-966, 1990.

315. Wellings SR, Wolfe JN: Correlative studies of the histological and radiographic appearance of the breast parenchyma, *Radiology* 129:299-306, 1978.

316. Wertheimer MD, Costanza ME, Dodson TF, et al: Increasing the effort toward breast cancer detection, *JAMA* 255:1311-1315, 1986.

317. Wheeler JE, Enterline HT, Roseman JM, et al: Lobular carcinoma in situ of the breast, *Cancer* 34:554-563, 1974.

318. Whitehead J, Carlile T, Kopecky KJ, et al: The relationship between Wolfe's classification of mammograms, accepted breast cancer risk factors, and the incidence of breast cancer, *Am J Epidemiol* 122:994-1006, 1985.

319. Whitehead J, Cooper J: Risk factors for breast cancer by mode of diagnosis: some results from a breast cancer screening study, *J Epidemiol Community Health* 43(2):115-120, 1989.

320. Willett WC, Stampfer MJ, Colditz GA, et al: Dietary fat and the risk of breast cancer, *N Engl J Med* 316:1174-1180, 1987.

321. Willett WC, Stampfer MJ, Colditz GA, et al: Moderate alcohol consumption and the risk of breast cancer, *N Engl J Med* 316:1174-1180, 1987.

322. Williams SM, Kaplan PA, Petersen JC, Lieberman RP: Mammography in women under age 30; is there clinical benefit? *Radiology* 161:49-51, 1986.

323. William RR, Horn JW: Association of cancer sites with tobacco and alcohol consumption and socioeconomic status of patients: interview study from the Third National Cancer Study, *J Natl Cancer Inst* 58:525-547, 1977.

324. Wolfe JN: Breast patterns as an index of risk for developing breast cancer, *Am J Roentgenol* 126:1130-1139, 1976.

325. Wolosin RJ: Effect of appointment scheduling and reminder postcards on adherence to mammography recommendations, *J Family Pract* 30(5):542-547, 1990.

326. Reference deleted in proof.

327. Wright CJ: Breast cancer screening: a different look at the evidence, *Surgery* 100(4):594-598, 1986.

328. Wright K: Breast cancer: two steps closer to understanding, *Science* 250:1659, 1990.

329. Yuan JM, Yu MC, Ross RK, et al: Risk factors for breast cancer in Chinese women in Shanghai, *Cancer Res* 48(7):1949-1953, 1988.

Chapter 3

QUALITY MAMMOGRAPHY: HOW TO IMAGE THE BREAST

This chapter provides an overview of the principal techniques for safe and effective mammography and reviews major concepts that we believe radiology professionals must accept and routinely apply. Clear and logical steps for performing mammography and for efficient monitoring of mammographic equipment should lead to the establishment and continued application of quality-control measures that ensure reliable mammography.

QUALITY MAMMOGRAPHY AND QUALITY MAMMOGRAPHIC SYSTEMS

The goal in establishing national mammography standards is to ensure that reliable mammography is available to all women. Discussion about mammography techniques and the proper use and maintenance of the equipment encourages those performing mammography to refine and maintain high quality-control efforts. Many leaders of radiology have pioneered important technical advances; they continue to stress that properly performed mammography will reduce breast cancer mortality. Radiology professionals continue to improve mammography standards and offer efficient, high-quality, and cost-effective service. Women themselves are developing new hope and the vision that mortality from breast cancer is effectively decreased through early detection of breast disease. Advances in medical knowledge and in techniques to diagnose and treat breast cancer earlier should assure women healthier and happier lives. Sophistication and precision of medical care rest on the professionals who perform the services.

Providing effective imaging and excellent breast health care depends on individual skill and judgment. While mammography service is now available in the vast majority of radiology departments, certain basic requirements for quality mammography are not always present. Generalization is a monster; however, it is important to counter a general misconception that mammography is easily incor-porated into routine radiology practice. Technically and professionally, mammography continues to undergo positive change. Committed radiology professionals use dedicated imaging systems, and for consistent and dependable analysis over time they direct their efforts to provide reproducible breast images. However, mammography performed solely by professionals dedicated to its practice is not yet a reality.

Webster characterizes a *professional* as "one having great skill or experience in a particular field or activity" and as "one who has assured competence."[1] To achieve this professional level of assured competence requires radiologists and technologists to develop their experience and skill through a special interest in the performance of mammography and requires an uncommon patience for meticulous detail.

Like other radiology examinations, mammography has a wide range of normal variance. An essential step in performing quality mammography lies in the ability to confidently determine breast normality and distinguish it from areas of abnormal-appearing breast tissue. Final examination interpretations must be linked to strategies that provide accurate and decisive reporting, including specific recommendations for continued evaluation when a worrisome mammographic finding is detected (see p. 130). Exemplary breast imaging and accurate and decisive reporting are most apt to occur in facilities where technologists and radiologists regularly perform and interpret a high volume of mammograms. These essential attributes promote advocacy for mammography "specialization."

COMMUNICATION: RANDOM VERSUS SYSTEMATIC

A 1977 Gallup study, conducted for the American Cancer Society, revealed that women were not getting regular breast check-ups, including mammograms, or routinely practicing breast self-examination (BSE). When asked why they did not have routine clinical breast evaluation and mammography, educated women, aware of breast cancer and of the importance of its early detection, responded: "Because my doctor never told me to." This familiar response is still much too common. Current research shows that little improvement has been made since 1977 in communicating to women the significance of three simple procedures: (1) clinical breast examination, (2) the importance of routine mammography examinations, and (3) BSE.[28,33,36] Physicians do not have to be *told* of the importance of early detection, but unfortunately some must be reminded of the importance of more effective "interfacing" of that information when caring for their female patients. Making strong recommendations to women to obtain and continue competent breast health care must become as routine for physicians as their measuring a woman's blood pressure and pulse.

Students of human behavior have long believed that people's thoughts influence their behavior. Persuasion is based on the assumption that changing people's beliefs or thoughts will lead to desired changes in their actions. While the concept is simple, persuasive efforts can often fail because the communicator does not fully appreciate exactly how a message will be understood by those to whom it is directed. Measuring the mental picture of any target audience is a distinct advantage. The mental image of a diagnosis of breast cancer is frightening to women. Identifying and understanding the fear and anger women have about breast cancer, and realizing that some women need to understand the topic more clearly, should assist physicians in measuring the beliefs some women hold about mammography. Once a "measurement" is made of a woman's emotional reaction to the technology designed to uncover this silent disease, it should be easier to design more effective and persuasive messages to communicate the importance of this life-saving technique.

The primary goals of well-organized mammography facilities center on promoting mammography for early detection and diagnosis of breast problems and on maintaining breast education and total breast health care programs. Women must also assume responsibility for their own breast health care, and their enthusiasm for mammography is growing. Data indicating that early detection of nonpalpable breast lesions does diminish mortality from breast cancer[4] should encourage physicians and women to meet the highest standards of breast evaluation.

Knowledge empowers and gives the chance to make intelligent choices. Enhancing women's knowledge about total breast health care should lead to increasing use of mammography.[26] The effective use of language lets knowledgeable physicians motivate and educate women about breast screening strategies and about general breast health care, and it further assists in establishing positive commitments between physicians and their patients. The real utility of quality breast health care and screening mammography must be made clear.

Cancer death is no longer inevitable. Facilitative health professional teams can contribute to its cure by performing the *first* step in quality mammography: achieve early detection of breast problems by having more women obtain mammograms.[37]

BREAST ANATOMY OVERVIEW

An appreciation of basic breast anatomy is critical to performing state-of-the-art mammography.

The breast, a skin gland of ectodermal origin on the ventral surface of an embryo, begins to develop in the sixth week of gestation by forming a line, known as a "milk ridge," from the armpit to the groin. At birth, breasts are comprised of a nipple and branching lactiferous ducts. In the female, the ducts eventually develop from breast buds into areas of more distinct and palpable connective breast tissue.[16,17,31]

Normal breast development occurs as complex hormonal stimulation takes place in the postpubescent female. Ovarian secretion of estrogen, the principal female sex hormone, begins the process of puberty, and pubertal changes contribute to breast development. From the onset of menarche (about age 12) to menopause (between the ages of 45 and 55), progressive changes in a woman's body include an increase in breast tissue with maturation and a reduction of dense breast tissue that occurs with aging. Complete breast maturation may not occur until a woman reaches her third decade. Individual female breast size is extremely variable.[15,17]

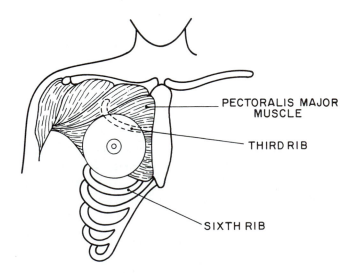

Fig. 3-1. The pectoralis major muscle lies adjacent to the ribs. The breast normally extends from between the second and third ribs to the sixth rib.

Normally the breast extends from the second or third rib to approximately the sixth rib, with nearly half the breast lying over the pectoralis major muscle (Fig. 3-1). A portion of this muscle is present on properly performed mammography. Breast tissue that extends into the axilla is referred to as the tail, or the tail of Spence. The breast is attached to the skin with bands of fibrous connective tissue known as Cooper's ligaments.

The mature female breast is composed of fatty and glandular tissue, supporting fibrous and connective tissue, and blood vessels and lymphatic channels. Except for the lymph channels, these structures are observed radiographically. Lymph nodes, however, are commonly observed in the superior and lateral portions of the breast. Fibrous tis-sue surrounds the lobes of the breast, with fatty tissue found in between. Collections of lobules form the breast's glandular lobes, and routinely each breast has a total of between 15 and 20 lobes that are distributed centrally and laterally[15,32] (Fig. 3-2). The lobule is the breast's smallest, epithelial-lined structure. Composed of the intralobular terminal duct and ductules, it is the simplest functioning unit of the breast (Fig. 3-3).[38] The small ducts are most often the site of carcinoma. Forming the breast's distal ductal system, small ducts leave the lobes, creating larger collecting ducts, the lactiferous ducts, and converge just beneath the nipple area (see Fig. 3-2). The nipple and its surrounding skin, the areolar area, contain smooth muscle and sebaceous glands. The areolar area is pigmented, and

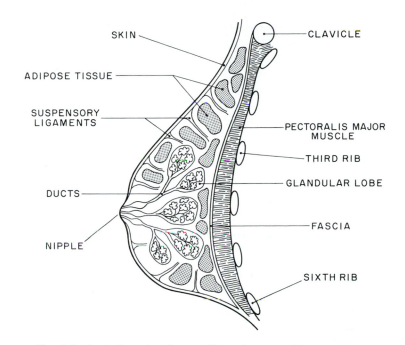

Fig. 3-2. Sagittal section diagram illustrating normal breast anatomy.

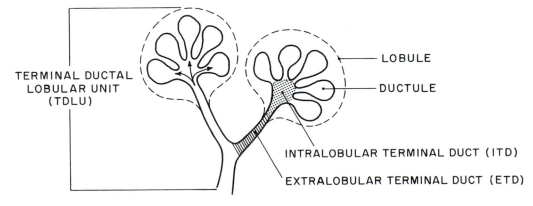

Fig. 3-3. Diagram illustrating the terminal ductal lobular unit (TDLU).

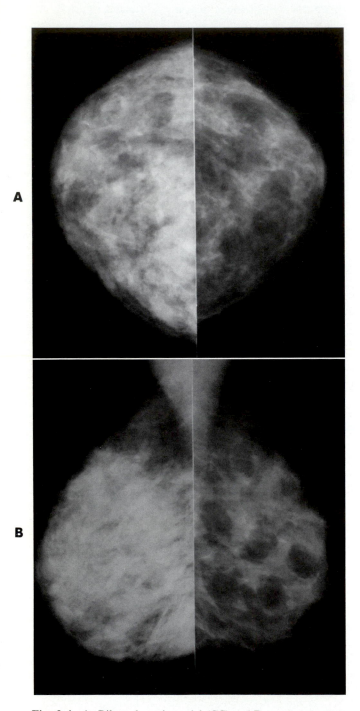

Fig. 3-4. A, Bilateral craniocaudal (CC) and **B,** mediolateral oblique (MLO) projections reveal dense parenchyma in lactating breasts. More prominent glandular enlargement is seen on the right, with well-delineated round densities representing prominent ducts. The diffuse, dense asymmetry of the right breast versus the left is secondary to lactation. NOTE: Postlactation follow-up examination is helpful to establish a nonlactating baseline for future mammography.

smooth muscles of the areola project the nipple of the lactating breast to assist infant feeding. Lactiferous ducts dilate just before emptying through the nipple, forming the lactiferous sinuses that serve as milk reservoirs. Milk flows through the ducts and empties to the outer surface of the breast through openings in the nipple.[15] Following cessation of lactation, while the glandular lobes may remain slightly more abundant than before a first pregnancy, there is overall regression of prominently enlarged glandular lobes (Fig. 3-4).[15,16]

Menopause also brings about progressive changes in breast tissue. The glandular lobes routinely undergo involution and convert into ordinary breast stroma. As the lobules diminish, the breast's connective tissue becomes more collagenized and less cellular.[17] Glandular tissue regresses and is replaced by normal fatty stroma. Although most women experience significant involutional change after menopause, some women do not. The persistence of mature and dense-appearing mammary glands is not entirely understood. Experienced mammographers, however, quickly acknowledge that all ranges of premenopausal breast appearance can also be seen in postmenopausal women and vice versa. It is most common for involution to occur gradually, and its progress is radiographically observed as less dense glandular breast tissue (Fig. 3-5).

An infrequent breast anomaly of relative unimportance medically is supernumerary nipple formation (Fig. 3-6). An extra nipple may be formed below the breast and frequently go undetected by a woman because it strongly resembles a common skin mole. Accessory breast tissue formation, with or without nipple, occurs rarely in or near the axilla (Fig. 3-7).[17,31]

The vascular system of the breast includes branches of the axillary, internal mammary, and intercostal arteries as well as venous drainage provided through the axillary internal mammary and external veins.

The importance of the lymphatic system of the breast was not recognized until late in the nineteenth century when a German surgeon, von Volkmann, showed the lymph system to be a place where existing cancer could spread.[13,31] Since that discovery, extensive research has broadened our understanding of the lymphatic system itself and our knowledge of the importance of the timing and the actual need for surgical lymph node removal.[11,16]

Lymph vessels serve to drain the fat portion of breast milk in lactating breasts and also serve as a transport system to filter infected and foreign cells, including cancer cells. One of the most important group of nodes, the axillary venous group, receives most of the lymphatic material.[16,27] Axillary nodes are easy to palpate and may be enlarged in the presence of infection or invasion of neoplastic cells from the breast. Surgically dissected nodes showing histologic evidence of invasion by neoplastic cells establish that the cancer cells are no longer isolated to the breast (Fig. 3-8).

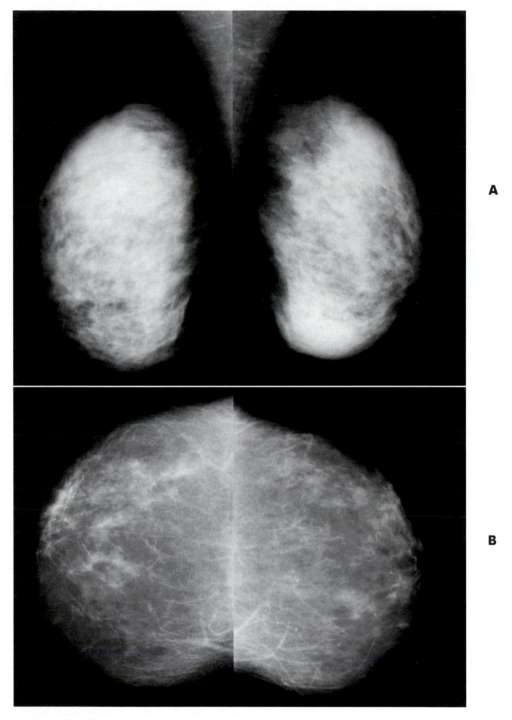

Fig. 3-5. A, Baseline mammogram of a 54-year-old postmenopausal woman showing markedly dense breasts bilaterally. **B,** 1989 images of a 45-year-old woman showing areas of uninvoluted glandular density.   *Continued.*

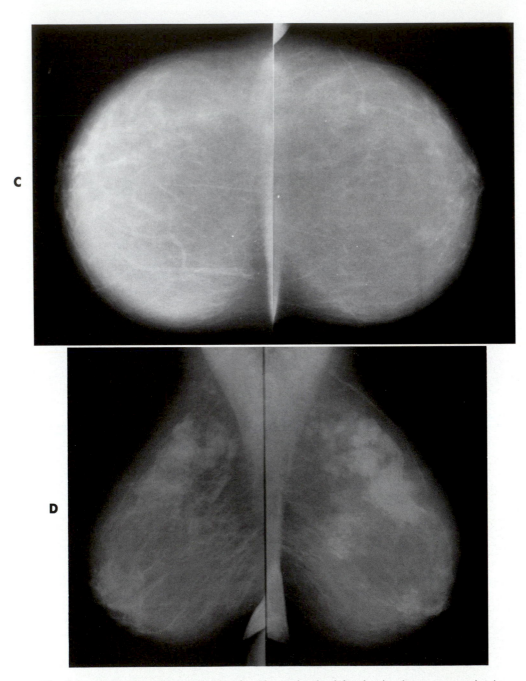

Fig. 3-5, cont'd. C, 1992 images showing change in glandular density due to progressive involution. **D,** This nulliparous, 78-year-old female discontinued hormone replacement therapy at age 60. Bilateral MLO projections show a combination of patchy, isolated dense breast tissue in otherwise fatty-replaced postmenopausal breasts. While the dense appearance is somewhat unusual for a woman this age, it is observed in nulliparous females.

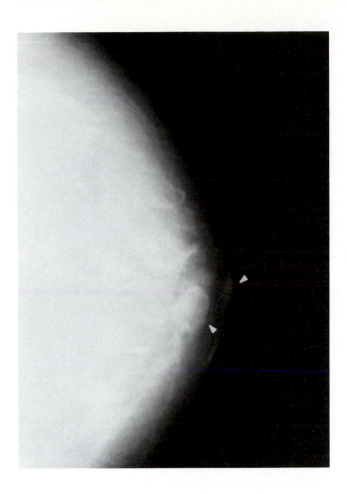

Fig. 3-6. Supernumerary nipple formation. This anomaly (polythelia) is seen in both sexes and may occur at any point along the "milk ridge." Rarely an accessory nipple may function during lactation.

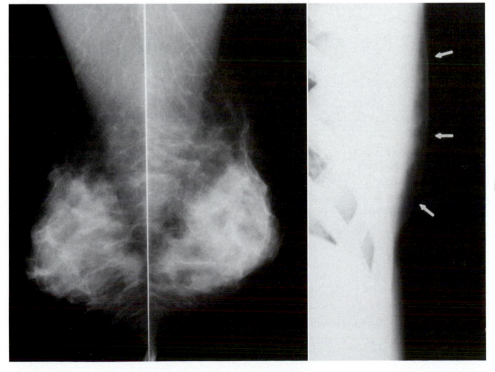

A

B

Fig. 3-7. Rarely do true accessory mammary glands develop. **A,** An increase in breast stroma is seen on the left MLO projection and axillary accessory breast tissue was palpated. **B,** A standard axillary projection demonstrates soft tissue shadow of residual breast tissue.

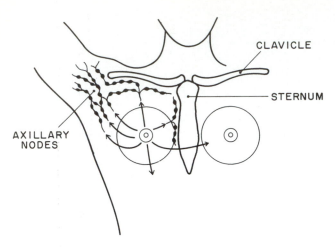

Fig. 3-8. Diagram of the axillary lymph node group and lymphatic channels.

TECHNICAL ASPECTS OF MAMMOGRAPHY

High-quality mammography requires two things: equipment and people (radiologist, technologist, and competent clerical personnel). Issues of quality and of patient safety routinely stimulate imaging product development. Image manufacturers have improved nearly every component of mammography equipment. It is often believed that there is little difference in performing mammography versus performing other routine radiology examinations. The thinking goes that if radiology service is offered, it is routine to provide mammography as part of a full-service package. This thinking has its drawbacks. In 1990, Brown et al. projected that 10,000 mammography machines would be installed to meet a growing service demand.[2] Offering mammography does require purchase of one of those thousands of machines. Offering *quality* mammography, however, requires a great deal more than simple purchase of a machine with advertised "state-of-the-art" status. It is critical to know the principles of mammographic imaging and to strictly adhere to operation recommendations to enhance the ability to detect subtle areas in the breast that may represent a cancer. Complete analysis is needed of the actual time and effort required by all members of an imaging team to achieve a quality mammography operation. It is critical to implement and maintain optimal exposure and film processing techniques and the established steps of quality assurance. These steps are necessary to produce high-resolution images that consistently demonstrate distinctive image contrast and resolution. In breast imaging, contrast is improved by adequate breast compression. Bringing the breast closer to the film reduces scatter and permits use of lower kVp. Superior film resolution allows identification of small objects that are close to one another. In mammography, high-resolution imaging is particularly significant in identifying microcalcific densities in breast tissue.[18]

X-ray absorption by the breast differs because of the characteristic composition and inherent variation of breast tissue. Since there is a limited range of contrast within breast tissue that can be seen mammographically, discovery of small, nonpalpable breast lesions requires high-resolution imaging.[19]

Equipment

Two important features, a high-voltage generator and a specifically configured x-ray tube, distinguish mammography equipment and influence the final mammographic image. Another crucial component is a specific screen-film combination or the so-called image receptor device.

To exclude variation in line voltage, the machine generator must be capable of constant potential output. Several types of single-phased and multiphased generators exist, and medium- and high-frequency converters help to achieve this constant potential output. Variation in voltage results in variation of the kV wave form, referred to as the "kV ripple effect." The greater the "ripple," the less efficient the photon energy.[3,10,19,32]

Mammography units with constant potential generators produce steady x-ray intensity and provide constant mA and kVp over time.[10,32] Steady x-ray intensity promotes shorter exposure times and thereby reduces radiation dose and diminishes the potential for unsharpness from image motion.

As a constant potential is placed across an x-ray tube, just before striking the anode, individual electrons gain energy and produce electron voltage. Once the electrons strike the anode, they convert a variable fraction of their energy (up to 100%) to an x-ray photon. Consequently, x-ray photons have a "range" of energy. The range of exiting photons is also filtered as the photons exit the x-ray tube. The tube anode target and filter combinations vary. Their combination determines the effective use of radiation dose and the ability to maximize breast image contrast. The preferred and commonly used anode-filter combination for mammography screen-film imaging is a molybdenum (Mo)-targeted tube with molybdenum (Mo) filter. This Mo/Mo combination is preferred because when the peak kilovoltage ranges between 26 and 30 keV, the target produces the correct "range" of keV photons to provide high-contrast imaging. A molybdenum filter removes both high- and low-energy photons. Since the k-shell absorption edge for a Mo filter is 19 keV, x-ray photons with energies below 15 and above 20 keV are absorbed by the filter. The remaining photons—between 17 and 20 keV—are of optimal energy for interaction with the soft tissues of the breast, making the Mo/Mo tube target and exit filter combination optimal for film-screen mammography.[3,10,32]

State-of-the-art mammography units feature an x-ray

tube with a rotating anode. A steady production of x-rays produces heat as the target angle of the rotating anode receives photons on the target surface. To overcome excessive tube heat storage, an effectively cooled environment is imperative to protect the life of the tube.[3] In high-volume breast screening programs, where 8 to 12 examinations per hour may be performed, the number of exposures in half-day screening sessions may range from 128 to 192. There is a direct relationship between heat dissipation and consistent high-quality imaging. Efficient heat dissipation is essential to ensure consistent x-ray production; consequently, it is an important feature, especially where high-volume screening is performed.

The special nature of mammography requires recognition of certain machine design parameters that directly influence quality. Automatic Exposure Control (AEC) systems digitally store and adjust all technique exposure factors to provide constant optical density across a wide range of breast tissue densities and breast sizes. This fully automated feature selects the proper mA, kVp, and mAs, reduces exposure times, and thus minimizes radiation exposure. Technical precision and the compensatory features of AEC should reduce the need to repeat breast images and serve to improve patient throughput. Manual control function must be available, however, to permit full manual selection of technique parameters, when warranted.

Overall image sharpness directly depends on focal spot size. Image sharpness is defined as low geometric blurring, and spatial resolution is the ability to define small objects that are in proximity.[18] Appropriate focal spot object-distance and object-to-image receptor distance contribute to image sharpness. Another way to diminish geometric blurring is use of a small focal spot. As a rule, focal spot size increases when mA is increased and decreases when kVp is decreased.[32] The National Electrical Manufacturer Association (NEMA) allows wide tolerance factors in actual focal spot size measurement, especially when compared to measurements that manufacturers quote as the "nominal" focal spot size of their various mammography units. Consequently, identical mammogram units, placed in the same work environment and quoted to feature the same dimensions and operation specifications, may produce images with varying degrees of sharpness because of variations in actual focal spot dimension and the ultimate distribution of x-rays.[16,32] The focal spot size is commonly measured by physicists, while performing routine quality control measures, by using a resolution pattern placed in the direct line of the x-ray beam. If questions or problems about focal spot size arise with any mammographic unit, this measurement may be easily obtained.

Dual focus tubes are a standard offering for state-of-the-art mammography units. They have small and large focal spots, ranging from 0.1 to 0.4 mm. Controversy exists about the appropriate geometry of the target angle of the

anode. The objective of angling the target is to minimize off-focus radiation. Off-focus radiation can be reduced by collimating the x-ray beam close to the focal spot. Collimation in mammography units limits the x-ray beam to the film size[32] (Fig. 3-9). Some manufacturers offer a variable aperture collimator, and its adjustable features help curtail scatter radiation and provide sharper images.

The source-to-image receptor distance (SID) also effects image sharpness; longer SIDs give better detail. Some units have variable SIDs. The SID for mammography—between 50 and 65 cm—is relatively short when compared to routine radiography examinations. Excessive SID would create the need to increase radiation exposure at an additional expense of losing spatial resolution. Good spatial resolution, also dependent on focal spot size, is important in mammography image magnification. For magnification technique, small focal spot capability is essential. A 0.1 mm sized focal spot is preferred for 2 × magnification. Imaging system magnification factors range from 1.5 × to 2 ×. Well-designed magnification platforms and spot

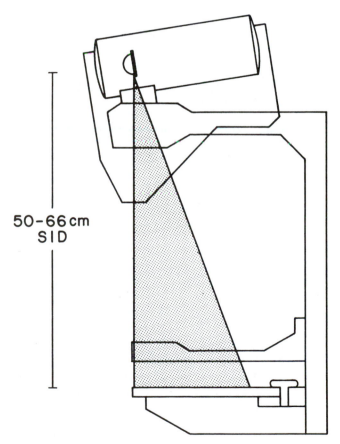

50-66 cm SID

Fig. 3-9. Diagram illustrating angled tube target. The SID of various machines can range from 50 to 60 cm. The importance of these variations (i.e., target angle, focal spot size, and SID) and their ultimate effect on breast imaging must be recognized. (Not drawn to scale.)

compression paddles help ensure greater breast stability and reduce motion unsharpness that results from patient or equipment motion. Efforts are being directed to designing more comfortable and adjustable compression devices and magnification equipment without loss of efficiency. Scrupulous attention to technical detail is required to improve the ability to definitively diagnose breast calcifications using magnification technique. Otherwise women will receive excessive radiation, compromised images, and too many equivocal film interpretations. One must properly determine exactly when magnification imaging is appropriate and maintain the highest image quality so that areas in the breast that are of concern may be effectively demonstrated (Fig. 3-10). (See Chapter 3.)

Users of medical equipment evaluate and emphasize the relevance of specific features of imaging units to manufacturers. Each manufacturer has talented professionals who work to communicate and analyze mammography and patterns of successful design improvements. Working together, users and manufacturers should address shortcomings of mammography. Comparative assessment of technical and diagnostic performance standards should assist those routinely involved with mammography to make selective decisions about equipment features that substan-

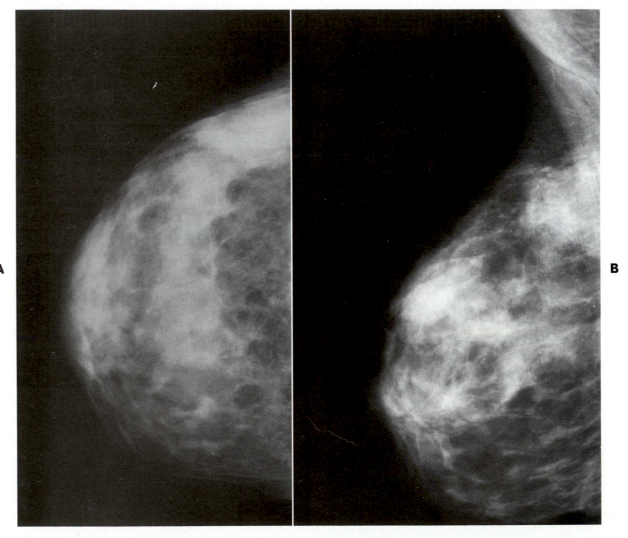

Fig. 3-10. **A** and **B,** Standard craniocaudal and mediolateral oblique projections revealed microcalcifications in the midposterior portion of the right breast tissue. **C** and **D,** Coned compression imaging in both the CC and MLO projection continued to demonstrate calcific densities in this woman's mammogram. **E** and **F,** Coned magnification imaging was also performed in the CC and MLO projections. The nature of the calcifications, their number, size, and configuration are more obviously well defined using the compressed magnification technique.

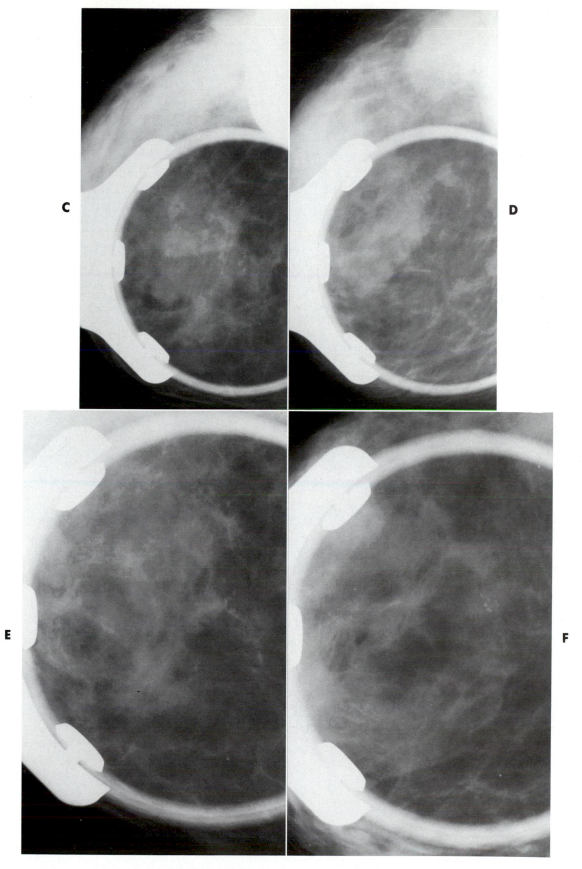

Fig. 3-10, cont'd. For legend see opposite page.

Table 3-1. Mammography systems specification matrix

Manufacturer model	G.E. Senographe 600T HF	Siemens Mammomat 2	Philips U.C.	Fischer Imaging Athena	Instrumentarium ALPHA III
X-ray tube assembly					
Anode type	Rotating	Rotating	Rotating	Rotating	Rotating
Anode heat capacity (HU)	90,000	405,000	266,000	300,000	300,000
Anode material	Mo + V	Mo	Mo compound with graphite	Mo	Mo
Anode HU control	No	No	No	Yes	Yes
Focal spot sizes, SF/LF (mm)	0.1/0.3	0.15/0.4	0.1/0.3	0.1/0.3	0.1/0.3
Window material	Be	Be	Be	Be	Be
Filtration (mm)	0.8 mm Be + 0.03 Mo for <36 kVp 1.00 A1 for >36 kVp	0.03 Mo for 25-40 kVp 1.5 A1 for 41-49 kVp	1.0 mm Be + (0.03 mm Mo or 0.5 mm A1)	0.03 Mo	0.03 Mo
Maximum load	Not specified	1,000 kHu/Hr	Not specified	Not specified	1,100 kHu/Hr
Collimation	Aperture cones for each SID and cassette size	Aperture cones for each cassette size and spot compression	Aperture cones for each cassette size and spot compression cone	5-bladed manually adjusted collimator	Diaphragm for each case size
X-ray general type	1-phase high-frequency converter	3-phase, high-frequency converter	1-phase, medical-frequency converter	High frequency	High frequency
kVp range	22-49 1kV steps	25-49 1kV steps	22-49 1kV steps	20-49 ½ kV steps	20-35 1kV steps
mAs range	4-600	2-220 SF, 2-710 LF, depending on selected kVp (12% steps)	5-400	4-750	4-600
Exposure time range	0.04-10 auto set	Determined by selected kVp and mAs	0.05-4 determined by kVp and mAs	0.04-10 auto set	0.04-6 auto set

Exposure factor indicators	kVp, mAs, focal spot, density, AEC	kVp, mAs, focal spot, density, film-screen	kVp, mA, focal spot, AEC, density	kV, mAs, time	kV, mAs, time
Automatic exposure control					
AEC controls	11 density steps, 5 film-screen combo	±8 density steps, 2 film-screen combo	7 density steps, 2 film-screen combo	11 density steps, 3 film-screen combo	11 density steps, 9 film-screen combo
Postexposure mAs indication	Yes	Yes	Yes	Yes	Yes
Exposure blocked, operator to reset when limit is exceeded	Yes	Yes	Yes	Yes	Yes
AEC sensor position selectable	Yes	Yes	Yes	Yes	Yes
Examination unit					
Rotation (degrees)	±180 degrees—manual	±105 degrees—manual	±105 degrees—manual	±180 degrees	±180 degrees
Source to image distance (mm)	Adj: 50,55,60,65 cm	60 cm	60 cm	66 cm	60 cm
Screen-film cassette sizes	13×18, 18×24, 24×30	18×24, 24×30	18×24, 24×30	18×24, 24×30	18×24, 24×30
Reciprocating grid (Bucky) ratio (lines per cm)	5:1,35	4:1,27	5:1,31	5:1,43	5:1,44
Magnification factor	1:5,1.85	2.0	1.7	1.5, 1.8	1.6, 1.8
Compression	Pneumatic	Auto/manual	Auto/manual	Auto/manual	Auto/manual
Power requirements					
Frequency (Hz)	50/60	50/60	50/60	50/60	50/60
Line voltage comp automatic compensation	Automatic	Automatic	Automatic	Automatic	Automatic

tially improve diagnostic accuracy of breast problems and favorably affect management decisions about a worrisome area in the breast. The specification matrix, representative of a limited number of vendors, lists certain features of state-of-the-art mammography systems (Table 3-1).

Screen-film mammography system

High-quality imaging requires the use of specifically designed, compatible mammography film and intensifying screens. There is no question that this combination has noticeably improved image quality, allowing as much as a 50% reduction in radiation dose within the past few years[24,30] (Fig. 3-11).

Overall improvement in breast imaging techniques makes us impatient to optimize all of the screen-film performance characteristics. System speed, image sharpness, and high contrast-to-noise ratio are interdependent imaging characteristics. Kitts et al. point out that with constant attempts to achieve ideal image quality, trade-offs still occur between these interdependent, yet discriminating, characteristics.[25] Fundamental limitations currently require selecting one characteristic over another because of their reciprocal and interdependent nature. Radiographic contrast depends on the differences in x-ray absorption. The wide range in breast thickness and the overall density of breast tissue affect both image contrast and overall image sharpness. Low x-ray energies used in mammography contribute to film granularity and increase system noise and thus decrease the ability to identify soft tissue lesions (i.e., lower contrast) from similar surrounding soft tissue structure. The range of film densities that give diagnostically

useful information in mammography is limited. The ability to radiographically visualize any area of interest is directly related to x-ray absorption of the area and to the exposure latitude of the x-ray film. Consequently, an increase in film contrast (e.g., film speed) necessary for breast imaging narrows the film's exposure latitude. Because of the glandular soft tissue of the breast, to optimally visualize breast structure, uniform tissue thickness must be achieved at imaging. Proper breast compression is therefore critical. Compression confines the breast tissue, separates overlapping structures, reduces radiation dose, and captures critical information within the narrow exposure latitude inherent in high-contrast film.[7,25]

Numerous film manufacturers have developed high-speed screen-film systems. The DuPont Microvision single-emulsion high-speed mammography film allows for increased film speed because of development of smaller grained silver halide coupled with minimum thickness coating on a single side of the x-ray film. This combination promotes superior film contrast, especially when extended processing conditions are applied.

Two additional elements complete the screen-film system: intensifying screens, designed to accommodate high-contrast single-emulsion film, and film processing. Achieving high x-ray absorption by the intensifying screen is directly related to the phosphor compound of the screen and the screen thickness. Intensifying screens must be very thin to reduce blurring of the image. Gadolinium oxysulfide, now routinely used in mammography screens as an intensifying phosphor and first introduced as the Min-R screen in the 1970s by Eastman Kodak, has become the

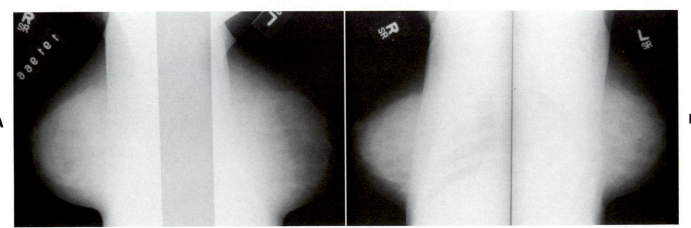

Fig. 3-11. In 1950 this woman had breast surgery for "a cancer lump my doctor said would kill me." **A,** Mammogram from 1974, 24 years after breast surgery. Attempted MLO projection. **B,** Attempt to include ribs, once thought to be necessary to visualize posterior breast tissue. One can only assume the high radiation dose experienced by this patient to produce images with little diagnostic information.   *Continued.*

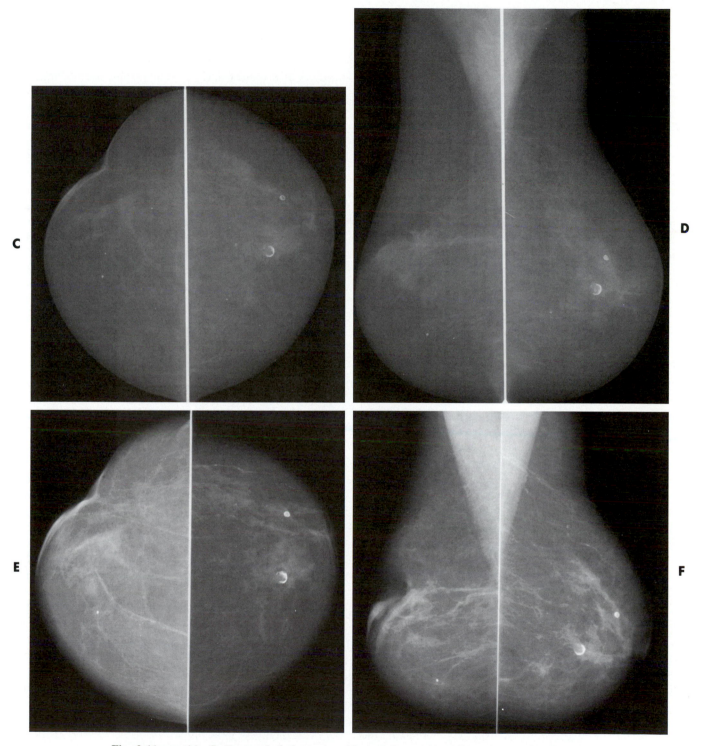

Fig. 3-11, cont'd. C, Postsurgical change is evident on the craniocaudal projection. **D,** The mediolateral oblique projection does not reveal postsurgical change. Seven years after her 1985 mammogram this 84-year-old woman continues to both survive her "cancer" and reap the benefits of improved mammography technique. **E** compares the 1985 mammography on the left to 1992 mammography techniques on the right. **F,** 1992 MLO projection demonstrating state-of-the-art mammography.

standard. In the 1980s, Kodak pioneered the improvement of mammography film and introduced the OM-1 product to be used with the Min-R screen cassettes. Since then, a great deal more attention has been directed to improving the quality of mammography and reducing radiation dose using appropriate screen-film combinations. With continuing improvements through the 1980s, mean glandular dose was reduced and is now less than 100 mrad per view.[35] Kodak's most recent contribution has been introduction of a dual-emulsion, dual-screen system. Current evaluation of the merits of the dual system reveal that overall image quality remains stable. Some compromise in image sharpness and resolution to visualize microcalcifications within the breast has been noted. However, the dual system permits a marked reduction in x-ray exposure dose.[22] Currently, efficient intensifying screen conversion of x-ray photons to light photons absorbs a high fraction, almost 75%, of the incident 20 keV x-ray photons used in mammography. Commercial improvement in the many aspects of mammography imaging continues, and it is likely that the future will bring even more sophistication to the technology.

Film processing

Film processing of single-emulsion film requires special attention. As previously discussed, high-speed mammography film has a specific coating weight of silver halide on a single side of the film, so it requires a longer time for the developer to penetrate and develop the image. A 20-second developer immersion time is typical of normal 90-second processing cycles. While developer immersion times depend on film manufacturers' recommendations, film processing can be extended from 90 to as long as 210 seconds.[29] If development time is not long enough to complete the developing process, contrast will be reduced and film background will be lighter. An increase in the developer temperature will increase developer activity. While developer temperature recommendations can range from 92° to 95° F, routinely 95° F (36° C) is advocated. Variations in excess of ± 2° *will* affect film quality and must be corrected. Consideration of extended processing cycles must also include consideration of the effect on developer replenishment rates. If overreplenishment occurs, a reduction in film bromides will extend developer activity and produce dark films with high base-plus fog. Sensitometric performance analysis to verify processor stability is critical in reinforcing quality assurance of the processor. Standard reference films must be established and compared with daily sensitometry test strips. Density and contrast on the radiograph must be continually reproducible.[23] Quality assurance must also include attention to film storage and handling techniques, cassette and screen monitoring, film-screen contact testing, darkroom procedures, and viewbox and automatic viewer maintenance.

Successful quality assurance programs, while under the direct supervision of a radiologist, depend greatly on the ability and enthusiasm of the mammography technologist. A wide range of major tasks is typically required of the technical staff. Standard methods of development and organization of mammography procedures stress the connection between a final result and a preceding event. Careful attention to patient care, mammography instrumentation, proper patient positioning, technique selections, quality control procedures, and impeccable record keeping is required. Attention paid to the critical details of mammography makes a well-defined difference in the final image quality. The technologist must assume responsibility for consistent high-quality mammograms. A technologist sensitive to patient care will enhance communication and increase the ability to extract and to impart important information related to the examination.

The American College of Radiology (ACR) Accreditation Program requires comprehensive documentation of a facility's (1) credentialed personnel, (2) type of equipment used, (3) existing quality control measures, and (4) phantom dose measurement. In addition, typical mammography images and a phantom test image must be submitted for evaluation.[21] The program has developed manuals recommending specific quality control procedures, including performance frequency plans and personnel descriptions. While ACR mammography accreditation is a voluntary program, the opportunity to improve and expand the practice of mammography rests with the radiologic community.[20] The ACR Program information is readily available and its contribution must be recognized. It is much more difficult, especially in medicine, to measure the impact of lack of appropriate measures to ensure quality care. Routine application of quality control standards is the *only* way to ensure that quality mammography becomes available to all women.

BREAST POSITIONING

The ultimate goals of mammography are to obtain optimal image quality and skillfully interpret the findings. In addition to selecting appropriate technical parameters, it is essential that precise patient positioning be achieved. As previously mentioned, the breast is an inherently low-contrast organ, making it difficult to distinguish problem areas from surrounding normal breast tissue. Factors that contribute to image contrast and resolution have been discussed, but the importance of breast compression is worth repeating.

Commonly, statements are made by women about the discomfort of compression during mammography. Eklund and Cardenosa have stressed that breast mobility should assist rather than restrict efforts to properly position breast tissue.[7] These authors wholeheartedly agree and also encourage technologists to take full advantage of individual variation in tissue elasticity and, in every possible instance, arrange breast tissue before compression is routinely applied. Attention to proper compression assists in adjusting and smoothing the breast skin and may reduce uncomfortable stretching. Oversight in careful positioning of the breast may result in an uncomfortable mammography examination. Positioning women for mammography requires patience and good judgment; application of these characteristics becomes evident on the final image product. The technologist must be prepared to explain that while compression need not hurt, it must be applied firmly and evenly. Women are more likely to cooperate and add to the success of the examination when they sense that both personal and technical consideration is given them and when they feel that they have input and therefore control during their examination. The all-too-common complaint that mammography is painful must become the exception, not the rule.

Premenstrual hydration affects breast tissue, and some women experience increased breast tenderness during the premenstrual phase. Attempting to apply appropriate breast compression when women are physically uncomfortable may be impossible and the resulting mammogram will often be of poor quality. When scheduling mammograms, information should be given to women about the possible influence of their menstrual cycle on their mammogram evaluation. Ideally, particularly sensitive women should be given the opportunity to be scheduled during their postmenstrual phase, when discomfort from breast compression is minimized. This simple consideration gives women the choice of appropriate examination time and encourages continued compliance with future mammographic screening. It is also more likely to result in optimal breast imaging (Fig. 3-12).

Clerical and technical personnel are critical members of the mammography health care team. Their interest and commitment to a mammography service are vital to its success. These personnel are often challenged by the patient before any mammography is performed and must be able to respond, advocating mammography, and answering questions that are often critical to gaining a women's confidence and cooperation. Some women suffer cancerphobia based on a family history of breast cancer, and some are fearful from myth or misinformation about either the disease or the mammographic process. Women pose questions to these personnel that they do not pose to their physicians and they must be appropriately assured of the importance of mammography.

The craniocaudal and mediolateral oblique projections are basic to both screening and diagnostic mammography evaluation. A woman's "routine" screening evaluation may result in discovery of a worrisome area requiring further mammography workup. The type of additional imaging will depend on the type and location of the area of concern and requires a sound problem-oriented approach. Reimaging may result in alternative positioning of the entire breast or may require spot compression or magnification projection of a limited area of breast tissue.

Mammography can be an anxiety-inducing examination, and being thorough and responsive to women's needs becomes even more important when she must return for additional evaluation. There should be quick and easy access to scheduling routine and special mammography appointments. Customized scheduling is as important a service as customized routine and follow-up mammography examinations. Facility preparedness and dedicated personnel reduce confusion and increase utilization.

Ideally, the end product of mammography positioning is the appropriate demonstration of breast tissue unique to a specified mammography projection. Whether two or more projections are acquired, reproducibility is key to differentiating normal variation from a "new" finding. Benign and cancerous patterns can be confused, and experienced radiologists and technical personnel have learned how to avoid many a diagnostic pitfall. Uncertainty can be reflected in suboptimal mammography. The frequency of performing procedures influences one's ability to compare many individual breast characteristics and use the mammographic information to further develop the concepts and the techniques of high-quality breast evaluation.

Breast positioning, essentially uncomplicated, can produce a diagnostic dilemma if those performing mammography are not familiar with the spectrum of simple, but subtle, positioning techniques.

Craniocaudal projection

Although mammography may be performed seated or standing it is facilitated in the standing position.

The craniocaudal view best demonstrates the subareolar, central, and medial portions of the breast.[16] While the patient is standing, the breast is gently lifted to meet the edge of the inframammary fold (IMF) and the cassette holder is placed under the breast. The breast tissue is smoothed away from the chest wall with a steady forward movement and the tissue is pulled onto the film. Compression is then firmly applied from the top of the breast. Normally the entire medial aspect of the breast can be viewed in the craniocaudal projection; however, the most lateral aspect of the breast tissue may be omitted initially. Compensatory inward placement of the lateral breast tissue includes both medial and lateral portions of the breast. Careful attention must be given to the inward placement of tissue to maintain overall image integrity and avoid omitting either medial or lateral tissue, which could result in missing a subtle breast lesion. As the lateral portion of the breast is eased onto the film, compression is applied[7,8,32] (Fig. 3-13).

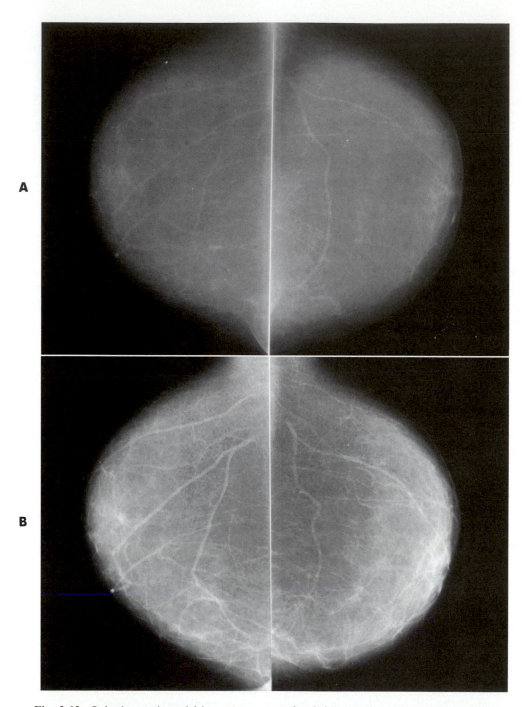

Fig. 3-12. Only the craniocaudal images were completed, in a woman with abundant breast volume during her premenstrual phase. **A,** Her extreme discomfort and lack of tolerance for appropriate breast compression resulted in poor mammography. Sensitivity to her discomfort led to rescheduling her examination. **B,** Craniocaudal projections in the postmenstrual phase show improved image quality. The woman admitted a change in her attitude about mammography and committed to routine follow-up examinations because of lessened discomfort at the second examination.

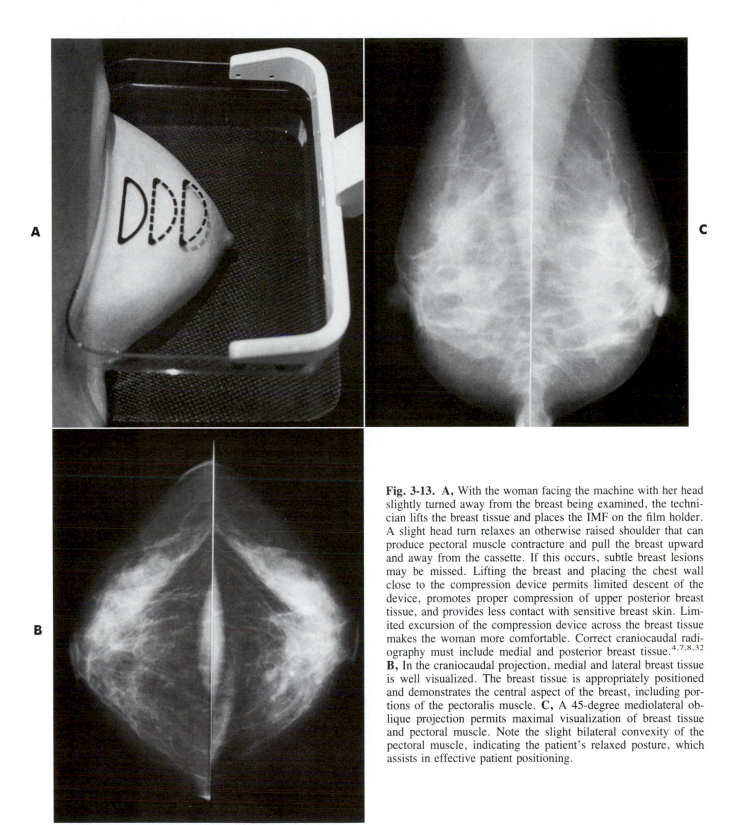

A

B

C

Fig. 3-13. A, With the woman facing the machine with her head slightly turned away from the breast being examined, the technician lifts the breast tissue and places the IMF on the film holder. A slight head turn relaxes an otherwise raised shoulder that can produce pectoral muscle contracture and pull the breast upward and away from the cassette. If this occurs, subtle breast lesions may be missed. Lifting the breast and placing the chest wall close to the compression device permits limited descent of the device, promotes proper compression of upper posterior breast tissue, and provides less contact with sensitive breast skin. Limited excursion of the compression device across the breast tissue makes the woman more comfortable. Correct craniocaudal radiography must include medial and posterior breast tissue.[4,7,8,32] **B,** In the craniocaudal projection, medial and lateral breast tissue is well visualized. The breast tissue is appropriately positioned and demonstrates the central aspect of the breast, including portions of the pectoralis muscle. **C,** A 45-degree mediolateral oblique projection permits maximal visualization of breast tissue and pectoral muscle. Note the slight bilateral convexity of the pectoral muscle, indicating the patient's relaxed posture, which assists in effective patient positioning.

Mediolateral oblique projection

The mediolateral oblique (MLO) is considered the ideal mammography projection because maximum visualization of the breast and the pectoral muscle can be achieved. In addition, the MLO projection permits maximum compression to be applied relatively easily. Of the two standard projections, CC and MLO, the MLO position is more often described by women as the more comfortable. The breast, because of its anterior relationship to the pectoralis major muscle, can be positioned with the glandular tissue completely visible. It is important that the pectoralis muscle be moved forward with the breast tissue, enabling appropriate compression.

The angle or degree of obliquity for the MLO projection can range from 30 to 60 degrees and depends entirely on a woman's body build.[4,8,14] When the patient's arm is raised to shoulder level and the cassette holder placed slightly posterior to the axilla, the breast is positioned with the long axis of the pectoralis muscle parallel to the cassette. It is incumbent on the technologist to review the patient's entire body position prior to exposure and to ensure that the arm and shoulder are relaxed. Arm and shoulder tension will be reflected in the pectoralis muscle and may prevent maximum forward movement of the breast tissue and the muscle (Fig 3-13, *C*).

These numerous technical elements must receive simultaneous consideration. In addition, the breast must be smoothed in an outward and upward fashion to keep the breast from drooping, which could produce superimposition of breast structures that could be mistaken for distortion caused by a breast lesion[34] (Fig. 3-14).

If the contralateral breast interferes with imaging the compressed breast, it may be necessary to have the patient gently secure the contralateral breast. Care must be taken, however, not to overzealously perform this maneuver and thus disturb the position of the compressed breast (Fig. 3-15).

Additional views

When a worrisome area is detected on only a single mammographic projection, it must be determined if there is real reason for worry or if the area represents superimposition of breast stroma or film artifact. If possible, before reimaging, the patient's breast skin should be carefully

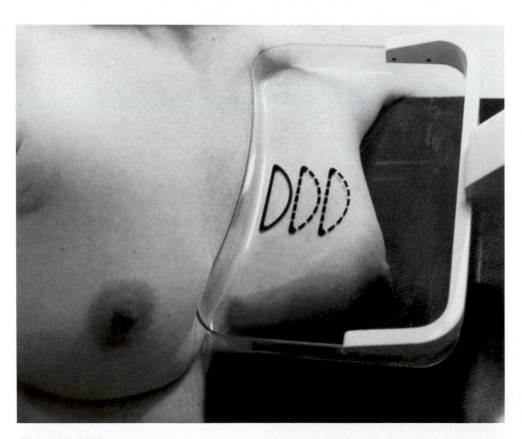

Fig. 3-14. MLO projection shows secure breast placement and compression. The compression device extends from the clavicular area to the inferior aspect of the breast. The breast and pectoral muscle are well placed medially, and the integrity of the position is not compromised after compression is applied.

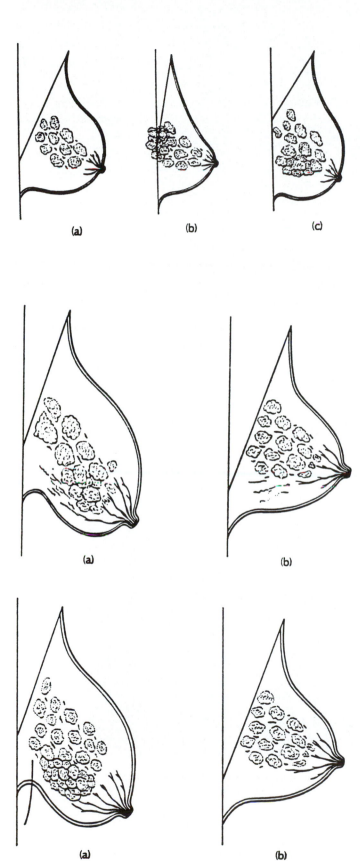

reexamined; a film or cassette artifact should also be considered as a possible contributing factor. Repeating a projection with simple rearrangement of breast tissue may clarify an area in question.

Mediolateral/lateromedial projection. To gain insight to the three-dimensional relationship of a lesion when there is confusion as to its exact location, a direct lateral view may be used. Either lateromedial or mediolateral projections, obtained 90 degrees to the craniocaudal projection, will provide accurate information.

If a lesion is located in the lateral aspect of the breast, a mediolateral projection, placing the lesion closer to the film, may confirm or deny its presence. Conversely, if a questionable area is located medially, a lateromedial projection is obtained (Fig. 3-16).

Rolled projection. Just as the mediolateral oblique and lateromedial projections help to diminish confusion of a lesion's location, the "rolled view" can also assist in diminishing confusion of an indeterminate mammographic finding.

When a lesion is seen only in a single standard view, rotation of breast tissue may determine in just which quadrant a lesion is located. This rotation maneuver may also help determine whether or not the lesion is real. Changing the orientation of breast tissue will vary the degrees of obliquity, separate superimposition of breast tissue, and confirm any portion of tissue that remains dense (Fig. 3-17).

Spot compression. The spot compression view is especially valuable to confirm the presence of a worrisome lesion, especially in dense breast tissue. The spot compression device is designed to enhance areas of breast tissue that may not be fully appreciated using standard compression. These variable-size compression devices, when efficiently applied, reduce breast thickness and reduce scatter radiation. A reduction in scatter radiation enhances image contrast and consequently provides more precise visualization of the area under evaluation. Before positioning the patient, one must localize a questionable area using the conventional mammogram images. For spot compression, the breast is positioned as in the routine mammogram, and the area of concern should be marked on the breast skin. If

Fig. 3-15. Mediolateral oblique projection. **A,** *a,* Correct position: axillary fold at 30 degrees down to nipple level. *b,* Incorrect position: cassette not high enough into the axilla. *c,* Incorrect position: patient leaning back or beam too vertical. **B,** *a,* Incorrect: the inferior markings are crowded. *b,* Correct: the breast has been lifted up during compression and the inferior markings are horizontal. **C,** *a,* Incorrect: a fold of skin inferiorly prevents good compression. *b,* Correct: the skin fold has been smoothed out and the breast lifted during compression. (From Roebuck E: *Clinical radiology of the breast,* Oxford, 1990, Heinemann.)

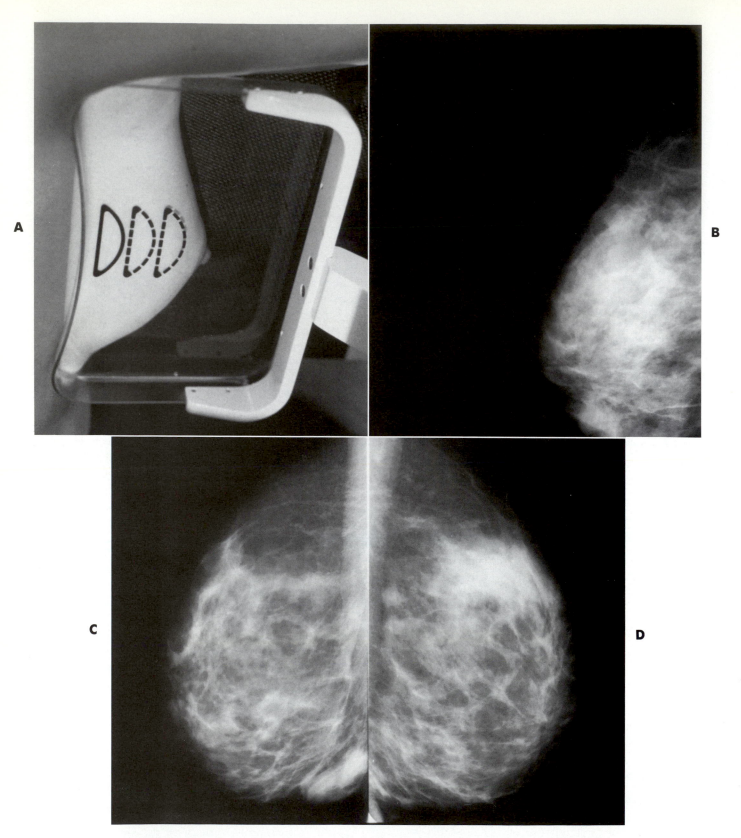

Fig. 3-16. The lateromedial projection will assist in evaluating a worrisome lesion on the medial aspect of the breast. **A,** Compression is applied while positioning the medial side of the breast against the recording device. In placing the side of the breast in question closer to the cassette, image sharpness is improved. As a rule, more breast tissue is evident on the mediolateral oblique projection than on the lateromedial. The LM projection may visualize a minimal amount of pectoralis muscle, or this muscle may be altogether absent. In **B,** no pectoral muscle is evident. **C,** This well-positioned lateromedial projection of the breast, obtained 90 degrees to the craniocaudal projection, reveals maximum visualization of breast tissue and pectoralis muscle. Body build and the actual amount of breast tissue affect the ability to position the woman to be able to visualize the most posterior aspect of breast tissue. Every effort must be made to pull the breast tissue as far forward as possible with compression firmly applied.

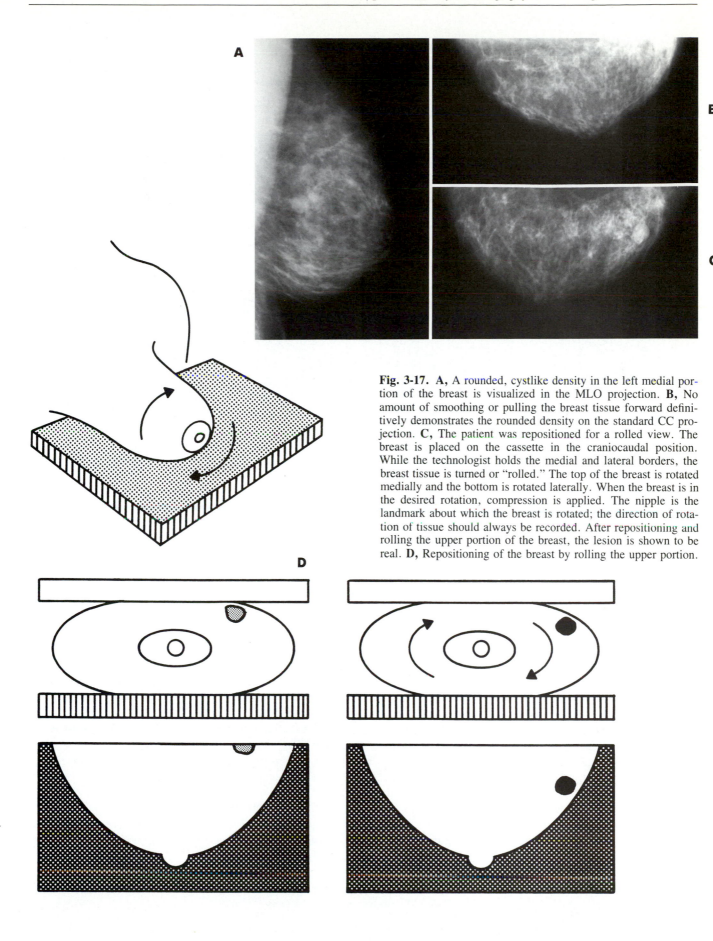

Fig. 3-17. A, A rounded, cystlike density in the left medial portion of the breast is visualized in the MLO projection. **B,** No amount of smoothing or pulling the breast tissue forward definitively demonstrates the rounded density on the standard CC projection. **C,** The patient was repositioned for a rolled view. The breast is placed on the cassette in the craniocaudal position. While the technologist holds the medial and lateral borders, the breast tissue is turned or "rolled." The top of the breast is rotated medially and the bottom is rotated laterally. When the breast is in the desired rotation, compression is applied. The nipple is the landmark about which the breast is rotated; the direction of rotation of tissue should always be recorded. After repositioning and rolling the upper portion of the breast, the lesion is shown to be real. **D,** Repositioning of the breast by rolling the upper portion.

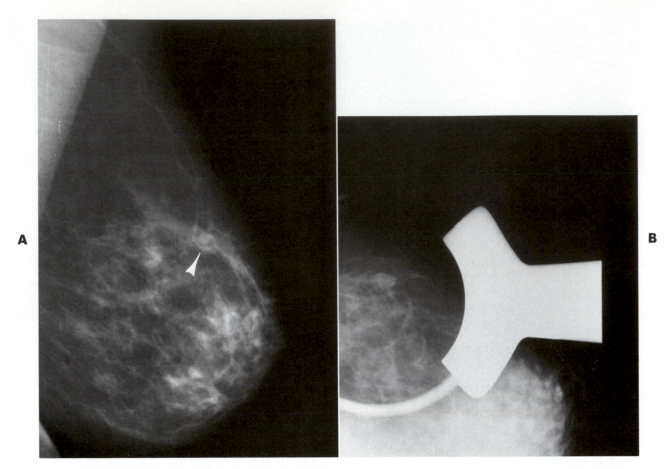

Fig. 3-18. A and **B,** A dense area was detected in this 65-year-old woman with a history of previous and multiple bilateral biopsies as well as lumpectomy performed in the right breast in 1986. Understandably anxious, this woman routinely undergoes follow-up care. **A,** Her overall mammographic pattern had not changed significantly over the years until a small rounded density in the superior portion of the left breast was believed to have changed in size and configuration. **B,** Once the overlying stromal structures were compressed, coned magnification of the density confirmed that the density had not changed substantially. Based on her medical history and the desire to avoid another surgical biopsy procedure, this woman requested stereotaxic evaluation of the nonpalpable cystic appearing lesion. SFNB was performed and cytology confirmed benign epithelial cells.

additional views are necessary, the same area or a change in breast position may be addressed using the original landmark. Magnification projection also relies on these strategies in addition to the use of a small focal spot size. Extremely small focal spot size is required to achieve high-resolution magnification imaging.

Calcifications and their specific subtle patterns and size can be difficult to detect or overlooked completely in the dense breast. Dense areas require vigorous compression and superimposed breast stroma may confirm or deny the presence of a lesion or define microcalcifications (Fig. 3-18).

Cleavage projection. A medial craniocaudal projection, or "cleavage" view, can image the upper medial

breast tissue. The patient faces the mammography unit, and her head is rotated away from the side of interest. The breasts are elevated and the cassette holder is placed at the level of the inframammary fold. The medial breast tissue is moved anterior and the upper portion of the breast tissue is placed over the machine detector. Compression is then applied to the area in question (Fig. 3-19).

Postsurgical imaging

Mammography is used to detect recurrent breast disease following excision of a cancer. The postsurgical changes are often difficult to evaluate. Asymmetric tissue formation resulting from biopsy or modified mastectomy procedure presents patterns of scar formation that require mam-

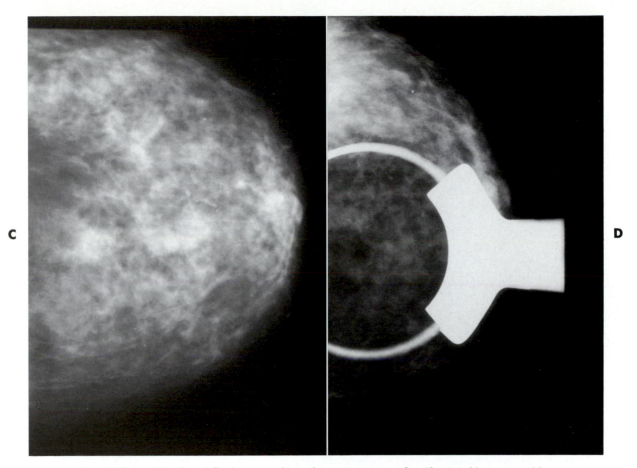

Fig. 3-18, cont'd. **C** and **D,** In comparison, the mammogram of a 48-year-old woman with a strong family history of breast cancer reveals mottled stromal architecture. **C,** In the craniocaudal projection, there is minimal irregularity evident in the mid-portion of the left breast. **D,** Because of her strong family history of breast cancer, coned compression projection was obtained. The breast stroma is effectively displaced and reveals no definitive lesion. In both of these cases, spot compression and spot magnification were helpful in differentiating dense breast areas, and an invasive technique was avoided.

mographic differentiation from possible underlying, preexisting lesions. Fat necrosis or fibrosis can occur, and retraction and increase in linear density resulting from surgical radial scar formation can mammographically appear as a stellate lesion (see Chapter 11). Surgical trauma may occur and be radiographically evident. It can also resemble significant breast disease. Consequently, it is essential to observe and indicate postsurgical changes on the patient's history sheet so that they will not be mistaken later for recurrent carcinoma. Equally important is careful scrutiny of the contralateral breast for clinically occult, yet mammographically evident, lesions.

A patient's history is the medical team's roadmap. Just as any map holds conventions and symbols, a mammography history format has developed in the same fashion. If we do not understand its importance or use the symbols

that depict the territory, the medical team, and worse, the patient, may get lost. A properly recorded mammography history should routinely provide consistently reliable information to any consultant. When divergent routes of care are taken, it is in the best interest of the health care team and the patient to record them. Defining and linking what we observe and selectively perform should provide a more efficient system of breast health care. Our best hope of reaching a common ground is to use the things we have in common (Fig. 3-20).

About 75% of women with positive nodes and 25% of those with negative lymph nodes treated with mastectomy experience recurrence within 10 years.[12] The risk for subsequent carcinoma in the contralateral breast varies and can depend on age at diagnosis.[5] Vigilance in subsequent follow-up screening mammograms, especially in the post-

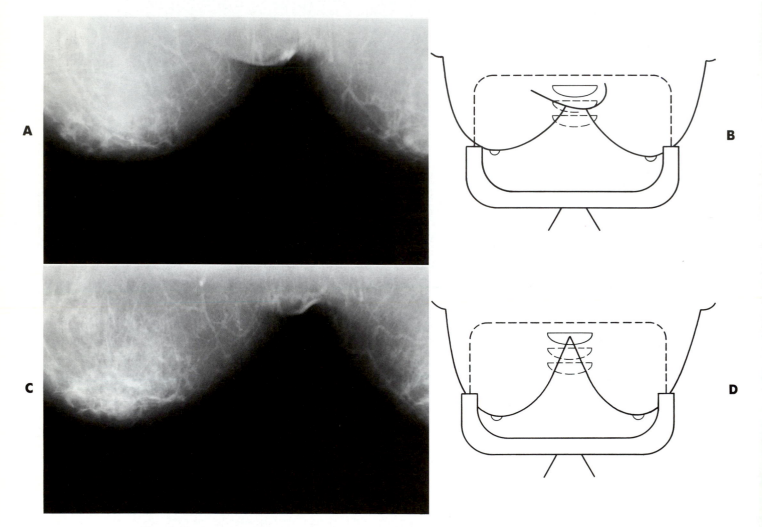

Fig. 3-19. A 41-year-old obese female reported for screening mammography complaining of breast tenderness, especially at the cleavage point of the right breast. Her mammograms revealed no definite mass and no abnormal calcifications. However, the patient pointed to an area of "fullness" on the medial aspect of the right breast. While there was no palpable mass, her complaint prompted additional imaging. **A** and **B,** The cleavage projection revealed an area of increased breast tissue on the right medial aspect. Because of the patient's obese condition, reexamination of the area was recommended with particular attention directed to precision positioning and compression of the medial portion of the right breast. **C** and **D,** The asymmetry seen on the first cleavage study was no longer apparent. The asymmetric finding was undoubtedly related to adipose tissue overlying the sternal area. No observable evidence of intrinsic breast abnormality is seen.

Mammography History

Name: ()   XRay: _____
Phys: Date:

VID#: 138715 ()

Baseline ___ Screening ___ Follow-up ___ Symptomatic ___
            Prev. Mam _____ Unavail: ___
Age: 0   Where _____

Fam. Hist: pre pst age   P/M pre pst age
   Mother ___ ___ ___ ___   Aunt ___ ___ ___ ___
   Daught ___ ___ ___ ___   Gdma ___ ___ ___ ___
   Sister ___ ___ ___ ___   Othr ___ ___ ___ ___
                                     ___ ___ ___ ___

Symptoms: Rt   Lf
   Tender: ___ ___   Comments: _____
   Dischrg: ___ ___   Color: _____
     Lump: ___ ___   Location: _____
                                   _____

Biopsy:
   Rt: _x_ Date: September 1991   Estrogen: _____ yrs.
   Lf: ___ Date:

Menstral/Pregnancy History
Age Menarche: ____   Age Menopause: ___   Pregnancies: ___ Live Births ___
Date Last Menstrual Period: _____   Age At First Pregnancy: ____
Pregnant Now? ___   Did You Nurse? ___   Age At Last Pregnancy: ____

Hormones/Surgeries/Miscellaneous
Birth Control ___ yrs. Now: ___   Thyroid ___ yrs.   Now: ___

Hysterectomy: Partial ___   Complete ___   Date: _____
Oophorectomy: Bilat. ___   Unilat. ___   Date: _____
Mastectomy: Bilat. ___   Rt ___ Lf ___ Date: _____

Had Cancer? _X_ Type _Lobular and intraductal carcinoma_ in situ-right breast
Caffeine User ___   Used Powder,Perfume,Deodorant? ___

Additional Comments
_____
_____
_____
_____

                             Mammographer: _____

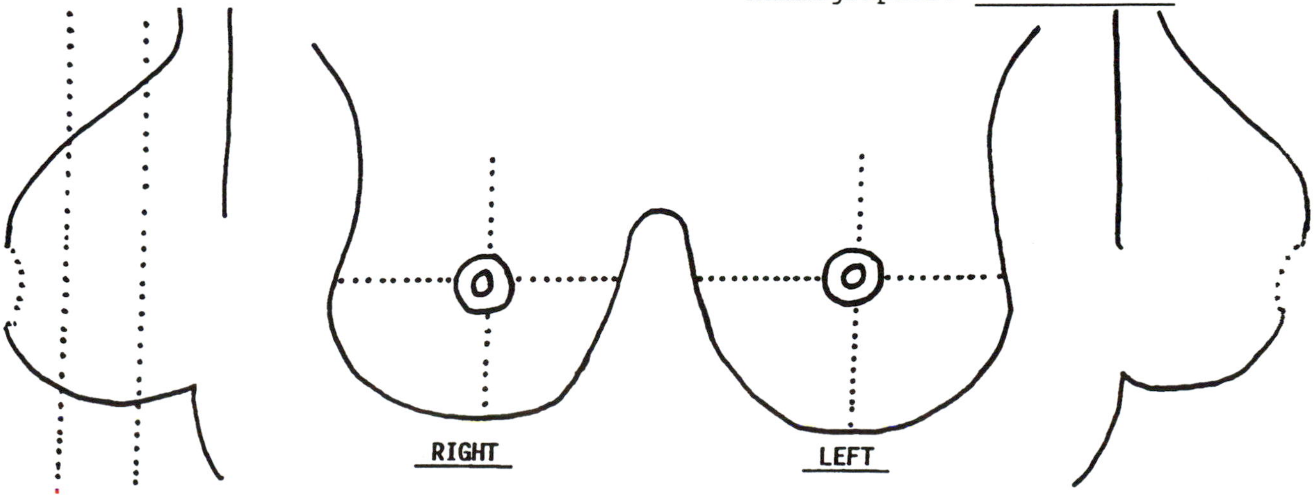

RIGHT   LEFT

Fig. 3-20. A, Mammography history sheet.   *Continued.*

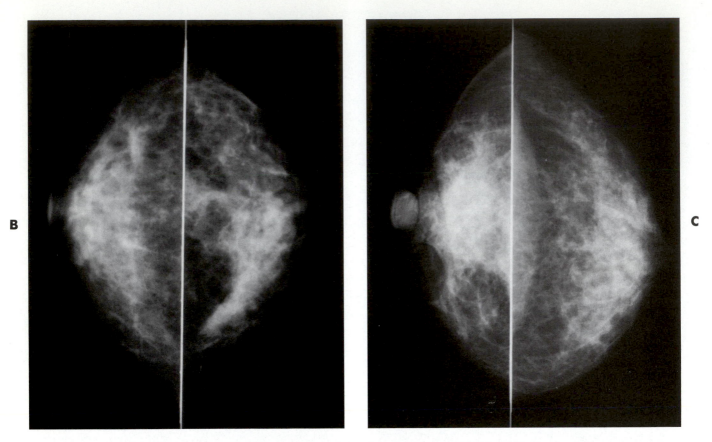

Fig. 3-20, cont'd. B, A 1989 mammography study reveals normal breast architecture in a 54-year-old woman with no breast symptoms and no family history of breast cancer. Between her 1989 and 1991 examinations, she developed a palpable mass. Surgical excision revealed intraductal and lobular carcinoma in situ. **C,** This woman's 1992 postlumpectomy mammograms reveal considerably less breast tissue and asymmetry of the remaining stromal architecture.

surgical breast, is crucial (Fig. 3-21). Different surgical procedures provide a range in mammographic appearance that requires the ability to note measurable differences over time. Interval progression of an abnormal finding demands prompt and clear-cut recommendation.

Augmented breast

The exact number of women having augmentation mammaplasty is unknown. It is currently estimated that over 1 million women in the United States have had breast augmentation implant surgery. The potential safety and approval of this surgical procedure have been widely debated.[9] Media attention and reports in the lay literature have added one more element of anxiety for all women who have had augmentation, for women who consider augmentation a procedure of choice, and for women diagnosed with breast cancer who consider postmastectomy reconstructive surgery essential.

There is no other time when expertise in the technique

to image the augmented breast is more essential. Women are confused and anxious about the efficacy of augmentation, and more so about the personal effect augmentation may have on their overall health.

With or without implants, the risk of cancer remains unchanged for women. Imaging the augmented breast presents a special challenge. It requires specific technical expertise to visualize a limited amount of glandular tissue that may be harboring a lesion obscured by an implant device.

The Eklund technique, described in 1988, is well recognized as the "gold standard" for implant imaging.[6] Using the Eklund procedure, breast tissue is manipulated over and anterior to the implant device itself. The implant is moved or "pinched" back toward the chest wall and compression is applied to the remaining breast tissue, allowing for visualization of tissue that is unaffected by the implant. While augmented breast evaluation requires more images (four per breast), it is critical to obtain all of the projec-

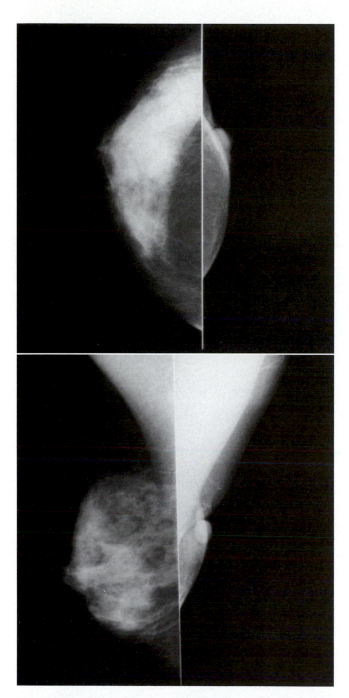

Fig. 3-21. This 59-year-old woman had a subareolar left mastectomy procedure in 1984 with preservation of underlying stromal tissue and the nipple. Occasional bilateral calcifications are noted; they were present on a previous examination. In some women with diminished glandular tissue, it is a challenge to obtain quality postsurgical images. Patience and persistence are needed by the technical staff. Quality images are critical since initial postsurgical mammogram evaluation sets a new baseline for subsequent breast imaging. Follow-up examination requires diligent attention from the patient, the referring physician, and the radiology mammography unit.

tions (Fig. 3-22). Standard imaging, without implant manipulation, reveals the relationship of the breast tissue as it surrounds the implant device and demonstrates posterior tissue that may be excluded on the implant compression views. This becomes of greater importance in the case of implant encapsulation.

The encapsulated implant poses yet another challenge, since implant pliability against the chest wall is absent. However, every effort must still be made to manipulate the breast tissue in front of the implant. Eklund et al. advise an additional 90-degree lateral projection be obtained. This projection permits greater visualization of posterior breast tissue above and below the implant that is not otherwise observed, especially in patients with rigid encapsulation[7] (Fig. 3-23).

MARKING OF RADIOGRAPHS

Critical to all radiography examinations is the proper marking of the examinations performed. Mammography is one radiologic examination in which a uniform system of film marking has been adopted and correct labeling of the mammogram is essential.

Routinely, the right and left markers are placed along the axillary portion of the breast in the craniocaudal projections and in the upper axillary area of the breast in the lateral projections (Fig. 3-24). Additional compression and magnification projections require similar identification. Many types of film labels are available to simplify recording critical information. Labels on which to record the projection and related tube angle and documented performance techniques, as well as the degree of obliquity and breast compression measurements, may be placed on the films. Brief and simple to use, a label provides an immediate reference source for subsequent evaluation that is most useful in reproducing the images (Fig. 3-25).

STEREOTAXIC FINE-NEEDLE BIOPSY

The stereotaxic fine-needle biopsy (SFNB) procedure, indicated for women with nonpalpable breast lesions, optimizes the precision with which lesions may be localized, needle-biopsied, and, when necessary, preoperatively marked. This system thus facilitates the diagnostic accuracy of worrisome breast areas.

When the *Mammotest* stereotaxic biopsy system is used, a patient lies prone on a padded, elevated table with the breast pendulant through an aperture in the table (Fig. 3-26). Controls accessible from both sides of the stereotaxic system permit movement of the table in the vertical, horizontal, and transverse directions. A breast compression device and x-ray tube, combined in a single arm, travel vertically.

Once the patient is positioned, the table is secured in place for the remainder of the procedure. Stereoradiographs are then acquired. The film cassette holder, located

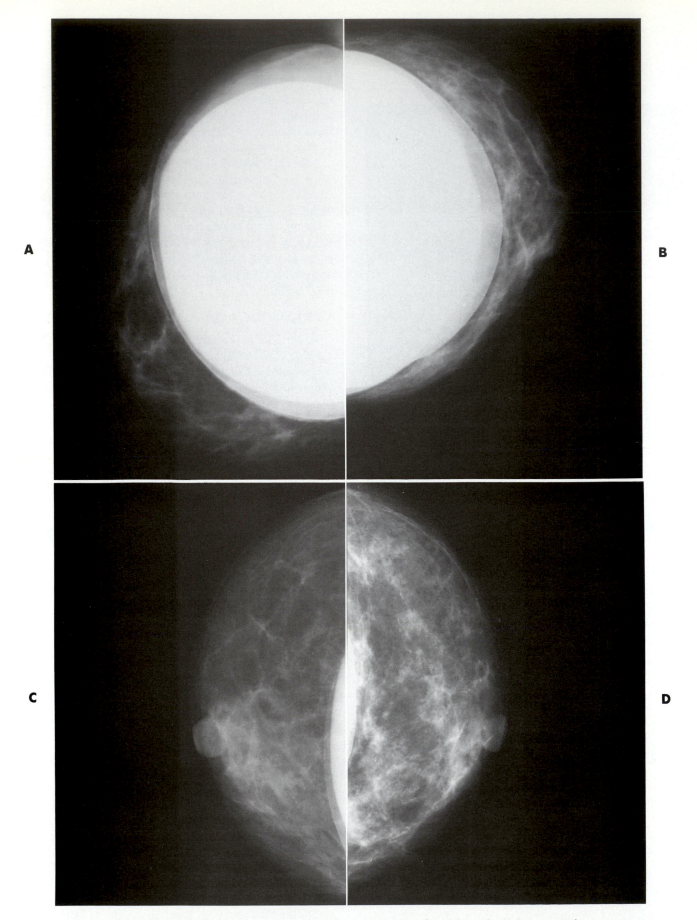

Fig. 3-22. A and **B,** These are standard craniocaudal images of a patient who had augmentation mammoplasty performed in 1988. **C** and **D,** Applying the Eklund technique, modified compression clearly delineates breast stromal architecture and precludes superimposition of glandular tissue by the implant device.

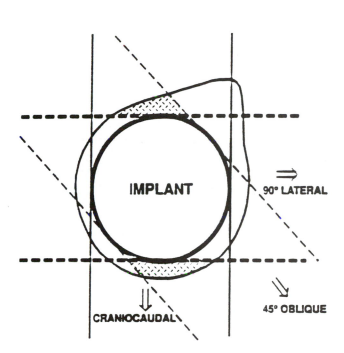

Fig. 3-23. In patients who have firm fibrous encapsulation, a 90-degree lateral view is needed to visualize posterior breast tissue directly above and below the implant *(shaded area)*. This tissue would not otherwise be seen on MLO and CC views. (From Eklund GW, Cardenosa G: *Radiol Clin North Am* 30[1]:21-53, 1992.)

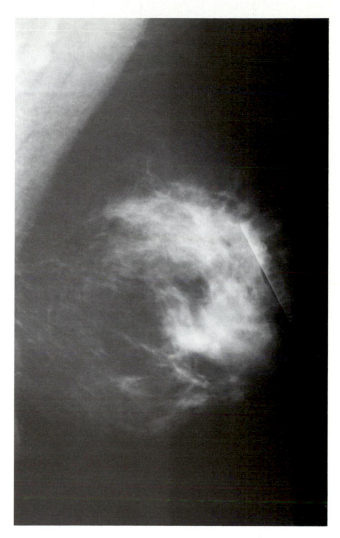

Fig. 3-24. Unacceptably careless and improper placement of markers.

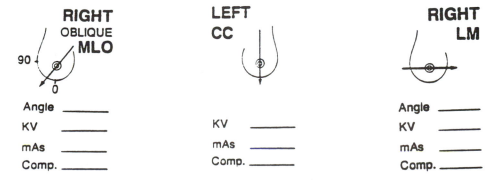

Fig. 3-25. Example of mammographic positioning labels. (Courtesy Advanced Radiographic Technologies, Inc., Peoria, IL.)

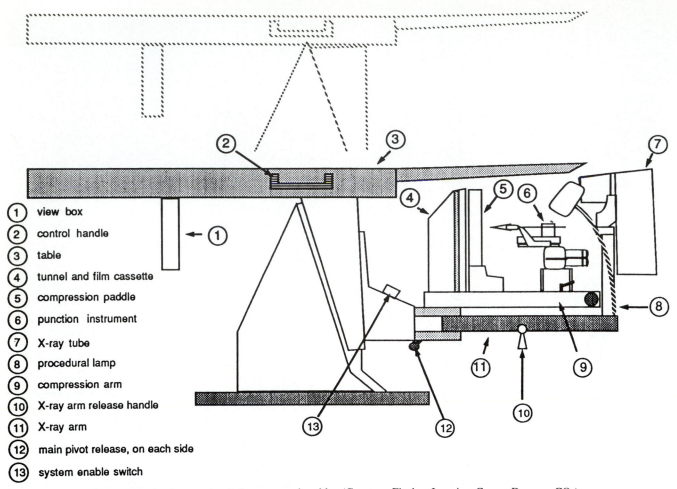

① view box
② control handle
③ table
④ tunnel and film cassette
⑤ compression paddle
⑥ punction instrument
⑦ X-ray tube
⑧ procedural lamp
⑨ compression arm
⑩ X-ray arm release handle
⑪ X-ray arm
⑫ main pivot release, on each side
⑬ system enable switch

Fig. 3-26. Components of the stereotaxic table. (Courtesy Fischer Imaging Corp., Denver, CO.)

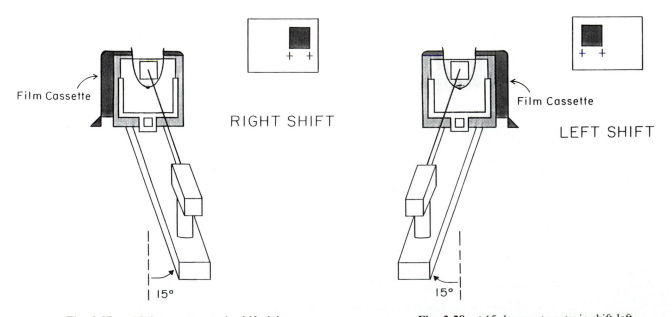

Fig. 3-27. −15-degree stereotaxic shift right.

Fig. 3-28. +15-degree stereotaxic shift left.

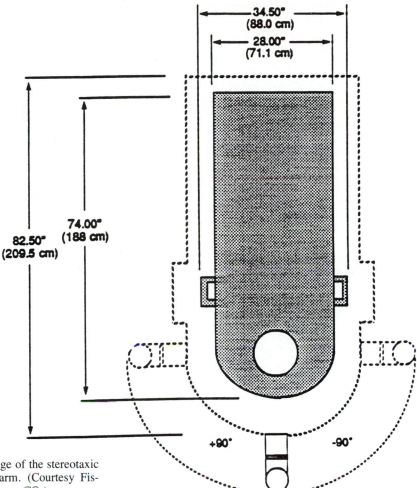

Fig. 3-29. Maximum range of the stereotaxic compression x-ray tube arm. (Courtesy Fischer Imaging Corp., Denver, CO.)

directly behind the compression device and accessible from either side, receives an 18 × 24 film cassette. The automatic exposure control (AEC) detector is located behind the film cassette holder. The tube arm, with a total movement of 30 degrees for stereotaxic imaging, is extended −15 degrees to the right for the first exposure (Fig. 3-27) and then +15 degrees to the left for the second exposure (Fig. 3-28). The entire compression arm has a radial movement with detents at −90, −45, 0 to +45, and +90 degrees. This motion versatility permits stereoimaging and biopsy in a craniocaudal position (0) and in 45-degree obliquity and 90-degree lateral positions (Fig. 3-29).

The punction instrument is mounted on the compression arm. This instrument includes the needle holder and guide, used to position the Rotex needle, as well as the vertical and horizontal controls and depth stop. The depth stop, adjusted by a thumbscrew, limits the forward travel of the needle.

Together the stereoscopic image and a cursor marking

device, located on the *Mammotest* console, provide the target calculation measurements (Fig. 3-30). The target area of the lesion is marked by the operator using both stereoscopic images by first placing and then engaging the marker device on the crosshairs found in the corner of each stereoimage and then on the lesion target area. This results in calculated coordinates that precisely define the position of the lesion.

Using the vertical and horizontal controls and the depth stop on the punction device, the specified stereotaxic target coordinates are registered. The ability to advance the needle to the center of the lesion can be accomplished with an accuracy of better than 1 mm. A printout of the data identifies the patient by name and records the date and time of the calculation and the exact location of the stereotaxic target. The needle is then placed in the holder and advanced to the calculated site.

The initial biopsy needle technique consists of a standard 22-gauge spinal aspiration needle that is attached to a

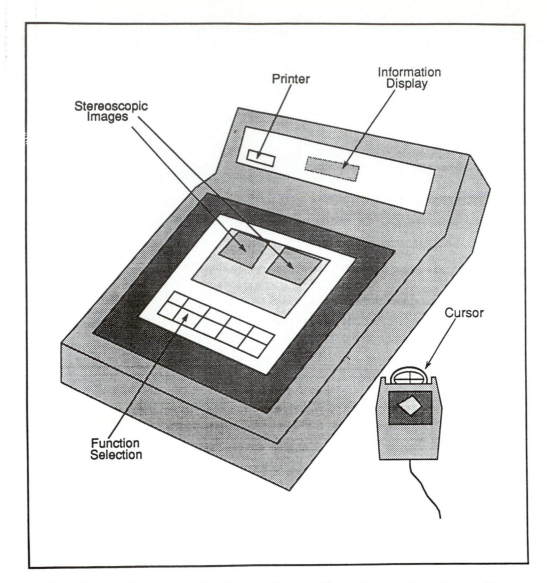

Fig. 3-30. Console control panel and cursor. (Courtesy Fischer Imaging Corp., Denver, CO.)

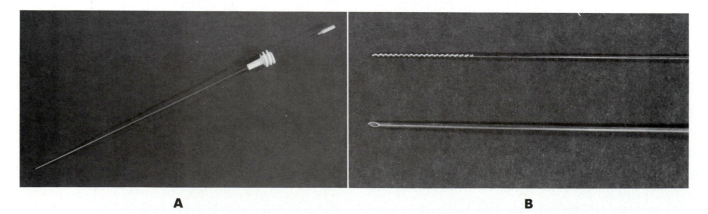

A   **B**

Fig. 3-31. A, Rotex II screw needle biopsy instrument. **B,** The 0.55 mm microscopically grooved end of the Rotex needle and the 172 × 0.8 mm Rotex cannula. (Manufactured in Stockholm, Sweden, by Ursus Konsult Co.)

10 ml multifit Luer-Lok syringe.* The syringe is then inserted into an INRAD, pistol-type, aspiration biopsy gun and the 22-gauge needle is advanced to the center of the lesion. Standard aspiration technique is performed. The 22-gauge needle is moved back and forth with the hub of the needle appropriately corresponding to the depth stop. Subsequent biopsy is performed using the Rotex II Screw Needle Biopsy instrument, which consists of a 172 × 0.8 mm thick cannula that covers a 0.55 mm thick inner needle (Fig. 3-31). The distal 17 mm portion of the Rotex

*Becton-Dickinson, Rutherford, NJ.

needle is microscopically grooved. The Rotex needle is placed in the needle holder on the punction instrument and the cannula is rotated off the grooved Rotex needle while simultaneously advancing the needle portion to the calculated center of interest. This grooved end, when inserted into the lesion and gently rotated, secures cellular material directly from the lesion site. Before removing the Rotex II biopsy instrument, the cannula is then rotated back over the Rotex needle to protect the cellular material. This cellular material and that obtained in the lumen of the aspiration needle are prepared on standard glass slides for final preparation of cytologic evaluation (Fig. 3-32).

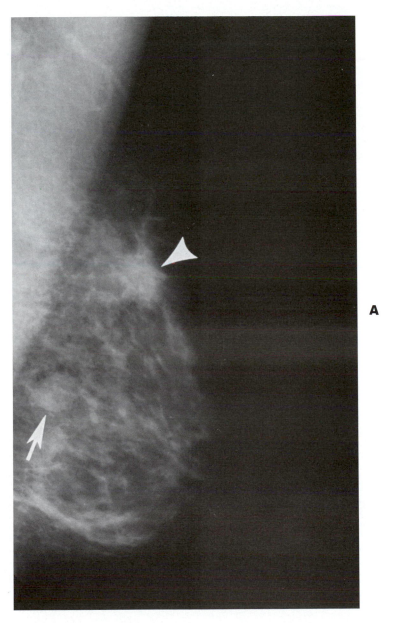

Fig. 3-32. A, Routine screening mammograms of the left breast revealed two areas of concern in a 47-year-old woman with a history of contralateral breast carcinoma.

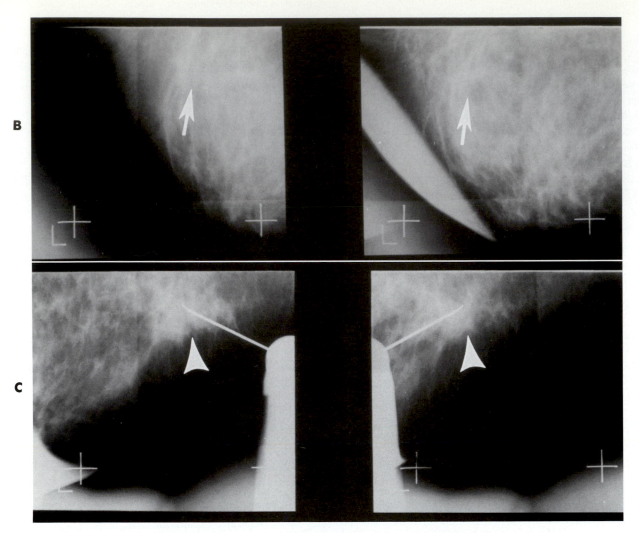

Fig. 3-32, cont'd. **B,** Stereotaxic evaluation performed with the breast in a craniocaudal position confirmed the density in the lower inner quadrant to be an area of superimposition of breast stroma with no frank lesion *(arrow)*. **C,** The second area, located in the upper outer quadrant, remained prominent on stereotaxic imaging *(arrowhead)*. Aspiration and Rotex biopsy revealed cytology negative for malignant cells.

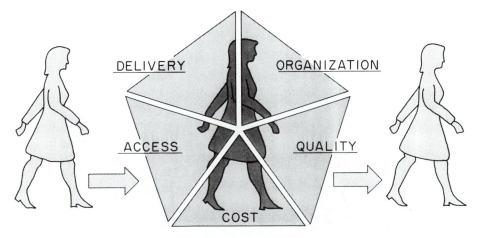

Fig. 3-33. Quality mammography includes access to organized, cost-effective delivery. Only with all five elements can proper diagnosis and management of breast disease be provided.

CONCLUSION

How can women make the best decisions for their breast health care when their physicians provide them with conflicting information? Quality health care for women must be provided. Consensus must be developed to provide consistent advice to women to participate in breast screening programs. High-quality, cost-effective mammography must be delivered to all women.

Incentive for women to seek mammograms will come more easily when mammography services are uniformly organized and performed effectively. We must replace current confusion about age of initiation, frequency of follow-up, and inconsistency of mammographic technique with a unified, supportive system that promotes and maintains a partnership of respect for health care experts and women alike. Diagnosis and management of breast disease depend on using the best single tool we have to the best advantage. Quality mammography is the current tool that can fully integrate high standards of early diagnosis and medical care of breast disease (Fig. 3-33).

REFERENCES

1. *American Heritage dictionary,* second College edition, Boston, 1982, Houghton Mifflin.
2. Brown ML, Kessler LG, Rueter FG: Is the supply of mammography machines outstripping need and demand? *Ann Intern Med* 113:547-552, 1990.
3. Bushong SC: What to look for when buying a mammography system, *Diagnostic Imaging,* Feb 1992.
4. deParedes E, Marsteller LP, Eden BV: Breast cancers in women 35-years of age and younger: mammographic findings, *Radiology* 177:117-119, 1990.
5. Dixon JM, Anderson TS, Page DL, et al: Infiltrating lobular carcinoma of the breast, *Histopathology* 6:149-161, 1982.
6. Eklund GW, Busby RC, Miller SH, Job JS: Improved imaging of the augmented breast, *Am J Radiol* 151:469-473, 1988.
7. Eklund GW, Cardenosa G: The art of mammographic positioning, *Radiol Clin North Am* 30(1):21-53, 1992.
8. Eklund GW, Cardenosa G: Art of positioning needs revival in mammography, *Diagnostic Imaging,* Sept 1991.
9. FDA hearings on silicone breast implants, Feb 1992.
10. Feig S: Mammography equipment: principles, features, selection, *Radiol Clin North Am* 25:897-911, 1987.
11. Fisher B, Anderson S, Fisher E, et al: Ten-year results of randomized clinical trials comparing radical mastectomy and total mastectomy with or without radiation, *N Engl J Med* 312:674-681, 1985.
12. Fisher B, Slack N, Katryck K, Wolmark N: Ten-year following results of patients with carcinoma of the breast in a cooperative clinical trial evaluating surgical adjuvant chemotherapy, *Surg Gynecol Obstet* 140:528-534, 1975.
13. Frykberg ER, Bland KI: Evolution of surgical principles for the management of breast cancer. From Blank KI, Copeland EM, editors: *The breast: comprehensive management of benign and malignant diseases,* Philadelphia, 1991, Saunders.
14. Gormley L, Bassett LW, Gold RH: Positioning in film-screen mammography, *Appl Radiol,* July 1988, pp 35-37.
15. Gray H: *Gray's anatomy,* ed 34 (DV Davies, editor), London, 1967, Churchill Livingstone.
16. Haagensen CD: *Diseases of the breast,* ed. 3, Philadelphia, 1986, Saunders.
17. Harris JR, Hellman S, Henderson IC, Kinne D: *Breast diseases,* Philadelphia, 1987, Lippincott.
18. Haus AG: Evaluation of image blur (unsharpness) in medical imaging, *Med Radiogr Photogr* 61:41-53, 1985.
19. Haus AG: Recent advances in screen film mammography, *Radiol Clin North Am* 25:913-928, 1987.
20. Hendrick RE: Standardization of image quality and radiation dose in mammography, *Radiology* 174(3):648-654, 1990.
21. Hendrick RE, Haus AG, Hubbard LB: American College of Radiology accreditation program for mammographic screening sites: physical evaluation criteria (abstract), *Radiology* 165:209, 1987.
22. Jackson VP, Harrill CD, White SJ, et al: Evaluation of a dual-screen, dual-emulsion mammography system, *Am J Roentgenol* 152:483-486, 1989.
23. Kimme-Smith C: Mammographic image receptors and image processing, *Curr Opinions Radiol* 2:719-725, 1990.
24. Kimme-Smith C, Bassett LW, Gold RH, et al: New mammography screen-film combinations: imaging characteristics and radiation dose, *Am J Roentgenol* 154:713-719, 1990.
25. Kitts EL Jr, Beutel J, Holland RS, Blank B: Relative doses in mammography: the future developments of film/screen mammography systems: recent results in cancer research, vol. 119, Berlin, 1990, Springer-Verlag.
26. Kopans DB: Analysis: years of study fail to quell breast screening controversy, *Diagnostic Imaging,* November 1988.
27. Kopans DB: *Breast imaging,* Philadelphia, 1989, Lippincott.
28. Kruse J, Phillips DM: Factors influencing women's decision to undergo mammography, *Obstet Gynecol* 70(5):744-748, 1987.
29. Law J, Kirkpatrick AE: Film processing for mammography, *Br J Radiol* 61:939-942, 1988.
30. Law J, Kirkpatrick AE: Further comparison of films, screens and cassettes for mammography, *Br J Radiol* 63:128-131, 1990.
31. Love S: *Dr. Susan Love's breast book,* Palo Alto, Ca, 1990, Addison-Wesley.
32. Peters ME, Voegeli DR, Scanlon KA: *Handbook of breast imaging,* New York, 1989, Churchill-Livingstone.
33. Rimer BK, Keintz MK, Kessler HB, et al: Why women resist screening mammography: patient-related barriers, *Radiology* 172:342-346, 1989.
34. Roebuck EJ: *Clinical radiology of the breast,* Oxford, 1990, Heinemann.
35. Rothenberg LN: Patient dose in mammography, *RadioGraphics* 10:739-746, 1990.
36. Selinger HA, Goldfarb NI, Perkel RL, Carlson BL: Physician compliance with mammography guidelines: a retrospective chart review, *Fam Med* 21:56-58, 1989.
37. Sierra AE, Potchen EJ: Use of mammography in screening for breast cancer, *Obstet Gynecol Clin North Am* 17(4):927-938, 1990.
38. Wellings SR, Wolfe JN: Correlative studies of the histological and radiographic appearance of the breast parenchyma, *Radiology* 129:299-306, 1978.

Chapter 4

HOW TO INTERPRET
A MAMMOGRAM

Mammography requires dedicated radiologists who see a sufficient volume of mammographic examinations to maintain their clinical skills and thus limit their rates of false-positive and false-negative interpretations. The interpretation of a mammogram, more than any other radiologic procedure, requires continual refinement in observer skills. The observer must constantly use experience to modify his/her judgmental criteria. To appreciate his/her own experience, the radiologist must be well informed of the implications of prior decisions. A major difference between the Karolinska system and the standard American approach to screening mammography is the form and certainty of feedback to the radiologist who interprets an indeterminant mammogram. In Sweden, stereotaxic fine-needle cytology specimens are obtained directly by the radiologist who observed the suspicious abnormality on the mammogram. With this experience, the radiologist can rapidly modify his/her criteria for suspicion when interpreting screening mammograms. This adjustment in diagnostic fidelity is based on knowing what pathology to expect from which mammographic presentation. The system forces constant iteration in the interpretative skills of the mammographers. To properly learn from experience, the radiologist must make a sufficient number of decisions over a short enough time to develop the feedback needed for effective clinical judgment.

Ciatto et al. reported the variation in observer performance in interpreting screening mammograms.[23] Their data reveal that the number of films read per year by each observer had little effect on true positive interpretations. However, when fewer than 1000 mammograms were read per year, the false-positive rate was markedly increased (Fig. 4-1).

Mammograms generally should not be interpreted along with other films. When mammograms are interpreted as part of a routine radiologic practice, the false-positive error rate increases markedly in comparison to a dedicated mammographic service where each mammographer interprets a large number of films. The proper interpretation of screening mammograms requires separate viewing facilities and dedicated equipment and personnel.

VIEWING SYSTEMS

Mammographic viewing systems require more light shading than is available in many radiologic imaging areas. Extraneous light is a problem in mammographic interpretation. Various shading techniques have been advocated. We have found hand-held shading devices to be the most effective means for rapid screening of large volumes of mammograms at the least cost. Screen-controlled shading systems, which limit extraneous light emanating from the viewing screen, are also effective.

Automatic viewing screens are more important in mammography than in other areas of diagnostic radiology. The rapid display of multiple images allows for a timely comparison between images and between patients. Goin et al. evaluated the contribution of viewing the radiographs of both right and left breasts simultaneously, as compared with viewing radiographs of the individual breasts alone.[39] In borderline cases, the noncancerous breast was occasionally identified as the most suspicious for cancer. When mammograms of the two breasts were compared, the false-positive rate was lower. We recommend that a screening mammogram be read by comparing the two breasts in both the mediolateral oblique and the craniocaudal projections. A lateral-medial examination should also be taken on the baseline screening examination. Special attention must be given to the presence of clustered microcalcifications.

NUMBER OF READERS

The quality of mammographic service depends in part on how many different radiologists interpret the mammograms in any single department. As the number of observers increases, interobserver disagreement also increases.

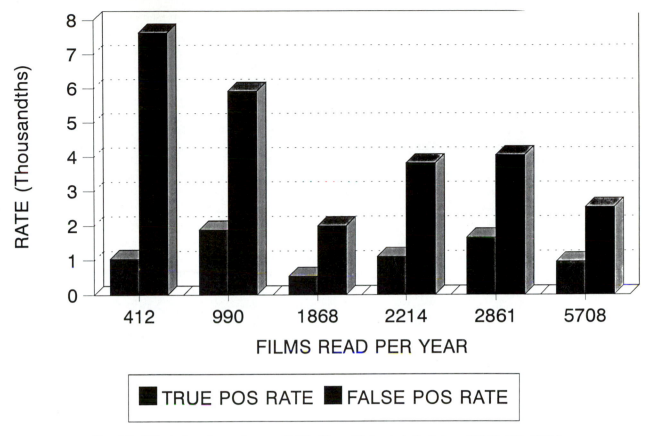

Fig. 4-1. Effect of reading volume on ROC. (From Ciatto et al: Radiology 165:99-102, 1987.)

The greater the number of radiologists who interpret mammograms, the less consist the reports in the eyes of the receiver of radiographic reports. Reporting consistency is extremely important in maintaining credibility and effective communication. When multiple observers report different mammograms on different patients to a single referring physician, credibility and communication may suffer. Vineis et al. studied interobserver agreement.[127] Eight radiologists interpreted the mammograms of 45 women for a total of 180 films per radiologist. These radiologists' experience varied from 100 to 4000 mammographic cases per year. Nine of the 45 women had breast cancer, 25 had benign disease, and 11 had normal breasts. Weighted kappa values were in the range 0.27 to 0.82 (median 0.60) for parenchymal patterns, 0.33 to 0.67 (median 0.48) for five classes of diagnosis, and 0.22 to 0.57 (median 0.38) for indications for further diagnostic tests.

The experience of the observer also markedly influences the quality of mammographic interpretation. Pamilo et al. studied the influence of the experience of the radiologist in the decision to recall for further studies 579 women who had screening mammograms.[85] The number of recalls for microcalcification decreased with experience, and the pro-

portion of breast cancer in this group increased over two screening rounds. They suggest that "a high ratio of malignancy in surgical biopsies can be expected when the radiologist undertaking primary screening also performed all further studies."

Moskowitz reviewed preoperative mammography reports provided by a pool of general radiologists.[74] Their series had high sensitivity (88%) but poor specificity (32%), with an overall accuracy of 46%. An experienced radiologist blindly reviewed the mammograms in retrospect and achieved a high sensitivity (100%), good specificity (73%), and an overall accuracy of almost 80%. They concluded that these results show the need for the most experienced radiologist available to be involved in deciding which of the difficult lesions require biopsy. This will reduce unnecessary surgery.

The amount of experience alone is not sufficient to identify the most skilled mammographic interpreter. Ciatto et al. reported the experiences of six different radiologists in interpreting screening mammograms.[23] His study was particularly interesting in that he reported indices of both the false positive and the false-negative interpretations. To infer whether there was an overcall (false-positive preponderance), he used the benign to malignant ratio based on the results of the biopsies each radiologist recommended. To assess whether cancers were being missed, he reported the cancer detection rate for each radiologist. Thus he was able to assess how many biopsies were being recommended for benign disease and how many cancers were detected per 1000 screening mammograms read.

The experience of each radiologist was evident from the number of films read in this study. The film reading volume ranged from 2883 to 39,955 over the 15-year period of analysis. The cancers detected per 1000 screening mammograms read ranged from 0.5 to 1.9, with a mean of 1.17 ± 0.46. The benign to malignant ratio ranged from 2.4:1 to 7.3:1 (mean 3.75 ± 1.64). Thus cancer was found in one out of every 3.4 biopsies recommended by one radiologist and one out of every 8.3 biopsies recommended by another radiologist who was reading mammograms from the same set of patients. The radiologists who read the most and the least films had significant differences in their benign to malignancy ratio, 2.7:1 versus 7.3:1 respectively. However, they had similar cancer detection rates, 0.9 verus 1.0. These observations suggest that while the number of films interpreted is extremely important in decreasing the number of biopsies recommended for benign disease, the independent skill of the observer is important in detecting cancer on a mammogram. Reading volume did not substantially affect the true cancer detection rate.

There is a distinct advantage to having more than one observer view each screening mammogram (dual reading). One can advocate dual reading and still limit the number of different radiologists who report mammograms from a single institution. The referring physician must be able to depend on consistent interpretations and communications. The communication chain is best maintained by having a limited number of radiologists responsible for a large volume of films. Currently, two radiologists are responsible for all the mammograms done at the Karolinska Institute. Each radiologist reads about 90 screening mammograms and 40 other mammograms each day. Screening mammograms are dual read. The large volume of mammograms is in part responsible for the radiologists' high sensitivity and specificity.

Bird et al. analyzed the mammographic reports of 58 nonpalpable breast lesions that were biopsied.[12] Sixteen of these were invasive or in situ carcinoma. Abnormal mammograms were reported by one of two independent radiologists during the normal course of practice and placed into one of five categories by each radiologist. Lesions scoring ≥3 were needle localized, excised, and examined histologically. All mammograms were later reviewed as unknowns by another radiologist and were similarly scored. A significant number of the cancers were scored differently by the two radiologists. These significant variations between radiologist interpretations reaffirm the need for double reading of screening mammogram films.

The need for dual reading does not require that each film be seen by two radiologists. Physician assistants can be taught to read screening mammograms. The initial screening of the films by trained physician assistants (PAs) can increase the volume of films read without sacrificing the quality of film interpretation. Hillman et al. studied the use of PAs for mammographic interpretation.[45] The interpretations by PAs were as sensitive and as specific as those made by six radiologists who interpreted the same cases. A relative operating characteristic analysis revealed the area under curves for PAs to be larger than the area under curves for radiologists. Interpretations by PAs took less time and cost less than did those by radiologists. The recommendations of the PAs were similar to those of the radiologists. They concluded that properly trained, evaluated, and supervised PAs can interpret mammograms. Legal, practical, and ethical considerations dictate that this can best be accomplished under the direction of radiologists well trained in mammography.

One possibility would be to have all screening mammograms read by two trained nonphysician readers. They would be instructed to pay special attention to microcalcifications, irregular densities, rounded lesions, and variations in regional breast density. They would be asked to set aside any film with anything even remotely suspicious. The intention is that they would only be asked to identify the truly normal case. This approach is similar to that advocated by Leo Rigler in the evaluation of screening chest films. The cases put aside may be as many as 50% of the screening films while the frequency of breast cancer is less than 1%. The radiologist would then review only these films. Each film would be examined with a higher index of suspicion. Someone else had already found something to be concerned about on these films. The expertise of the radiologist would then be used to provide what amounts to a second opinion on suspicious films. The radiologist would be better able to withstand the complacency induced by the reading of so many normal films. A system such as this may decrease both the false-negative and false-positive interpretations.

HOW TO REPORT A SCREENING MAMMOGRAM

The primary purpose of the mammographic report is to communicate observations and their implications. However, there are other important uses of the report that are often forgotten in the need to get the work done. For example, the radiologic report forms the basic data needed to evaluate the observer and the mammographic system. Without knowing what thoughts went from the interpreter of the image to the individual ultimately responsible for the care of the patient, it is difficult to test the implications of mammography to patient care. Thus individual radiologists would not be able to develop accurate relative operating characteristic (ROC) or receiver operating characteristic curves were they not held to some rigorous reporting system, whereby one could evaluate what was said and what was communicated.

ROCs are derived from signal detection theory and are used to describe how any system responds to a signal. Thus "receiver operating characteristic" has historic precedence. "Relative operating characteristic" is context independent and is therefore usually preferred.[125] Relative operating characteristics and receiving operating characteristics are essentially synonymous and are therefore used interchangably. ROCs refer to symptoms, signs, and laboratory values used in making a diagnosis. When both the graded diagnostic decisions and the ultimate proof of the presence or absence of a disease are available, ROC analyses can be carried out. Without graded diagnostic decisions, it is virtually impossible for individual radiologists to appreciate whether they are erring on the false-positive or false-negative side.[97]

Gohagan et al. used a comparative analysis of ROC curves in the BCDDP project to illustrate the clear superiority of mammography over clinical palpation as an individual screening modality and the further superiority of the combination of the two techniques.[38]

If a radiologist constantly hedges on the impression and recommendations in the report, it will be impossible to measure that radiologist's false-positive and false-negative rate in comparison with normal values. It will not be possible to develop an ROC curve unless one has an estimation of the "a priori" probability obtained at the moment of the radiologic interpretation. In order to obtain this ROC curve, it is necessary to have a reporting system that adheres rigorously to a standard formula. We must be able to evaluate the intention of the observer at the moment of observation.

At some time in the evaluation of screening mammograms, someone must make a firm decision. If the radiologist is unable to decide on the basis of the observation, then someone else must eventually do so. It is perfectly reasonable to manifest a level of uncertainty. However, if one is uncertain in all cases observed, it will be difficult for the radiologist to learn from experience and for a quality assurance system to know the contribution of screening mammography. It is important to know what mammography can contribute to the care of patients in an ever-changing medical care system.

Timing the communication

The timing of information flow from the mammographic interpreter to the clinician caring for the patient is important from the medical and legal standpoint. If there is a significant finding on the mammogram that warrants urgent attention, direct verbal communication of the report is necessary. Usually this would be done by a telephone call. Obviously, anything that can enhance the dialogue between the individual interpreting the radiograph and the clinician ultimately responsible for the care of the patient would eventually go to benefit the patient care and the system of mammography.

A written report is the traditional means of communication. This is sufficient as long as the chain linking the initial dictation of the report to the ultimate reception by the referring physician is adequate. For legal purposes, it is important to have a standardized business practice that effects a quality control on the flow of the dictated report from the observer to the receiver of the information.

Robertson and Kopans have identified a significant problem in communicating the information from radiographs.[95] In their study they observed a substantial delay between dictation of the report and the time something was done for the patient. In most cases of breast cancer detection this level of delay may not have much clinical significance. However, the prolongation of patient anxiety and uncertainty is a major problem in obtaining compliance with a system for the early detection of breast cancer. Anything we can do to decrease the uncertainty in the patient and to provide the earliest possible reassurance of normality in the worried may well have a substantial impact on ultimate use of screening mammography.

Communication system

There are many ways in which radiologists dictate their reports. One is the automatic dictation system where one identifies on a computer a series of possible attributes that are ultimately put into the sentences for the written report. If one uses this technique, it is important to appreciate the implications of alternative writing styles. Automatic reports range from a very clear to a noninformative confused writing style. There is nothing wrong with reporting "normal" when normal is what is apparent. However, it is useful to present a discussion of the ranges of normality envisioned when interpreting a radiograph. The report should convey to the reader some index of the certainty of observation. A normal mammogram in a dense breast is quite different from a normal mammogram in an entirely radiolucent breast. The possibilities of masked cancer in the dense breast are considerably greater. Bongiorni et al. emphasized the structurally dense breast as an intrinsic factor limiting mammographic accuracy.[16] Depending on the risk factors and other concerns, an individual with a dense breast may be a candidate for more vigilant observation. The radiologist can be more certain of the absence of early breast cancer in women with a relatively radiolucent breast. Automatic dictating systems that merely state "normal" may not clearly delineate variations in normality that may affect patient care. The same holds true for the presence or absence of calcifications, most of which appear to be benign. It is important to describe the appearance of calcifications in order to convey the possibility of malignancy.

A more traditional system is a customized dictation for each patient. Experienced mammographers have a wide reference base for a normal screening mammogram. Many different mammographic appearances are entirely normal. Most screening mammograms are normal. A wide range of normal variations must be recognized and appreciated as normal if screening mammography is to provide useful clinical information.

A hybrid reporting system uses customized dictation for variation of the normal and an automatic report for a truly high-certainty normal. In each instance a probability estimate or a scaling system should be used so that the referring physician can appreciate the certitude with which the a priori impression is made. Unfortunately, proper a priori probabilities in screening mammography are so low that it may be difficult to assign a number that represents the true probability without confusing the referring physician. Less than 1% of screening mammograms will reveal breast cancer. If one limits this probability to nonpalpable cancers, this number is even less. Therefore the probability of a screening mammogram being normal is 99+%. If that number were put on most mammogram reports, the prediction of normality would be correct and highly accurate, but not very useful.

A callback system for screening mammography may not require that any report be issued in response to the screening mammogram. At the Karolinska Institute the examinations are considered to be normal if the patient is not called back for further diagnostic studies. A callback implies that this screening mammogram warrants that further evaluation be done. It does not assert normal or abnormal, nor does it necessarily provoke an undue concern for cancer. This system merely says that the radiologist is sufficiently uncertain at the present time to conclude that this screening mammogram is normal. Further evaluation is warranted. When using a simple callback system without further description or a report, it is important that the referring physicians and the patients be aware of the system in order to reduce undue anxieties.

Style of communication

A standard style of radiologic communication is needed for mammograms. Typically, a description of the objective observations is communicated initially so that the reader will be able to appreciate the basis on which the ultimate interpretation is made. The issues of age, risk factors, and other attributes of the mammogram, including benign calcifications and irregular mottling, are all factors affecting the diagnosis of normality. Thus they should be included in the descriptive narrative that precedes the interpretation.

The description is then followed by an interpretation that combines the elements of observation with the implications for the patient. An interpretation in screening mammography would most often read "this mammogram is normal." It is easier to interpret a mammogram as normal when a previous normal mammogram is available for comparison.

Many physicians read only the interpretation portion of the report. Therefore the clarity of this part of the report is most important. In our opinion, all written mammographic reports should conclude with a recommendation. *The mammographer is uniquely aware of the certitude of the mammographic interpretation.* While it is important to share the level of certainty in reading screening mammograms, the radiologist is responsible for the interpretation and its implications in the care of the patient. Thus a concluding recommendation is most appropriate.

A report therefore contains a description of the objective observation and an interpretation of what those observations mean for that patient followed by a recommendation for subsequent care of that patient. In the United States, recommendations usually suggest follow-up mammograms according to the American Cancer Society's guidelines. These guidelines are usually considered appropriate for the timing of subsequent screening mammograms. This approach allows for variation in individual recommendations and ultimate care.

Once the observation, interpretation, and recommendations are imparted, it is important for purposes of communication to have a classification of the mammogram so that a subsequent audit can assess the implication of this mammogram relative to a normal standard.

A practice audit is an essential component of quality control in mammography. The mammographer must have the data needed to constantly learn by experience. It is almost impossible for a radiologist to be fully aware of the experiences he/she has had in mammography without having some system to collect and analyze the experience in a sufficient number of interpretations. Therefore, one could evaluate for an excess in either false-positive interpretations or missed breast cancers.

We support the standard international classification in mammographic interpretation. If all mammographers used the same standard reporting system, it would be much easier to compare the various international studies intended to assess the value of mammography under specific circumstances. The international system is essentially a five-part interpretation that is important for both data gathering and standardization between different radiologists and different institutions.

The standard international classification uses six categories: Category 0   No breast
Category 1   Normal

Category 2   Abnormal, but not malignant. For example: a fibroadenoma, extensive number of benign microcalcifications, unusual density, apparent benign cystic disease, etc.

Category 3   Abnormal, doubtful. Warrants further attention. For example: callback or a fine-needle aspiration.

Category 4   Probably malignant, will need surgery.

Category 5   Definitively malignant. (Tell the pathologist to recut the tissues if no cancer is found on the first analysis.)

Categories 3, 4, and 5 most often require follow-up and attention by the referring physician. Most screening mammograms will be read as a category 1. However, some near-normals will be read as category 2. The differences between categories 1 and 2 are not usually clinically significant. The abnormalities seen with category 2 do not warrant further attention. Their importance is that there is no reason for further concern by the patient or the referring physician. An awareness of the abnormality, however, may be important to the patient's care, particularly since future observers may conclude that this benign abnormality has a probability of malignancy, which would affect the patient (Table 4-1).

Category 3 patients will usually benefit from fine-needle aspiration as a prerequisite to consideration for surgical biopsy. Category 3 patients will infrequently need a surgical biopsy (percentages), whereas all category 4 patients will require a surgical biopsy. In the Karolinska experience, 1.2% of screening mammograms were interpreted as category 3. All underwent fine-needle aspiration. Only 25% of those category 3 patients or 0.27% of the total screening mammograms ultimately had a surgical biopsy. If mammographic interpretation alone had been used as the criterion for surgical biopsy, all category 3 patients would have had a surgical biopsy. The interposing of stereotaxic fine-needle aspiration between the mammographic interpretation and the surgical biopsy decreased the number of surgical biopsies by 75% in this group of patients. Their mammograms were disconcerting but did not contain evidence of definite cancer. Some 3% of screening mammograms eventually led to a fine-needle aspiration, but less than 1% led to surgical biopsies in a population of women whose prevalence rate of breast cancer approaches that of the surgical biopsy rate.

Even in category 4, the prebiopsy information as to the possible pathologic findings obtained by FNA is useful to effect the most appropriate surgical strategies. If we do a fine-needle aspiration on a category 4 patient and find malignancy, we can be sufficiently certain of the diagnosis that a one-stage surgical biopsy becomes a feasible initial surgical approach. Category 5, when observed in nonpal-

Table 4-1. Karolinska experience in interpretation of 18,987 screening mammograms from August 1989 to June 1991

	Classified mammogram		Cytology		Surgical	
	No.	%	No.	%	No.	%
Category 1	226	1.19	19*	0.10	0	0
Category 2	163	0.96	98	0.52	7	0.03
Category 3	228	1.2	228	1.2	51	0.27
Category 4	34	0.18	34	0.18	34	0.18
Category 5	84	0.44	84	0.44	83†	0.4
TOTAL	716	3.7	567	2.99	175	0.92

735 (3.87%) females recalled (without classifying mammograms).
*FNA because the patient and/or physician "thought" they felt something.
†One patient refused surgery.

pable breast cancer, is the type of mammographic observation that we would diagnose as cancer independent of what the fine-needle aspirate reveals or what the pathologist may find on the initial histologic examination.

TYPES OF ERROR IN SCREENING MAMMOGRAPHY

The types of errors found in mammographic interpretation are important to understand if one is to seek and appreciate the implications of an individual ROC curve.[125] The quality of screening mammography is measured by comparing an individual's experience with the behavior of a large number of observers. In order to know whether we are doing as good a job as we can or as good as others do, it is necessary to have adequate data on the experience of individual observers or individual systems of breast system screening. A major problem in evaluating breast cancer screening is the inconsistent measures in reporting the experience of individual observers or systems of observation. Without consistent and uniform data collection, we cannot conclude which system or individual observer is preferable to another. It is possible, through appropriate data base management and auditing of mammographic practices, for radiologists to closely monitor their proclivity toward either missing cancers or suspecting cancer where none is present.

The false-negative, "the missed cancer," is the most common concern of individuals interpreting screening mammograms (see Chapter 2). This has been a legal basis for malpractice litigation. A missed cancer is considerably more likely to result in litigation in the United States than is a request for a surgical biopsy that turns out to be benign. Most physicians practice conservatively. "The worst thing to do would be to miss a cancer." This conclusion is not necessarily valid. Some cancers will not be observed on a mammogram no matter what is done. In other instances, a false-positive examination can result in harm to the patient. A tension between false-positive and false-negative interpretations is an expected outcome of the uncertainty induced in interpreting examinations. This can be as subjective or as judgmental as mammography. It is important that we define parameters in interpreting mammography. We should seek to increase the objective elements in mammographic interpretation.

There are many measures of the quality of mammographic interpretations that relate to the type of error, i.e., false positive or false negative. Positive predictive value equals the true positive divided by the true positive plus the false positive (PPV = TP/[TP + FP]). Thus PPV equals the number of cancers diagnosed per number of biopsies recommended. The negative predictive value equals the true negative divided by the true negative plus the false negative (NPV = TN/[TN + FN]).

The measurement of sensitivity of a diagnostic procedure is the index that indicates whether the procedure will be able to identify the abnormality. Sensitivity equals the true positive divided by the true positive plus the false negative (Sensitivity = TP/[TP + FN]). Sensitivity equals the number of breast cancers detected by the screening system in relation to the number of breast cancers existing in the population being screened. Specificity equals the true negative divided by the true negative plus the false positive (Specificity = TN/[TN + FP]). Accuracy equals the true positive plus the true negative divided by the total number of patients. Most radiologists are fully familiar with the issues of sensitivity, specificity, and accuracy. However, it is not apparent that they routinely apply these when they develop their experiential data appropriate to their own practice of radiology.

Another measure used is the false-positive rate. The false-positive rate equals the false positive divided by the false plus the true positive (FPR = FP/[FP + TP]). Of these measures, the accuracy of a diagnostic test has the least utility. Accuracy does not define what should be changed to improve on our ability to detect disease and, at the same time, does not include normal patients into the prospective diseased population. For example, Sener et al. reported results on 321 patients who had excisional biopsies of nonpalpable mammographic abnormalities.[106] Their mammographic impression had a sensitivity of 0.64 (48/75) and specificity of 0.898 (221/246). They had a false-positive rate of 0.34 (25/73) and false-negative rate of 0.07 (10/141).

It is important in screening mammography to do whatever we can to decrease the number of patients who are subjected to "unnecessary" surgical biopsies and/or breast surgery. Unnecessary surgical biopsies expose patients to

the risk of error in pathologic diagnosis, excessive surgical intervention, and the psychologic trauma that goes with unwarranted mastectomies. While we seek to eliminate unnecessary surgical biopsies, we must keep in mind the need to detect breast cancer as early as possible so that breast-conserving surgery can be used to decrease breast cancer mortality.

Mammographic sensitivity

How many mammograms miss a cancer? What is an expected false-negative rate? There are three ways to estimate the false-negative rate or sensitivity of a system or system component designed to detect breast cancer. These are (1) the comparative incidence rate, (2) the interval cancer rate, and (3) the "gold standard comparison," a comparison with an alternative diagnostic method or known disorders. How good is screening mammography in detecting breast cancer? It is easy to know how many breast cancers are detected per screening mammograms done. We just compare cancers found with the number of examinations done. If we knew the annual incidence rate of breast cancer *in the population being screened*, it would be relatively easy to estimate how many of the total cancers were detected by mammography. We could also estimate how many were missed and thereby obtain a false-negative rate.

To reliably use this approach, we must have a thorough understanding of the risk profile of the patient population versus the population from which the incidence figures were derived. Local population and risk-specific incidence figures are usually not available. Despite these limitations, the cancer detection rate of a breast cancer detection system can provide a useful index of the sensitivity of the system. For example, the first year of the Karolinska breast cancer screening program detected 7.3 cancers per 1000 women screened. These women were not selected on the basis of risk other than age. The screen was limited to women between the ages of 50 and 69 years. Since this was the first year of the program, most of these women were exposed to a prevalence screen.

We estimate the prevalence of breast cancer in Stockholm to be about 8.0 per 1000 women of this age. The numbers for this population are derived from the country as a whole, though some local differences may exist. The mammographic screen detected breast cancer at approximately the same rate estimated for the population under study. It seems unlikely that many breast cancers were missed. However, in view of the lead time bias, the number of cancers detected on a mammographic screen may exceed that established by clinical prevalence data.

Clinical prevalence data are often obtained on the basis of symptomatic breast cancer. The mammographic detection of "preclinical" breast cancer may appear to have detected all the cancers when indeed a different population of cancers was detected. The system may have missed some cancers and picked up others that would not have been identified yet in a traditional prevalence study that included all symptomatic patients. At the Karolinska Institute, every suspicious mammogram leads to a callback and additional diagnostic studies including a clinical examination. However, some clinically detectable subtle breast cancers may have been missed on the screen and not be noted as missed by an incidence or prevalence comparison study.

A second way to determine missed cancers is to study comparative interval cancer rates (see Chapter 2). If we wish to compare two proposed systems of breast cancer diagnosis that involve periodic screening, we can attempt to evaluate the number of breast cancers missed in the screen by observing the number of cancers diagnosed in the interval between screens. As discussed in Chapter 2, interval cancers are due to more than just the ability of the screen to detect cancer. Some 58% of interval cancers are true interval cancers.[88] When all other factors are held constant, the interval cancer rate depends on the incidence rate, growth rate of the cancer, observer error, and technical flaws. Only the last two can be considered as contributing to a false-negative diagnosis.

Bartl et al. found that 15% of breast cancers in his series were not mammographically detectable.[8] False-negative mammograms do occur in patients whose breast cancer is first found in metastatic axillary nodes. Haupt et al. found abnormal mammograms in only 11 of 31 patients (35%) with metastatic cancer in axillary nodes who were subsequently found to have primary cancer in the ipsilateral breast.[42] In order to identify how many breast cancers are not mammographically detectable, it is necessary to detect the breast cancer by some other means. These breast cancers are usually interval cancers, or those detected clinically. Thus relatively few good studies have truly assessed the mammographic sensitivity in detecting nonpalpable breast cancers. Most reports of false-negative mammograms have been women with normal mammograms who have palpable breast cancers. Mann et al. reviewed the effects of the normal mammogram on the treatment of 36 women with palpable breast cancers during a 2-year period. On the 17 patients who had biopsies within 1 month of a normal mammogram, three (17.6%) had extension of disease to axillary nodes. Of 19 patients whose biopsy was delayed for 3 to 24 months, cancer was found in axillary nodes of 11 (57.9%).[67]

These observations are responsible for the widely held shibboleth that mammography should not be used to exclude the presence of cancer in a newly palpable breast lump. For purposes of this discussion, however, we are emphasizing *nonpalpable* breast cancer. Concern for the palpable cancer is only related to the limitations of the mammogram in diagnosing such cancer.

The inability to detect some palpable cancers on the mammogram has often been considered an issue of mammographic error. However, we will limit our discussion to those failures to detect breast cancer that could have been, and perhaps should have been, detected on the initial mammogram. The sensitivity of the mammographic system in detecting nonpalpable breast cancer depends on a number of factors. These include:

1. The population being studied. The risk factors or ambient frequency of the disease in the population will affect the sensitivity of the breast cancer detection system.
2. The technique used in the mammographic procedure. The accuracy of the prebiopsy impression will be better in a system where substantial effort is directed toward the quality of the mammographic image. Poor mammograms more often result in missed lesions and a large number of unnecessary surgical biopsies.
3. The interpretive skills of the observer. Observer performance has received considerable attention in quality control systems designed to enhance the usefulness of mammography for detection of early breast cancer. While mammographic interpretive skills substantially influence the ability of the system to detect early breast cancer, interpretative accuracy will vary substantially depending on how early the cancer is to be recognized.

Kopans points out that in measuring the positive predictive value (PPV) of a diagnostic system, it is important to consider the stage at which the diagnosis was made.[52] If the observer seeks to detect the smallest of cancers, there will be an increasing false-positive rate. If one limits the detection to large cancers that have already spread to the axillary nodes, the interpretation of the mammogram will yield a high proportion of true-positive cases. The question of sensitivity is directed toward false-negative diagnoses. The smaller the lesion being sought, the more likely there will be false-positive interpretations. Conversely, if we seek to detect only large lesions, the accuracy of the detection system will increase. Small lesions will more likely be missed when the observer limits the observation to obvious breast cancers.

As Kopans discusses, the usefulness of any specific PPV depends heavily on a number of elements.[52] Therefore, it has been difficult to define a specific PPV to be applied in all cases. He notes that the risk factors and prevalence rates are essential data in identifying which PPV we should attain. The size of the cancer, the histologic type, and the stage are important considerations. In order to compare one interpreter to another, it is necessary to appreciate the nature of the false-negative mammograms that have occurred. We must distinguish among those that are not visible, those masked by normal breast tissue, and those visible in retrospect.

PATHOLOGIC BASIS OF SCREENING MAMMOGRAPHY

The major distinction observed between the customary mammographic interpretation and mammographic interpretation that excels in distinguishing normality from significant pathology resides in the radiologist's understanding of the normal anatomy and ranges of pathologic entities found in the human breast. A radiologist must clearly understand the possible pathologic constraints or anatomic variations that may create the mammographic image. If a density cannot be explained on the basis of anatomic or pathologic entities, then it will usually be meaningful. Any radiologist who assumes responsibility for the interpretation of mammograms has a duty to be conversant with breast disorders. When a suspected abnormality is detected on a mammogram, the radiologist must seek to ascertain its anatomic or pathologic correlate. The mammographer must seek to translate a density into a possible pathologic representation.

To better appreciate the mammographic features of nonpalpable cancer, it is reasonable to begin with a review of what is known about the histologic basis for the mammographic image of nonpalpable breast cancer. We then discuss the scientific grounds for the features of breast cancer seen on screening mammograms.

In the simplest terms, the breast is composed of fat and stroma. The stroma is composed of connective tissue and glandular structures in varying phases of development and activity. These lobules and ducts, with their intervening septa, account for the stromal structure seen in a mammogram. Normally, the vessels of the breast are also clearly seen. What then are the pathologic changes in the breast that we are seeking to identify in screening mammograms?

Correlation of mammography to histology

The correlation of mammographic detectability to the histology of the lesion was studied by Bartl et al. in 52 women with stage I breast cancer.[8] They had a mammographic sensitivity of 85% of the breast cancers they studied. In tumors with a large amount of connective tissue (scirrhous or invasive cancer) the sensitivity was 94%, whereas in tumors with little connective tissue (solid, medullary, adenomatous, papillary) the sensitivity decreased to 69%. This helps to explain the different ability of mammography to detect certain types of breast cancer. Holland et al. identified histologic characteristics of invasive lobular carcinomas to explain why they are mammographically occult even in the advanced stage.[46] They reviewed the pathology and radiology of 15 mammographically occult breast cancers, 3 of which were preinvasive and 12 invasive. In addition, they studied 52 breast cancers that showed only microcalcifications without an associated tumor shadow (33 preinvasive and 19 invasive). They observed that invasive lobular cancers have a diffuse distribution and frequently a poor desmoplastic reaction, in contrast to invasive ductal cancers, whose greater desmoplastic reaction makes them more visible on mammography.

The correlation of mammographic size to the size of the lesion found by the pathologist is necessary to measure tumor growth and to stage tumors by size. Geppert et al. compared the mammographic appearance to the pathology in 24 patients with minute breast cancers (diameter of 0.5 cm or less) with the mammographic appearance of infiltrating cancers with diameters ranging from 1.8 to 2.4 cm.[36] Larger cancers showed a good correlation between the microscopic and radiologic diameter of the tumor. In the smaller cancers, the radiologic size was greater than the microscopic diameter. The covering tissue of these minute tumors was rich in fibroblasts and poor in fibers. This is responsible for this difference in apparent size as seen on the mammogram.

Owings et al. studied how thoroughly a needle localization biopsy should be sampled for microscopic examination and developed guidelines for specimen sampling by prospectively studying 157 consecutive needle localization breast biopsies.[82] Microscopically, 32% of the cases showed cancer, 12% demonstrated atypical hyperplasia, and 56% were benign breast tissue without atypia. All were performed because of mammographic microcalcifications without a soft tissue density. The macroscopic examination in each case failed to reveal a gross lesion. Forty-nine of 50 cancers (98%) and 14 of 19 atypical hyperplasias (74%) were associated with mammographic microcalcifications. Thirty-eight percent fewer blocks would have been processed if the histologic examination were restricted to areas with microcalcifications and not included the remaining breast tissue removed at surgery. They conclude that restricting histologic examination to areas of radiographic calcifications and fibrous parenchyma results in a high level of detection of clinically significant lesions and a considerable reduction in the amount of tissue processed.

Andersen et al. observed a histologic distinction between three different growth patterns: (1) microfocal, (2) tumor forming, and (3) diffuse.[2] This was based on a prospective study of 40 consecutive patients with in situ carcinomas of the breast and two with atypical ductal hyperplasia (ADH) who underwent an operation during a 2-year period at a single hospital. In situ carcinomas made up about 9% of all newly diagnosed breast cancers. With the exception of one case, the 26 microfocal growths (2 ADH, 13 LCIS, 11 DCIS) were accidental findings in otherwise benign breast biopsies. The tumor-forming and diffuse ductal carcinoma in situ were diagnosed clinically and/or by mammography. Of the tumor-forming and diffuse DCIS, 25% were demonstrated solely by mammography.

Mammograms have been used to demonstrate the presence or absence of an extensive intraductal component in early infiltrating ductal carcinoma. This information is important to determine the extent of surgical resection needed before radiation therapy. Healey et al. reviewed the preoperative mammographic findings in 105 cases of stage I and stage II infiltrating ductal carcinoma.[43] Cancers with an extensive intraductal component were significantly more likely to show microcalcifications with or without a mass compared to those without an extensive intraductal component (83% versus 27%, p < 0.0001). The presence of microcalcifications without a mammographic mass was more common for cancers with an extensive intraductal component (34% versus 5%, p = 0.0002). Conversely, a soft tissue mass without microcalcifications was seen mammographically in 56% of patients without an extensive intraductal component, compared to only 10% of cases with an extensive intraductal component (p < 0.0001). The presence of microcalcifications in the absence of a mammographic mass has a 73% likelihood that the cancer will have an extensive intraductal component (95% confidence interval = 39% to 94%). Microcalcifications without a mass are more commonly associated with an extensive intraductal component of the cancer.

Mammography and hormone receptors. Broberg et al. studied the relationship between mammographic pattern and estrogen receptor content in the breast.[18] He divided the mammograms obtained from 184 patients with cancer into five radiologic subgroups:

A. Mass with spicules
B. Diffuse
C. Clusters of calcifications without mass
D. Circumscribed
E. Not visible at mammography

The estrogen receptor (ER) content of the 121 group A tumors was higher than that of the other subgroups in both pre- and postmenopausal women. Eighty percent of group A tumors were ductal cancers. The tumors in groups B and C had very low ER values and those of groups D and E had intermediate values. The likelihood of finding a high ER content of a tumor is thus greater when the tumor is seen radiographically as a mass with spicules than when it appears to be clusters of microcalcifications. It is suggested that patients with tumors belonging to group A should have a more favorable prognosis than patients with tumors belonging to groups B and C.

Conversely, Ainge et al. compared hormone receptors to mammographic appearance in patients with breast cancer.[1] In 210 patients with unilateral breast cancer, they found no statistically significant association between tumor morphology and progesterone receptors.

Axillary metastasis/faster growing cancers. Schwartz et al. observed that women who had invasive cancers that appeared as clustered calcifications were just as likely to have axillary metastases as women who had nonpalpable mammographic masses.[108] Tinnemans et al. reported on 153 consecutive patients with clusters of at least five microcalcifications without palpable findings as the only indications for biopsy.[126] One hundred and seventy-three groups of microcalcifications were excised and 51 malignancies were detected (29.5%). Most of the malignant lesions were noninfiltrating (56%). Axillary or distant metastases occurred in 11% of the cases that were fully evaluated.

Colbassani et al. reported 55 patients with isolated microcalcification clusters and no palpable tumor.[24] Fifteen of these patients had malignant lesions at biopsy. Ten of these cancers were noninvasive. Only one of the five invasive cancers had axillary metastases (20%). Prorok et al. reported 62 women who had excisional breast biopsy for microcalcification and no associated palpable mass. Carcinoma was discovered in 20 (32%).[93] These cancers ranged in size from 0.6 to 14 mm in greatest diameter. Six patients had multicentric carcinoma, including one with synchronous bilateral lobular carcinoma. Axillary metastasis was present in three patients (15%), each with multicentric lesions.

Heuser et al. defined fast cancers as those surfacing between two screening mammograms.[44] He divided these fast cancers into two subsets: fast 1 and fast 2. The faster cancers were discovered in younger patients and had a smaller 5-year survival rate. Fast 1 had a 74% (±9%) 5-year survival rate, while slower growing cancers had a 94% (±4%) 5-year survival rate. Faster growing cancers had a significant lack of mammographic microcalcifications. The absence of microcalcifications and the presence of lymphatic invasion around the primary cancer site were associated with axillary metastases. Other factors associated with axillary metastases were higher mitotic index, poor cellular differentiation, and larger size of the cancer at diagnosis. These authors confirm that interval cancers are biologically different and not comparable to cancers discovered by scheduled screens. Cancers that metastasize to lymph nodes while very small have properties similar to true interval cancers, which are presumably faster growing cancers.

Meyer et al. reported on 500 preoperative guided localizations for occult lesions over a period of 5 years.[71] They had a PPV of 23.4%. In their series the biopsy was prompted by abnormal calcifications in 41% and by occult masses, areas of architectural distortion, or asymmetry in 59%. Seventy-four of the 117 patients with carcinoma had axillary node dissection. Twenty-two percent had axillary metastasis.

Marrujo et al. studied 237 radiologically suspicious nonpalpable lesions. In this series they found 64 nonpalpable, 25 invasive, 16 minimally invasive, and 23 noninvasive cancers.[68] Their PPV was 28.7%. The noninvasive and minimally invasive cancers tended to occur in younger women, average age 52 and 51 years respectively. These almost always appeared as clustered microcalcifications. Invasive cancers affected an older population (average age 65), and in a majority of cases the mammographic appearance was that of a mass. A review of surgical specimens revealed that 27% had residual disease at the biopsy site. Of the patients who underwent mastectomy, 34% had an unsuspected focus of cancer on another quadrant of the breast. An additional 14% had an unsuspected focus of epithelial atypia.

No patient with either noninvasive or minimally invasive cancer was found to have axillary lymph node metastases, whereas 29% with invasive tumors had axillary metastases. Marrujo et al. believe that treatment must address the high incidence of residual disease at the biopsy site, the multicentricity, and the proved capacity for invasive lesions to metastasize to the axillary lymph nodes, regardless of the size of the primary tumor.[68]

Ronay et al. reviewed 1048 breast cancer patients operated on from 1969 to 1985 at the University of Erlangen Clinic.[98] Bilateral simultaneous disease occurred in 17% (6.1% invasive forms, 10.6% in situ) of the patients. Contralateral nonpalpable breast cancers detected by mammography averaged 9 mm in diameter; axillary metastasis occurred in 20% of these. Palpable breast cancers with positive mammograms averaged 17 mm in diameter, and 41% of cases had axillary metastasis.

Bongiorni et al. observed that the increased proportion of breast cancers diagnosed by mammography alone has increased the proportion of comedocarcinoma from 5% to 14%.[16] Comedocarcinoma now ranks second in breast cancer incidence. This increase is in part due to the earlier diagnosis of breast cancer, which has intraductal calcifications. Most comedocarcinoma can be diagnosed mammographically by the characteristic intraductal calcifications (Table 4-2).

Carcinoma in situ: its clinical and radiologic implications

Understanding of the radiology, pathology, and biology of carcinoma in situ is a prerequisite to appreciating the implications of the various efforts designed to detect early breast cancer. Although the issues relevant to carcinoma in situ have been clarified in the literature, they do not seem to be widely appreciated by clinicians. Most invasive carcinomas of the breast begin as a proliferation of potentially malignant cells within the lumen of the ductal lobular system. Carcinoma in situ appears to arise from the same region of the breast as do invasive carcinomas. There may be a continuum between epithelial atypia, carcinoma in situ, and invasive carcinoma.

Carcinoma in situ of the breast is divided into two

Table 4-2. Histologic diagnoses for 121 ductal carcinomas that were biopsied on the basis of microcalcifications alone, without a visible tumor shadow

Diagnosis	Number
Comedocarcinoma	60
Fine papillary/cribriform carcinoma	11
Mixed forms (comedo and cribriform)	40
Ductal carcinoma (further differentiation was not possible retrospectively)	10
TOTAL	121

From Lanyi M: *Diagnosis and differential diagnosis of breast calcifications,* New York, 1986, Springer-Verlag.

types, lobular carcinoma in situ (LCIS) and ductal carcinoma in situ (DCIS). These two entities differ on the basis of histology, clinical presentation, biology, and management (see Chapter 2). The distinction between the two entities is extremely important in the mammographic diagnosis of early breast cancer. Indeed, screening mammography has been largely responsible for the increasing recognition of these entities and has occasioned a number of recent reviews.[25,35,107] The distinction between LCIS and DCIS is usually not difficult based on the mammographic appearance and the histology. Occasionally, however, the two entities will exist together.

The frequency of in situ carcinoma of the breast has been identified in necropsy studies in Denmark. Nielsen reported that about 25% of all women develop in situ cancer of the breast without coexisting invasive growth.[77,78] Usually this is only seen after painstaking histologic examination of the entire breast. Of 110 women 20 to 54 years of age who were autopsied for medicolegal reasons not related to the possibility of breast cancer, 18% had occult breast cancer. Thus the prevalence of in situ carcinoma in the human breast is clearly different from that which is diagnosed during life. It has been estimated that there is a 0.53% risk of having in situ breast cancer diagnosed between the ages of 20 and 75 years when mammographic screening is not available.[15] Thus, only a small fraction of in situ lesions are ever diagnosed clinically. In the Danish epidemiologic study, when mammography was routinely used for all symptomatic patients, in situ cancers comprised 6% of all newly diagnosed breast cancer.

Lobular carcinoma in situ (LCIS). Lobular carcinoma in situ (LCIS) was first described and named by Foote and Stewart in 1941.[33] The clinical significance of LCIS is no longer controversial. Most investigators believe that this lesion represents a risk factor for invasive cancer but is not to be considered a cancer as such. Haagensen et al. insisted on calling this lesion "lobular neoplasia," rather than "lobular carcinoma in situ."[40] since they worried that the designation of carcinoma would imply an inappropriate degree of malignancy.

LCIS predominantly occurs in premenopausal women and is most often an incidental finding in breast tissue excised for some other reason. LCIS is not associated with any radiologic abnormalities. While Sigfusson et al. claimed a type of calcification associated with LCIS, most other authors have refuted the contention that LCIS is associated with any specific form of calcification.[116] Lanyi et al. assert that it is no longer appropriate to evaluate calcifications histologically on the chance that lobular neoplasia (LCIS) may be associated with them.[59] They completely agree with Lewison, who says "some enthusiastic radiologists . . . claim that (lobular) carcinoma in situ can be recognized by mammography. In my opinion, this is a 'triumph of hope over experience.' "[63]

LCIS is characterized by small, noncohesive cells filling and expanding a lobule. They may occasionally spread to the ducts. The biology of this lesion has been evaluated by Rosen et al. and Haagensen et al.[40,100] Rosen followed 99 patients with LCIS for an average of 24 years. Eighteen percent of his patients developed an ipsilateral invasive cancer. A contralateral invasive cancer was eventually diagnosed in 13.5 of these patients. It took more than 15 years after the initial biopsy for these invasive cancers to become evident. Almost 40% were not detected until after 20 years.

Haagensen did a retrospective review of 5560 patients with an original diagnosis of benign disease.[40] In these he found 211 cases of LCIS. Sixty-three percent of these LCIS patients were followed for at least 10 years (mean 14 years). Carcinoma eventually developed in 36 of these patients (17%) and was likely to recur with equal frequency in either breast. Thus LCIS represents a risk factor for the subsequent development of invasive carcinoma anywhere in either breast. This risk has been estimated at approximately 1% per year and is present for the lifetime of the patient.[25]

Rusnak et al. suggest that LCIS will have as high as a 20% incidence of cancer after a 15-year follow-up, with each breast being equally at risk.[103] LCIS is a ubiquitous lesion often found in otherwise normal breasts. It may be part of a continuum from normal epithelium to epithelial atypia to lobular carcinoma in situ to invasive lobular cancer. The lesion is often multifocal but will usually not develop into invasive cancer. The appropriate management is to do no more than maintain vigilant observation by periodic mammograms seeking evidence of invasive cancer. However, the mammogram is notoriously insensitive in lobular carcinomas for the reasons discussed previously. Blichert-Toft emphasized that lobular carcinoma in situ is an incidental finding of a pathologist and does not have radiologic characteristics.[14]

Whether lobular carcinoma in situ is to be considered as a true cancer becomes an important consideration in reviewing the accuracy of various diagnostic maneuvers recommended in detecting breast cancer. Considering LCIS a normal risk variant is very different from including LCIS with invasive breast cancer in studies designed to evaluate the effectiveness of various diagnostic regimens. The failure to clearly separate these pathologic conditions has resulted in confusion about the most effective means to limit the number of "unnecessary surgical biopsies" induced by a false-positive mammographic interpretation.

Ductal carcinoma in situ (DCIS). Ductal carcinoma in situ (DCIS) is considered to be a true cancer in its earliest stages. If not treated, these lesions may well become invasive. DCIS is an entirely different disease than LCIS in terms of its biology, natural course, and appropriate treatment. Indeed, the radiologic detection of ductal carcinoma in situ is a major objective of screening mammography. This disease is being diagnosed with increasing frequency by the presence of mammographic microcalcifications. Connolly et al. found microcalcifications in 85% of DCIS cases.[25]

Ikeda et al., in a retrospective study of mammograms in 190 women with biopsy-proven DCIS, found that 117 (62%) of the women had mammograms that showed suspicious clustered microcalcifications.[50] Of the remaining 73 (38%) of the women, 30 (16%) had negative mammograms, and 43 (23%) of these DCIS patients had mammographic manifestations of breast cancer other than microcalcifications.

The pathology of DCIS is characterized by the proliferation of a single cell population. Different cell types may be involved, and these are responsible for the different patterns identified in DCIS histology. These distinguishing characteristics have very little clinical significance other than the comedo type, which may have a faster rate of proliferation than other DCIS cell populations.

The natural history of DCIS has been difficult to assess. Rosen et al. and Page et al. attempted to study the natural history of DCIS by reexamining biopsy specimens originally categorized as benign.[84,99] Because of the way the cases were selected for these studies, the more malignant (comedo-type) cancers were excluded from consideration. These obvious cancers would usually not have been considered as benign at the time of the original biopsy. In cases where DCIS was identified in retrospect in biopsy specimens previously called benign, a subsequent ipsilateral carcinoma appeared in some 25% to 30% of the patients. Thus not all cases of DCIS will progress to invasive carcinoma. When DCIS does become invasive, the ipsilateral breast is involved, whereas LCIS is a marker for prospective future disease in either breast. In DCIS the subsequent invasive cancer is usually found in the same area of the breast where the previous in situ cancer occurred.

This local recurrence of invasive cancer in DCIS may be related in part to a failure to identify a microinvasive component of what was mistakenly interpreted as DCIS. Lagios et al. found an occult invasive component in 46% of lesions that were initially termed DCIS.[54] Therefore, the possibility of an occult invasion may be related to the frequency with which DCIS subsequently develops invasive cancer. The size of the initial lesion is related to the probability of microinvasion. Lagios et al. found occult invasion in 70% of 13 DCIS cases larger than 50 mm.[54]

Dershaw et al. studied 51 women with ductal carcinoma in situ. Mammograms, specimen radiographs, and pathology reports were reviewed. Mammographic patterns of DCIS were microcalcifications in 37 of 54 (68%) lesions.[26] The calcifications were within a mass in 16 patients (30%). Multifocal DCIS was evidenced radiographically by patterns of more than one mass, more than one cluster of microcalcifications, or irregular parallel linear intraductal calcifications. They found multifocal lesions in 35 of 54 (65%) breasts. The multifocal nature of the disease was only evident on specimen radiographs in 11% of these patients.

In a collected series of 80 patients with DCIS followed for 10 years, a subsequent ipsilateral invasive carcinoma developed in 39% of the patients.[103] DCIS represents the classic early cancer seen as microcalcifications on mammograms. The advent of mammographic screening has increased the proportion of ductal carcinoma in situ. Before mammography, twice as many lobular as ductal carcinomas in situ were identified. There are now twice as many ductal as lobular lesions being diagnosed. Blichert-Toft made a distinction between three histologic growth patterns that they termed microfocal growth, diffuse growth, and tumor-forming growth.[15] Microfocal growths are limited to a few lobules or ducts without any particular changes in the surrounding stroma. These usually measure less than 1 mm in diameter. Diffuse growth affects a larger portion of the breast without interrupting the normal glandular pattern. There may be inflammation and fibrosis in the stroma. The lesions are usually small, 5 to 10 mm in diameter, although they may be considerably larger. Tumor-forming growth, on the other hand, is characterized as densely arranged glandular elements separated by strands of confluent fibrotic stroma, often with an inflammatory reaction. These lesions are at least 5 mm in diameter, but may be as large as 6 to 7 cm. Diffuse and microfocal growths usually are not palpable, while tumor-forming growths are often found by palpation. In their experience, ductal carcinoma in situ distributes approximately evenly among each of the three types.

Blichert-Toft studied in situ carcinomas with special reference to histologic growth patterns.[15] They found in situ carcinoma in its pure form in roughly 6% of all newly diagnosed breast cancers. In the most thorough mammographic screening series, the incidence rate is from 8% to 16%. This excess in diagnosis comprises the ductal type in particular, primarily in its most aggressive forms, while the lobular type is no more common than in published series of palpable breast cancer.

Today, in situ cancers occur chiefly as nonpalpable lesions shown on mammography or as small changes accidentally discovered by the pathologist in a meticulous examination of an otherwise benign specimen.

WHAT TO LOOK FOR IN A MAMMOGRAM

The broad range of normal mammographic patterns makes mammography more challenging and more interesting than many other radiologic procedures. The "borderlines of normal" are so broad that specific cues must be sought to observe an abnormality.

Screening mammography has an advantage over many other diagnostic procedures in radiology. Periodic examinations of apparently healthy women allow for frequent comparisons with a previous study. A review of previous films, when available, is essential for responsible interpretation of screening mammograms. To appreciate subtle changes in the mammogram over time, it is necessary to appreciate the normal changes that occur during the menstrual cycle and with age (see Chapter 7).

Each woman's breasts are a unique signature. There are numerous patterns of normal breast architecture; some are related to specific benign processes (e.g., fibrocystic changes). However, when seeking to identify a nonpalpable breast cancer, one must be attuned to a limited number of specific diagnostic attributes.

The features of nonpalpable breast cancer, published in the literature, include regional increase in breast density, isolated dense masses with or without microcalcifications, irregular or lobulated rounded densities, spiculated densities, clustered microcalcifications, asymmetry, skin thickening, and prominent regional vasculature as indices of increased regional blood flow. Skin thickening and vascular change are usual signs of a palpable breast cancer. Roebuck et al. described the appearance of a subcutaneous reaction to cancer.[96] When this sign was used as the sole indicator of malignancy in a series of 273 consecutive biopsy cases, a specificity of 96% and a PPV of 89% were observed. They conclude that in cases not investigated by Tru-cut needle or cyst aspiration and in the absence of infection or lymphedema, malignancy should be considered a highly likely cause of a subcutaneous reaction. Most patients will have symptoms, so this is not a significant feature of nonpalpable breast cancer.

When using screening mammograms to find nonpalpable breast cancer, only a few features warrant particular attention. Clustered microcalcifications, asymmetric densities, a rounded density with an irregular border or spiculations, focal stromal retraction, and mass lesions of greater

Table 4-3. Positive predictive value of mammographic signs of nonpalpable breast cancer

Sign	PPV
Parenchymal distortion	0.11
Opacities with undefined borders	0.35
Strongly suspect microcalcifications	0.56
Stellate opacities	0.76

density than the surrounding normal breast stroma are the mammographic features of nonpalpable breast cancer. The most valuable of these are clustered microcalcifications, stromal retraction, and mass lesions. Asymmetry alone, as a feature of neoplasia, is less effective in detecting early breast cancer. Irregular masses, stromal distortions, and focal increase in stromal density may be considered manifestations of a mass lesion. Thus the principal features reported in the literature revolve around microcalcifications or a mass, or both. If one limits the cues for further diagnostic evaluation merely to the presence of clustered microcalcifications, or a mass that is denser than surrounding structures, one markedly increases the PPV screening mammography.

However, this increased specificity in diagnostic acumen comes at a slight cost for a decreased sensitivity. Somewhat more cancers may be missed by limiting one's observational concern to clustered microcalcifications and mass lesions than would be the case if additional attributes, such as subtle asymmetry, are added to the diagnostic criteria. However, adding a concern for subtle asymmetry leads to more false-positive screening mammograms.

Ciatto et al. reviewed 512 consecutive cases where biopsies were performed on mammographically detected nonpalpable lesions.[23] They advised biopsy in the presence of parenchymal distortion, opacities with undefined borders, strongly suspect microcalcifications (rodlike or branching morphologic features, high spatial density), and stellate opacities (Table 4-3).

Schwartz et al. studied 1059 women who underwent 1132 breast biopsies for nonpalpable lesions to determine whether these cancers should be staged separately from those detected in the traditional manner.[108] Their PPV was 29.1%; 58% were invasive ductal carcinoma, 4% invasive lobular carcinomas, 25% in situ ductal cancers, 8% microinvasive ductal carcinomas, and 6% lobular carcinomas in situ.

Microcalcifications

Microcalcifications of malignancy. The most characteristic mammographic features of the early nonpalpable breast cancer are the microcalcifications of malignancy. Rosselli-Del-Turco et al. reviewed the frequency with which mammographic microcalcifications led to a surgical biopsy.[102] They reported a remarkable difference in the probability that the biopsy would be positive for cancer between women having screening mammograms and self-referred women (presumably with symptoms) (Table 4-4). These results indicate that there is a greater tendency to overcall benign calcifications in screening mammograms than in symptomatic or self-referred women.

The use of the magnification view to evaluate microcalcification has been extremely important in clarifying the nature of the calcification and whether it has a "malignant appearance." The radiologic appearance and clinical features of these microcalcifications are discussed in the next section.

Before the use of mammograms to diagnose clinically occult breast cancer, the relationship of microcalcifications to breast cancer diagnosis was not appreciated. Wilkinson et al. examined radiographs of 658 paraffin blocks obtained from 119 breast biopsies, done prior to the use of mammography.[132] These biopsies were initially interpreted as benign. They sought to determine the frequency and relevance of significant calcifications. The presence of occult cancer in breast biopsy specimens originally interpreted pathologically as benign has been reported in up to 2.4% of cases. The paraffin block radiographs revealed some calcifications in 87.4% of the cases; 19.3% contained cal-

Table 4-4. Frequency of microcalcifications evidenced at mammography by pathologic diagnosis and population examined (screening or self-referred)

	Screening	Self-referred	Total
Women examined	21,801	25,296	47,097
Biopsies recommended	355	2,771	3,126
Positive predictive value	.44	.34	.36
Cancer detected	157	953	1,110
Percent with microcalcifications	19.7	19.5	19.5
Benign lesions detected	198	1,818	2,016
Percent with microcalcifications	14.5	4.5	5.5

From Rosselli-Del-Turco M et al: *Radiol Med* 72:7-12, 1986.

cifications considered to be significant. These blocks were then sectioned in steps and no malignant neoplasms were demonstrated. Suspicious calcifications were commonly found in the paraffin block radiographs, but this finding did not lead to the identification of more cases of breast cancer.

The postoperative handling of the breast specimen is very important, since the histopathologic diagnosis should be correlated to the preoperative radiologic observation. Azavedo et al. believed that every radiologist performing mammography should insist that the radiologist's role and responsibility in breast imaging and diagnosis does not end with the reading of a mammogram.[4] The case must be followed until the final diagnosis is reached. This integration of disciplines is essential to address the problem of false-negative pathology reports. An integral part of the Swedish breast cancer screening program is regular interdisciplinary meetings and close teamwork in the management of nonpalpable breast cancer.

The microcalcifications of malignancy are found in the cancerous ducts and the surrounding epithelial cells. Calcifications in breast epithelial cells were studied by Zimmerman et al., who looked for intracytoplasmic calcifications in nipple aspirate specimens.[134] Cytologic abnormality was significantly associated with the presence of calcifications, and marked cellular changes were found four times as often in this group as in the total population with satisfactory cytology. Calcific deposits were found in six of fourteen available tissue specimens, four of which contained breast cancer. Calcifications were noted in only 23% of 97 available mammograms. Further investigation revealed other significant radiologic findings. They found cytologic calcifications more frequently in aspirates from women between the ages of 41 and 60, and these were often associated with clinical findings of breast disease. There was an increased prevalence of breast cancer in patients with cytologic calcifications in epithelial cells obtained by nipple aspiration.

Chemistry of microcalcifications. Many investigators have sought to clarify the chemical nature of breast calcifications. Frappart et al. extracted microcalcifications previously located by radiography from 25 fresh specimens.[34] Two principal types of microcalcifications were distinguished:

> Type I microcalcifications were amber in color and generally crystalline on scanning electron microscopy, with only one calcium peak on microprobe analysis. X-ray diffraction revealed that weddellite (calcium oxalate) was involved.
>
> Type II microcalcifications were whitish, nonbirefringent under polarized light, and generally ovoid or fusiform, with two peaks, one calcium and the other phosphorus, on microprobe analysis. These microcal-

cifications are composed of calcium phosphate, the most characteristic form of which is hydroxyapatite. They commonly form needles arranged in rosettes on transmission electron microscopy.

Frappart et al. found type I in four of eight benign lesions, two of three in situ lobular carcinomas, and no intraductal adenocarcinomas or infiltrating carcinomas.[34] Type II calcifications were present in all infiltrating carcinomas and intraductal adenocarcinomas and in four of eight benign lesions; they were even associated with type I microcalcifications in one in situ lobular carcinoma. They concluded that the presence of weddellite is a strong indication that a lesion is benign or at most an in situ lobular carcinoma.

It has been long recognized that not all calcifications seen on radiographs are readily found by the pathologist on examination of the tissue specimen. Radi noted that it has not been emphasized in the literature that calcium oxalate can produce radiopacities and yet is easily overlooked in tissue sections.[94] He studied 78 biopsy specimens obtained because of suspicious calcification detected by mammography. Nine (11.5%) contained only type I microcalcifications, 9 (11.5%) contained both types I and II microcalcifications, and 48 (61.5%) contained only type II microcalcifications. In 12 (15.4%), microcalcifications were not identified. The overall incidence of type I calcifications was 17.3% (22/127), but the incidence in those specimens obtained because of calcifications detected by mammography was 23.1% (18/78).

Radi's experience was similar to Frappart's in that type I microcalcifications were found only in benign lesions, such as cysts, and not associated with carcinoma or epithelial hyperplasia, whereas type II microcalcifications were associated with benign or malignant lesions. They suggested that type I microcalcifications are a product of secretion, while type II microcalcifications are a result of cellular degeneration or necrosis. In biopsies in which microcalcifications are not identified by the usual histologic stains, examination of sections under polarized light may reveal the presence of calcium oxalate crystals. It may be possible to remove small calcifications by needle aspiration and identify type I calcifications as benign.

Location of microcalcifications in relation to the cancer. The anatomic relation of microcalcifications to the breast cancer is important to assess the extent of surgical excision needed to remove the cancer. Frequently the malignancy cannot be felt even at surgery. We rely on specimen radiography to determine if the calcifications have been removed. Oppedal et al. studied 87 breast biopsies with signs of microcalcification or tissue condensation.[80] Fourteen malignant lesions (16.1%) were found, and atypical intraductal proliferations were seen in an additional 14 biopsies. The calcifications were mostly located in the atypical epithelium. In nine cases, however, calcifications were located at a distance from the atypical epithelium. They therefore concluded that an open biopsy is mandatory in such cases.

Lobular carcinoma in situ (LCIS) is usually an incidental finding independent of the mammogram. Both Hutter et al. and Pope et al. found calcifications to be adjacent to the lesion, rather than within the lesion in LCIS.[49,90] These experiences may have been due to the incidental finding of LCIS, which had nothing to do with the mammographically detected calcifications.

Price et al. studied microcalcifications in 20 women with in situ carcinoma of the breast.[92] All had microcalcifications on the mammogram, and in half there was also mammographic evidence of disruption of the breast structure. Multifocal carcinoma was found in seven patients, and histology suggested that not all foci would progress to extensive duct infiltration or invasion. Calcification occurred in both carcinoma and adjacent benign breast lesions. In three cases no calcification was found in the carcinoma but it was present in adjacent epitheliosis. They observe that microcalcifications are not specific to breast cancer but are a product of increased cellular activity and may be extruded into the surrounding interstitial tissue. They imply that microcalcification on the mammogram, particularly if sparse, demonstrates a high-risk area of the breast rather than carcinoma.

Similarly Roses et al. found cancer in 17 (33%) of 52 patients operated on for clustered microcalcifications.[101] In four of these the microcalcifications corresponded to fibrocystic disease, with the cancer being found only in adjacent tissue with little or no calcification.

Prorok et al. reported 62 women who had excisional breast biopsy for microcalcification and no associated palpable mass.[93] Carcinoma was discovered in 20 (32%) of the patients. Six patients had multicentric carcinoma, including one with synchronous bilateral lobular carcinoma. Axillary metastasis was present in three patients (15%), each with multicentric lesions. In six patients (30%) with cancer, the microcalcification was present only in adjacent tissue and ducts.

The location of the calcifications in relation to the cancer is of special importance in cytologic sampling based on mammographic detection of suspicious microcalcifications. In an attempt to better appreciate the location of suspicious microcalcifications in relation to breast cancer, Homer et al. reviewed 40 consecutive cases of nonpalpable breast cancer presenting as microcalcifications without an associated mass.[48] In 25 (63%) of the cases, the mammographic calcium was confined to the tumor and in 13 (33%) the calcification was present both within the tumor and contiguous to the tumor margin. In two cases (5%), the calcium was not contained within the tumor but was located next to it. In one of these cases, the calcium was within 4 mm of the malignant neoplasm; in the other it

was within 13 mm. No difference was seen between calcifications located within the tumor and those next to the tumor. Precise histologic analysis revealed that the microcalcifications that had prompted biopsy were confined to the tumor in 63%, within and contiguous to the tumor in 32%, and within 13 mm of the tumor in 5%.

Lagios et al. found the distribution of the mammographic microcalcifications closely approximated the extent of the disease confirmed histologically in 53 breasts resected for biopsy diagnosis of DCIS.[54] Owings et al. went further and sought to define how thoroughly a needle localization biopsy should be sampled for microscopic examination.[82] Owings et al. developed guidelines for specimen sampling by prospectively studying 157 consecutive needle localization breast biopsies. Microscopically, 32% of the cases showed cancer, 12% demonstrated atypical hyperplasia, and 56% were benign breast tissue without atypia. All biopsies were performed because of mammographic microcalcifications without a soft tissue density. Macroscopic examination in each case failed to reveal a gross lesion. Forty-nine of 50 cancers (98%) and 14 of 19 atypical hyperplasias (74%) were associated with the radiographic calcifications. They concluded that restricting histologic examination biopsy tissue to areas of radiographic calcifications and fibrous parenchyma results in a high level of detection of clinically significant lesions and a considerable reduction in the amount of tissue processed.

It is interesting to consider whether breast tissue in proximity to breast cancer differs from breast tissue surrounding benign abnormalities. Lanyi reviewed associated histologic findings from 762 cases in which the area surrounding the primary abnormality was adequately described by the pathologist.[59] Proliferative processes, ranging from type II cystic disease to lobular neoplasia, were evenly distributed among malignant and benign lesions (36.3% and 36.5% respectively). Lobular neoplasia occurred regularly, regardless of the nature of the primary abnormality. Sclerosing adenosis in the vicinity of carcinoma was noted in almost 13% of the malignant cases (Table 4-5).

Technical aspects in demonstrating microcalcifications. The mammographic demonstration of microcalcification requires a rigorous adherence to careful mammographic technique. Some investigations have sought to apply computer technology in both detection and evaluation of mammographic calcification. Wee et al. developed a computer pattern recognition program to evaluate calcifications seen on mammograms.[130] The approximate length, the average internal gray level, and the contrast were used as criteria to assess calcifications. Some 84.3% of the lesions studied were correctly identified as benign or malignant with this computer approach. These investigators established that computer programs may be eventually useful to evaluate breast calcifications. Interest in computer anal-

Table 4-5. Abnormalities found in breast tissue surrounding microcalcifications removed at surgical biopsy

	Malignant (315/499)*	Benign (447/645)*
Sclerosing adenosis	12.7%	23%
Type II cystic disease	1.6%	13%
Papillomatosis without atypia	16.2%	13%
Papillomatosis with atypia	7.9%	1.8%
Type III cystic disease	0.6%	2.2%
Lobular neoplasia	10.5%	7%

*Numbers in parentheses represent the number of cases with accurate histologic description of surrounding area and the total number of cases examined.

From Lanyi M: *Diagnosis and differential diagnosis of breast calcifications*, New York, 1986, Springer-Verlag.

ysis of mammographic calcification was revisited in 1988 in the work of Oestman et al. and Fam et al.[31,79] Fam's group used a computer algorithmic process to detect and mark clustered microcalcifications in digitized screen film mammograms.[31] In 49 of 50 cases they were able to detect and accurately locate suggestive clusters found by radiologists in a screening program. In five cases, additional clusters were found by the computer process that were not identified by radiologists. These additional clusters were subsequently considered to be mammographic calcifications that were missed by radiologists.

Smathers et al. compared the visualization of microcalcifications using xeromammography, screen film, and digital techniques.[118] In this study they used phantoms with pulverized bone fragments and aluminum oxide specks. They found that the bone speck size that corresponded to the 50% detectability level for each technique was as follows: xeromammography, 0.550 mm; digitized film, 0.573 mm; and screen film, 0.661 mm. They postulate that electronic magnification with edge enhancement can improve the ability of screen film mammography to detect microcalcifications.

Oestman et al., on the other hand, studied the detectability of malignant tumor–derived microcalcifications using conventional mammography and compared this with digital images.[79] The digital images were 2000 × 2510 pixels × 10 bits, which were derived from a storage phosphor-based digital radiography system. This system was capable of 5 line-pair/mm resolution at identical exposure factors. Microcalcifications (50 to 800 μm in diameter) were randomly superimposed on a preserved breast specimen. The authors attempted an ROC analysis based on 480 observations by four readers. They indicate that the ability to detect calcifications with digital images (ROC area = 0.871 ± 0.066) was equivalent to conventional mammography (ROC area = 0.866 ± 0.075). This equivalent detectability was evident despite the lower spatial resolution with

the digital system. The ability of a digitized system to discern microcalcifications despite its lower resolving capacity suggests that a substantial factor in attaining this equivalency was the ability of the digital system to effect greater contrast control. In this study with digital mammography, 62% of all clusters were localized, but only 23.6% of the individual calcifications were counted. With conventional mammography, 61% of all clusters were correctly localized; significantly more of the individual calcifications (31.5%) were identified.

Sickles and his colleagues have had a long-time interest in appraising the technical attributes for optimal mammographic identification of breast calcifications.[110] They did a prospective study to evaluate the ability of single microfocal magnification (1.5×) mammogram to assist in the diagnosis of isolated clustered breast microcalcifications. In 117 pathologically proven cases, the conventional contact mammogram resulted in equivocal interpretation. The superior image quality of the additional magnification caused an improved visualization of microcalcifications in every instance. This permitted a definite and correct radiologic interpretation (benign or malignant) in over 70% of the cases.

Sickles compared a wide variety of state-of-the-art mammography techniques in a study of microcalcifications.[111] These included conventional and microfocal spot x-ray tubes, screen film, and xeroradiographic recording systems, contact and magnification techniques. The results in this study confirmed their previous observations that geometric unsharpness is a limiting factor in microcalcification detectability for most conventional mammography systems.

In 1986 Sickles' group evaluated high-contrast mammography with a moving grid.[114] In this study they evaluated 1000 unselected screen film mammography patients. In approximately 60% of these patients, a high-contrast moving grid resulted in improved films. However, in only 20% did this translate into clinically useful information. Based on this study, Sickles and Weber suggested that the use of grid techniques be restricted to patients with such dense or thick breasts that they are difficult to evaluate with standard screen film mammography.[114] They believed that only in these women can one justify the increase in radiation dose needed for moving grid mammography.

Kimme-Smith et al. matched and evaluated contact and microfocal-spot-magnified images of 31 breasts. Each contained a cluster of microcalcifications within a biopsy-proved benign (n = 21) or malignant (n = 10) lesion.[51] Each matched set consisted of one image magnified 1.5× or 2.0× by microfocal spot, one contact screen film mammogram, and one televised-digitized, enhanced, and optically magnified contact screen filmed mammogram. The average area under the ROC curve for the experienced mammographers was 0.60 for contact radiographs, 0.61

for the television-digitized images, and 0.69 for the micro-focal-spot-magnified radiographs. The less experienced senior residents scored 0.44 for the television-digitized images (below random choice), 0.51 for contact radiograph, and 0.69 for the microfocal-spot-magnified radiographs.

They concluded that when evaluating microcalcifications, radiologists without extensive experience in mammography should not substitute television-digitized and enhanced contact mammograms for microfocal-spot-magnified mammograms. Rigorous clinical evaluation is needed before this system is accepted for clinical use.

Experience using mammographic microcalcifications to detect breast cancer. Groups of microcalcifications have been considered as characteristic for breast cancer since the earliest days of mammography. Salomon observed highly visible spots on an x-ray print of an amputated breast.[104] These were the first microcalcifications of the breast to be seen radiographically. Salomon described these as "small, black spots" at the center of a cancer, and he interpreted them as "intraductal cancerous masses undergoing cystic degeneration."[104]

Leborgne described carcinomatous calcifications as "resembling fine grains of salt, generally clustered."[61] These, he believed, were almost pathognomonic of breast cancer, as opposed to the larger and fewer calcifications seen in benign disease.

The mere detection of breast calcifications became the grounds for many "unnecessary" surgical biopsies. Lanyi has written a definitive text on the subject of breast calcifications.[59] He had previously questioned whether microcalcifications are a blessing or a curse.[58] He thinks that 70% to 90% of the biopsies performed because of microcalcifications on mammograms are unnecessary. "Most of the time, descriptions of diagnostic criteria are irrelevant and vague. It is confusing that lobular carcinoma in situ is considered to be a real cancer, as happens frequently; and that historically dissimilar ductal carcinomas and benign abnormalities of different origin are simply considered as malignant or benign, and subsequently reported as such." This opinion results from an analysis of articles on microcalcifications published between 1951 and 1984. Obviously, he believes that the use of proper mammographic criteria to identify malignant microcalcifications would dramatically reduce the number of needless biopsies.

The expected frequency of mammographic microcalcifications is difficult to estimate. The reported experiences vary considerably. Some reports limit their evaluation to cases with calcification without clearly stipulating the criteria by which the calcifications were considered suspicious for cancer. If strict criteria are used, "suspicious calcifications" will be correlated with more cancers. We will review a number of reported series involving a correlation of suspicious microcalcifications with cancers found. We seek to illustrate the various ways investigators have

sought to evaluate the likelihood that cancer will be found with different patterns of microcalcifications (Table 4-6).

The distinction between calcifications found on screening mammograms and those found in pathology specimens is particularly important in reviewing these series. Zimmerman et al. found calcific deposits in 6 of 14 available tissue specimens obtained from patients he was evaluating for the presence of intracytoplasmic calcifications in nipple aspirate specimens.[134] Four of these six tissue samples contained breast cancer. He noted calcifications in only 23% of 97 available mammograms obtained from the same group of patients. Stomper et al. studied 27 consecutive, clinically occult, noncalcified breast cancers.[122] Forty-one percent of these malignancies contained microscopic calcifications, even though they were not seen at mammography.

Menges studied the diagnostic value of mammographic signs of malignancy in clinically occult breast cancer.[69] In 72%, microcalcification was the major feature that led to the correct diagnosis; in 48%, it was the only sign. Murphy et al. found cancer in 35% of 30 consecutive cases of mammographically isolated clustered microcalcifications that prompted breast biopsy.[76] Half of these were noninvasive. Roses et al. found cancer in 17 of 52 patients operated on for clustered microcalcifications (33%).[101] In four of these the microcalcifications corresponded to fibrocystic disease, with the cancer found only in adjacent tissue that contained little or no calcification. Prorok et al. found cancer in 20 of 62 women (32%) who had excisional breast biopsy for microcalcification and no associated palpable mass.[93] Colbassani et al. found cancer in 15 of 55 patients (27%) with isolated microcalcification clusters and no palpable tumor.[24] They reported that a careful study of the microcalcifications did not show significant differences between the malignant and the benign group. Since the clustered microcalcifications were so nonspecific, these authors recommended that all patients with isolated microcalcification clusters should have a biopsy. Lanyi concludes that Colbassani's opinion cannot be taken seriously, since he based it on the analysis of too few cases to draw a meaningful conclusion.[59] Subsequent investigators have presented more specific criteria to identify which of these clustered microcalcifications are more likely to be associated with malignancy.

The refinement in the mammographic criteria for the use of microcalcifications, as indices of malignancy, can be seen in reports in the literature. Different investigators have reported differing results largely based on their criteria for considering that a calcification pattern was suspicious for malignancy. Gisvold et al. observed calcification on the mammograms of 51% of 343 nonpalpable mammographic lesions; 27% of these 343 lesions were malignant.[37] Bahnsen et al. reported suspicious microcalcifications in 87% of 116 cases of early ductal cancer.[5] Tinne-

Table 4-6. Published series of nonpalpable breast cancers detected by the presence of mammographic calcifications

Authors	Biopsy	Cancer	Positive predictive value (PPV)	Biopsy/ cancer	Invasive	Tubular	DCIS	LCIS	Other
Murphy (1978)	15	7	.467	2.1	3		4	0	
Rogers (1972)	46	19	.413	2.4	5		11	3	
Murphy (1978)	31	11	.355	2.8	5	6		5	0
Roses (1980)	52	17	.327	3.1	10		6	1	
Prorok (1983)	62	20	.323	3.1	15		3	2	
Rosenberg (1987)	497	159	.320	3.1	93		56	10	
Schwartz (1984)	328	104	.317	3.2	56		40	8	
Hall, F. (1988)	213	64	.300	3.3					
Tinnemans (1986)	173	51	.295	3.4	21		22	7	173
Colbassani (1982)	55	15	.273	3.7	8		7	0	
Lanyi (1981)	135	36	.267	3.8	0		33	3	
Solmer (1980)	31	8	.258	3.9					
Hallgrimsson (1988)	52	13	.250	4.0					
Egan (1980)	468	115	.246	4.1	42		46	12	
Chetty (1983)	103	25	.243	4.1					
Rowen (1986)	202	49	.243	4.1					
Bigelow (1984)	50	12	.240	4.2					
Ciatto (1987)	263	63	.240	4.2					
Silverstein (1989)	521	122	.234	4.3					
Wilhelm (1986)	203	46	.227	4.4					
Meyer (1984)	203	45	.222	4.5					
Landercasper (1987)	113	25	.221	4.5					
Landstrom (1989)	80	17	.213	4.7					
Grisvold (1984)	125	26	.208	4.8					
Rusnak (1989)	112	22	.196	5.1					
Hicks (1983)	162	31	.191	5.2					
Lang (1987)	23	4	.174	5.8					
Powell (1983)	282	47	.167	6.0	11		26	10	
Graham (1988)	261	36	.138	7.3					
Skinner (1988)	60	8	.133	7.5					
Petrovich (1989)	51	6	.118	8.5					
Ostrow (1987)	81	9	.111	9.0					
Lang (1987)	21	2	.95	10.5					
Chourcair (1988)	44	2	.45	22.0					
TOTAL	5118	1236	.24	4.14					

mans et al. reported 153 consecutive patients who had clusters of at least five microcalcifications and no palpable findings as the only indications for biopsy.[126] One hundred and seventy-three groups of microcalcifications were excised and 51 malignancies were detected (29.5%). Sickles observed clustered microcalcifications as the primary mammographic abnormality in 42% of 300 consecutive nonpalpable breast cancers.[112] Only 23% demonstrated the rod, curvilinear, and branching shapes considered to be characteristic of malignancy.

Landercasper et al. found malignancy in 44 of 203 specimens taken from 174 patients who had nonpalpable breast lesions.[55] Sixty percent of the malignant lesions were in situ and 34% were invasive carcinoma. The chance of a biopsy containing a malignant lesion was 17.5% if the biopsy was done because of discrete density on mammography and 22.1% if the biopsy was indicated by the presence of microcalcifications. If both a density and microcalcifications were present, 29.6% of the patients had cancer. Landstrom et al. found 21 cancers in 211 preoperative needle localization–directed biopsies of nonpalpable breast lesions.[56] Seventeen (81%) were invasive and four (19%) noninvasive. Forty-three percent of the cancers were minimal (in situ or an invasive cancer less than 5 mm with negative axillary nodes), and 48% were less than 1 cm. Mammographic microcalcifications were found in 81% of the malignant group and 33% of the benign group. The combination of microcalcifications with an irregular density was only found in the malignant group.

Lanyi stated that almost half (43% to 49%) of clinically occult breast cancers are detected by the presence of microcalcifications.[59] Menges et al. observed well-defined microcalcifications in 72% of 220 clinically occult breast cancers discovered by mammography.[69] Dense, irregular foci could be seen in only 28% of their early cancers. In most cases mammographic microcalcification was the major feature leading to the diagnosis of cancer. Mammographic microcalcification was the only sign in 48% of the patients, where even a specimen radiograph failed to show an infiltrative focus. Meyer et al. published a series of 500 mammographically discovered breast lesions, of which 117 (23.4%) turned out to be malignant.[71] Biopsy was prompted by abnormal calcifications in 41% (203 of 500) of the cases.

Petrovich et al. reported a 48% incidence of microcalcifications as the mammographic abnormality associated with malignancy in 106 biopsies taken from 104 patients.[89] Meyer et al. observed microcalcifications as the dominant mammographic feature in 50.4% or 635 of 1261 occult breast abnormalities.[70] Two hundred and thirty-seven (18.8%) of these 1261 abnormalities proved to be cancerous. Eighty-five were ductal carcinoma in situ.

Owings et al. prospectively studied 157 consecutive needle localization breast biopsies performed because of mammographic microcalcifications without a soft tissue density.[82] Microscopically 32% of the cases showed cancer, 12% demonstrated atypical hyperplasia, and 56% were benign breast tissue without atypia. Forty-nine of 50 cancers (98%) and 14 of 19 cases of atypical hyperplasia (74%) were associated with the mammographic calcifications. Papatestas et al. found cancer in 149 (31%) of 475 nonpalpable mammographic lesions.[86] Cancer was found in 69 (33%) of 206 patients with clusters of microcalcifications. When the calcifications were associated with densities, cancer was more likely to be found at biopsy (16 of 39 cases, or 41%). Cancer occurred in 64 (28%) of 230 with nonpalpable masses.

From these series it can be seen that the probability of a cancer being found when biopsies are performed for suspicious microcalcifications depends entirely on the type and character of microcalcifications. The criteria used in identifying which calcifications are to be considered suspicious vary in the different series. Over time, however, there is an increasing consensus as to the mammographic manifestation of "suspicious microcalcifications."

Microcalcifications and in situ carcinoma. Part of the problem in identifying the probable yield from biopsies performed for microcalcifications relates to whether the cancers identified were carcinomas in situ. Lobular in situ carcinomas may be found in otherwise normal breasts where biopsies were performed for what were, in reality, benign calcifications. Thus in some instances, lobular carcinoma in situ may be a mere fortuitous finding. On the other hand, ductal carcinomas in situ are often associated with microcalcifications. In some series, the failure to clearly differentiate the noninvasive cancers leads to considerable confusion when attempting to assess the relationship between the finding of a cancer and the presence of "suspicious" microcalcifications. Thus it is reasonable to discuss in greater depth the relationships of microcalcification to in situ carcinoma.

Murphy et al. reported on 30 consecutive cases of mammographically isolated clustered microcalcifications that prompted biopsy, 15 of which were in situ.[76] They did not distinguish whether these noninvasive cancers were ductal carcinoma in situ or lobular carcinoma in situ.

Sener et al. reported 321 patients with excisional biopsies of nonpalpable mammographic abnormalities.[106] Twenty-eight of 36 (78%) noninfiltrating carcinomas displayed microcalcifications alone. As the number of microcalcifications increased, so did the incidence of carcinoma. Only 11 out of 75 cancers appeared as a mass with microcalcification. Eleven of the 21 masses with calcifications were cancer. Tinnemans et al. performed biopsies on 153 consecutive patients with clusters of at least 5 microcalcifications and no palpable findings.[126] One hundred and seventy three groups of microcalcifications were excised, and 51 malignancies were detected (29.5%). Most of the malignant lesions were noninfiltrating (56%).

Marrujo et al. used screening mammograms and physical examination to discover 237 radiologically suspicious nonpalpable lesions.[68] In this they found 64 nonpalpable cancers, 25 invasive, 16 minimally invasive, and 23 noninvasive. Of the noninvasive lesions, 7 were 10 mm or less in diameter, and 14 were 11 to 20 mm. The noninvasive and minimally invasive cancers tended to occur in younger women. These almost always appeared as clustered microcalcifications.

Landercasper et al. found malignancy in 44 of 203 specimens biopsied, and only 34% of these were invasive cancer.[55] In Landstrom et al.'s series, only 19% of the cancers were noninvasive.[56]

If the noninvasive cancers are restricted to ductal carcinoma in situ, then the importance of mammographic microcalcifications becomes readily apparent. Dershaw et al. studied 51 women with ductal carcinoma in situ (DCIS).[26] Mammograms, specimen radiographs, and pathology reports were reviewed. In 68% (37 of 54) of the lesions microcalcifications were the sole manifestation of DCIS. In an additional 30% (16 of 54), calcifications occurred within a mass.

Stomper et al. reported 100 consecutive cases of clinically occult DCIS detected by mammography.[121] Seventy-two percent of the lesions appeared as microcalcification only, 10% as soft tissue abnormalities, and 12% as a combination of the two. Six percent of the lesions were found incidentally in the biopsy specimen. On the basis of mammography measurements, 22% of the lesions were 5 mm or smaller, and 75% were 20 mm or smaller. Thirty-five percent of the microcalcification clusters were categorized as predominantly linear casts, 52% as granular, and 13% as granular with casts. These authors concluded that there is a wide spectrum of mammographic appearances of clinically occult DCIS. Sneige et al. found mammographic calcifications in 6 of 12 patients with DCIS.[119]

Price et al., although not clearly distinguishing DCIS from LCIS, made some interesting observations concerning the relationship of microcalcification to lobuloductal dysplasia and noninvasive carcinoma.[92] They reviewed 20 women with in situ carcinoma of the breast. All had microcalcification on the mammogram, and in half there was also mammographic evidence of disruption of the breast structure. Three quarters of these women presented with breast symptoms. Multifocal carcinoma was found in seven patients. The histology suggested that not all foci may progress to extensive duct infiltration or invasion. Calcification occurred both in carcinoma and in adjacent benign breast lesions. In three cases, no evidence of calcification was found in the carcinoma, but it was present in adjacent epitheliosis. They believe that microcalcifications are not specific to breast cancer but represent a product of increased cellular activity. The calcifications may be extruded into the surrounding interstitial tissue. This implies that microcalcification on the mammogram, particularly if sparse, demonstrates a high-risk area of the breast.

Based upon the available evidence in the literature, it is reasonable to conclude that mammographic microcalcifications are an important, and at times the only, indication of DCIS. On the other hand, when LCIS is found on a biopsy occasioned by the presence of mammographic microcalcifications, the correlation may well be mere coincidence. LCIS is probably not associated with typical clusters of microcalcifications characterized as "suspicious for cancer." It is important to also appreciate that mammographic microcalcifications are not limited to nonpalpable breast cancers. Rosselli-Del-Turco et al. found mammographic microcalcifications in 19.7% of 157 breast cancers diagnosed in a mammographic screening program conducted on asymptomatic women and in 19.5% of 953 breast cancers diagnosed in self-referred women (most with symptoms).[102]

Criteria of malignant microcalcifications. Most mammographic calcifications are benign. What features are useful to distinguish benign from malignant calcifications? Various investigators have attempted this distinction. Roselli-Del-Turco et al. used three features to distinguish benign from malignant microcalcification[102]: (1) size, shape, or density of the calcifications, (2) size or shape of the "cluster," and (3) number of microcalcifications.

Size, shape, or density of individual microcalcifications. Le-Gal et al. wrote a classic paper on microcalcifications.[62] They excised 227 cases of breast microcalcifica-

tions without palpable tumor. Ninety-nine were benign, 27 were borderline lesions, and 101 were cancer, of which 58 were in situ. They identified five types of calcifications based on their morphology:

Type 1: Annular—100% were benign
Type 2: Regularly punctiform—22% were malignant
Type 3: Too fine for presizing shape—40% were malignant
Type 4: Irregularly punctiform—66% were malignant
Type 5: Vermicular—100% were malignant

Rosselli-Del-Turco et al. also classified microcalcifications on the basis of morphology.[102] They used dotlike, sticklike, or ramified architecture of the individual calcification and whether the shape was regular or irregular. They also evaluated radiologic density. Their analysis of the morphologic criteria, which led to a distinction between benign and malignant biopsy results, is one of the most thorough that has been published (Table 4-7). The distribution, number, concentration, morphology, shape of the calcifications, and presence or absence of an associated mammographic opacity all played a part in distinguishing benign from malignant biopsy outcomes. The radiologic density was not a useful criterion.

Ciatto et al. defined strongly suspected microcalcifications as those with rodlike or branching morphologic features and high spatial density.[23] Stomper et al. classified 35% of the microcalcifications as predominantly casts (linear), 52% as granular, and 13% as granular with several casts.[121] Sickles found clustered calcifications as the primary mammographic abnormality in 42% of 300 breast cancer cases,[112] but only 23% demonstrated the rod, curvilinear, and branching shapes characteristic of malignancy.

In his initial study, Lanyi found only one cancer in four to five biopsies performed to evaluate clustered microcalcifications.[59] However, by paying specific attention to the character of the microcalcifications, Lanyi was able to double the yield of cancer in cases biopsied for microcalcifications. He went from 13.8% to 27% during the period 1974 to 1983. Using his criteria between 1983 and 1985, Lanyi identified 12 ductal carcinomas in 23 cases biopsied solely on the basis of clustered microcalcifications. Thus by defining clearly the character of the microcalcifications that were suspicious for cancer, Lanyi was able to substantially reduce the number of surgical biopsies so that some 50% of the cases biopsied for microcalcifications yielded ductal carcinoma. He increased his PPV to 0.50.

Lanyi points out that three diagnostic features define whether or not a microcalcification is suspicious for cancer. These objective criteria are the shape of the microcalcification cluster, the shapes of the individual calcifications, and the number of calcifications. He found a fourth feature—intensity of calcifications on the radiographic

Table 4-7. Distribution of mammographically evidenced microcalcifications by morphologic criteria in 217 cancers and in 111 benign lesions: positive predictive value (PPV) of each radiologic criterion

Mammographic morphologic criteria	Cancers N.	%	Benign N	%	PPV (%)
Total evaluated cases	1,110		2,016		
Cases with microcalcifications	217		111		66.2
Spatial disposition					
Isolated	40	18.4	42	37.8	48.8
Clustered	146	67.3	69	69.2	67.9
Widely diffused	31	14.3	0	—	100.0
Total number					
1 to 4	145	66.8	81	72.9	64.2
5 to 10	22	10.2	25	22.5	46.8
Over 10	30	23.0	5	4.5	90.9
Number/cm^2					
1 to 10	34	15.7	27	24.3	55.7
11 to 20	44	20.3	27	24.3	62.0
21 to 50	87	40.0	48	43.2	64.4
Over 50	52	24.0	9	8.2	85.2
Morphology					
Dotlike	151	69.6	93	83.8	61.9
Sticklike	33	15.2	16	14.4	67.3
Ramified	33	15.2	2	1.8	94.3
Shape					
Regular	25	11.5	62	55.8	28.7
Irregular	192	88.5	49	44.2	79.7
Radiologic density					
Low	103	47.5	60	54.0	63.2
High	114	52.5	51	46.0	69.1
Mammographic capacity					
Abent	61	28.1	67	60.4	47.7
Next to the microcalcification	33	15.2	4	3.6	89.2
Microcalcifications inside opacity	121	55.8	36	32.4	77.1
Microcalcifications at border	2	0.9	4	3.6	33.3
Maximum diameter					
0.1-0.3 mm	47	21.7	27	24.4	63.5
0.6-0.9 mm	64	29.5	42	37.8	60.4
Over 0.9 mm	106	48.8	42	37.8	71.6
Average diameter					
0.1-0.3 mm	48	22.1	27	24.3	64.0
0.4-0.5 mm	88	40.5	56	50.4	61.1
0.6-0.9 mm	51	23.5	9	8.1	85.0
Over 1 mm	30	13.8	18	16.2	62.5

From Rosselli-Del-Turco et al: The significance of mammographic calcifications in early breast cancer detection, *Radiol Med* 72:7-12, 1986.

image—not to be useful because it would require microdensitometry to be quantitatively assessed. The apparent density of microcalcifications depends more on the radiographic technique and the scattering principles of the breast than on an intrinsic attribute of the calcification. The apparent density of a mammographic calcification depends on whether the breast is fatty or involuted or has a dense, glandular pattern. In the opinion of Lanyi, the relative density of the various calcifications is too subjective to be of much value.

Lanyi distinguishes four shapes of malignant calcifications (see Chapter 7). The well-defined calcifications in breast carcinoma are:

1. Punctate calcifications of variable size
2. Bean- or comma-shaped calcifications
3. Wavy (wormlike) or linear calcifications of variable length (so-called vermicular calcifications)
4. Branched calcifications resembling the letters V, W, X, Y, and Z.

Lanyi analyzed 7028 cases of microcalcifications in 121 intraductal carcinomas. He found that monomorphism of the punctate calcification was rare and most apt to occur in papillary/cribriform carcinomas. He uses the "principles of polymorphism," which state: if the number of calcifications exceeds 15, only polymorphous microcalcifications can be demonstrated in ductal carcinomas. Approximately 50% of all carcinoma calcifications are of the punctate type. As the number of calcifications increases, the punctate form tends to become less prevalent. Polymorphism is the greatest in comedocarcinomas. *Since polymorphism increases with the number of calcifications, this can be a useful feature in assessing multiple punctate calcifications that are monomorphic. When they are widely dispersed, they are almost always benign.*

Size or shape of cluster. Lanyi's book on breast calcifications remains the most comprehensive treatise on the subject.[59] His system for the differential diagnosis of benign and malignant lesions was largely based on the radiologic patterns of grouped microcalcifications. The value of this system has been tested in a blinded study of 297 mammograms with grouped microcalcifications in which the diagnosis had been verified by operation and histology. This system saved 63% of the biopsies. Among 42 carcinomas, only one was erroneously regarded as benign. The sensitivity of the study was 97.6%, and its specificity was 73.3%. The radiologic symptoms associated with the correct and false diagnoses were analyzed. Lanyi teaches that the shape of the cluster of calcifications is a relevant feature in ascertaining the probability for malignancy. "Cluster mapping" entails drawing a line around the periphery in two mammographic planes in order to evaluate the shape of the "cluster." This shape is an important criterion for malignancy, since it is related to the anatomic correlates of the microcalcifications. Calcifications in a ductal carcinoma have characteristic distributions that depend upon ductal anatomy. A "swallow-tail" is a characteristic shape of clustered microcalcification related to malignancy.[59] This may be difficult to appreciate. More often, large char-

acteristic clusters take on a globular shape (Fig. 4-2). Because of the nature of the ductal anatomy, which is laden with calcifications in some early cases of intraductal carcinoma. A triangular or trapezoid distribution, evident on both of the planes, occurred in over 50% of cases where carcinoma was found.

Lanyi classifies the cluster maps into six different categories, which were observed in 97% of cases in breast carcinoma. These are (1) triangular or trapezoidal, (2) square or rectangular, possibly with tapered ends, (3) bottle or club shape, (4) propeller or butterfly shape, (5) rhomboid or kite shape, and (6) linear or branched. The occurrence of nontriangular configurations depends on the degree in which the particular duct segment is filled with calcifications and on the projection. The shape of the cluster map depends on the shape of the pyramid-shaped ducts and thus of the carcinoma. Muir et al. revealed that the size of the mammographic lesion was important in ascertaining the probabilities of malignancies.[75] They found that if the mammographic lesion was more than 150 mm^2, was associated with an irregular density, and contained five or more calcifications, it was very likely to be an invasive carcinoma.

Stomper et al. also observed that the size of the cluster was an important consideration.[121] In their series 22% were less than 5 mm and 75% less than 20 mm.

Number of microcalcifications. Le-Gal et al. found that the number of calcifications was greater in breasts with carcinoma.[62] Fifty-six percent of the cases with more than 50 calcifications were malignant. Fifty percent of the malignant lesions had more than 10 calcifications within a 5 mm diameter. When several clusters were found, 70% of the cases were malignant. This does not argue against the principle of polymorphism, inasmuch as the probability of polymorphism increases as the number increases. In 321 patients who had excisional biopsies of nonpalpable mammographic abnormalities, 28 of 36 noninfiltrating carcinomas presented with microcalcifications alone.[106] Sener et al. noted that as the number of calcifications increased, so did the incidence of carcinoma. Skinner et al. noted that

---

Fig. 4-2. Clustered microcalcifications. **A** and **B** reveal a craniocaudal and mediolateral projection of a mammogram performed in a 80-year-old women in 1988. The breast are unusually dense for a patient this age. This patient had been on estrogen therapy for osteoporosis. Extensive vascular calcification can be seen in both breasts. Some benign ductal calcification is also seen in the right breast. There are no clusters of malignant appearing microcalcifications. **C** and **D,** only 2 years later, the patient demonstrated a large cluster of pleomorphic microcalcifications involving the upper outer quadrant of the left breast. These calcifications are clearly distinguishable from the background normal calcifications present on the prior film. These calcifications demonstrate a triangular configuration in the mediolateral view and is a somewhat more globular configuration in the craniocaudal projection. These calcifications are characteristic of malignancy. The many factors that makes this mammogram a category 4 relate to the risk factor in the age of the patient, dense breasts at this age, and the pleomorphic nature of a large group of clustered microcalcifications. Fine needle aspiration cytology revealed malignant cells.

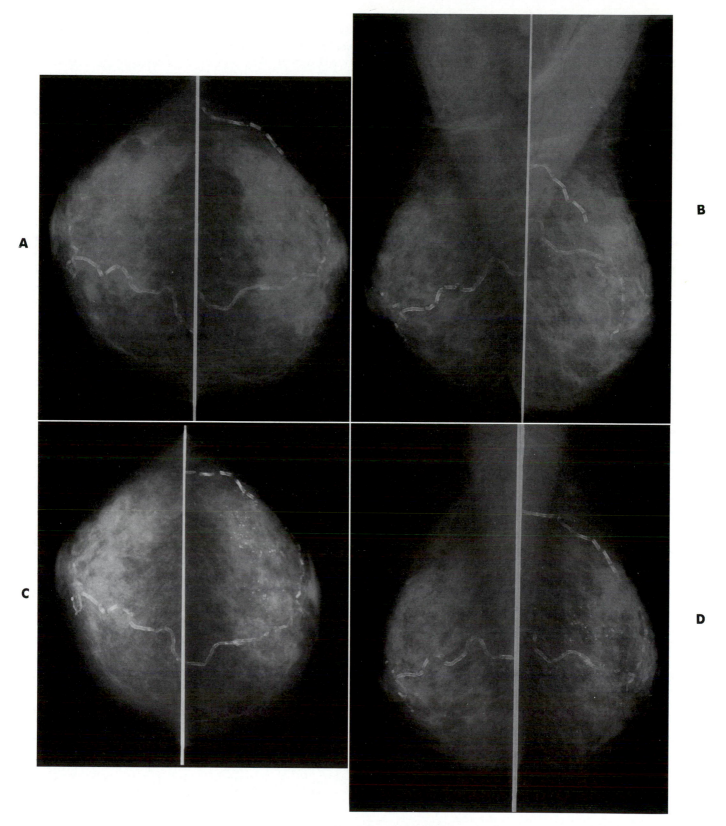

Fig. 4-2. For legend see opposite page.

the presence of 10 or more microcalcifications in a lesion markedly increased the probability that the lesion was malignant.[117] Bongiorni et al. demonstrated that comedocarcinomas have had an increasing detectability when one pays attention to extensive polymorphic microcalcifications.[16] Most comedocarcinomas can be diagnosed by the characteristic intraductal calcifications. Comedocarcinoma relates to extensive intraductal carcinoma in that when one sees a mammogram with an extensive intraductal carcinomas, it is more likely to be demonstrated by the presence of microcalcifications in the absence of a mammographic mass. When cancer is found, the presence of microcalcifications in the absence of a mammographic mass conveys a 73% likelihood that the cancer will have an extensive intraductal component.[43]

The relevance of the number of calcifications relates significantly to their degree of monomorphism or polymorphism. Even five microcalcifications may be suspicious with any degree of polymorphism, if the patient is at high risk, or if no microcalcifications were seen in a suspicious area 6 months previously.

A major problem in the mammographic detection of nonpalpable breast cancer relates to the analysis and management of multicentric calcifications. Usually this is not difficult, since the calcifications are widely dispersed and appear benign. However, at times there can be multiple clusters of microcalcifications, any one of which could be caused by cancer. Do we biopsy all of them? Is there any recourse but total mastectomy? Can we safely follow them with serial mammograms to look for a change as evidence of a malignant nature?

Multicentric microcalcifications. Bahnsen et al. reviewed 116 cases of early ductal cancer. Suspicious microcalcifications, occurring in 87% of the patients, were the most important mammographic signs in the diagnosis of early ductal carcinoma.[5] Multicentricity occurred in 26% of the 65 noninvasive cancers in this series. Of the 37 cases with early stromal invasion, multicentricity occurred in 26%. Lagios et al. studied 53 breasts resected for biopsy diagnosis of ductal carcinoma in situ.[54] The frequency of occult invasion and multicentricity was 21 and 32%, respectively. For lesions with associated microcalcifications, the distribution of the mammographic microcalcifications closely approximated the extent of the disease confirmed histologically.

Marrujo et al. reported 237 radiologically suspicious nonpalpable lesions.[68] A review of surgical specimens revealed that 27% had residual disease at the biopsy site. Of patients who underwent mastectomy, 34% had an unsuspected focus of cancer on another quadrant of the breast. An additional 14% had an unsuspected focus of epithelial atypia. These studies suggest that needle aspiration biopsy and vigilant follow-up mammograms, in cases where the cytology is benign, may be an appropriate way to manage this difficult problem.

Age and microcalcifications. Rosselli-Del-Turco et al. studied microcalcifications in patients who underwent a surgical biopsy.[102] They observed a significant relation between the age of the patient and the probability that suspicious microcalcifications would have been the mammographic clue that led to the biopsy (Table 4-8).

Similarly, Papatestas et al. observed that while microcalcifications are more likely to represent neoplasms in younger women, masses more frequently represented invasive tumors.[86] Stomper and Gelman noted that women aged 49 years or less with DCIS were more likely to have microcalcifications and less likely to have a soft tissue mass than women aged 50 years or more (P = 0.04).[123]

Mass with microcalcifications. In 321 patients with excisional biopsies of nonpalpable mammographic abnormalities, only 11 out of 75 cancers (14%) presented as a mass with microcalcification.[109] Dershaw et al. studied 51 women with DCIS.[126] In 68% (37 of 54) of the lesions, microcalcifications were the sole manifestation of DCIS. In an additional 30% (16/54) of the lesions, calcifications occurred within a mass. Papatestas et al. reported localized nonpalpable lesions detected on mammogram in 475 women.[86] Cancer occurred in 149, for a PPV of .31. Sixteen (41%) of 39 with calcifications associated with densities had cancer. Sixty-four (28%) of 230 with nonpalpable

Table 4-8. Frequency of microcalcifications according to pathologic diagnosis and age

		Age group				
		1-39	40-49	50-59	60+	Total
Cancers	Cases	70	245	315	480	1,110
	% with microcalcifications	19.5	22.1	16.5	19.2	19.5
Benign	Cases	768	712	349	187	2,016
	% with microcalcifications	0.5	8.9	5.2	13.6	5.5
PPV		0.08	0.26	0.47	0.71	0.36

From Rosselli-Del-Turco M et al: *Radiol Med* 72:7-12, 1986.

masses had breast cancer. Among patients with invasive, malignant neoplasms with calcifications, 39% had positive axillary nodes.

Microcalcifications and the irradiated breast. Libshitz et al. studied calcifications in therapeutically irradiated breasts of 81 patients.[64] Malignant calcifications may remain stable, diminish, or completely disappear following irradiation. The persistence of calcifications need not indicate residual cancer. After irradiation calcifications can develop that are similar to either intraductal or secretory calcifications. Unusual calcifications may develop at the site of an irradiated cancer. It is important to recognize that benign calcifications can develop so that they will not be confused with malignancy.

Buckley et al. studied mammographic changes in 57 patients following radiation therapy by doing serial mammograms.[20] Residual tumors were identified on the basis of remaining malignant-type microcalcification. Local recurrence was identified on mammography. The most useful sign was the development of a mass lesion and the increase or development of malignant-type microcalcifications. Buckley notes that a distinction between radiotherapy effect and recurrence of carcinoma can be made when a reaction that is normally caused by radiation therapy occurs to an inappropriate degree or with inappropriate timing.

Stomper et al. studied mammographic detection of recurrent cancer in the irradiated breast of 45 patients.[124] Of the 23 biopsy-proven recurrences, eight (35%) were detected by mammography only, nine (39%) were detected by physical examination only, and six (26%) were detected by both. Mammographic findings in recurrent malignancy include microcalcifications in six, microcalcifications associated with a mass in four, soft tissue masses in three, and inflammatory changes in one. These results show that mammographic follow-up is complementary to physical examination in the detection of local recurrence in women who have undergone radiation therapy for early breast cancer.

Solin et al. studied new calcifications in the postirradiated breast.[120] In 19 patients they found new mammographic calcifications without palpable or mammographic mass after breast-conserving surgery and definitive irradiation for early breast cancer. The postradiotherapy interval was 9 to 96 months, with a median of 34 months. Eleven biopsy specimens (58%) were positive for recurrent breast cancer and eight were negative. Calcifications that developed in a quadrant different from the initial tumor tended to be malignant, with four of five having a positive biopsy result. Microcalcifications were not commonly associated with the initial tumor, with only 5 of 19 having microcalcifications. These results show that the development of new calcifications in the postirradiated breast is associated with a PPV of 58% and that the tumors found tended to be early and potentially salvageable. Solin notes that a positive biopsy rate of 58% in the postirradiated breast is in marked contrast to the lower positive biopsy rate for microcalcifications in the nonirradiated breast reported in the literature.

Mass lesions, stromal distortions, and local increase in breast density

Lanyi observed that the best yield for mammographically detected breast cancer was provided by rounded shadows in radial structures, which were found to be positive for cancer in every second or third biopsy.[59]

Sener et al. observed that 27 of 39 (69%) patients with infiltrating carcinomas demonstrated a mass alone.[109] The size of the mass was not a reliable guide for predicting carcinoma. Only 11 of 75 cancers had a mass with microcalcification. Eleven of the 21 calcified masses were cancer. They found infiltrating cancers and positive nodes significantly more often in palpable than in nonpalpable masses. Infiltrating cancers were generally associated with a mass, whereas noninfiltrating cancers were generally diagnosed by the presence of microcalcifications.

Stomper et al. used serial radiologic/pathologic correlations on specimens in 27 occult, noncalcified breast cancers to determine the frequency and correlation of mammography appearance and pathologic diagnoses.[122] Mammography revealed a well-defined round mass in one case; a well-defined lobular mass in two cases; an indistinct round, oval, or lobulated mass in seven cases; irregular or mixed lesions in seven cases; spiculated masses in nine cases; and architectural distortion in one case. Histologic margins of infiltrating and intraductal carcinomas created several types of tumor-fat interfaces, and surrounding reactive fibrosis correlated with these radiographic appearances.

Ikeda et al. did a retrospective study of mammograms in 190 women with biopsy-proven DCIS.[50] They excluded 117 (62%) of the women whose radiographs showed suspicious clustered microcalcifications. Of the remaining 73 (38%) of the women, 30 (16%) had negative mammograms, and 43 (23%) of these DCIS patients had mammographic manifestations of breast malignancy other than microcalcifications. Of the DCIS patients with mammographic abnormalities other than microcalcification, 15 (35%) had circumscribed masses, and 12 (28%) had various focal nodular patterns. The remaining 37% (16 patients) showed other mammographic signs of malignancy, including asymmetry (n = 1); dilated retroalveolar ducts (n = 2); ill-defined, rounded tumor (n = 2); focal architectural distortion (n = 4); subareolar mass (n = 3); and developing density (n = 4).

Interval changes

As more women are obtaining screening mammograms, the number who have already had a baseline mammogram is increasing. Therefore an increasing proportion of the breast cancers detected are incident rather than prevalence cancers. Interval changes will become increasing important in the mammographic detection of early breast cancer.

Wilhelm et al. reported on breast cancers found on the second of two serial mammograms.[131] They found interval mammographic changes may become the major indications for biopsy. Four hundred and fifty-two needle localizations were carried out for microcalcification, mass, asymmetric density, or a combination of calcification with mass or asymmetric density that became apparent on the second of two serial mammograms. Of the 95 cancers detected, interval mammographic changes were seen in 35 patients. This mammographic sign had a PPV of 0.21 (4.8 biopsies per cancer). Invasive cancers constituted 51% of the initial group but only 34% of the cancers detected because of interval change. Benign breast disease occurred in 160 of 195 women who had undergone biopsy because of interval changes. Hyperplasia and/or atypia were found in 35% (57/160) of this group.

Mammographic features of a benign breast biopsy

What causes a poor specificity in mammographic recommendation for surgical biopsy? An appreciation of the mammographic patterns that have led to a benign biopsy may lead to an improved specificity of mammographic diagnosis of breast cancer.

In reviewing a series of 138 benign breast biopsies, Skinner et al.[117] observed that the mammographic abnormalities most commonly associated with benign disease included:

1. Well-defined densities without calcifications
2. Asymmetric densities without calcifications
3. Abnormalities consisting solely of a focus of fewer than 10 mammographic calcifications

When these criteria were used, malignancy occurred in only 5.5% of the patients who had a surgical biopsy. This compares to a positive biopsy rate of 23% in the total series.

Kopans et al. did a prospective study to evaluate the significance of asymmetric breast tissue (asymmetric volume of breast tissue, asymmetrically dense breast tissue with preserved architecture, or asymmetrically prominent ducts) on mammograms.[53] Of 8408 mammograms obtained in 1985, 221 (3%) demonstrated asymmetric breast tissue. Follow-up was 36 to 42 months after the initial mammographic study. During this time, none of the patients underwent biopsy on the basis of these mammographic findings, although 20 underwent excisional biopsy because of clinical findings. Breast cancer was diagnosed in two patients and breast lymphoma in one. The remaining 17 biopsies were benign. They conclude: "An asymmetric volume of breast tissue, asymmetrically dense

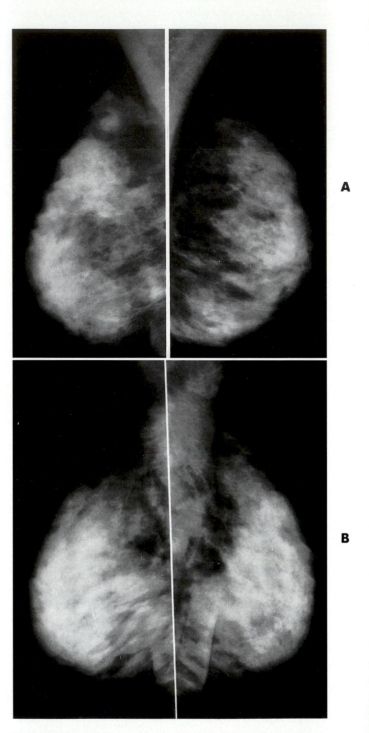

A

B

Fig. 4-3. Normal asymmetric mammogram. The relative prominence of the right axillary tail has been present for a number of years and is unchanged from prior mammograms. **B,** A normal asymmetric mammogram in a patient who also has accessory left axillary breast tissue. The axillary tail is clearly spearate from the accessory breast tissue. The asymmetric axillary tail and the axillary accessory breast are both located on the left. Prominent asymmetry of the axillary tail may be related to a form fruste of accessory mammary tissue.

breast tissue, or asymmetrically prominent ducts that do not form a mass, do not contain microcalcifications, or do not produce architectural distortion should be viewed with concern only when associated with a palpable asymmetry and are otherwise normal variations." This asymmetric breast tissue is to be distinguished from an asymmetric density that is one representation of a mass lesion and may well be malignant (Fig. 4-3).

Barnard et al. studied histologic features of benign breast disease diagnosed after biopsy of nonpalpable mammographic abnormalities.[7] The incidence of sclerosing adenosis and microcalcifications was considerable higher in the group of nonpalpable mammographic lesions. Fibrous disease of the breast and radial scar (infiltrating epitheliosis) were also more common. There was no difference in the incidence of epithelial hyperplasia between the two groups. Correlation with mammographic appearances showed that microcalcification was most often associated with blunt duct adenosis and that stromal distortion or masses were most often caused by fibrous disease.

Weber et al. studied 20 patients with biopsies that revealed atypical hyperplasia of the breast.[129] The mammographic appearance included rounded, clearly delineated opacities with benign appearances or spiculated masses possibly associated with microcalcifications, stellate opacities, and isolated foci of microcalcifications. Obviously, in this series the appearance could not be distinguished from the mammographic features of breast cancers.

Rosselli-Del-Turco et al. observed that when subsequent histologic examination revealed a benign pathology, the microcalcification was more frequent in those cases coming from the screening program (14.5% of 198 cases) than among self-referred cases (4.5% of 1818 cases).[102]

Fibroadenoma. The most common of the benign lesions still often mistaken for breast cancer on mammograms is fibroadenoma. The mammographic distinction between fibroadenoma and breast cancer can usually, but not always, be made. Fibroadenomas are usually circumscribed and, when associated with calcifications, are usually coarser, larger, and more dense than the microcalcifications in malignancy. Fibroadenomas may be multiple and, as such, should be distinguished from multicentric carcinoma (Figs. 4-4 and 4-5).

Deschenes et al. observed that, in the National Breast Cancer Screening, prevalence of fibroadenoma was 8.3 per 1000.[27] The peak age of women at the time of diagnosis of a fibroadenoma is in their twenties, while those with a fibroadenoma containing a carcinoma is in the forties. For patients under 25 years, excision can be postponed a few months since spontaneous regression may occur and risk of breast cancer is small at that age.

Wilkinson et al., in a retrospective study of 134 patients with a clinical diagnosis of fibroadenoma of the breast, indicated that the histologic confirmation of this diagnosis is made in only 50%.[133] The majority of the others have a diagnosis of benign mammary dysplasia. Eight patients had an unsuspected carcinoma, all but one being above the mean age for the fibroadenoma group. The natural history of fibroadenoma is not known precisely. In this study, women with a clinical diagnosis of fibroadenoma were carefully observed provided they were less than 35 years of age and fine-needle aspiration cytology revealed no malignant cells.

Traumatic fat necrosis. Another benign breast abnormality that may be mistaken for cancer is fat necrosis. Usually the distinction is readily apparent on mammograms. However, Bassett et al. presented five cases with features of traumatic fat necrosis seen on mammograms.[9] The appearances vary from one indistinguishable from carcinoma to single or multiple lipid-filled cysts, with or without calcified walls. Branching, rodlike, or angular microcalcifications associated with fat necrosis may resemble the calcifications associated with carcinoma. A review of these cases led them to the conclusion that while breast cancer in some cases has characteristic radiographic findings, there are no pathognomonic findings.

Orson et al. reported eight cases of fat necrosis of the breast. They showed a spectrum of mammographic appearances, from mimicking other benign diseases to suggesting a malignant lesion.[81] Three of the eight cases showed the benign ringlike calcification associated with fat necrosis; this is a higher percentage than reported in previous series. Typical fat necrosis has a characteristic radiologic presentation, and biopsy of these lesions is not necessary unless other clinical or radiologic signs suggest malignancy.

Benign calcifications. The spontaneous disappearance of breast calcification has not been reported in the microcalcifications associated with malignancy. The use of the term "microcalcification" should be reserved for calcifications most likely to be associated with malignancy change. Benign calcifications, in general, have another connotation and can usually be readily differentiated from the microcalcifications of malignancy. A major problem in breast cancer detection has been the lack of adequate recognition of which calcifications should be considered benign and warrant no further diagnostic concern.

Fewins et al. observed the spontaneous disappearance of both coarse and fine calcification in the breast in 11 patients who presented either with breast symptoms or to a screening unit.[32] Parker et al. reported 17 patients aged 47 to 67 years of age with 20 foci of disappearing breast calcifications.[87] The most common configuration of disappearing calcifications was round or oval. All calcifications but one were found in dense glandular areas of the breast. Dense glandular tissue within 1 cm of the border with the stroma was the most common location. One of 20 foci suggested malignancy.

So-called microcystic adenosis is the most common histologic finding in cases of benign microcalcifications observed in the breast stroma on a mammogram. Lanyi et al. found a 10% incidence of microcystic (blunt duct) adenosis in 135 breast biopsies carried out because of microcalcifications.[60] These microcalcifications have a characteristic radiographic pattern. Chronic cystic mastitis was found by Prorok et al. to be the most common finding associated with benign microcalcifications (55%)[93] (Figs. 4-6 and 4-7).

Milk of calcium, in tiny benign cysts, is responsible for the characteristic "teacup" appearance of many benign microcalcifications.[113] The milk of calcium settles to the bottom of multiple tiny benign cysts, producing a mammographic picture of clustered linear and curvilinear calcifica-

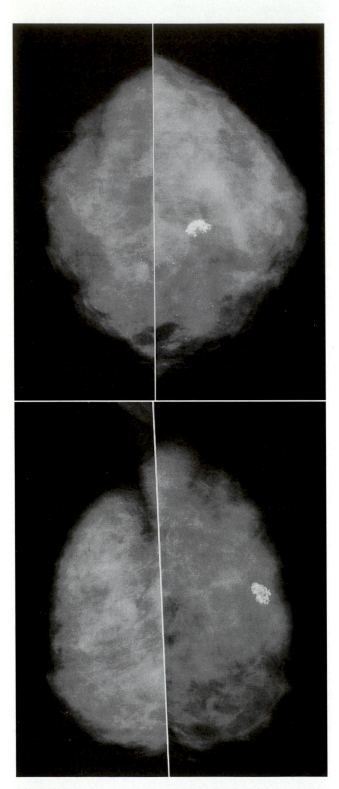

Fig. 4-4. Characteristic mammographic appearance of a calcified fibroadenoma. The benign nature of the lesion is obvious from the mammogram. No further study needs to be done.

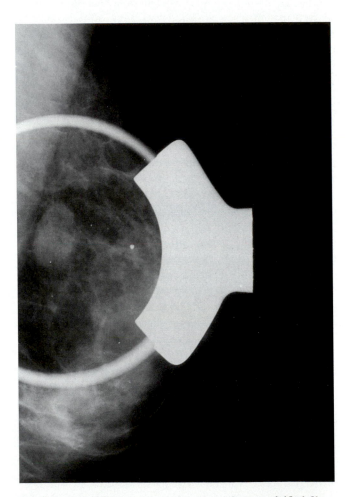

Fig. 4-5. Coned-down compression view of a noncalcified fibroadenoma in a premenopausal woman. Note the calcification outside the fibroadenoma is in no way connected with it. This ovoid density has clearly defined margins and some evidence of fatty replacement within the structure of the lesion. The pattern is typical for a benign fibroadenoma without calcification. This is characteristically a lesion of younger women. Lesions like this are infrequently seen on postmenopausal screening mammograms.

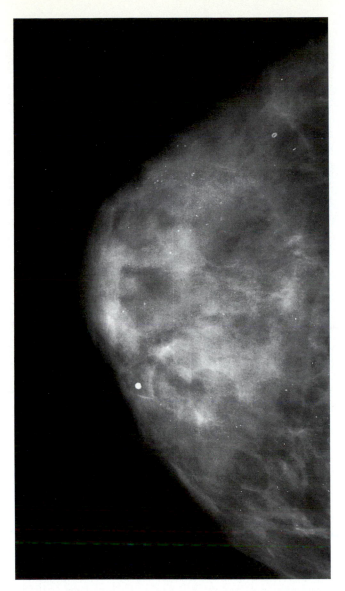

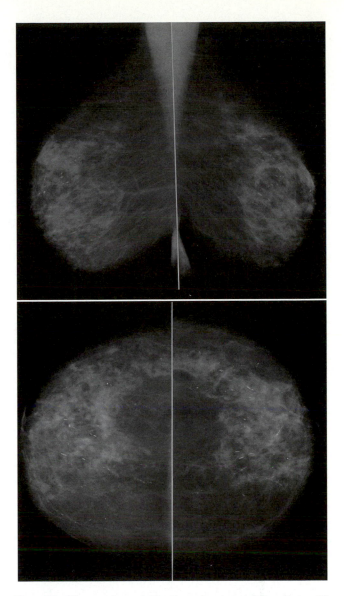

Fig. 4-6. Craniocaudal magnification view of a 40-year-old woman with multiple benign calcifications. This illustration represents a case of multifocal calcifications that are entirely benign. If only one of these calcifications existed in isolation, it might appear to be a microcalcification of malignancy. However, on close scrutiny of each of these calcifications, it can readily be appreciated that they are typical of totally benign calcifications.

Fig. 4-7. These microcalcifications located within ducts diffusely distributed throughout the breast are common and are entirely benign, they should never give rise to concern for malignancy. While these linear calcifications are typically termed radiologically as intraductal calcifications, the histologic correlate is lacking. These may well be stromal in origin. The capacity radiologically to distinguish the pathologic locale of many of these normal calcifications is so deficient that we prefer to refer to them simply as benign calcifications without attempting to assign anatomic or pathologic correlate. The same holds true for so-called plasma cell mastitis with calcifications. This is never associated with inflammatory cells in histologic sections. We conclude that it merely represents another form of benign calcifications found within normal human breasts. Thus far, there have been no adequate mammographic pathologic correlations of what has usually been termed plasma cell mastitis. At one time this was a popular diagnosis; currently it is not in vogue. When we assert that the benign residual calcifications in the breast are normal, we do not mean that they do not represent an attribute within 1 standard deviation of the norm. Rather, in this context normal means that the observation per se has no clinically relevant significance to the patient. The presence or absence of this normal variation will not affect whatever would happen to the patient now or in the future. This may adversely affect the patient only if people who interpret mammograms find some of these normal calcifications and consider them to be of malignant origin. This false-positive mammography is to be avoided, since most of these benign calcifications can readily be detected mammographically as benign in origin.

tions when imaged in the lateral projection with a horizontal x-ray beam. Milk of calcium is found much more frequently in small breast cysts than anywhere else in the body. It is not at all uncommon, occurring in more than 4% of women undergoing diagnostic mammography.

Skin calcifications are another important origin of benign breast microcalcifications. Calcifications that lie within the breast skin may be mistaken for intraparenchymal calcifications on mammograms as they are projected over the breast tissue in two views. Tangented views may reveal the true nature of these calcifications. However, it may be difficult to get the correct part of the skin in tangent when seeking to clarify the cause of these calcifications. Linden et al. developed a simple, reliable technique using commercially available stereotaxic localization in six patients to demonstrate the breast skin calcifications.[65]

Bruwer et al. observed intranodal gold deposits simulating microcalcifications on mammography in the axillary nodes.[19] Breast cancers that are manifested as extensive punctate calcifications very rarely occur in this pattern in metastatically involved axillary lymph nodes. Such punctate densities are much more indicative of intranodal gold deposits that occur almost invariably in patients with rheumatoid arthritis who have undergone prolonged chrysotherapy.

Artifacts may occasionally be mistaken for breast microcalcification. The most common problem is caused by deodorant powder that the patient applied prior to the mammogram. Simple precautions and a proper history can eliminate this potential confusion.

CALLBACK

The initial decision on screening mammography is whether or not to call the patient back for additional views. At the Karolinska Institute we have a 3.87% callback rate.[3] Mammographic views other than the routine craniocaudal and mediolateral-oblique (MLO) views are often needed to define an area of concern sufficiently to reach a diagnostic conclusion. Additional views are often needed as a prerequisite to recommending fine-needle aspiration and/or a surgical biopsy. At the Karolinska Institute, the additional views confirm normality in 28% (that is, 272 of the 735 patients called back from a pool of 18,987 had prevalence screens) (see Table 4-1).

In women with dense breasts or mottled stromal architecture, the possibility of a mass may be difficult to exclude on the initial craniocaudal and mediolateral-oblique projections. In these instances, it may be necessary to have the patient return for additional views to see whether the stromal architecture is sufficiently separated with compression to reveal the absence of an underlying mass lesion. Coned-down compression views are particularly useful to clearly define subtle abnormalities warranting further attention. The use of a coned-down compression view will

markedly diminish the number of unnecessary surgical biopsies that result from a false-positive mammographic interpretation.

Many rounded masses on the mammogram may be further evaluated by ultrasound. However, the variations in ultrasonic technique and interpretation are such that many screening mammographers today would recommend a needle aspiration to resolve a question of a cystic mass. This not only decreases the prospect that a cyst is obscuring a subtle cancer but also allows us to obtain cells from the area of concern to decrease the possibility that the dense area is cancer. In experienced hands ultrasonic evaluation of rounded densities in the breast is an appropriate adjunct to screening mammography. However, in many instances simple needle aspiration will reduce the density sufficiently that further mammograms will more clearly view the normal breast and stromal architecture.

Criteria for call-back

The basic principle of screening mammography is that most patients will be considered normal and can therefore return for follow-up care according to standard guidelines. However, a certain percentage of patients will require further examinations and must be "called back" for these studies. The frequency of callback varies with the techniques that were performed. Sickles et al. studied the relationship of one- or two-view mammography to the frequency of the need to do additional mammographic examinations.[115] They found that their two-view interpretation not only identified more cancers than the one-view reading (27 versus 25 from 22,500 asymptomatic women undergoing prevalence mammograms) but also that two-view initial screening mammograms required fewer additional mammograms to evaluate potential abnormalities (179 versus 642, or 7% versus 26%). Thus the additional data gleaned from an initial two-view mammogram decreased the need for callback in some 19% of Sickles' patients. The cost of callbacks far exceeds the money saved by having a one-view rather than a two-view initial screening examination. The rate for callback varies considerably in different published series.

Pamilo et al. studied the reasons for recall and the influence of experience in recall in 579 (3.21%) women for mammography screening.[85] The proportion of recall for further studies was greatest (6.3%) at the onset of screening. With increased experience, the proportion decreased by stages. In the second screening round it was only 2.04%. The proportion of cases referred for surgical biopsies in the first screening round was 0.7%, and the proportion of screening-detected breast cancers was 0.52%. These changed little with increased experience. In the second screening round, the proportions of referrals for surgical biopsies (0.43% of those screened) and of screening-detected breast cancers (0.3%) were both low. A tumor-like density was the most common finding causing recall. The number of recalls caused by superimposition of normal parenchymal structures decreased with experience, while the proportion of breast cancer and benign tumors increased. The proportion of cases with parenchymal distortion resulting in recall for further studies was similar in both screening rounds, but the number of those referred for biopsy fell dramatically in the second screening round. The number of recalls for microcalcification also fell with experience, and the proportion of breast cancer in this group increased over two screening rounds. Pamilo asserts that a high ratio of malignancy in surgical biopsies can be expected when the radiologist undertaking primary screening also performed all further studies.

The standard approach to Category I mammographic diagnoses is to recommend that the patient return in 1 year, or according to the ACR guidelines. In each case a recommendation must be made for the future care or screening. For normal examinations, the patient should return to the pool of screening patients for future screening at an appropriate interval.

For Category II patients, those who have abnormal mammograms but no evidence of malignancy, most should return to the pool of patients for subsequent routine screening. The mere fact that a nonmalignant abnormality has been identified does not mean that the patient cannot get a malignancy sometime in the future. Occasionally, a possible consequence of diagnosing a benign abnormality in the breast is that the patient may be lost to further follow-up since the abnormality has been identified as benign. Thus it is imperative that Category II patients routinely undergo subsequent screening mammograms at appropriate intervals.

Some Category II patients may be called back for further diagnostic procedures even though the presumption on the original mammogram is that of a benign abnormality. This amounts to 22% in the most recent Karolinska series (Table 4-1). For example, in some obvious fibroadenomas, calcifications may require further diagnostic evaluation. In those instances, it is important that the patient return for a magnification view to better delineate the calcifications and/or for coned-down compression film to further delineate the boundaries of what may be a mass.

All borderline situations, between benign and malignant abnormalities, should be labeled as Category III. They warrant further evaluation in each instance. At the Karolinska Institute some 30% of patients called back for a screening mammogram are Category III. When the patient returns, the procedure most appropriate to delineate the suspected abnormality will depend on the abnormality identified on the initial image. The abnormalities of concern can be separated into microcalcifications, rounded masses with ill-defined borders, questionable spiculated masses, and varying degrees of asymmetry. The appropri-

ate response to the suspected abnormalities in part depends on the nature of the breast under examination.

What to do on callback

Microcalcifications. A Category III patient is frequently called back because of microcalcifications that are not clearly benign on the initial examination. The most appropriate clarification study is a coned-down magnification view. The magnification view will usually identify the nature and structure of the microcalcifications. In classifying calcifications, it is relatively easy to identify many as benign—for example, the typical rounded calcifications of sclerosing adenosis or linear blood vessel calcification. Magnification films will allow clearer delineation of the nature of these benign calcifications. At other times, however, there continues to be lingering doubt as to the cause of the calcification, especially if it is linear or branching. In those instances, further cytologic clarification of that region of the breast would be imperative (see Chapter 7). In some breasts, multiple calcifications throughout the entire breast are persistently disconcerting. These small microcalcifications may well represent multiple foci of malignancy, and it is very difficult to identify a specific area that would warrant sampling for histologic assessment. In some of these instances, random surgical biopsies have resulted in the identification of carcinoma in situ (see Chapter 2).

Meyer et al. point out the need for competent mammographic interpretation to decrease the need for callback and "unnecessary" surgical biopsy in patients with microcalcifications.[70] They studied x-ray-guided biopsies in 1261 occult breast abnormalities of which 49.6% or 623 had masses, 50.4% or 635 had calcifications as the dominant feature, and 18.8% or 237 had cancer including 85 cases of ductal carcinoma in situ. The biopsy results of mammograms from other facilities yielded a PPV of 0.167 (164/981) versus 0.261 (73/284) in Brigham and Women's Hospital interpretations. This is a statistically significant difference and lends support to the value of second opinions in patients with biopsy recommendations for occult breast lesions, especially when findings are inconclusive.

Suspicious masses, stromal distortion, and focal density. The typical spiculated mass in a radiolucent breast is categorized as IV or V. Cytologic assessment is necessary. However, many suspicious masses, areas of stromal distortion, or areas of focal density require clarification before cytologic sampling can be recommended. A common reason for callback is to clarify questionably rounded or irregularly rounded lesions (Fig. 4-8). Often, these are small cysts or aggregates of stromal structure that have the appearance of early carcinoma. Usually, they will not be as dense as carcinoma. If the density of the abnormality is the same as normal surrounding stroma, it is more likely benign. The density of the suspect abnormality is an impor-

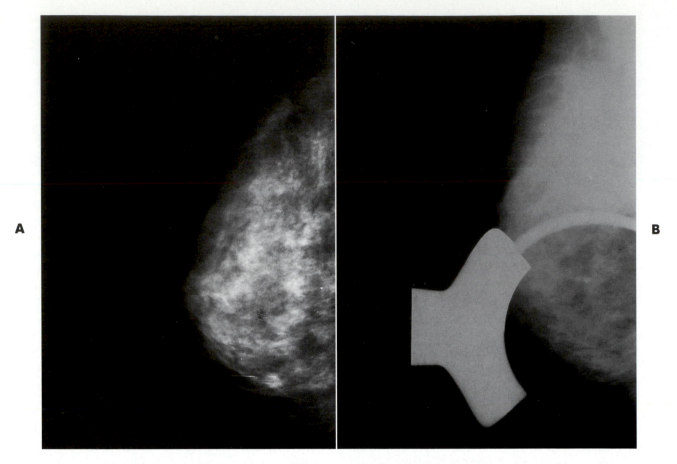

Fig. 4-8. An irregular density on the inferior margin of a mediolateral mammogram. This "lesion" may be spiculated and requires that the patient have additional views even though it was not seen in the craniocaudal view. **B,** coned-down compression view of the area of concern seen in **A.** It is important to be sure that the coned-down view clearly includes the area of concern. In this the density was "compressed away" by the coned-down technique. The area of initial concern represented a fortuitous superimposition of stromal architecture, which gave the appearance of a spiculated density.

tant feature in identifying whether one should be concerned for malignancy. On callback, however, these problems can usually be clarified by using a coned-down compression view, which will usually define the boundaries of a totally benign lesion. If irregular borders persist on coned-down compression view, then cytologic assessment of that region of the breast is warranted.

A second aspect of irregular or potentially rounded densities is that frequently these densities are so ill defined that it is difficult to be sure that there is a mass within the stromal structure. In these instances, the coned-down compression view may displace normal stromal architecture such that the fortuitous superimposition that resulted in the initial impression of a mass lesion can be overcome. Coned-down compression views allow for an adequate delineation of the breast architecture when local stromal density suggests the possibility of a mass lesion. Often a coned-down compression view can eliminate further concern for the presence of a mass within the breast. Occasionally, a stereotaxic image can reveal when an apparent density or mass is caused by a superimposition of normal breast stroma (see Chapter 3).

At times it is possible to further evaluate a questionable mass lesion evidenced by possible stellate configuration of the stromal architecture by merely *rolling* the breast and having a different cranial caudal projection. A rolled view of the breast may displace superimposed stromal structures by changing the position of the breast within the image. Therefore a rolled-breast image is frequently helpful in addition to or in lieu of a coned-down compression view if one must distinguish between a mass lesion in the breast and a fortuitous superimposition of stromal structures. A rolled-breast image in a craniocaudal projection is a useful supplement when a patient is called back (see Chapter 3).

Asymmetry. Breast asymmetry has been a frequent reason to call the patient back for more definitive evaluation. Asymmetry is the weakest among the criteria traditionally used to identify nonpalpable breast cancer. Asymmetry may be a normal variant. It is therefore important to clearly delineate whether asymmetry is a normal degree of stromal variation or is potentially related to a neoplasm. In these instances, on callback, the most useful diagnostic procedure is usually a coned-down compression view to displace the normal stromal structures as much as possible to identify whether there is an underlying mass lesion. Lateromedial and rolled views may also assist in ascertaining normality in breast asymmetry. When microcalcifications occur in asymmetry, the usual recourse is to obtain a magnification mammogram. If the calcifications are suspicious, cytologic assessment will be necessary, especially if microcalcifications are not clearly benign. Suspicious microcalcifications in asymmetric dense tissue in the breast are usually indications for further diagnostic studies.

DIFFICULT BREAST IMAGE

The patients on callback who are eventually found to have benign processes are often those who initially had a difficult breast image because of the widely varying patterns of normal breast stroma. Usually, the stroma can be seen to converge at the nipple and be dominant in the upper outer quadrant of the breast.

Mottled stroma

Sometimes breast stroma may be irregularly distributed throughout the breast, giving the appearance of multiple breast masses that are isodense to normal stroma. This so-called *mottled stroma* may be confused with suspicious masses (Fig. 4-9). Additional views obtained on callback may not eliminate concern for the possibility of a mass lesion. A coned-down compression view will reveal that the density is indeed present. Magnification views will usually reveal irregular or ill-defined borders of the questionable mass. However, mammographic features allow one to de-

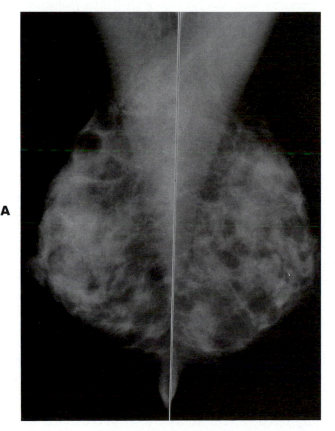
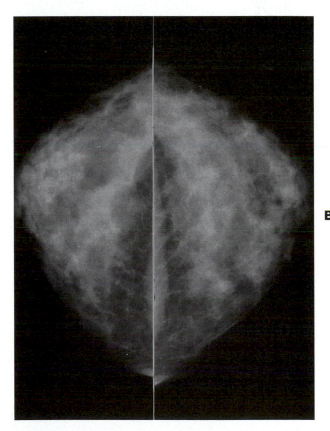

Fig. 4-9. Craniocaudal projection of a mammogram on a 47-year-old woman. This mammogram has a "mottled" appearance of the stroma. The irregular density is in part related to the irregular fatty replacement of normal stroma of a dense breast **B,** Craniocaudal projection of the same patient taken at the same time as **A.** Both images may suggest multiple irregular densities, any one of which may hide an occult cancer. It is important not to over interpret these cases. Serial imaging after progressive fatty replacement of the breast is most useful in distinguishing between normal "model" stromal architecture and focal malignancy.

cide which if any of these areas may represent normal stromal mottling or malignancy and thus warrant further attention. These features include (1) differential density, (2) total breast pattern in this patient, (3) location of the area in question, and (4) comparison with a previous mammogram. In such situations, the principal distinguishing feature is the *relative density* in the region of concern. Malignant masses are characteristically more dense than normal breast stroma. This differential density may be difficult to distinguish in already dense breasts.

A second feature useful to assist in distinguishing normal stromal mottling from malignancy is the total breast pattern. Does the other breast have a grossly irregular distribution of stroma? Is the pattern symmetrical in character if not in distribution? Normal stromal mottling will usually be evident in both breasts since both breasts are of similar genetic makeup responding to a similar hormonal milieu. Bergkvist et al. have shown that the characteristics of the reproductive lives of women have a significant and lifelong impact on their mammographic parenchymal pattern.[11] They classed the patterns according to Wolfe and found that the P2 and DY patterns increased regularly with increasing age at first birth and was highest in nulliparous women. This association was present for all age groups and was most pronounced in the oldest women. Fajardo et al. subsequently showed that radiologists were less confident in their interpretation of mammograms with P2 and DY parenchymal patterns than they were for other mammograms.[29] These researchers also showed a significant correlation between decreasing diagnostic certainty and increasing complexity of the mammographic patterns.[29] The areas of concern in patients with a pattern of mottled stroma are those that are grossly dissimilar in distribution and in density.

One important consideration is that the medial portion of the breast usually contains relatively little stroma in older women. Any appearance of a density in the medial half of the breast in the craniocaudal projection warrants greater vigilance than would a similar density located in the outer half of the breast. Similarly, a density located inferiorly in the mediolateral view is also of increased concern. Most normal stroma tends to be toward the upper outer quadrant of the breast (Fig. 4-10).

A fourth useful diagnostic test is the presence of a previous examination, where the appearance may be essentially unchanged between two serial mammographic studies. Obviously, this assistance is not available on the initial baseline mammogram. When these patients are first seen, there is often some concern as to whether some of these rounded densities are neoplastic. In these instances, the distinction of tissue density between cancer and normal stromal structure is the most important criterion used to make the distinction. Regional differences in densities of the rounded masses may be a criterion for identifying those patients who warrant a fine-needle aspiration biopsy.

Dense breasts

Dense breasts pose a significant problem in detecting early breast cancer. In such cases, the density of normal stroma or cysts may mask an underlying malignancy. The mammographic detection of early breast cancer relies heavily on the discovery of abnormal breast density or calcification. Holland et al. suggested that most preinvasive cancers without microcalcifications are mammographically occult, while even invasive cancers situated in dense

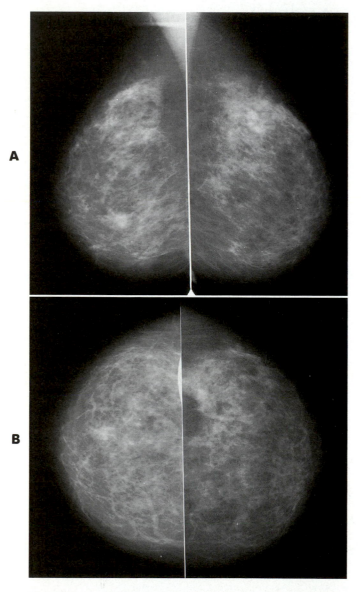

Fig. 4-10. A, Mediolateral mammogram in a postmenopausal woman who is not receiving estrogen therapy. The inferior irregular density in the right breast is typical of invasive ductal carcinoma. **B,** Craniocaudal view reveals the lesion to the retroareolar and somewhat separated from the normal lateral stroma.

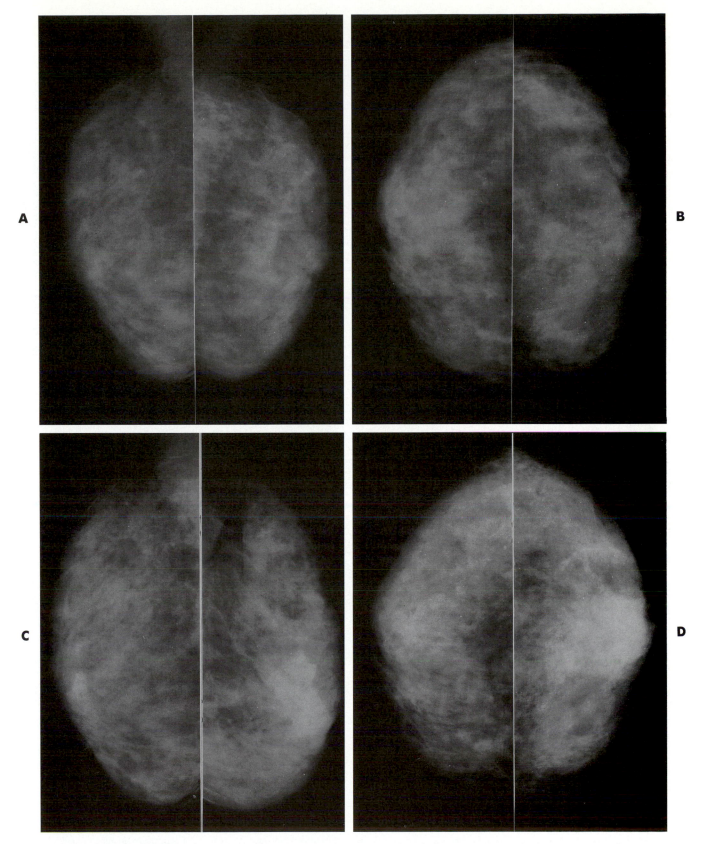

Fig. 4-11. A and **B,** Mediolateral and craniocaudal mammograms in a woman who has mottled irregular stromal distribution. The irregularity makes it difficult to define the specific areas for occult cancers. The left breast has greater periareolar density than the right. The irregular mottling of the stromal architecture, however, makes it difficult to identify a specific area where one would suspect malignancy at this time. **C** and **D,** Films taken of the same patient 2 years later. In this instance, the periareolar density is considerably more obvious and turned out to be an invasive ductal carcinoma. In this case, the change in the mammographic appearance is an important feature to distinguish the presence of cancer in a dense breast with irregular stromal architecture.

breasts may be mammographically occult.[46] Cahill et al. studied features of mammographically negative breast tumors.[21] A total of 9.3% of 323 consecutive patients with operable breast cancer had negative mammographic reports. Misinterpretation of carcinoma as a benign lesion and diagnostic difficulties in dense dysplastic breasts were found to be the main causes of error.

If the breast is normally very dense, subtle differences in regional density may be difficult to detect. While overall breast density may make it difficult to detect cancer, malignant lesions, even in dense breasts, will usually appear denser than the surrounding normal stroma. Fortunately, normal breast involution patterns occur in the age group with increasing risk for breast cancer. However, most young women and many older women, especially those with prior fibrocystic patterns, will have dense breast stroma that may obscure malignancy.

Mammographic features of malignancy may allow for the detection of breast cancer in even very dense breasts. These features are (1) architectural distortion and asymmetry, (2) stromal retraction, and (3) malignant calcifications. Even in dense breasts, normal stroma is usually located in the upper outer quadrant. A local area of distortion of this pattern may indicate early cancer (Fig. 4-11). A density appearing posterior to dense normal stroma should be of concern, especially if it is not contiguous with the normal stroma (Fig. 4-12).

A second feature to search for in dense breasts is the pattern of stromal retraction. Evidence for retraction can be discerned by noting a convergence of stromal elements toward a focus rather than toward the nipple. Sometimes this apparent convergence away from the nipple can be clarified by coned-down compression views.

In many dense breasts, microcalcification may be the only indicator of early cancer. The analysis of microcalcifications in dense breasts is no different than the usual analysis of microcalcifications. However, in the dense breast, the vigilance of search for microcalcifications is even more important than in a relatively radiolucent breast, where the microcalcifications may be more easily visualized. In addition, overall breast density will make it more difficult to detect a mass in association with the calcifications and thereby remove one of the distinguishing features in the mammographic detection of breast cancer. The discovery of an associated mass as an aid in ascertaining which microcalcifications should be considered suspicious for cancer is often not possible in very dense breasts. Thus, we lose one of the possible features of malignant microcalcifications.

Cystic breasts

Another difficult breast is the breast with multiple cysts. Women with multiple breast cysts may also have underly-

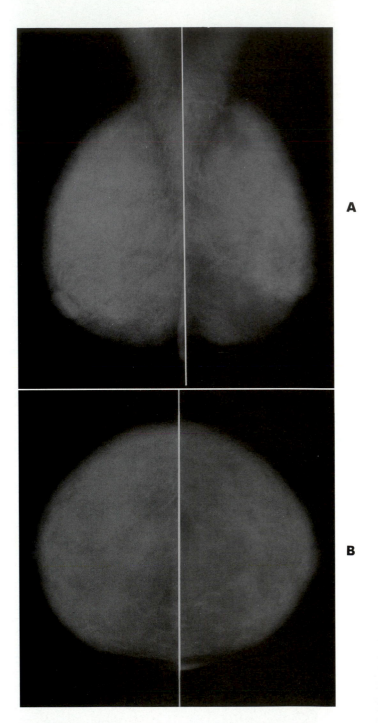

A

B

Fig. 4-12. Mediolateral and craniocaudal mammograms of very dense breasts in a woman who had been lactating. In this case, there is no portion of the breast where the stroma is absent. Thus there is no density posterior to the stroma that is more suspicious. These are normal densities in a women who had been lactating. Obviously, a subtle carcinoma may well be obscured by the homogeneously dense breasts.

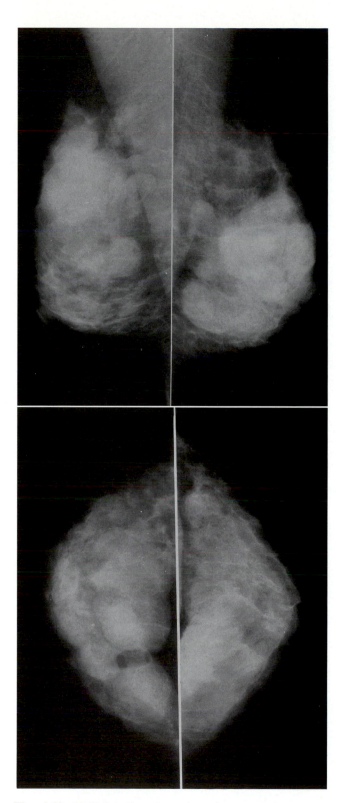

Fig. 4-13. Mediolateral and craniocaudal mammograms in a woman with multiple rounded and irregular densities caused by multiple cysts. These "densities" are of a similar density to surrounding normal breast stroma. Cancer will usually be more dense than adjacent stroma.

ing cancers. Breast cysts alone are not risk factors for breast cancer. Women with cystic breasts require vigilant mammographic observations in an effort to detect early breast cancer partially obscured by an unrelated cyst. At times it may be necessary to drain the cysts by needle aspiration to more appropriately observe the underlying breast architecture. In women with high-risk factors and multiple cysts that obscure the mammographic delineation of the breast tissue, it may be appropriate to clarify the underlying breast stroma following the needle drainage of at least some of the cysts. Nonpalpable cancers do occur in patients who have multiple palpable lumps related to a cystic breast (Figs. 4-13 and 4-14).

Multiple small cysts may lead to a "snowflake" appearance where there are multiple small rounded and irregular masses within the breast. Although these can be confusing, they are relatively easy to identify because of the homogeneous nature of the densities throughout the breast. To distinguish this from the mottled breast, where the densities are nonhomogeneous in size and in their distribution, is relatively easy when compared to other difficult breast images.

SOURCES OF ERROR IN MAMMOGRAPHIC INTERPRETATION
Interval cancer*

Cancers diagnosed on the latter of two serial screening mammograms reveal much about the reasons for a missed breast cancer diagnosis. Some of these cancers were not present on the prior mammogram. The cancer may have developed in the interval between the examinations, at least to the point that it may become visible on mammographic films. Traditionally, interval cancer is defined as those cancers that occur during the interval between two serial mammograms and, therefore, is diagnosed because of symptoms and not as a result of screening. Cancers that develop between two serial screening studies—that are not visible at all on the initial study but found on a subsequent incidence mammogram—could also be considered interval cancers. These two types of interval cancers may differ, however. Those that develop symptoms are usually not diagnosable by mammography. That is, they may have been occult cancers on the initial study and only developed symptoms (i.e., palpable mass) during the interval. Breast cancers diagnosed on the second of two serial mammograms that were not on the initial mammogram were more likely cancers that truly developed in the interim. This is especially true when their diagnosis would not have been obscured by some overlapping normal breast tissue on the initial examination. These latter cancers (i.e., those diagnosed on the second of two serial mammograms and

*See also Chapter 2.

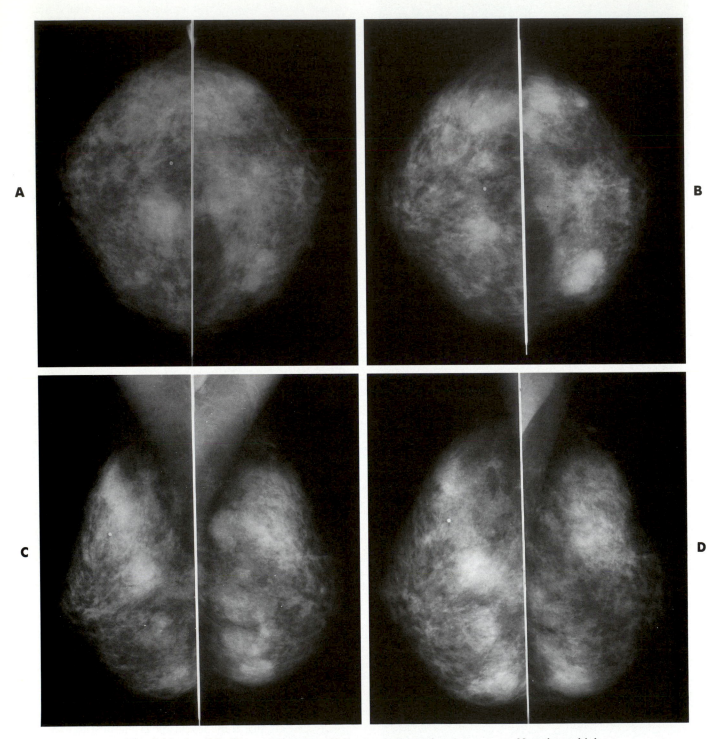

Fig. 4-14. A and **B,** Two serial craniocaudal mammograms taken 1 year apart. Note the multiple rounded densities that have changed substantially in the intervening year. Some have gotten larger and some became smaller. There was no intervening therapy. **C** and **D,** Similar changes are seen in the mediolateral views. These all represent benign cysts. The rapidly changing size, configuration, and density of these cysts makes it very difficult to distinguish which, if any, may be due to carcinoma.

clearly not present on the initial mammogram) are more likely to be rapidly growing cancers. These may have a different diploid/aneuploid ratio than the prevalence breast cancers detected on the initial screening and mammogram from the ambient population.

Holland et al. analyzed 64 interval cancers from a series of 209 cancers detected at regular mammographic screening in Holland.[47] In 19 of 64 patients, direct or indirect signs of the tumor were seen on previous screening mammograms on review. These were observer error. In four cases, the site of the tumor lay outside of the imaging field. These they considered to be a technical error. In 41 cases, no signs of tumor could be seen on the mammogram, even on review.

Further analysis of these 41 cases was affected by calculating the tumor doubling times. Twenty of the 41 cases were probably too small to be detected at the last screening. These they considered "real" interval cancers. However, 21 cases were probably large enough but somehow were masked from radiologic detection. They found that the main reasons for masking proved to be (1) a dense breast, (2) a poorly outlined tumor mass of diffuse infiltrated type, mainly invasive lobular carcinoma, and (3) intraductal localization. Based on this study, these authors suggested that women with dense breasts should be screened more frequently using more views and modalities and with broader criteria for advising surgical biopsy. The issue of growth rate and interval cancers was further explored by Heuser et al.[44] They studied the breast cancers detected in the BCDDP at Louisville over a 5-year period in order to better understand the propensity to grow fast or slow and to metastasize or not to metastasize. They divided fast cancers into two subsets, fast 1 and fast 2, and stipulated that these were the cancers surfacing in the interval between mammograms. The faster cancers exhibited significant absence of calcification and were discovered in younger patients. These patients had a shorter 5-year survival (fast one $= 74 \pm 9\%$, to slow $= 94 \pm 4\%$). These authors noted that, in addition to growth rates, another index of the virulence of the small cancers was the early appearance of axillary lymph nodes. They found that the absence of microcalcifications and the presence of lymphatic invasion around the primary cancer site were significantly associated with axillary metastases. These authors are of the opinion that interval cancers are biologically different and not comparable to cancers discovered on scheduled screening mammograms. These interval cancers metastasize to lymph nodes while very small and should be considered especially virulent.

Fallenius et al. used DNA morphometry to assess the prospective virulence on fine-needle aspirates of small cancers.[30] In this instance, they found cancers detected by mammography to be of a different DNA configuration than those detected by palpation. Using DNA analysis, they suggest that the nonpalpable cancers detected by mammography and confirmed by stereotaxic fine-needle aspiration biopsies are less virulent than those detected at the palpable stage. These views do not necessarily differ from those of Heuser et al.[44] who studied cancers occurring in the interval and did not necessarily separate palpable from nonpalpable lesions. Fallenius suggested that nonpalpable cancers are naturally less virulent than cancers discovered at the time of palpation.[30] Nonpalpable cancers discovered by screening mammography should have a slow growth rate when detected by prevalence mammograms. Truly new cancers developing between two screening mammograms will be more rapidly growing than the average cancer detected on a prevalence screen. The latter cancer may have been relatively stable within the breast for many years before detection.

When discussing missed breast cancer, it is important to appreciate the distinction between a missed breast cancer and an interval cancer of either type. Another traditional form of missed breast cancer is that which is not detectable by mammography but found only on clinical examination.

Most true interval cancers will have been identified by clinical examination simply because screening mammograms are not usually performed between two standard screening mammographic examinations. It is important to distinguish the interval cancer diagnosed on clinical examination from that identified by mammography alone. The number of breast cancers that will not be detectable on mammography depends in part on published series under analysis. Azavedo and Svane's report used the Karolinska system, where women considered to be asymptomatic are drawn to screening mammography without consideration of potential clinical findings.[3] Recalled women who have abnormal mammograms have a subsequent clinical examination performed by a member of the breast cancer diagnosis team. In this system, the initial concern was developed by the screening mammogram and only subsequently did the palpation reveal a lesion. These patients were considered to be essentially asymptomatic, in that they did not initiate the breast cancer diagnostic encounter on the basis of their concerns. In this series, 19% of cancers were clinically detectable in addition to being mammographically observable.

Missed cancer

The inability to detect some palpable cancers on the mammogram has often been considered mammographic error. However, we will limit our discussion to those failures to detect breast cancer that could have been, and perhaps should have been, detected on the initial mammogram. There are three major reasons for this problem. The first is the technical aspects of the procedure, whereby appropriate technique may well have detected a missed breast cancer. The second relates to the masking of lesions by surrounding breast stroma or density. The third is the more customary concern of observer error.

Technical error. Schmitt et al. demonstrated that most breast cancers missed by a technical flaw result from the inability to get the posterior portion of the breast on the film.[105] They studied the ability to visualize the retromammary space and ribs or both sites using adequate technical factors in 186 patients with breast cancer. All cancers were analyzed for position on the film, number of films required for visualization, relationship of the tumor to the posterior edge of the film, number of occult tumors, tumor size, histologic type, sensitivity of detection method, and number of interval cancers. They found 6% of their cancers within 1 cm of the posterior edge of the film. With adequate technique, all cancers were visualized in the mediolateral view, but three were not visualized on the craniocaudal view. Thus it is possible to miss up to 6% of cancers if sufficient retromammary space in the area of the ribs is not demonstrated on film. This type of technical error can be overcome by rigorous attention to detail in mammographic technique. Breasts in which the posterior portion cannot be observed because of the patient's anatomy should be reported as such.

Pagani et al. evaluated mediolateral and craniocaudal film-screen mammograms and a mediolateral noncontact xeromammogram alone and in combination in 53 women.[83] Four mammographers interpreted the films in a blinded randomized fashion. Cancer detection was improved when a greater number of views was evaluated. Certain cancers, by virtue of their position in the breast, could be obscured by superimposed stroma in one-view projection.

Another technical basis for missed breast cancer relates to films that are of insufficient technical quality to demonstrate the cancer. This is particularly true where the cancer is of insufficient density to clearly be seen on the initial film. Often this type of error in detection is related to a failure in observer performance. However, there are times when even the most diligent observer would not be able to detect the lesion, which has insufficient contrast against the normal tissue background. Films that are underpenetrated or overpenetrated and those with insufficient contrast are the cause of these problems. It is possible to have calcifications detected on the second of two serial mammograms and not readily visible in retrospect on the initial film unless one uses unusual procedures, such as film digitization to contrast the calcification to the surrounding breast. When there is insufficient contrast between calcific and normal tissue, it is possible to obscure subtle microcalcifications on screening mammograms. This may result in an error in film technique, causing failure to observe nonpalpable breast cancer. Most technical errors leading to missed nonpalpable breast cancer can be overcome by rigorous adherence to mammographic technique.

Masked lesions. A *masked lesion* is a lesion that, in retrospect, may have been detectable on the initial examination, but it would not have been reasonable to expect detection until it became more apparent on the subsequent study. Certain signals, when observed on a mammogram, should lead radiologists to consider the possibility of a masked cancer. These include asymmetry, dense stroma, mottled stroma, or "spiculated" stroma strands. When breasts are identified with any of these four features, the radiologist must approach the mammogram with an increased vigilance, seeking to detect an underlying breast cancer that may be obscured. In mottled or dense stroma, observing the relative density of the normal breast may be all that is necessary to detect a breast cancer. Sometimes the relatively subtle density of some early carcinomas may preclude our ability to detect them in dense or mottled breasts. The masking of the lesion is often due to overlying dense stromal structures or a mottled appearance of the breast, where one would have great difficulty discerning the cancer from normal stroma. The irregular distribution of normal stroma throughout a fatty breast can frequently lead to an interpretation that all areas of irregular stroma are indeed normal stroma, rather than early cancer. On a subsequent film, one of those areas may become considerably more dense and thereby lead to the diagnosis of cancer, though the area was not evident as cancer on the initial mammogram.

When one detects asymmetric density, a callback examination with coned-down and magnification views is necessary. These views should clarify whether a mass is responsible for the relative asymmetry between the breasts. "Spiculated" stromal strands, a common feature in some breasts, can lead to failure in the radiologic detection of breast cancer. In these patients there may be many areas in which cancers can be hidden, since many of the spiculations may resemble early cancer (Fig. 4-15). The distinction between normal stromal strands and early cancer can be extremely difficult in some patients. Multiple areas of spiculated stroma may numb the radiologist into suggesting that all are normal in this patient. Spiculated stroma, masking as a lesion, is most appropriately managed by additional compression views in areas of concern. The displacement of overlying stroma strands will no longer appear as unified and thereby suspicious for cancer. A second approach to the spiculated stroma image is to do a rolled mammogram in a craniocaudal projection. This technique changes the plane through which the beam penetrates the breast, which separates layers of stroma that may appear as a unified mass on an initial examination. A coned-down compression or rolled-breast view in patients with spiculated stromal patterns is usually necessary.

An approach to possible masking. When observing a breast with possible masking of a nonpalpable breast cancer, callback for coned-down compression and/or rolled

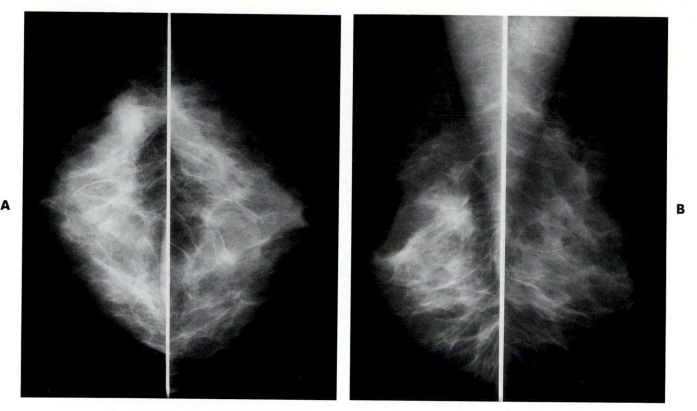

Fig. 4-15. Benign and malignant spiculations seen in craniocaudal and mediolateral mammograms of a 48-year-old woman. **A,** On the craniocaudal view there is a density with suggestive spiculation in the medial portion of the left breast. This is not seen in the mediolateral view (**B**), since the density on the craniocaudal view is due to a fortuitous superimposition of the normal, albeit mottled, stromal architecture seen in the mediolateral view. A coned-down compression view eliminated the left breast density as the area of concern. However, there is an obvious mass in the lateral portion of the right breast. The right breast mass is spiculated, with a irregular outline quite characteristic for carcinoma. The possibility of other areas of stromal retraction, however, tend to confuse the overall image. The carcinoma is better seen on the mediolateral projection, where the upper portion of the right breast clearly depicts an area of increased density with multiple spiculations.

projections is appropriate. If one is still in doubt, a stereotaxic view may be more definite about whether an abnormality requires further diagnostic procedures such as FNA. In the dense breast with possible cystic lesions, an ultrasound examination can further delineate whether dense structures are cystic or solid. In some cases of multiple cystic lesions or large cysts, it is appropriate to use needle puncture to drain the cyst, so that one can better evaluate underlying breast architecture.

Observer error. Classic observer error occurs when an obvious cancer, which "should" have been seen, is noted in retrospect. The missing of an obvious cancer, which "everyone" readily detects in retrospect, is usually due to a lapse in concentration, inattention to detail, or a distraction during the original interpretation. Occasionally, an obviously erroneous mammographic report is due to procedural

error in communication. If the report gets identified with the wrong patient, it may appear as if there were observer error, when the correct observation was made by the radiologist. If the failure to observe such a lesion or a failure to communicate the observation occurs, the radiologist and/or hospital in the United States may be subjected to malpractice litigation. This litigation should not be successful unless there is harm caused to the patient by the delay in diagnosis. There is controversy over whether substantial harm can be shown to occur from a brief delay in diagnosis. How long a delay must be to become negligence is usually left up to a court to decide on the merits of an individual case (see Chapter 2).

The missing of an obvious cancer does not present as much of a problem as the recognition of a subtle abnormality in retrospect, which most radiologists would not

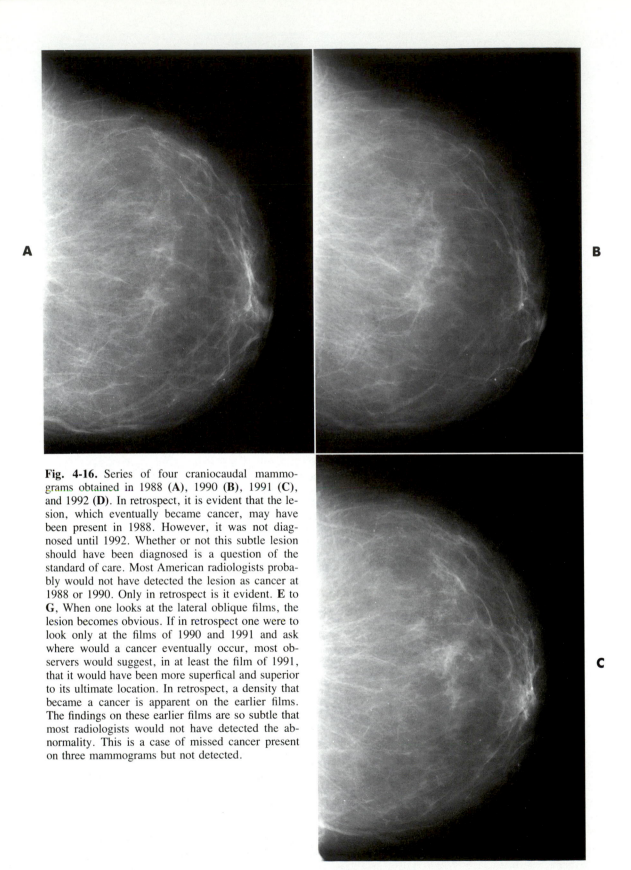

Fig. 4-16. Series of four craniocaudal mammograms obtained in 1988 (**A**), 1990 (**B**), 1991 (**C**), and 1992 (**D**). In retrospect, it is evident that the lesion, which eventually became cancer, may have been present in 1988. However, it was not diagnosed until 1992. Whether or not this subtle lesion should have been diagnosed is a question of the standard of care. Most American radiologists probably would not have detected the lesion as cancer at 1988 or 1990. Only in retrospect is it evident. **E** to **G**, When one looks at the lateral oblique films, the lesion becomes obvious. If in retrospect one were to look only at the films of 1990 and 1991 and ask where would a cancer eventually occur, most observers would suggest, in at least the film of 1991, that it would have been more superfical and superior to its ultimate location. In retrospect, a density that became a cancer is apparent on the earlier films. The findings on these earlier films are so subtle that most radiologists would not have detected the abnormality. This is a case of missed cancer present on three mammograms but not detected.

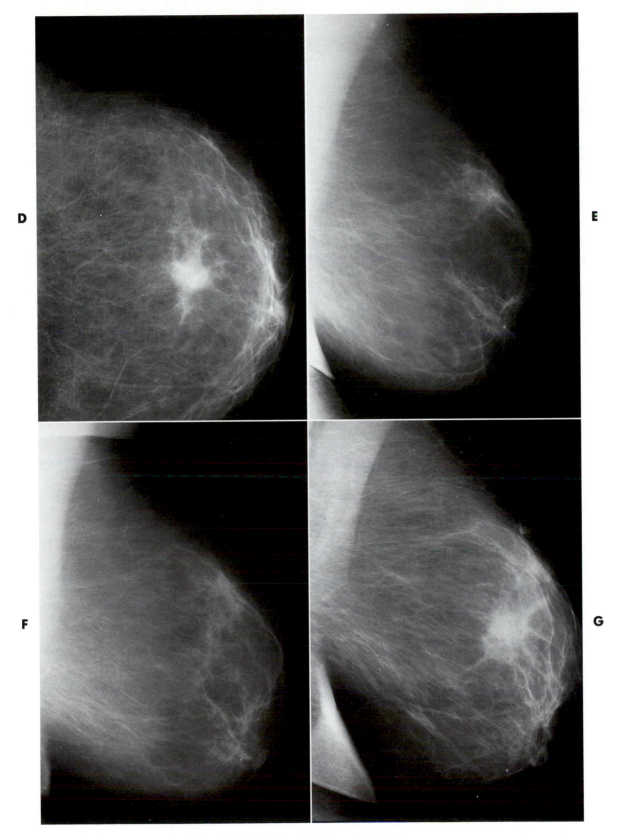

Fig. 4-16, cont'd. For legend see opposite page.

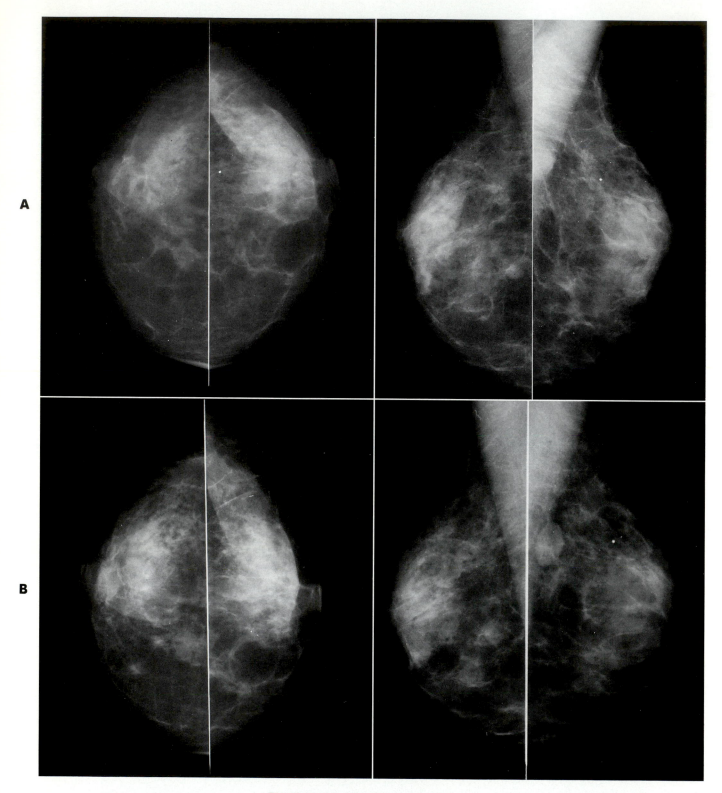

Fig. 4-17. For legend see opposite page.

have been expected to identify in prospect. We use three typical examples to demonstrate such issue (Figs. 4-16 to 4-18).

False negative. The missed breast cancer, which "should" have been observed, is a major problem in mammographic diagnosis. This "miss" may be due to a failure to detect the abnormality or a failure to properly interpret an abnormality that was detected. A failure to adequately communicate an observation to a physician or a patient will have the same effect as a false-negative observation or interpretation. Thus the sources of a missed breast cancer resulting from observer error are threefold: failure to detect, failure to correctly interpret that which was detected, or failure to adequately communicate an observation.

Failure to detect. Most observer error studies are concerned with the missed lesion—a cancer not detected by the observer. Another observer at another time, or even the same observer on subsequent viewing of the same film, may observe the cancer. This is the observer error that we all try to overcome in training ourselves to better diagnose nonpalpable breast cancers. One way to decrease the prospect of missing a lesion is to increase the number of false-positive overcalls. If the observer raises the threshold of suspicion for possible abnormalities, he/she may force an excessive number of surgical biopsies per breast cancer detected. This, of course, is not an appropriate approach to cancers missed because of observer error. False-negative observer errors are of two types: failure to detect the abnormality or failure to correctly interpret a detected abnormality. The failure to interpret is a judgmental call. It relates to the threshold of concern about things that are observed.

The most common observer error in early breast cancer detection relates to the detection of subtle microcalcifications. This is most often missed. Obviously, the capacity to observe subtle microcalcification depends in part on the inherent ability of the film system and the radiologist to note subtle differences in regional contrast. One must have a meticulous approach to looking at each mammogram, with specific attention to possible subtle microcalcifications. Different observers have a remarkably different ability to find and identify subtle microcalcifications on standard mammograms. Shading systems and magnifying lenses are helpful in many instances. Many things influence the observer's ability to discern subtle microcalcifications, including the intensity of the light system. Subtle microcalcifications must not be washed out by excessive light on the film. The viewing system should maximize the contrast between calcifications and normal breast parenchyma.

A major problem in identifying subtle microcalcifications is the attention and concentration of the observer. If mammograms are read in a place where there is considerable commotion or interruptions, it may not be possible to give full attention to looking for subtle microcalcifications. No other radiologic diagnosis is as dependent on intense scrutiny of the film. Distractions have a major influence in missed subtle microcalcification. *A lack of concentration is the most common reason for missing microcalcifications.*

A quality image is obviously necessary to detect microcalcification. The film density, contrast, etc. must exhibit calcifications to their best advantage. Some investigators have suggested that digitization of films to enhance contrast inherent in the image would assist in detecting microcalcifications. Digitization, while helpful for contrast, has had limitations in spatial resolution. Despite limitations in resolution, digitization may permit easier detection of subtle microcalcification. The ability to detect calcifications may not be as dependent on the size of the calcification as it is on its contrast against background breast tissue. In dense breasts, digitization appears to be of benefit by enhancing the contrast between the calcifications and other

Fig. 4-17. Craniocaudal and mediolateral screening mammograms in an asymptomatic 42-year-old woman. There is a subtle change in density along the inferior portion of the pectoralis muscle on the left. **A,** The ovoid lesion is masked by the pectoralis muscle shadow in the 1990 films. This rounded density is seen in the films of 1991 (**B**), which are taken with a slightly greater degree of obliquity. The lesion in the upper posterior portion of the breast—which turned out to be fibroadenoma—is well delineated as a ovoid lesion on the films of 1991. It is not visualized on the craniocaudal views in either year. The craniocaudal views vary considerably in positioning. The posterior benign calcification seen in the 1990 film is not seen in the 1991 craniocaudal view. Less breast is seen in the 1991 craniocaudal view than was visualized in 1990. The failure to observe the ovoid lesion in the left breast in 1991 represents a classic case of a masked lesion where the conspicuity is diminished by overlapping normal structures. In this instance, it is the pectoralis muscle. This abnormality is masked because of technical aspects of breast positioning. The rounded density in the posterior inferior portion of the right breast is a benign cyst.

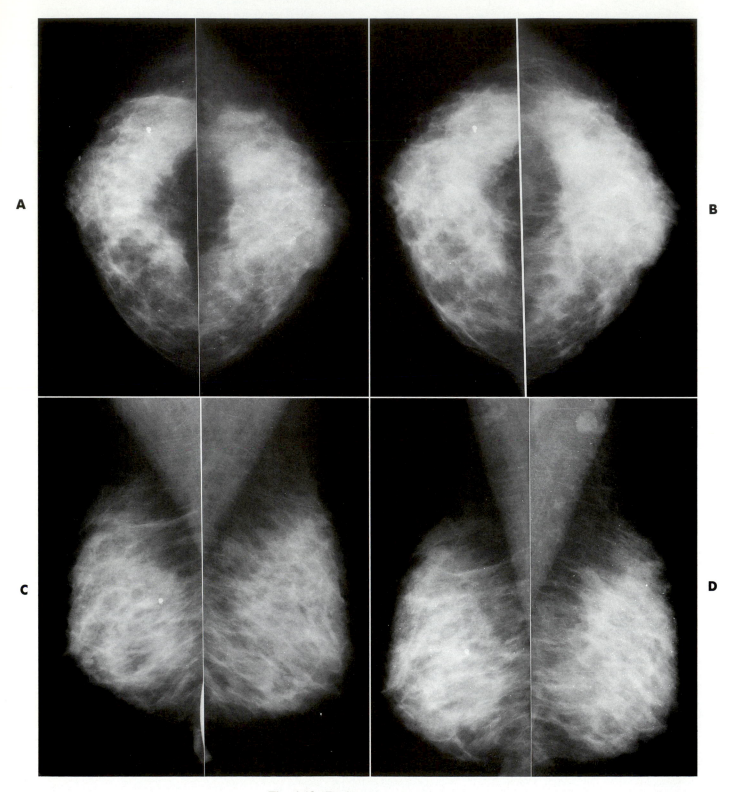

Fig. 4-18. For legend see opposite page.

breast density. In those instances, digitization of films may be able to improve observer performance in mammography.

Other techniques have been used to improve detection of subtle microcalcifications. In the dual-energy approach, one image is taken for soft tissue densities and a second image is designed to optimize imaging of subtle calcifications. Some of the more recent computed imaging systems (e.g., Fuji) will allow for dual imaging of various intensities on the same image, so that one may be able to evaluate the calcifications on one image and the breast stroma on another image taken at the same time.

Failure to correctly interpret a detected abnormality. This problem is most noted when rounded densities are misinterpreted as benign cysts. This is especially common in mottled breasts. These benign densities may resemble early cancers, which may be of a similar density to normal mottling of the breast stroma. It may not be possible to detect the difference in some instances. When they are not seen in retrospect, they are considered masked cancer. However, at other times differential densities of mottled breast stroma are such that the observer fails to appreciate a distinction between densities. *The missed cue of increased tissue density is the most common reason for observer error that is not related to microcalcifications.*

An asymmetric breast can at times result in observer error. One tends to be influenced by the fact that most recommended biopsies in an asymmetric breast will yield a benign result. If a radiologist finds that all of the recent biopsies recommended for asymmetric breasts have been benign in nature, the observer ROC curve will change in recognition of diminished concern for asymmetric breasts as an indication of early breast cancer. It is important that obvious breast asymmetry be further evaluated. When additional images suggest that there is no underlying masked lesion, then one can readily conclude that the asymmetry is a normal variant for this patient. However, relying on limited recent experience to ignore the possible significance of asymmetric breast density may result in missing an early breast cancer.

Wilkinson et al. found eight patients with breast cancer in 134 patients with a clinical diagnosis of fibroadenoma.[133] All but one of these patients with cancer were the mean age for the fibroadenoma group. This failure to correctly interpret an observed lesion was due to a lack of appropriate risk factor consideration. Here age was a factor being given inadequate emphasis. Mitnick et al. found 13 of 350 cases of intraductal carcinoma had mammographic features similar to benign tumors.[73] These may well result in false-negative mammographic interpretations. The carcinomas were sharply circumscribed, round, or oval lesions that contained microcalcifications. These calcifications were smaller and more likely to be asymmetrically located within the lobule than those of the fibroadenomas that they mimicked.

Baines et al., in a study of the Canadian trial of 44,718 women, found that a sensitivity of screening mammography in the total series was 0.75, with a specificity of 0.94, a PPV of 0.07, and the negative predictive value of 0.998.[6] Chamberlain et al. compared first and subsequent screens in a group of high-risk women and suggested that sensitivity of screening declines between the first and second visits but that specificity increases.[22] Despite improved specificity, the ratio of benign biopsies to cancer was worse at the repeat screening (21:1) than at the first screening (6:1), because the yield of cancers between the first and subsequent screens fell to a greater extent than the yield of benign disease.

Goin et al. did an ROC curve analysis of mammography.[39] They evaluated the accuracy of mammography in 38 incidence cancer cases. Their incidence cases were those that develop in a patient after the initial visit and at least one additional annual visit before biopsy was performed. They used 40 normal subjects; a sensitivity of 72% was attained at a 28% false-positive rate. Moskowitz retrospectively studied 17 carcinomas found in 69 breast

Fig. 4-18. A and **C,** Films in a 44-year-old woman who had mammograms in 1990 that were interpreted as normal mammograms in dense breasts. This patient has a twin sister who developed breast cancer at age 42. **B** and **D,** Screening mammograms were repeated in November of 1991. When these films were initially read and compared to the previous film, they were erroneously interpreted as no evidence of substantial change. In retrospect, however, there is an increase density in the upper outer quadrant of the left breast. Even this observation is controversial. Although the posterior contour of the stromal silhouette in the upper position of the breast had changed, this was initially thought to be due to the change in mammographic positioning. There is a benign calcification evident in the left breast. Some 3 months after the 1991 mammograms, this patient developed a palpable mass in the upper outer quadrant of the left breast, which was found to be invasive ductal carcinoma. These mammograms represent a masked lesion where the interval cancer was not detected on the mammogram. It may well have been in the image, but it was not discerned. This false-negative mammogram is one that would not have been necessarily corrected by improved technique or improved observer performance.

biopsies.[74] He reviewed the preoperative mammography reports provided by a pool of general radiologists. He observed a high sensitivity (88%), but poor specificity (32%), with an overall accuracy of 46%. Cahill et al. studied the features of mammographically negative breast tumors.[21] They found a total of 9.3% of 323 consecutive patients with operative breast cancer had a negative mammogram. Warren et al. studied the sensitivity, specificity, predictive value, and accuracy of film-screen mammography.[128] They analyzed 312 breast biopsies done at the University of Kentucky over a 3-year period. Each of the mammograms was classified as true positive, true negative, false positive, or false negative, based on the final pathologic diagnosis. Mammography had a sensitivity of 84%, specificity of 59%, PPV of 40%, negative predictive value of 92%, and accuracy of 65%. Bird reviewed 21,716 mammograms at a low-cost screening center.[13] A total of 142 cancers were discovered, 12 of which gave false-negative results at mammography. His prevalence rate was 6.5 per 1000, sensitivity 91.5%, and specificity 90%. PPV for lesions categorized as suspicious for malignancy was 54%. Thirty-one percent of the cancers were minimal, in other words, in situ or less than 1 cm in diameter with no tumor-positive nodes.

A reason for some failure to detect is a concern for excessive false-positive rates. The best approach to this problem is for each individual radiologist to know his/her current ROC curve. This should be evaluated in relation to the ambient frequency of abnormalities detectable in the patients under study.

Radiologists who read mammograms must know of their false-positive or false-negative rates. Constant feedback and follow-up of cases are essential to quality mammography.

False positive. The false-positive mammogram is a major problem of screening mammography. In the United States the most common causes of false-positive mammograms relate to excessively cautious interpretations, fear of malpractice litigation (defensive medicine), and a failure to appreciate the distinction between variants of normal and subtle cancer. Potchen et al. and Brennen discussed the concerns for mammography and malpractice.[17,91] Since defensive medicine is a real problem only in the United States, our discussion will emphasize only the concern for distinguishing normal variants from nonpalpable cancer. The most common normal variants mistaken for breast cancer are microcalcifications, mottled breast stroma, and asymmetric breast tissue. Barnard et al. showed that microcalcifications that led to a benign biopsy were most often associated with blunt duct adenosis.[7]

Lanyi dealt eloquently with the false-positive interpretation of mammographic microcalcifications.[58] He claims that 70% to 90% of the biopsies performed because of to microcalcifications on mammograms are unnecessary.

"Most of the time, descriptions of diagnostic criteria are irrelevant and vague. It is confusing that lobular carcinoma in situ is considered to be a real cancer, as happens frequently; and that historically dissimilar ductal carcinomas and benign abnormalities of different origin are simply considered as malignant or benign and subsequently reported as such." This opinion results from an analysis of articles on microcalcifications published between 1951 and 1984. Lanyi's opinion is that the number of needless biopsies can be reduced drastically. The microcalcifications of malignancy have typical characteristics; if applied properly to the analysis of mammograms, they should diminish false-positive interpretations. "Microcalcifications should now result in excessive' false positive interpretations only in situations where the radiologist is either not aware of the characteristic features of analysis, or he/she doesn't apply them correctly."[58]

While the overreading of "normal" microcalcification is the most common cause of "unnecessary" surgical biopsy, the second most common cause is the overinterpretation of "normal" asymmetry. Kopans et al. did a prospective study to evaluate the significance of asymmetric breast tissue on mammograms.[53] They studied patients with (1) asymmetric volume of breast tissue, (2) asymmetrically dense breast tissue with preserved architecture, or (3) asymmetrically prominent ducts. Of 8408 mammograms obtained in 1985, 221 (3%) demonstrated asymmetric breast tissue. Follow-up was 36 to 42 months after the initial mammographic study. During this time, none of the patients underwent biopsy on the basis of mammographic findings, although 20 had clinical findings that led to excisional biopsy. Malignancy was diagnosed in 3 patients. The remaining 17 biopsies were benign.

Based on this study, Kopans concluded that "an asymmetric volume of breast tissue, asymmetrically dense breast tissue, or asymmetrically prominent ducts that do not form a mass, do not contain microcalcifications, or do not produce architectural distortion, should be viewed with concern only when associated with a palpable asymmetry and are otherwise normal variations."

There are other causes of asymmetric breast tissue that are not cancer or normal anatomy. For example, Logan et al. revealed that insulin-dependent diabetes may cause mammographically dense, asymmetric stroma and benign breast masses that clinically resemble cancer.[66] They identified 36 patients, aged 20 to 54, with diabetic fibrous breast disease. For this diagnosis, they require that the patient have a long-term history of IDDM, radiographically dense glandular tissue, and one or more hard, irregular, easily movable, discrete, painless, palpable breast masses with strong ultrasonographic acoustical shadowing and firm resistance to the back-and-forth motion of the needle used for fine-needle aspiration cytology (FNAC). They conclude that patients meeting all criteria can be monitored with serial FNAC procedures to prevent them from undergoing multiple surgical biopsies. No breast cancer was found during an average of 6 years of monitoring these 36 women.

It is possible to find a suspected abnormality in many, if not most, routine mammograms. Most radiologists are aware of the effect of too many biopsy recommendations. Excessive biopsies markedly decrease the credibility of mammography as a tool to detect nonpalpable breast cancer.[57] An excessive number of false-positive mammograms has as much of a negative effect on the ability to detect early breast cancer as do lesions missed by observer error. The radiologist must walk a narrow line between the problem of missed cancer and the false-positive overcall. Patient acceptance of mammography depends in part on their ability to rely on the mammogram as a tool to foster further appropriate care and not lead to an unnecessary surgical biopsy or breast deformity where none would be warranted. Excessive false-positive rates have an effect on patient and public acceptance of screening mammography. The frequency of follow-up examinations that ultimately yield benign results influences the overall cost of recommending mammographic screening to detect early breast cancer.

A confirmation of normality in the worried well is an appropriate concern of medical care. We should do what we can to decrease unnecessary anxiety in otherwise well women. Excessive false-positive rates may induce more disease than the benefits of screening mammography may attain. These medicosocial implications of mammography are important as one seeks to maximize the usefulness of mammography to detect early nonpalpable breast cancer.

INDICATIONS FOR SURGICAL BIOPSY

The range of recommended surgical biopsies per cancer found in the United States is truly amazing. What is a reasonable PPV? The answer to this question is not clearly known. Kopans discusses the difficulty in ascribing a single appropriate PPV.[52] He believes that a number of data elements are necessary to assess the significance of any reported PPV. These include the risk profile of the population being discussed, the cancer rate, the size and stage of cancers detected, and the cause of the false-negative mammograms. These data are not readily available in most of the series reporting the PPV of screening mammography.

The number of breast biopsies per cancer ranges from 25:1 to 8:7.[4,57] The PPV, therefore, ranges from 0.004 to 0.875. In 1989 there were approximately 16 biopsies per breast cancer found in the city of Chicago (PPV = 0.063). The number has dropped from 9:1 to 6:1 (PPV = 0.111 to 0.167) over the past 5 years in Detroit. Hall et al. suggested that it would be possible to go as low as 2:1 (PPV = 0.500).[41] Ciatto et al. saw a similar objective,

feasible using mammography alone.[23] It has been difficult to obtain a biopsy rate of much less than 4:1, and in no instances less than 3:1, without markedly increasing the number of false-negative examinations. Obviously, if we were to attain a 1:1 correlation between biopsies and cancer, we meet the limitation of the procedure itself. Mammography is imperfect. That imperfection will always lead to some false-positive mammograms. False-positive examinations are easy to measure: simply observe the number of biopsies performed per cancer diagnosed and calculate the PPV. False-negative measures are much more difficult to estimate. We do not always know when we miss a cancer in a breast cancer screening program. In addition to finding missed cancers on subsequent examinations, it is possible to estimate the number of missed cancers by keeping records that allow for the determination of how many cancers are found in the population being screened. Ciatto et al. have shown an ability to reduce missed breast cancers at the cost of decreasing the PPV. With the addition of fine-needle aspiration, however, we can reach an almost 1:1 ratio. The closest that has ever been obtained to that desired goal has been seen in the published series from the Karolinska Institute.[4] They reported 1.14 surgical biopsies per cancer found (PPV = 0.875).

Meyer et al. reported 603 patients scheduled for biopsy who were referred from other facilities. After further study the procedure was canceled in 53 (8.8%) women.[72] An analysis of initial mammograms on those biopsies terminated included (1) no mass present (n = 22), (2) aspiration of a mass (n = 13), (3) skin calcifications (n = 9), (4) random calcifications (n = 4), (5) skin artifacts (n = 3), and (6) other (n = 2). Radiologists should adopt rigid criteria for recommending biopsy. Meyer et al. urged follow-up radiology when low-suspicion abnormalities are detected.

We have reviewed some 60 published series of patients with nonpalpable breast cancer. The PPVs range from 0.004 to 0.875. This remarkable range warrants a close scrutiny. We will analyze the available literature to appreciate those features of breast cancer detection that yield the maximum benefit to patients in screening mammography. Thus, we will review each publication on the subject of PPV of mammography in the detection of nonpalpable breast cancer.

EFFECT OF TOO MANY "UNNECESSARY" SURGICAL BIOPSIES

The number of surgical biopsies per cancer found, or its reciprocal—the PPV of the diagnostic strategies used to decide whether a surgical biopsy is warranted—has become an increasingly important consideration in the diagnosis of nonpalpable breast cancer. Nonpalpable breast cancer was traditionally an uncertain diagnosis before the surgical biopsy. Many patients are subjected to a surgical biopsy that yields a benign lesion. If the diagnostic process were perfect in predicting the presence or absence of malignancy, every surgical biopsy would yield a malignant tissue. If we attempt to detect every possible subtle cancer in a woman's breast, then biopsies or mastectomies may be needed for most women to exclude any remote possibility of cancer. Some surgeons and some radiologists believe that frequent surgical biopsies are the only way to be sure that we identify as many cancers as possible at a stage where they can still be cured. However, when this argument is carried to its extreme, an excessive number of unnecessary surgical biopsies will occur.

What is the effect of too many surgical biopsies? The direct cost of surgical biopsies, were they to be excessive, could be prohibitive in applying a diagnostic strategy appropriate for the early detection of nonpalpable breast cancer. The cost of the diagnostic system would be excessive. Any system that can obtain the same diagnostic accuracy and/or yield of breast cancer cure at a lower cost is a reasonable object.

In addition to the direct cost, there are indirect opportunity costs of a surgical biopsy. If one envisions a finite resource pool for the diagnosis and management of breast cancer, it is reasonable to consider that money spent on biopsies for benign breast disease could be better spent to provide access to mammography for more women. This could be obtained by decreasing the expenditures on surgical biopsies and increasing the total expenditures toward early detection through more widely applied mammography (e.g., to indigent patients). The opportunity cost of unnecessary surgical biopsies is an important factor in the United States. Consideration of cost to society is necessary when advocating any system to improve on the early diagnosis of breast cancer.

In addition to the direct and opportunity costs involved, unnecessary surgical biopsies have an effect on women's use of mammography as a diagnostic tool. We constantly attempt to increase the appropriate use of screening mammography in the population that is at a sufficient risk for breast cancer. Women whose friends had anxiety induced by a false-positive suspicion of breast cancer that went to surgical biopsy are less likely to want to become involved in the system (see Chapter 2). Women aware of unnecessary surgery induced by screening mammography may not have screening mammograms done.

Another cost of unnecessary surgical biopsies relates to the credibility of the diagnostic system. If screening mammography has a near random ability to select those patients who will benefit from surgical biopsy, then patients and physicians will not believe that it is an appropriate way to control breast cancer. In the early days of screening mammography, this was a major problem in the United States. Improved interpretive skills of radiologists and mammographic technique combined with a wider awareness of alternatives to surgical biopsy to increase accuracy of the system and thereby to increase appropriate use of screening mammography. The credibility of screening mammography is increasing. This is evident by the increased compliance rates of women seeking screening mammograms.

In addition to the cost of unnecessary surgical biopsy, there are risks involved. There is the risk of error induced by the additional diagnostic procedure. The risk of the surgical biopsy itself is very low. However, there is entailed morbidity involved in having an "unnecessary" surgical biopsy. Kopans points out that "biopsy is an extremely safe procedure. A recommendation for breast biopsy, with implied possibility of breast cancer, induces high anxiety in patients. The procedure itself results in a lost of productivity during the surgical and recuperative time, creates varying degrees of surgical trauma and cosmetic alteration, and generates increased cost for the health care system."

In addition to the direct effect of the surgical biopsy procedure, there is always the residual concern that a surgical biopsy may result in an error in the pathologic interpretation of the tissue. Beahrs reviewed 1810 breast biopsies performed in the Breast Cancer Detection and Demonstration Program.[10] Of these, 592 were less than 1 cm in size and therefore considered minimal. A retrospective review by a panel of pathologists was obtained in 506 of these patients. In 64 cases, or 3.5% of the 1810 breast biopsy cases, the pathologic features were not sufficient for the diagnosis of cancer. On further review 16 of these 64 cases turned out to be cancer. This left 48 cancers in doubt, a false-positive pathology report of 9.4%. When one calculates the cost of a surgical biopsy based on a mammographic impression, the possibility of a false-positive pathology report must be considered. Elston, in the United Kingdom, did a similar study on the pathology quality control in interpreting breast cancer from breast biopsy specimens.[28] They had four consistency surveys. They were 83% in agreement. In the United Kingdom series they found no errors at a benign and malignant border.

The exact frequency of false-positive pathology interpretations is uncertain. It will obviously vary with the experience, care, and concern of the individual pathologists performing the examination. Use of multiple observers seems a reasonable approach to reduce this possibility. Many pathologists have quality control measures that substantially decrease the possibility of false-positive pathology reports. Nevertheless, such reports do occasionally occur.

Finally, the risk of unnecessary surgical biopsy, pointed out by Kopans and others, is primarily directed toward the induced anxiety in patients as we attempt to diagnose breast cancer at an early stage.[52] As has been stated many times throughout this book, a major issue for concern is to develop a diagnostic system based on screening mammography that will not cause as much disease as it cures. The purpose of any appropriate medical recommendation is to decrease that component of human misery induced by disease. As we focus on a relatively narrow aspect of medical care—the early detection and possible cure of breast cancer—we must keep in mind that everything we advocate may cause as much harm as it could cause benefit. Everything possible must be done to induce the potential for injury envisioned in advocating a diagnostic system. Primo non nocere; first cause no harm.

REFERENCES

1. Ainge GR, Choplin RH, Bechtold RE, et al: Relationship between mammographic features and hormone receptor content in patients with breast cancer (review). *South Med J* 82(12):1506-1511, 1989.

2. Andersen J, Blichert-Toft M, Dyreborg U: In situ carcinomas of the breast. Types, growth pattern, diagnosis, and treatment, *Eur J Surg Oncol* 13(2):105-111, 1987.

3. Azavedo E, Svane G: Radiologic aspects of breast cancers detected through a breast cancer screening program, *Eur J Radiol* 13:88-90, 1991.

4. Azavedo E, Svane G, Ringertz H: The role of the radiologist in screening for nonpalpable breast tumors in Sweden, *Invest Radiol* 26:174-178, 1991.

5. Bahnsen J, Warneke B, Frischbier HJ, Stegner HE: Intraductal breast carcinoma. Clinical, x-ray and histological findings and their therapeutic consequences, *Geburtsh Frauenheilk* 45(7):488-493, 1985.

6. Baines CJ, McFarlane DV, Miller AB: Sensitivity and specificity of first screen mammography in 15 NBSS centres, *Can Assoc Radiol J* 39(4):273-276, 1988.

7. Barnard NJ, George BD, Tucker AK, Gilmore OJ: Histopathology of benign non-palpable breast lesions identified by mammography, *J Clin Pathol* 41(1):26-30, 1988.

8. Bartl W, Euller A, Pfersmann C, et al: Diagnosis of breast cancer in the clinical stage T1. Zur Diagnose von Mammakarzinomen im klinischen Stadium T1, *Wien Klin Wochenschr* 96(19):722-727, 1984.

9. Bassett LW, Gold RH, Cove HC: Mammographic spectrum of traumatic fat necrosis: the fallibility of "pathognomonic" signs of carcinoma, *Am J Roentgenol* 130(1):119-122, 1978.

10. Beahrs OH, Smart CR: Diagnosis of minimal breast cancers in the BCDDP: the 66 questionable cases, *Cancer* 43(3):848-850, 1979.

11. Bergkvist L, Tabar L, Bergstrom R, Adami HO: Epidemiologic determinants of the mammographic parenchymal pattern. A population-based study within a mammographic screening program, *Am J Epidemiol* 126(6):1075-1081, 1987.

12. Bird D, Hart S: Early experience with needle localization and biopsy of mammographic lesions [see comments], *Aust NZ J Surg* 60(5):337-340, 1990.

13. Bird RE: Low cost screening mammography: report on finances and review of 21,716 consecutive cases, *Radiology* 171(1):87-90, 1989.

14. Blichert-Toft M, Andersen J, Dyreborg U: Breast carcinoma in situ. Diagnostic and therapeutic aspects with special reference to growth patterns (review), *Ugeskrift Laeger* 152(25):1803-1806, 1990.

15. Blichert-Toft M, Graversen HP, Andersen J, et al: In situ breast carcinomas: a population-based study on frequency, growth pattern, and clinical aspects, *World J Surg* 12:845-851, 1988.

16. Bongiorni G, Marchisio V, Bragaja S: Comedocarcinoma: a tumor histotype to be reevaluated, *Radiol Med (Torino)* 79(6):590-592, 1990.

17. Brenner RJ: Medicolegal aspects of screening mammography, *AJR* 153:53-56, 1989.

18. Broberg A, Glas U, Gustafsson SA, et al: Relationship between mammographic pattern and estrogen receptor content in breast cancer, *Breast Cancer Res Treatment* 3(2):201-207, 1983.

19. Bruwer A, Nelson GW, Spark RP: Punctate intranodal gold deposits simulating microcalcifications on mammograms, *Radiology* 163(1):87-88, 1987.

20. Buckley JH, Roebuck EJ: Mammographic changes following radiotherapy, *Br J Radiol* 59(700):337-344, 1986.

21. Cahill CJ, Boulter PS, Gibbs NM, Price JL: Features of mammographically negative breast tumours, *Br J Surg* 68(12):882-884, 1981.

22. Chamberlain J, Clifford RE, Nathan BE, et al: Repeated screening for breast cancer, *J Epidemiol Comm Health* 38(1):54-57, 1984.

23. Ciatto S, Cataliotti L, Distante V: Nonpalpable lesions detected with mammography: review of 512 consecutive cases, *Radiology* 165(1):99-102, 1987.

24. Colbassani HJ Jr, Feller WF, Cigtay OS, Chun B: Mammographic and pathologic correlation of microcalcification in disease of the breast, *Surg Gynecol Obstet* 155(5):689-696, 1982.

25. Connolly JL, Boyages J, Schnitt SJ, et al: In situ carcinoma of the breast (review), *Annu Rev Med* 40:173-180, 1989.

26. Dershaw DD, Abramson A, Kinne DW: Ductal carcinoma in situ: mammographic findings and clinical implications, *Radiology* 170(2):411-415, 1989.

27. Deschenes L, Jacob S, Fabia J, Christen A: Beware of breast fibroadenomas in middle-aged women, *Can J Surg* 28(4):372-374, 1984.

28. Elston CW: Pathological aspects of the UK Breast Screening Project with special reference to minimal and "borderline" lesions, *Aust NZ J Surg* 54(3):201-204, 1984.

29. Fajardo LL, Hillman BJ, Frey C: Correlation between breast parenchymal patterns and mammographers' certainty of diagnosis, *Invest Radiol* 23(7):505-508, 1988.

30. Fallenius AG, Askensten UG, Skoog LK, Auer GU: The reliability of microspectrophotometric and flow cytometric nuclear DNA measurements in adenocarcinomas of the breast, *Cytometry* 8(3):260-266, 1987.

31. Fam BW, Olson SL, Winter PF, Scholz FJ: Algorithm for the detection of fine clustered calcifications on film mammograms, *Radiology* 169(2):333-337, 1988.

32. Fewins HE, Whitehouse GH, Leinster SJ: The spontaneous disappearance of breast calcification, *Clin Radiol* 39(3):257-261, 1988.

33. Foote FW, Stewart FW: Lobular carcinoma in situ: a rare form of mammary cancer, *Am J Pathol* 17:490-496, 1941.

34. Frappart L, Boudeulle M, Boumendil J, et al: Structure and composition of microcalcifications in benign and malignant lesions of the breast: study by light microscopy, transmission and scanning electron microscopy, microprobe analysis, and X-ray diffraction, *Hum Pathol* 15(9):880-889, 1984.

35. Frykberg ER, Santiago F, Betsill WL, O'Brien PH: Lobular carcinoma in situ of the breast, *Surg Gynecol Obstet* 164:285-301, 1989.

36. Geppert M, Schmitt W: Minute carcinomas of the breast in a histologic and mammographic comparison, *Geburtsh Frauenheilkd* 43(11):674-678.

37. Gisvold JJ, Martin JK Jr: Prebiopsy localization of nonpalpable breast lesions, *AJR* 143:477-481, 1984.

38. Gohagan JK, Spitznagel EL, McCrate MM, Frank TB: ROC analysis of mammography and palpation for breast screening, *Invest Radiol* 19(6):587-592, 1984.

39. Goin JE, Haberman JD, Linder MK, Lambird PA: Analysis of mammography: a blind interpretation of BCDDP radiographs, *Radiology* 148(2):393-396, 1983.

40. Haagensen CD, Lane N, Lattes R, Bodian C: Lobular neoplasia (so called lobular carcinoma in situ) of the breast, *Cancer* 42:737-769, 1978.

41. Hall WC, Aust JB, Gaskill HV, et al: Evaluation of nonpalpable breast lesions. Experience in a training institution, *Am J Surg* 151:467-469, 1986.

42. Haupt HM, Rosen PP, Kinne DW: Breast carcinoma presenting with axillary lymph node metastases. An analysis of specific histopathologic features, *Am J Surg Pathol* 9(3):165-175, 1985.

43. Healey EA, Osteen RT, Schnitt SJ, et al: Can the clinical and mammographic findings at presentation predict the presence of an extensive intraductal component in early stage breast cancer? *Int J Radiation Oncol Biol Physics* 17(6):1217-1221, 1989.

44. Heuser LS, Spratt JS, Kuhns JG, et al: The association of pathologic and mammographic characteristics of primary human breast cancers with "slow" and "fast" growth rates and with axillary lymph node metastases, *Cancer* 53(1):96-98, 1984.

45. Hillman BJ, Fajardo LL, Hunter TB, et al: Mammogram interpretation by physician assistants, *Am J Roentgenol* 149(5):907-912, 1987.

46. Holland R, Hendriks JH, Mravunac M: Mammographically occult breast cancer. A pathologic and radiologic study, *Cancer* 52(10):1810-1819, 1983.

47. Holland R, Mravunac M, Hendriks JH, Bekker BV: So-called interval cancers of the breast. Pathologic and radiologic analysis of sixty-four cases, *Cancer* 49(12)2527-2533, 1982.

48. Homer MJ, Safaii H, Smith TJ, Marchant DJ: The relationship of mammographic microcalcification to histologic malignancy: radiologic-pathologic correlation, *Am J Roentgenol* 153(6):1187-1189, 1989.

49. Hutter RV, Snyder RE, Lucas JC, et al: Clinical and pathologic correlation with mammographic findings in lobular carcinoma in situ, *Cancer* 23:826-839, 1969.

50. Ikeda DM, Andersson I: Ductal carcinoma in situ: atypical mammographic appearances, *Radiology* 172:661-666, 1989.

51. Kimme-Smith C, Bassett LW, Gold RH, Gormley L: Digital mammography. A comparison of two digitization methods, *Invest Radiol* 24(11):869-875, 1989.

52. Kopans DB: The positive predictive value of mammography, *AJR* 158:521-526, 1992.

53. Kopans DB, Swann CA, White G, et al: Asymmetric breast tissue, *Radiology* 171(3):639-643, 1989.

54. Lagios MD, Westdahl PR, Margolin FR, Rose MR: Duct carcinoma in situ, Relationship of extent of noninvasive disease to the frequency of occult invasion, multicentricity, lymph node metastases, and short-term treatment failures, *Cancer* 50(7):1309-1314, 1982.

55. Landercasper J, Gundersen SB Jr, Gundersen AL, et al: Needle localization and biopsy of nonpalpable lesions of the breast, *Surg Gynecol Obstet* 164(5):399-403, 1987.

56. Landstrom J, Osgood G, Young SC: Needle localization in occult breast lesions, *J Surg Oncol* 40(1):1-3, 1989.

57. Lang NP, Talbert GE, Shewmake KB, et al: The current evaluation of nonpalpable breast lesions, *Arch Surg* 122(12):1389-1391, 1987.

58. Lanyi M: Microcalcifications in the breast—a blessing or a curse? A critical review, *Diagn Imaging Clin Med* 54(3-4):126-145, 1985.

59. Lanyi M: *Diagnosis and differential diagnosis of breast calcifications,* Berlin, 1986, Springer-Verlag.

60. Lanyi M, Citoler P: The differential diagnosis of microcalcification. Micro-cyst (blunt duct) adenosis, *ROFO* 134(3):225-231, 1981.

61. Leborgne R: Diagnosis of tumors of the breast by simple roentgenography, *Am J Roentgenol* 65:1-11, 1951.

62. Le-Gal M, Chavanne G, Pellier D: Diagnostic value of clustered microcalcifications discovered by mammography (apropos of 227 cases with histological verification and without a palpable breast tumor), *Bull Cancer* 71(1):57-64, 1984.

63. Lewison EF: Lobular carcinoma of the breast. The feminine mystique, *Milit Med* 129:115, 1964.

64. Libshitz HI, Montague ED, Paulus DD: Calcifications and the therapeutically irradiated breast, *Am J Roentgenol* 128(6):1021-1025, 1977.

65. Linden SS, Sullivan DC: Breast skin calcifications: localization with a stereotactic device, *Radiology* 171(2):570-571, 1989.

66. Logan WW, Hoffman NY: Diabetic fibrous breast disease, *Radiology* 172(3):667-670, 1989.

67. Mann BD, Giuliano AE, Bassett LW, et al: Delayed diagnosis of breast cancer as a result of normal mammograms, *Arch Surg* 118(1):23-24, 1983.

68. Marrujo G, Jolly PC, Hall MH: Nonpalpable breast cancer: needle-localized biopsy for diagnosis and considerations for treatment, *Am J Surg* 151(5):599-602, 1986.

69. Menges V, Busing CM, Hirsch O: The diagnostic value of mammographic signs of malignancy in clinically occult breast carcinoma, *ROFO* 135(4):482-489, 1981.

70. Meyer JE, Eberlein TJ, Stomper PC, Sonnenfeld MR: Biopsy of occult breast lesions. Analysis of 1261 abnormalities, *JAMA* 263(17):2341-2343, 1990.

71. Meyer JE, Kopans DB, Stomper PC, Lindfors KK: Occult breast abnormalities: percutaneous preoperative needle localization, *Radiology* 150(2):335-337, 1984.

72. Meyer JE, Sonnenfeld MR, Greenes RA, Stomper PC: Preoperative localization of clinically occult breast lesions: experience at a referral hospital, *Radiology* 169(3):627-628, 1988.

73. Mitnick JS, Roses DF, Harris MN, Feiner HD: Circumscribed intraductal carcinoma of the breast, *Radiology* 170(2):423-425, 1989.

74. Moskowitz M: Screening for breast cancer: how effective are our tests? A critical review, *CA* 33(1):26-39, 1983.

75. Muir BB, Lamb J, Anderson TJ, Kirkpatrick AE: Microcalcification and its relationship to cancer of the breast: experience in a screening clinic, *Clin Radiol* 34(2):193-200, 1983.

76. Murphy WA, DeSchryver-Kecskemeti K: Isolated clustered microcalcifications in the breast: radiologic-pathologic correlation, *Radiology* 127(2):335-341, 1978.

77. Nielsen M, Jensen J, Andersen J: Precancerous and cancerous breast lesions during lifetime and at autopsy, *Cancer* 54:612-615, 1984.

78. Nielsen M, Thomsen JL, Primdahl S, et al: Breast cancer and atypia among young and middle-aged women: a study of 110 medical legal autopsies, *Br J Cancer* 56:814-819, 1987.

79. Oestmann JW, Kopans DB, Linetsky L, et al: Comparison of two screen-film combinations in contact and magnification mammography: detectability of microcalcifications, *Radiology* 168(3):657-659, 1988.

80. Oppedal BR, Drevvatne T: Radiographic diagnosis of non-palpable breast lesions. Correlation to pathology, *Acta Radiol Diagn (Stockh)* 24(3):259-265, 1983.

81. Orson LW, Cigtay OS: Fat necrosis of the breast: characteristic xeromammographic appearance, *Radiology* 146(1):35-38, 1983.

82. Owings DV, Hann L, Schnitt SJ: How thoroughly should needle localization breast biopsies be sampled for microscopic examination? A prospective mammographic/pathologic correlative study, *Am J Surg Pathol* 14(6):578-583, 1990.

83. Pagani JJ, Bassett LW, Gold RH, et al: Efficacy of combined film-screen/xeromammography: preliminary report, *Am J Roentgenol* 135(1):141-146, 1980.

84. Page DL, Dupont WD, Rogers LW, Landenberger M: Intraductal carcinoma of the breast: follow up after biopsy only, *Cancer* 49:751-758, 1982.

85. Pamilo M, Anttinen I, Soiva M, et al: Mammography screening—reasons for recall and the influence of experience on recall in the Finnish system, *Clin Radiol* 41(6):384-387, 1990.

86. Papatestas AE, Hermann D, Hermann G, et al: Surgery for nonpalpable breast lesions, *Arch Surg* 125(3):399-402, 1990.

87. Parker MD, Clark RL, McLelland R, Daughtery K: Disappearing breast calcifications, *Radiology* 172(3):677-680, 1989.

88. Peeters PH, Verbeek AL, Hendriks JH, et al: The occurrence of in-

terval cancers in the Nijmegen screening programme, *Br J Cancer* 59(6):929-932, 1989.

89. Petrovich JA, Ross DS, Sullivan JW, Lake TP: Mammographic wire localization in diagnosis and treatment of occult carcinoma of breast, *Surg Gynecol Obstet* 168(3):239-243, 1989.

90. Pope TL Jr, Fechner RE, Wilhelm MC, et al: Lobular carcinoma in situ of the breast: mammographic features, *Radiology* 168(1):63-66, 1988.

91. Potchen EJ, Bisesi MA, Sierra AE, Potchen JE: Mammography and malpractice, *Am J Roentgenol* 156:475-580, 1991.

92. Price JL, Gibbs NM: The relationship between microcalcification and in situ carcinoma of the breast, *Clin Radiol* 29(4):447-452, 1978.

93. Prorok JJ, Trostle DR, Scarlato M, Rachman R: Excisional breast biopsy and roentgenographic examination for mammographically detected microcalcification, *Am J Surg* 145(5):684-686, 1983.

94. Radi MJ: Calcium oxalate crystals in breast biopsies. An overlooked form of microcalcification associated with benign breast disease, *Arch Pathol Lab Med* 113(12):1367-1369, 1989.

95. Robertson CL, Kopano DB: Communication problems after mammographic screening, *Radiology* 172:443-444, 1989.

96. Roebuck EJ: The subcutaneous reaction: a useful mammographic sign, *Clin Radiol* 35(4):311-315, 1984.

97. Rombach JJ, Collette BJ, de-Waard F, Slotboom BJ: Analysis of the diagnostic performance in breast cancer screening by relative operating characteristics, *Cancer* 58(1):169-177, 1986.

98. Ronay G, Tulusan AH, Willgeroth F, et al: Die Rolle der Mammographie bei der Diagnose von simultanen Zweitkarzinomen in der kontralateralen Brust [The role of mammography in the diagnosis of simultaneous second cancers in the contralateral breast], *Geburtsh Frauenheilkd* 48(8):579-583, 1988.

99. Rosen PP, Braun DW Jr, Kinne DW: The clinical significance of preinvasive breast carcinoma, *Cancer* 46:919-925, 1980.

100. Rosen PP, Liberman PH. Braun DW, et al: Lobular carcinoma in situ of the breast, *Am J Surg Pathol* 2:225-250, 1978.

101. Roses DF, Harris MN, Gorstein F, Gumport SL: Biopsy for microcalcification detected by mammography, *Surgery* 87(3):248-252, 1980.

102. Rosselli-Del-Turco M, Ciatto S, Bravetti P, Pacini P: The significance of mammographic calcifications in early breast cancer detection, *Radiol Med* 72(1-2):7-12, 1986.

103. Rusnak CH, Pengelly DB, Hosie RT, Rusnak CN: Preoperative needle localization to detect early breast cancer, *Am J Surg* 157(5):505-507, 1989.

104. Salomon A: Beitrage zur pathologie und klinik der mammakarzinome, *Arch Clin Chir* 103:573, 1913.

105. Schmitt EL, Threatt BA: Effective breast cancer detection with film-screen mammography, *J Can Assoc Radiol* 36(4):304-307, 1985.

106. Reference deleted in proof.

107. Schnitt SJ, Silen W, Sadowsky NL, et al: Ductal carcinoma in situ (intraductal carcinoma) of the breast, *N Engl J Med* 318:898-903, 1988.

108. Schwartz GF, Feig SA, Patchefsky AS: Significance and staging of nonpalpable carcinomas of the breast, *Surg Gynecol Obstet* 166(1):6-10, 1988.

109. Sener SF, Candela FC, Paige ML, et al: Limitations of mammography in the identification of noninfiltrating carcinoma of the breast, *Surg Gynecol Obstet* 167(2):135-140, 1988.

110. Sickles EA: Further experience with microfocal spot magnification mammography in the assessment of clustered breast microcalcifications, *Radiology* 137(1 Pt1):9-14, 1980.

111. Sickles EA: Mammographic detectability of breast microcalcifications, *Am J Roentgenol* 139(5):913-918, 1982.

112. Sickles EA: Mammographic features of 300 consecutive nonpalpable breast cancers, *Am J Roentgenol* 146(4):661-663, 1986.

113. Sickles EA, Abele JS: Milk of calcium within tiny benign breast cysts, *Radiology* 141(3):655-658, 1981.

114. Sickles EA, Weber WN: High-contrast mammography with a moving grid: assessment of clinical utility, *Am J Roentgenol* 146(6):1137-1139, 1986.

115. Sickles EA, Weber WN, Galvin HB, et al: Baseline screening mammography: one vs two views per breast, *Am J Roentgenol* 147(6):149-153, 1986.

116. Sigfusson BF, Andersson I, Aspegren K, et al: Clustered breast calcifications, *Acta Radiol* 24:273-281, 1983.

117. Skinner MA, Swain M, Simmons R, et al: Nonpalpable breast lesions at biopsy. A detailed analysis of radiographic features, *Ann Surg* 208(2):203-208, 1988.

118. Smathers RL, Bush E, Drace J, et al: Mammographic microcalcifications: detection with xerography, screen-film, and digitized film display, *Radiology* 159(3):673-677, 1986.

119. Sneige N, White VA, Katz RL, et al: Ductal carcinoma-in-situ of the breast: fine-needle aspiration cytology of 12 cases, *Diagn Cytopathol* 5(4):371-377, 1989.

120. Solin LJ, Fowble BL, Troupin RH, Goodman RL: Biopsy results of new calcifications in the postirradiated breast, *Cancer* 63(10):1956-1961, 1989.

121. Stomper PC, Connolly JL, Meyer JE, Harris JR: Clinically occult ductal carcinoma in situ detected with mammography: analysis of 100 cases with radiologic-pathologic correlation, *Radiology* 172(1):235-241, 1989.

122. Stomper PC, Davis SP, Weidner N, Meyer JE: Clinically occult, noncalcified breast cancer: serial radiologic-pathologic correlation in 27 cases, *Radiology* 169(3):621-626, 1988.

123. Stomper PC, Gelman RS: Mammography in symptomatic and asymptomatic patients (review), *Hematol/Oncol Clin North Am* 3(4):611-640, 1989.

124. Stomper PC, Recht A, Berenberg AL, et al: Mammographic detection of recurrent cancer in the irradiated breast, *Am J Roentgenol* 148(1):39-43, 1987.

125. Swets JA, Getty DJ, Pickett RM, et al: Enhancing and evaluating diagnostic accuracy, *Med Decision Making* 11(1):9-18, 1991.

126. Tinnemans JG, Wobbes T, Lubbers EJ, et al: The significance of microcalcifications without palpable mass in the diagnosis of breast cancer, *Surgery* 99(6):652-657, 1986.

127. Vineis P, Sinistrero G, Temporelli A, et al: Inter-observer variability in the interpretation of mammograms, *Tumori* 74(3):275-279, 1988.

128. Warren DL, Stelling CB: Sensitivity, specificity, predictive value and accuracy of film/screen mammography. A three-year experience, *J Ky Med Assoc* 87(4):169-173, 1989.

129. Weber J, Tournemaine N, Audouin AF, et al: Borderline lesions of the breast: clinical and radiological study of 20 cases, *J Belge Radiol* 73(2):89-96, 1990.

130. Wee WG, Moskowitz M, Chang NC, et al: Evaluation of mammographic calcifications using a computer program, *Radiology* 116(3):717-720, 1975.

131. Wilhelm MC, de-Paredes ES, Pope T, Wanebo HJ: The changing mammogram. A primary indication for needle localization biopsy, *Arch Surg* 121(11):1311-1314, 1986.

132. Wilkinson EJ, Gnadt JT, Mibrath J, Clowry LJ: Breast biopsy evaluation by paraffin-block radiography, *Arch Pathol Lab Med* 102(9):470-473, 1978.

133. Wilkinson S, Forrest AP: Fibro-adenoma of the breast, *Br J Surg* 72(10):838-840, 1985.

134. Zimmerman AL, King EB, Barrett DL, Petrakis NL: The incidence and significance of intracytoplasmic calcifications in nipple aspirate specimens, *Acta Cytol* 21(5):685-692, 1977.

Chapter 5

DEFINING WHEN SURGICAL BIOPSY IS NECESSARY

Diagnostic examinations in asymptomatic women are intended to identify disease before it becomes clinically apparent. Each step in the diagnostic process seeks to confirm the presumption of normality. Once uncertainty is induced by the process of diagnosis, it is important to reaffirm existing normality as soon as possible. When presented with an uncertain mammogram, some physicians urge a surgical biopsy. Others seek additional mammographic studies to confirm or refute the presence of normality, while still others follow the additional mammographic views with a stereotactically derived cytologic or histologic assessment before initiating a surgical biopsy. These diagnostic tests seek to answer one question: If you perform surgery on this patient, what is the chance of finding a cancer? This is the role of preoperative diagnosis.

A pathologist examining the breasts of asymptomatic women being screened for breast cancer would find LCIS in some 5% of the patients, depending on the risk factors involved. Thus, if surgery was performed randomly without regard to preoperative tests, such as screening mammography, many cases of LCIS and an occasional invasive cancer would be discovered. Preoperative mammography and cytology are used to decrease the number of normal women subjected to surgical invasion in the course of breast cancer diagnosis. How many normal women must undergo surgical biopsy to control breast cancer in asymptomatic women? Can mammographic detection of breast cancer be improved with or without cytology?

HISTORY OF FINDINGS

The number of biopsies performed per cancer detected ranges from 28 biopsies per cancer to 1.15 biopsies per cancer, which is a PPV from .036 to .871.[5,30] In these series, many approaches attempted to diminish the frequency of "unnecessary" surgical biopsies. The criteria for surgical biopsy in 61 published series (published from 1973 to 1991) involving the diagnosis of nonpalpable breast can-

cer. In total, they represent 22,485 biopsies in which 5647 carcinomas were found. The PPV of the entire group was .251 for a biopsy per cancer rate of 3.98. Of the 3254 cases where the histology was reported, there were 1135 in situ carcinomas and 2119 invasive carcinomas for an in situ percentage of 34.9%. Of the 1135 in situ carcinomas, 800 were DCIS and 245 were LCIS. Thirty-seven were a combination of DCIS and LCIS, and in 53 cases the type of in situ cancer was not identified. Thus, in those cases where histology was reported, 7.5% were LCIS, which today is not considered in the same category as invasive carcinomas. This is an important distinction, since the proportion of LCIS varied substantially in the reports. Where it is not distinguished, it is possible that LCIS could represent a substantial portion of the total cases reported. Since there are no prebiopsy clues to the presence of LCIS, the occasions it is found are probably not due to a relevant mammographic observation. Perhaps the pathologic finding of LCIS is a random event independent of any criteria of surgical biopsy. This warrants continued study because the overall 7.5% of LCIS in these series is slightly higher than the 5% prevalence of LCIS in the population. When microcalcifications are the sole criterion for biopsy, there is an increased incidence of LCIS detected. Eight articles reported only calcifications as the criterion for surgical biopsy. These series were selected from a larger population of patients where surgical biopsy was done for other mammographic signs. The series of biopsies performed because of microcalcifications had a PPV of .262. Eight hundred and twenty biopsies found 215 cancers. These series reported a higher proportion of in situ carcinomas. Of the 164 cases in which the histology was reported, some 109 were in situ and 55 were invasive, which is an in situ percentage of 66%. Of these in situ carcinomas, 90 were DCIS and 19 were LCIS. LCIS was found in 21% of the biopsies that were done for the presence of microcalcification only compared with a 7.5% rate when all of the reports are combined. Thus, in those series reporting microcalcifications as the sole criterion for surgical biopsy, the frequency for LCIS is considerably greater than the average frequency for LCIS. Obviously, more cases of LCIS will be uncovered when microcalcification is used as the sole criterion for biopsy. Does LCIS cause microcalcifications that can be distinguished from the microcalcifications of malignancy? Further study needs to be done to clarify this issue.

The PPVs of the series reported in the 1970s were optimistic. Of the three series reported in the 1970s, there were 236 biopsies resulting in 127 cancers for a PPV of .538. In the 1980s there were 52 reported series encompassing 19,804 biopsies, which reveal 4694 carcinomas for a PPV of .236. This has improved remarkably in the 1990s, when the 7 reported series of 2445 biopsies yield 826 cancers for a PPV of .338. The differences in these three decades is striking. In the 1970s, some of the cases were reported on the basis of malignant-appearing calcifications only. The higher PPV, seen in reports from the

1970s, is largely due to the early publications reporting the role of microcalcification in breast cancer detection. In this population there is an increase in the proportion of LCIS. Table 5-1 lists the series reviewed in the order of their PPV. These data are illustrated in Fig. 5-1.

Effect of SFNA

In the reported series, where fine needle aspiration (FNA) cytology was added to screening mammography to decide which patient should have a biopsy, there was a remarkable improvement in the PPV. These series were reported over the 3 decades: 1 in the 1970s, 5 in the 1980s, and 2 in the 1990s. A total of 1885 biopsies yielding 988 carcinomas was reported for a PPV of .524. Table 5-2 lists those series where FNA data contributed to the PPV.

In the 332 cases where the histology was reported, there were 81 cases of in situ carcinoma and 251 cases of invasive carcinoma, for a 24% in situ carcinoma. Thirty-two of the in situ carcinomas were DCIS and eight were LCIS. LCIS was found in only 2.4% of the surgical biopsies that

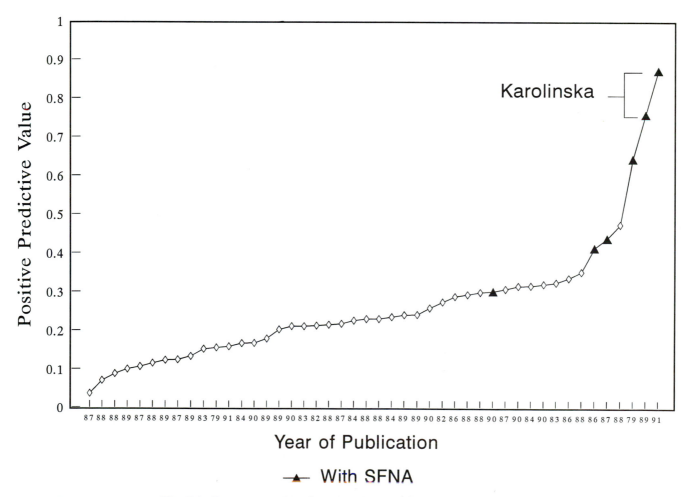

Fig. 5-1. Breast cancer detection systems: comparison of published series.

Table 5-1. Series reviewed by order of PPV

Author	Year	Biopsy	Cancer	PPV	Biopsies per cancer
Lang et al	1987	56	2	.036	28.00
Choucair et al	1988	103	9	.087	11.44
Landstrom et al	1989	211	21	.010	10.05
Lang et al	1987	66	7	.106	9.43
Proudfoot et al	1986	56	6	.107	9.33
Graham and Bauer	1988	678	78	.115	8.69
Petrovich et al	1989	106	13	.123	8.15
Ostrow et al	1987	121	15	.124	8.07
Hall WC et al	1986	70	9	.129	7.78
Siemssen et al	1981	115	16	.139	7.19
Rowen et al	1986	595	84	.141	7.08
Poole et al	1986	148	21	.142	7.05
Galakhoff et al	1983	33	5	.150	6.67
Kessler et al	1991	57	9	.158	6.33
Bigelow et al	1985	150	24	.160	6.25
Oppedal et al	1983	87	14	.161	6.21
Lefor et al	1984	18	3	.167	6.00
Powell et al	1983	282	47	.167	6.00
Molly et al	1989	213	38	.178	5.61
Egan et al	1980	6431	1161	.181	5.54
Hicks et al	1983	419	85	.203	4.93
Silverstein et al	1989	1014	206	.203	4.92
Albert et al	1990	100	21	.210	4.76
Wilhelm et al	1986	452	95	.210	4.76
Chetty et al	1983	190	40	.211	4.75
Hoehn et al	1982	66	14	.212	4.71
Knaus et al	1988	98	21	.214	4.67
Landercasper et al	1987	203	44	.217	4.61
Kehler et al	1984	182	41	.225	4.44
Skinner et al	1988	179	41	.229	4.37
Meyer et al	1984	500	117	.234	4.27
Rusnak et al	1989	200	48	.240	4.17
Lanyi and Citole	1981	135	36	.267	3.75
Gisvold and Martin	1984	343	92	.268	3.73
Marrujo et al	1986	237	64	.270	3.70
Colbassani et al	1982	55	15	.273	3.67
Solmer et al	1980	40	11	.275	3.64
Blichert-Toft et al	1982	45	13	.289	3.46
Rosenberg et al	1987	927	270	.291	3.43
Schwartz et al	1988	1132	330	.292	3.43
Hann et al	1989	96	28	.292	3.43
Ciatto et al	1987	512	152	.297	3.37
Hall F et al	1988	400	119	.298	3.36
Fajardo et al	1990	100	30	.300	3.33
de Waal et al	1987	183	56	.306	3.27
Papatestas et al	1990	475	149	.314	3.19
Schwartz et al	1984	557	175	.314	3.18
Owings et al	1990	157	50	.318	3.14
Prorok et al	1983	62	20	.323	3.10
Roses et al	1980	52	17	.327	3.06
Tinnemans et al	1987	359	118	.329	3.04
Hermann et al	1987	220	77	.350	2.86
Hallgrimsson et al	1988	128	45	.352	2.98
Murphy et al	1978	31	11	.355	2.82
Arnesson et al	1986	314	129	.411	2.43
Rogers and Powell	1972	46	19	.413	2.42
Lamb et al	1987	397	173	.436	2.29
Andersson et al	1979	159	97	.610	1.64
Azavedo et al	1989	567	429	.757	1.32
Azavedo et al	1991	70	61	.871	1.15

Table 5-2. Series where FNA contributed to PPV

Author	Year	Biopsy	Cancer	PPV	Biopsies per cancer
Andersson et al	1979	159	97	.610	1.64
Kehler et al	1984	182	41	.225	4.44
Arnesson et al	1986	314	129	.411	2.43
Lamb et al	1987	397	173	.436	2.29
Azavedo et al	1989	567	429	.757	1.32
Hann et al	1989	96	28	.292	3.43
Fajardo et al	1990	100	30	.300	3.33
Azavedo et al	1991	70	61	.871	1.15

used stereotactic FNA (SFNA) cytology to complement the mammographic findings. When FNA was used as an adjunct to the selection of patients for surgical biopsy, a considerably greater proportion of invasive carcinomas were detected than in those cases where FNA was not used. Indeed, considerably fewer LCIS patients were included in the series reporting the use of stereotactic FNA as an adjunct to mammographic observations in selecting patients for surgical biopsy. Thus the use of stereotactic FNA as part of the diagnostic strategy in selecting patients for surgical biopsy, markedly increases the PPV from .226 without FNA to .524 using FNA. Without FNA, 20,600 biopsies yielded 4659 cancers; when SFNA was added to the diagnostic strategy, 1885 surgical biopsies yielded 988 cancers.

SFNA decreased the proportion of patients who have LCIS in the reported series. In series that reported the histology, there were 237 cases of LCIS in 2922 biopsies, which were done without the assistance of SFNA for an 8.5% LCIS. If the series reporting microcalcification as the sole mammographic criterion for surgical biopsy are excluded, the percent of LCIS decreases to 7.9% (218/2758). The inclusion of those eight publications, which limited their report to surgical biopsies based only on mammographic microcalcifications, is responsible for the large proportion of LCIS seen in patients where SFNA was not used. Even when the microcalcification publications are excluded, there is still a higher proportion of LCIS in published series that do not use SFNA than in those series that report on the use of SFNA. LCIS was found in only 2.4% (8/332) of the histologic specimens from biopsies based on mammography plus SFNA.

Fig. 5-1 represents the total reported series, indicating if the series added SFNA cytology. Quite obviously, there is a marked improvement in the PPV when stereotactic aspiration cytology is used as an adjunct to the mammographic and clinical criteria to select patients for surgical biopsy (Table 5-3).

Published reports

Published materials are reviewed in the order of increasing PPV, which may provide some progressive insight into strategies that have been used to diminish the number of "unnecessary" surgical biopsies. Historical sequence, from the oldest to the more recent publications, is not reviewed, since there is almost a random relationship between when the studies were performed and the ultimate results. The most recent publication has a PPV of .158[25]; many earlier studies had much better PPVs. When seeking to diminish the number of biopsies per cancer, increasing the number of false-negative cases is important. Where possible, we report what the literature found about the false-negative rate.

Lang et al compared the PPV of mammography in two separate institutions in the same city.[30] These patients were evaluated from January, 1985 to November, 1986; 122 women with suspicious nonpalpable lesions detected at mammography who had a needle localization breast biopsy were reported. Routine specimen mammography confirmed the removal of calcifications. Four categories report the mammographic interpretation. These categories were benign, cannot rule out cancer, highly suspicious, or malignant neoplasm. The categories of benign, highly suspicious, or malignant were correct 80% with no false-negative results and only 4 false-positive results in 20 cases. When they used the phrase, "cannot rule out cancer," no cancers were found in 102 surgical biopsies. Obviously, a mammogram cannot be used to "rule out" cancer. A report that states that the mammogram cannot rule out cancer will be true for every mammogram; this statement is not useful and should not be used in mammography reports. This approach led to substantial variation in the two institutions. One hospital had a positive biopsy rate of 2 out of 56 (PPV = .036), whereas the other hospital had 7 out of 66 (PPV. = .106). This difference in two institutions in the same town related in part to the frequency with which the highly suspicious or malignant category was assigned at

Table 5-3.   Series reporting the histology of nonpalpable lesions

Author	Year	Biopsy	Cancer	PPV	Biopsies per cancer	Invasive	In situ	DCIS	LCIS	Other
Rogers and Powell	1972	46	19	.413	2.42	5	13	11	3	—
Murphy et al	1978	31	11	.355	2.82	6	5	5	0	—
Andersson et al	1979	159	97	.610*	1.64	129	18	16	2	—
Solmer et al	1980	40	11	.275	3.64	7	3	3	0	—
Siemssen et al	1981	115	16	.139	7.19	12	4	1	2	—
Lanyi and Citole	1981	135	36	.267	3.75	0	36	33	3	—
Colbassani et al	1982	55	15	.273	3.67	8	7	7	0	—
Powell et al	1983	282	47	.167	6.00	11	36	26	10	—
Chetty et al	1983	190	40	.211	4.75	22	18	—	—	—
Prorok et al	1983	62	20	.323	3.10	15	5	3	2	—
Oppedal et al	1983	87	14	.161	6.21	6	8	5	3	—
Schwartz et al	1984	557	175	.314	3.18	116	59	45	14	—
Gisvold and Martin	1984	343	92	.268	3.73	75	14	14	1	—
Lefor et al	1984	18	3	.167	6.00	3	0	—	—	—
Meyer et al	1984	500	117	.234	4.27	88	29	24	5	—
Bigelow et al	1985	150	24	.160	6.25	17	6	5	1	—
Proudfoot et al	1986	56	6	.107	9.33	3	3	3	0	—
Marrujo et al	1986	237	64	.270	3.70	41	23	—	—	—
Poole et al	1986	148	21	.142	7.05	16	3	3	—	2
Rowen et al	1986	595	84	.141	7.08	60	24	—	—	—
Wilhelm et al	1986	452	95	.210	4.76	43	52	28	24	—
Arnesson et al	1986	314	129	.411*	2.43	89	40	—	—	—
Hall WC et al	1986	70	9	.129	7.78	7	2	0	2	—
Ciatto et al	1987	512	152	.297	3.37	126	26	—	—	—
Tinnemans et al	1987	359	118	.329	3.04	59	10	32	8	2
Rosenberg et al	1987	927	270	.291	3.43	188	81	63	18	1
Landercasper et al	1987	203	44	.217	4.61	15	29	13	11	5
Ostrow et al	1987	121	15	.124	8.07	13	2	1	1	—
Choucair et al	1988	103	9	.087	11.44	7	2	2	0	—
Graham and Bauer	1988	678	78	.115	8.69	51	25	20	5	—
Hall F et al	1988	400	119	.298	3.36	72	47	34	13	—
Skinner et al	1988	179	41	.229	4.37	31	9	9	0	0
Schwartz et al	1988	1132	330	.292	3.43	228	101	81	20	1
Silverstein et al	1989	1014	206	.203	4.92	90	115	86	29	1
Petrovich et al	1989	106	13	.123	8.15	8	5	2	3	—
Landstrom et al	1989	211	21	.100	10.05	17	4	1	3	—
Rusnak et al	1989	200	48	.240	4.17	38	10	8	2	—
Molloy et al	1989	213	38	.178	5.61	30	8	6	2	—
Hann et al	1989	96	28	.292*	3.43	15	13	8	4	1
Fajardo et al	1990	100	30	.300*	3.33	18	10	8	2	—
Albert et al	1990	100	21	.210	4.76	16	4	3	1	—

SFNA was used as an adjunct to mammography in selecting patients for surgical biopsy.

one hospital versus the other. One of the institutions had mostly benign screening mammograms in which the report said "cancer could not be ruled out."

The data led the institutions to change their criteria for selecting patients for surgical biopsy. The PPV was increased from .074 to .150. Their specific recommendations include (1) delete the phrase "cannot rule out malignancy" from radiology reports; (2) do not perform a biopsy on a low-density mass less than 1 cm in diameter; (3) do not perform a biopsy for asymmetric density or questionable mass; (4) do not perform a biopsy for secondary signs of malignancy, such as skin thickening or asymmetric vasculature; and (5) biopsy is indicated for clustered calcifications, a dominant mass greater than 1 cm in diameter, stellate lesions, or interval changes from a previous mammogram.

Using this worst-case scenario as a starting point, we will progress through a series of articles on this and related subjects. The improvement of doubling the PPV in this series by changing the mammography reports and the criteria for biopsy suggests that it is possible to use improved mammographic criteria to diminish "unnecessary" surgical biopsies.

Low yield in surgical biopsies. Choucair et al reported on a series of 99 patients where the needle-directed surgical biopsies were performed for nonpalpable breast lesions.[9] Nine cancers were detected. In this series, all but one patient had an in situ or stage I disease. These patients underwent 103 biopsies, of which 94 revealed benign lesions (PPV = .087). Mammographic findings leading to a surgical biopsy showed calcification in 41% of the patients, mass in 44%, distorted glandular pattern in 4%, mass and calcifications in 4%, mass and distortion in 4%, and calcification and distortion in 2%. In this series, an unusually high number of patients had a history of prior breast cancer. Nine of the patients had a history of contralateral breast cancer and one of ipsilateral cancer. The authors argued that part of the reason for the low yield in biopsy is that the risk factor of prior breast cancer increased the vigilance for early biopsy of even the most remotely suspicious lesions.

These authors attempted to understand the basis for so many false-positive mammograms leading to surgical biopsies. They submitted 71 mammograms for independent review by a panel of four radiologists. Of these, 8 were malignant and 63 benign. The radiologists used 4 categories. These included benign, slightly suspicious, highly suspicious, and malignant. In 24% of the cases the same lesion was interpreted as both benign and highly suspicious by different radiologists. The 4 radiologists unequivocally agreed on their interpretation in only 11 of the 71 patients (15.5%). However, 3 of the 4 radiologists agreed 42% of the time, and in 35% of the patients, 2 radiologists agreed on the interpretation. They noted the trend toward aggressively screening women for subtle lesions of the breast and biopsy of suspicious lesions when found. Therefore the practicing surgeon is operating on smaller and smaller lesions, which are usually benign. While the PPV was .087, they argued that more recent series show a trend toward decreasing true-positive rates.

We believe that nationwide it is likely that radiologists and surgeons, in an effort to avoid missing potentially curable lesions, are over-reading these subtle lesions. . . . The average surgeon is looking at a positive biopsy rate for needle directed biopsies of 10 percent or less. . . . Mammography for subtle occult lesions is quite sensitive but poorly specific. Demonstration of a slightly suspicious lesion does not rule out carcinoma, nor does the lack of change in the lesion over a period of months or years ensure a benign process.

Choucair et al concluded that (1) surgical biopsy of nonpalpable breast lesions has a false-negative rate of approximately 90%; (2) variation in interpretations of mammograms is significant; (3) risk factors that ordinarily would increase the probability of breast cancer should be considered when deciding on whether or not to biopsy a nonpalpable lesion (chief among these is the history of prior breast cancer); (4) given the current state of the art, all lesions found on mammography, which are not determined unequivocally benign by more than one radiologist, should be biopsied; and (5) until further refinements are made for screening, surgeons should accept a low yield, approximately 10%, for biopsies of nonpalpable lesions.[9]

This is a rather typical paper from a surgical viewpoint, published as recently as 1988. These authors advocated what most would consider to be an excessively high false-positive rate for mammogram-induced surgical biopsies. They put relatively little emphasis of the specific mammographic criteria responsible for the concern that resulted in a breast biopsy. Simply, this paper points to a need for greater attention to the mammographic criteria that resulted in an eventual breast biopsy.

Specific mammographic criteria useful. Landstrom et al reported on needle localization in occult breast cancers in 1989.[29] They evaluated 211 patients who underwent biopsy in which 21 were found to have cancer (PPV = .100). Of the malignant cases, 17 were invasive and 4 were noninvasive, 3 of which were LCIS. Characteristic microcalcifications occurred in 17 of the 21 patients who were eventually shown to have cancer (PPV = .810). Microcalcifications were seen in only 63 of 190 benign breast biopsies (33%). Microcalcifications were found with an irregular density in 8 patients who had cancer and in none of the 190 patients found to have benign biopsies. They conclude that use of microcalcifications alone would have increased their PPV in detecting cancer. Their PPV would have increased from .100 to .189 (17/90), if they had operated only on the basis of characteristic microcalcifications. When microcalcification was associated with an irregular mass, the distinction between benign and malignant outcome was remarkable (PPV = 1.00). Microcalcification with "dysplasia" or asymmetry had a PPV of .250 (4/16). Neither microcalcification nor an irregular density was found in 106 women. The biopsies were suggested on the basis of some other criteria, and none were found to have cancer.

This paper clearly points out the utility of microcalcifications and irregular density as the specific mammographic criteria warranting surgical biopsy. When this is observed, it should be coded as a 4 or a 5. If these authors had eliminated surgical biopsy in patients who presented with neither microcalcifications nor an irregular density, they would have done surgical biopsies on only 105 patients, and 21 of these women would have had cancer (PPV =

.210), which would result in a biopsy-to-cancer ratio of 5 to 1, rather than their 10 to 1 ratio. In this case, 106 "unnecessary" biopsies could have been eliminated with no increase in the false-negative rate.

Increased false-positive rate. Graham and Bauer reported their experience with 678 needle localization biopsies in a community hospital.[17] Cancer was detected in 78 patients for a PPV of .115. Five of these 78 cases were LCIS (6.4%). The following four mammographic observations ultimately led to the biopsies:

1. A cluster of or suspicious microcalcifications: 261 of the 678 patients had suspicious microcalcification as the indication for biopsy. Of those patients, 36 had cancer for a PPV of .138. They do not define what they mean by "suspicious" microcalcifications. To obtain this PPV they must have included what others would see as normal calcifications in their definition of "suspicious."

2. Nodules or masses: the second most common indication for surgery was present in 31.1% (211/678) of the women. Malignancy was identified in 16/211 (PPV = .076). Again, a number of obviously benign lesions must have been included in this group to attain such a low PPV.

3. Density or asymmetry: the third leading mammographic criterion for surgical biopsy. This was present in 173/678 patients or 25.2%. Malignancy was found in 10/173 (PPV = .058). This PPV is similar to what has been found by other investigators.

4. Spiculated lesions: found less often. However, they proved to be the most specific finding in anticipating cancer on the biopsy. While present in only 33/678 or 4.9% of the total biopsies, 16 of those 33 patients with spiculated lesions had cancer (PPV = .485). Their definition of spiculated density is not clear. Overlying stromal elements may simulate spiculations, but this confusion can usually be resolved by compression or repositioning the breast. Classical spiculated densities have a PPV that approaches 1.00. The only confusion rests with some cases of radial scars.

Seventy percent of this series were minimal breast cancer, and 96% were node free. This hospital increased their mammography procedures from 253 in 1980 to 7570 in 1985. During this time, while seeking to detect nonpalpable breast cancer, they increased their false positives. This resulted in a reduction of their cancers found per needle biopsy from .300% in 1980 to .098% in 1985. They argue that this change in biopsy rate increased their capacity to detect the more subtle lesions and thereby improve the potential for patient survival.

PPV rate of .123. Petrovich et al reported 104 patients who had undergone 106 biopsies over a 14-month period.[43] Thirteen patients had breast cancer (PPV = .123). Three of these 13 patients had LCIS. The mammograms were performed during large-scale screening or as part of a routine examination of asymptomatic patients. Mammographic findings considered appropriate for biopsy included a mass, abnormal parenchymal density, or microcalcifications deemed suspicious carcinoma by the radiologist. Eight patients (7.7%) had a prior history of biopsy for benign breast disease. An additional 5 patients (4.7%) had a previous biopsy with finding of breast cancer, one ipsilateral and four contralateral. Mammographic findings that effected the biopsy were clustered or linear microcalcifications in 48% (51/106), a mass or abnormal-appearing density in 43% (46/106), and a calcified mass in 9% (9/106). They do not report the relationship between mammographic finding and the surgical yield.

These authors reviewed 17 previous series of mammographic wire localization for the biopsy of occult breast tumors. This represents data from 3980 patients who underwent a surgical biopsy procedure based on screening mammography. The aggregate PPV was .219 in these series, ranging from .007 to .333. Thirty percent of the carcinomas found were described as either noninvasive or minimal. The overall incidence of axillary lymph node metastases in patients with nonpalpable breast carcinoma undergoing axillary dissection was 15.3% (122/800) with a range of 0% to 57%.

More frequent association of mammographic mass lesion than macrocalcification with breast cancer. Ostrow et al. reported on their experience with 121 needle-localized breast biopsies done between 1982 and 1985.[38] Fifteen of the biopsies revealed carcinoma (PPV = .124). One of the 15 carcinomas was DCIS and one was LCIS. All mammograms were reviewed by a board-certified radiologist who had a special interest in mammography. He considered mammographic signs suggesting malignancy to be a discrete mass with ill-defined or spiculated margins in whole or in part, grouped microcalcifications, and a discrete mass with microcalcifications.

The 121 needle-localized biopsies were done on 113 women of whom 30 (24.8%) had a family history of breast cancer. A positive family history did not affect the frequency of cancer in these patients. Patients with a positive family history had the same rate of cancers as did those without a family history of breast cancer in this small series.

Eleven patients (9.7%) had previous breast carcinoma. A history of previous breast carcinoma substantially increased the probability that the biopsy would be positive. Four of the 15 patients with a positive biopsy had a previous history of breast carcinoma (PPV = .267). This was present in only 6 of the 98 patients with a negative biopsy (PPV = .061).

Carcinoma was ultimately diagnosed in 9 of 81 patients

with microcalcifications alone (PPV = .111). Forty patients had a mass lesion with or without microcalcifications; 6 of these biopsies revealed carcinoma (PPV = .150). In this series a mammographic mass lesion was more frequently associated with breast cancer than were microcalcifications alone.

Nontraditional screening pool. Hall et al reported a series of 70 needle-directed surgical biopsies that yielded 9 malignant lesions (PPV = .130).[19] Two of these were carcinoma in situ. The authors do not define whether they were LCIS or DCIS. These patients were selected for mammography because of breast pain, nipple discharge, high-risk profile (family history or prior surgery), or because the physical examination was difficult (i.e., previous biopsies, diffuse nodularity, or large breasts). These cases did not derive from a traditional screening mammography pool. The patient-selection criteria influence the PPV. A mammographic determined mass had a PPV of .083 (4/48). Microcalcification had a PPV of .011 (4/35). Four of the seven invasive carcinomas had axillary metastasis (57%). The fact that these patients did not derive from a screening mammography pool possibly accounts for the high axillary metastasis rate. Many mammograms were obtained because of a high-risk profile or difficult physical examination. However, all 7 patients with invasive ductal carcinoma had primary lesions less than 1.5 cm in diameter.

More than half of the 61 benign cases had fibroadenoma (18) or fibrocystic disease (14). Normal breast tissue occurred in 8 cases with the negative surgical biopsies. The other negative biopsies revealed fibrosis in 10 cases, sclerosing adenosis in 3 cases, papillomatosis in 4 cases, dysplasia in 3 cases, and normal lymph node in 1 case.

Palpable versus nonpalpable cancers. Poole et al. (1986) reported a series of 137 women with nonpalpable breast lesions discovered by mammography.[44] They underwent 148 biopsies that yielded 21 cancers (PPV = .142). These women represented an unselected population of referral patients and did not reflect a routine screening program. One hundred and sixteen were completely asymptomatic and had mammograms as part of the routine physical examination. Of the 127 biopsies that yielded benign lesions, 12 were fibroadenomas, 1 was a lymph node, and the rest were described as mammary dysplasia. Eighty biopsies were done for microcalcifications without an associated mass, and 68 were noncalcified mass lesions or architectural distortion. Although the incidence of carcinoma was higher in the group with the noncalcified mass lesions or architectural distortion, the difference was not significant.

These authors compared their experience in nonpalpable cancer with that of palpable cancer. During the same period there were 282 cancers found in 1285 women who underwent biopsy for palpable lesions (PPV = .219). In the

148 biopsies of patients with nonpalpable lesions, 28 had cancer (PPV = .142). However, the tumor dimension was 2 to 25 mm in nonpalpable lesions and 5 to 140 mm with palpable lesions. The mean dimension was 9 mm for nonpalpable and 31 mm for palpable lesions. The frequency of minimal cancer for nonpalpable lesions was 11/22 (52%), whereas for palpable lesions it was 14/282 (5%). More important, axillary metastases were present in only 3 of 19 for nonpalpable cancers (15.8%), while they were found in 131 of the 282 palpable cancers (46.5%). In this series, distant metastases at diagnosis were found in 1 out of 21 nonpalpable cancers (4.8%) and 24 out of 282 (8.5%) palpable cancers. This series, contrasting the diagnosis of palpable versus nonpalpable breast cancers, shows remarkable improvement in the clinical stage of the cancer when the diagnosis is made by mammography alone.

Needle localization. Galakhoff et al discussed in detail their technique used in needle localization of nonpalpable breast cancers.[14] They reported 33 nonpalpable breast lesions detected over a 6-month period that yielded 5 malignant tumors (PPV = .150).

Work-site service. Kessler et al recently reported on a breast cancer screening program sponsored by a corporation at a work site.[25] They did 3627 mammograms and recommended 63 biopsies (1.7%). This compares to 9.4% biopsies recommended in the Arizona BCDDP Study.[23] Kessler et al performed 57 biopsies and found 9 cancers (PPV = .158).[25] Their cancer incidence of 2.5 per 1000 screening mammograms is consistent with ambient incidence rates. They emphasize the corporate cost and the relative economics effected by work site mammography using a mobile program. Screening mammography is cost effective in this setting when viewed in relation to total health cost savings occasioned by earlier diagnosis.

PPV correlation with degree of suspicion. Bigelow et al retrospectively reviewed a series of 146 women who underwent 150 preoperative localizations of mammographically suspicious but nonpalpable breast lesions.[7] They found 24 cancers (PPV = .016). The mammographic lesions were divided into the following three classes: (1) calcification only; (2) areas of increased density, parenchymal asymmetry, or abnormal configuration; and (3) both density and calcification. Thirty-three percent of the patients had calcification only, whereas 55% showed a density only and 12% had both calcification and a density. The radiologist classified the mammograms as highly suspicious, moderately suspicious, and low suspicious lesions. The highly suspicious lesions were densities or calcification with definite malignant characteristics, such as spiculation, distortion of adjacent breast architecture, or bizarre calcifications. Moderately suspicious lesions were densities, or calcifications, believed to have a definite potential for malignancy but not the truly characteristic features. Low suspicious lesions were those that had a benign radiographic appearance, such as rounded densities with sharp borders or diffuse calcification. Of their 146 lesions, 11 (8%) were considered highly suspicious for cancer, 45 (31%) moderately suspicious, and 90 (61%) minimally suspicious. A high degree of suspicion on mammography had a PPV of .667. Moderately suspicious mammograms had a PPV of .250. When those patients with mammograms having a low index of suspicion had surgery, the PPV was .045.

These authors continue to do biopsies on the low suspicious lesions, since the 4.5% of cancers that would have been missed would have an excellent chance of cure if discovered early. The cost of increasing the discovery of cancer in 4 patients was 90 additional biopsies. Although the authors do not report the number of LCIS, 25% of the total had noninvasive carcinomas.

Calcifications as sole basis for biopsy. Powell et al reported on the use of x-ray calcifications alone as the basis for breast biopsies.[45] They performed 282 biopsies in 251 patients for multiple calcifications. These were a subset of a larger series of 4615 breast biopsies that yielded 974 cancers (PPV = .209). Mammographic calcifications alone were responsible for 6% of the total biopsies (282/4615) performed during the period under study. They found 47 cancers in 45 patients (PPV = .167). Twenty-six out of 47 cancers were DCIS and 10 were LCIS. When calcifications were the only criterion for biopsy, 77% of the malignant biopsies were noninvasive. However, if we were to exclude LCIS as nonmalignant cancer, then the PPV of microcalcifications in this series would be .131 (37/282).

Those patients with cancer who had x-ray calcifications alone as the indices of the cancer had excellent recurrence-free survival. Of the 45 patients, 20 have been followed for 5 years of whom 17 had recurrence-free survival. Of those followed for 5 to 10 years, 13 of 15 are free of disease, and 1 patient died from recurrence of this breast cancer. Of those who have been followed for 10 to 18 years, 10 of 10 are free of disease. The authors did not exclude LCIS from this analysis.

They evaluated the number of calcifications in the cluster in relationship to the probability of malignancy (Table 5-4).

They found no instances of cancer in the cluster of calcifications numbered less than 5. Cancer was most likely if the calcifications were numerous but not countable. The subjective impression of the radiologist who rated the calcifications improved the predictive value (Table 5-5).

The authors do not report the specific criteria used in formulating the degree of suspicion. The PPV of .167 in Table 5-4 is lower than that accomplished by other authors who evaluated the PPV of mammographic microcalcifications.[46,49] However, if the radiologist was highly suspicious of the calcifications, there was an increase in PPV to .315. If they had not operated on the patient with "benign"-appearing calcifications, they would have done 21 fewer biopsies and missed one cancer out of the 42 found. They do not report the criteria used to define "highly" suspicious. The films were analyzed for size, shape, and radiographic density of the individual calcifications, in addition to the size of clustering and the degree of clustering. These authors found no significant difference in these attributes between benign and malignant biopsies.

The calcifications found in benign biopsies were commonly due to blunt duct adenosis and papillomatosis. In two thirds of the 35 ductal carcinomas the calcium was located in the necrotic centers of the malignant ducts. In the remaining ductal cancers, the calcium was found in the lumen or between viable cancer cells. Thus ductal carcinomas were likely to have calcifications that have the pattern of casts in small ducts. The calcifications found in lobular carcinomas may have been coincidental to the cancer, as they were usually found in adjacent adenosis or stroma. The calcifications due to breast cancer are related to ductal carcinoma. When there is no associated mass, the carcinomas are frequently noninvasive and have an excellent prognosis. This paper reveals that when calcification alone is the criterion for biopsy of suspicious breast lesions, there is a high probability of long-term survival and rela-

Table 5-4. Positive predictive value of the number of calcifications in a cluster

Calcifications (No.)	Total biopsies	Malignant	Benign	PPV
	282	47	235	.167
1-4	14	0	14	.000
5-14	123	22	101	.179
15-25	68	11	57	.162
>25 countable	65	9	56	.139
Uncountable	12	5	7	.417

From Powell RW et al: *Ann Surg* 1975(5):555, 1983.

Table 5-5. Positive predictive value of the radiologist rating of the calcifications

Suspicion	Total biopsies	Malignant	Benign	PPV
	249	42	207	.189
1 (benign)	21	1	20	.048
2	86	3	83	.035
3	84	15	69	.179
4	30	17	22	.349
5 (malignant)	19	6	13	.315

From Powell RW et al: *Ann Surg* 1975(5):555, 1983.

tively benign breast disease. Microcalcification, as the sole indictor for surgical biopsy, resulted in a higher proportion of in situ carcinomas than would be found for other mammographic criteria. The degree of radiologic suspicion is important to distinguish those calcifications that warrant biopsy from those that do not.

Mass versus microcalcification PPV rates. Lefor et al reported a small series of needle localization of occult breast lesions.[31] They studied 18 lesions; 11 appeared as masses and 7 as areas of microcalcifications without a demonstrable mass. The mammographic mass lesions had a PPV of .091, while the cases with mammographic microcalcification had a PPV of .286 for an overall PPV of .167.

Nonpalpable lesions more likely to reveal a cancer. Molloy et al reviewed the clinical records of 477 consecutive patients who underwent open breast biopsies in 1985 and 1987.[34] They identified cancer in 38 of 213 needle localization biopsies (PPV = .178) for mammographically detected nonpalpable lesions and in 34 of 256 biopsies of palpable lesions (PPV = .133). The patients with palpable lesions tended to be younger with a mean age of 45.8 years for palpable and 51.5 years for nonpalpable lesions. Eight of the 38 cancers identified by needle localization were preinvasive lesions, whereas only 1 of 34 malignancies identified by biopsy of a palpable lesion was preinvasive. In this series, nonpalpable mammographically detected lesions were more likely to reveal a cancer at surgical biopsy than were those lesions detected by clinical palpation.

Sensitivity of mammography vs physical examination. Hicks et al compared the sensitivity of mammography and physical examination in detecting breast cancer.[23] They studied 725 breast biopsies in the 10,117 women screened in the Arizona BCDD Program. Four hundred and nineteen of these biopsies were done in asymptomatic women on the basis of the screening studies. Eighty-five cancers were found in this group (PPV = .203). Breast biopsies were recommended in 9.4% of the women screened (948/10,117). They reported 725 surgical biopsies and 31 breast aspirations. Breast cancer was discovered in 113 of the 725 women who underwent biopsy (PPV = .156). They detected 11 cancers per 1000 patients screened. This is higher than the ambient prevalence rate, suggesting some degree of self-selection in the screening population. Self-discovered breast abnormality resulted in 42% of the biopsies being performed between screening examinations. These 306 symptomatic patients and this group had 28 of the 113 cancers (PPV =.092). Of these cancers, 75% were found in asymptomatic women and were detected by the screening process (85/113). The screening process found 85 cancers in the 419 patients biopsied (PPV = .203)

To determine the cause for the large number of interval cancers in this series, the mammograms were reviewed

retrospectively. Seven mammograms in these 306 patients showed suspicious lesions that were initially overlooked. The remainder (299/306) were still interpreted as negative or probably benign. The average time interval between previous screening and the diagnosis of interval cancer was 8 months with a range of 2 months to 2 years.

Metastatic lymph nodes were found in 26 (23%) of these breast cancer patients. Of the cancers found by self-examination and interval biopsy 28% (8 of 28) demonstrated lymph node metastases compared with 18 of 85 (21%) of those cancers detected in the screening process. Relatively fewer axillary metastases were found in women whose breast cancer was asymptomatic.

The mammographic findings in 673 cases were reviewed and compared with the biopsy results. The mammograms were classed as mass, density, or calcification. Mammographic masses were classified as benign, suspicious, or cancer. Mammographic densities and calcification were classified only as benign or suspicious. There were 109 patients with cancer in these 673 patients whose mammograms were reviewed. Mammography revealed a mass in 309, a density in 202, and calcifications in 162. One hundred and thirteen of the 309 masses were interpreted as mammographically benign. In this group, 10 cancers were found on surgical biopsy (PPV = .088). When the mass was interpreted as suspicious there were 28 cancers out of 183 (PPV = .153). When the mammographic interpretation was "malignant mass," they found 6 cancers in 13 patients (PPV = .461). Their ability to distinguish a benign from malignant mass on a mammogram was considerably worse than presently applied mammographic criteria.[5]

Density was the primary mammographic clue that resulted in a biopsy. Carcinoma was found in 24 of 175 densities classified as benign (PPV = .137) and in 10 of 27 densities classified as suspicious (PPV = .370). When calcification was the primary motivating factor, cancer was found in 7 for a surgical breast biopsy of 41 patients classified (PPV = .146) as benign calcifications and 24 of 121 patients classified as having suspicious calcifications (PPV = .198). The various mammographic features were compared with physical examination in terms of sensitivity, specificity, and PPV. In the whole series of both symptomatic and asymptomatic women, the physical examination had a sensitivity of .24, a specificity of .95, and a PPV of .490. Mammography, however, had an overall sensitivity of .62, specificity of .51, and PPV of .203. When a density was present, it was more likely to yield a positive biopsy. However, an abnormal mammographic density was often not present in the presence of cancer.

Of the 85 breast cancers detected solely by screening mammography or physical examination, 48 (42%) were detected by abnormal mammographic findings alone. An additional 8 cases (7%) had suspicious physical examination and benign mammography. Of the 37 small cancers (less than 1 cm) in this series 30 (81%) were detected by the screening program. These small cancers comprise 35% (30 of 85) of the cancers detected by screening. These authors quote the HIP experience, where approximately 31% of the cancers were diagnosed between screenings or after the last screening. They point out that in the HIP study the 5-year mortality for women with breast cancer detected by screening was 13% (17 of 132) and those not detected by screening was 32% (53/167). Hicks et al suggest that these smaller cancers detected by screening account for the improved survival.[23]

Indices of suspicion improve PPV. In 1989, Silverstein et al updated their previous 1987 series.[54] Their 1989 article reported a total of 1014 cases of nonpalpable breast lesions where the diagnosis was made by slightly overpenetrated mammography. They used a hookwire surgical biopsy technique. In this series, 899 women aged 26 to 87 years underwent 1014 hookwire breast biopsies. Mammographic indications for biopsy were 521 clusters of microcalcifications (51%), 359 masses (35%), 58 architectural distortions (6%), and 76 combinations of these signs (7%). Out of 521 biopsies, 122, done for calcification alone, revealed cancer (PPV = .234). Similarly, 58 of 359 biopsies for mass revealed cancer (PPV = .162). When distortion alone was used as the criterion, cancer was found in only 7 out of 58 patients (PPV = .121). When mass and calcification were cues for surgical biopsy, cancer was found in 13 of 47 (PPV = .277); when distortion and calcification were the mammographic criteria for biopsy, cancer was found in 6 of 29 patients (PPV = .207). They further refined mammographic calcification by separating the mammograms into minimally suspicious and truly suspicious groups. These indices of suspicion improved the PPV of all criteria (Table 5-6).

When minimally suspicious distortion and calcification were the criteria, only 1 in 10 had cancer for PPV of .100. These authors identified radiologic indices or suspicion that can increase the PPV of the preoperative indices for surgery. The total number of biopsies for suspicious lesions was 458. One hundred and sixty-eight had cancer (PPV = .368). Only 38 cancers were found in 558 biopsies of minimally suspicious lesions (PPV = .068). If they had not biopsied minimally suspicious lesions, they would have increased their total PPV from .203 to .368.

In this series of 206 patients with cancers, 29 had lobular carcinoma in situ and 86 had ductal carcinoma in situ. Thus 14% percent of the 206 patients had LCIS. If minimally suspicious lesions were not biopsied, 7% of the cancers would have been missed. These authors do not report if these minimally suspicious lesions were more likely to be LCIS. This is a common problem with many of the published series of diagnostic criteria for asymptomatic breast cancer.

Albert et al attempt to correlate mammographic features in nonpalpable breast lesions.[1] They studied 3063 mammograms taken from 1984 to 1986 and identified nonpalpable lesions in 100 instances. These 100 cases went to biopsy. They classed the mammographic observations into definitive or indecisive, 79 being definitive and 21 indecisive. Of the definitive readings, they classed 48 as most likely benign and 31 as most likely malignant. In the benign cases, they were correct in each instance, whereas in the 31 most likely malignant cases, 19 were malignant (PPV = .613). Of the indecisive readings, 2 were malignant (PPV = .095). Smooth irregular masses with well-defined borders proved to be noncystic on the ultrasound examination with or without well-circumscribed, generally coarse, calcifications, which were most likely benign. The most likely malignant group were lesions with ill-defined borders or irregular microcalcifications. Indeterminant features of malignancy were (1) apparent asymmetry between both breasts with a focal architectural distortion; (2) fairly uniform and "regular clustered calcification," which progressed in the number of calcifications, increasing nonuniformity of calcifications, or the size of the area involved; and (3) increase in the size of what was originally interpreted as a certainly benign lesion.

Table 5-6. Distribution of cancers by suspicious versus minimally suspicious mammographic findings

Mammographic finding	Suspicious lesions	Cancers	PPV	Minimally suspicious lesions	Cancers	PPV
Calcification	300	107	.357	221	15	.068
Mass	94	44	.468	265	14	.053
Distortion	15	1	.067	43	6	.140
Mass and calcification	28	11	.393	19	2	.105
Distortion and calcification	19	5	.263	10	1	.100
TOTAL	456	168	.368	558	38	.068

From Silverstein MJ et al: *Radiology* 171:633-638, 1989.

Four of the 21 malignant lesions were in situ carcinomas. One was lobular in situ carcinoma and 3 were intraductal. LCIS was found in 5% of the biopsies.

Of these 100 patients, 42 presented with microcalcifications. These microcalcifications had a PPV of .286. This compares with the overall PPV of .210. If they had not performed surgery on patients whose mammograms were read as most likely benign, they would have increased their PPV from .210 to .404 and not had any increase in their false-negative rate. None of those patients with mammograms, which read as most likely benign, had cancer revealed on surgical biopsy.

An indecisive reading occurred in 21% of their patients. Only 10% of these lesions will be malignant. They conclude that the surgeon has little option to proceed with the biopsy when the radiographic interpretation states, "although benign appearing, the lesion may be malignant" or "benign characteristics, but recommend biopsy to rule out malignancy." This situation may have occurred in this series because multiple radiologists, in rotation, interpreted the mammograms. They suggest that the pattern of benign microcalcifications needs to be better defined to identify the group in whom close follow-up, rather than surgical biopsy, may be permissible. They conclude that evaluation of other modalities, such as FNA, may be useful to define which patients in the indecisive group need surgical biopsy rather than repeated examinations.

Nonpalpable mammographically detected tumors more likely noninvasive. Chetty et al reported from Scotland on 190 nonpalpable mammographic abnormalities considered to be suspicious for malignancy.[8] These lesions were surgically excised using a needle localization technique. These patients were seen between 1976 and 1982. Of these 190 patients, 142 were asymptomatic women referred from the Edinburgh Breast Screening Clinic. During that time, 19,000 women had been screened.

The criteria for suspicion of malignancy leading to surgical biopsy were the following:

1. Areas of microcalcification usually consisting of more than six elements
2. Irregular opacities
3. Areas of altered architecture
4. Lesions previously considered to be benign, but on which repeated mammograms were shown to have changed

Of the 190 lesions, 40 were malignant (PPV = .210).

As seen in Table 5-7, all of the in situ carcinomas were found at surgical biopsies, which were done for the presence of microcalcifications. Only three of these 18 patients had a complex lesion with calcification; the remainder had only microcalcification as the mammographic abnormality leading to surgical biopsy. In the 22 patients with invasive carcinoma, 10 presented with microcalcifications, 4 with circular opacities, 4 with spiculated opacities, 1 with architectural disturbance, and 3 with complex lesions with calcification.

They compared these 40 patients with cancer, who presented with nonpalpable tumors, with a group of patients treated at the same time, who presented with palpable tumors. Nonpalpable and mammographically detected tumors were more likely to be noninvasive, of small size, and associated with negative nodes.

Intraductal cancer presentation of microcalcifications only. Hoehn et al reported on nonpalpable breast lesions.[24] From 1970 to 1980, 62 patients underwent 66 needle-localized surgical biopsies. Fourteen of these patients had cancer (PPV = .212). The histologies of the cancer included four intraductal, seven infiltrating ductal, two tubular, and one mucinous. One of the patients with tubular carcinoma was the only patient in this series who had axillary metastases. All of the "noninvasive" intraductal cancers presented only with microcalcifications.

Selective screening mammography based on risk profile. Knaus et al did 100 needle-localized breast biopsies on 89 patients drawn from a group of 1110 gynecol-

Table 5-7. Comparison of mammographic abnormality and histopathology of nonpalpable lesions excised by needle localization

| Histology | No. | | Mammographic abnormality | | | |
		Microcalcification	Circular opacity	Spiculated opacity	Disturbance of architecture	Complex lesion with calcification
Benign	150	78	41	3	17	11
Cancer						
In situ	18	15	0	0	0	3
Invasive	22	10	4	4	1	3
PPV	.211	.243	.089	.571	.056	.353

From Chetty U et al: *Br J Surg* 70(10):607-610, 1983.

ogy office patients who had screening mammography based on risk profiles.[26] Eight percent of these office gynecology patients had a surgical breast biopsy. There were 21 nonpalpable breast cancers diagnosed in 18 patients in this group of 89 patients. Their technique included a repeat of the radiograph within 1 month to clarify an indistinct or suspicious finding on the initial mammogram. This "callback" was done at the request of the radiologist in 173 screening mammograms (15.5%). Two of their 18 breast cancer patients (11%) were diagnosed from this group who were called back for repeated mammograms in 1 month. The histology of these 21 cases was invasive ductal carcinoma in 17, DCIS in 2, and LCIS in 2.

Mammograms were done on the basis of a risk profile. Of the 18 patients with cancer, 6 had their mammography due to a positive first-degree family history of breast cancer. In 6 patients with a negative family history and positive biopsy, 4 (22%) had persistent, subjective symptoms of pain or soreness, and 2 (11%) had vague, objective findings. Six of the 18 patients with cancer had initial mammography using age as the only risk factor. These women were over 50 years of age. They did mammograms on women over 50 years of age and younger women with a positive family history or breast symptoms.

Density and microcalcifications as biopsy criteria. Landercasper et al performed hookwire-guided biopsies for nonpalpable lesions in 174 patients over a 3-year period.[28] They found cancer in 44 of 203 specimens taken for biopsy (PPV = .217). In this series, 66% of the lesions were in situ. Of the 29 in situ carcinomas, 11 were lobular, 13 were intraductal, and 5 were both. Of the 15 invasive carcinomas, 3 were lobular and 2 were ductal. This is an unusual number of invasive lobular carcinomas. Invasive lobular carcinoma would be expected to have a different mammographic appearance than invasive ductal carcinoma.

The mammographic criteria for biopsy included microcalcifications, density, or both. Of the 113 patients with microcalcification alone, 25 had cancer (PPV = .221). The authors did not define how many of these were in situ carcinomas. Eleven of the 63 patients with density alone had cancer (PPV = .175). In patients with both density and microcalcifications, the PPV for cancer was .296.

Architectural distortion found to be the most reliable characteristic. Skinner et al reported that between June 1984 and July 1986, 178 women had a needle-guided surgical biopsy of asymptomatic nonpalpable breast lesions.[55] Mammograms of 7 patients were unavailable for review, and the pathology of another 3 patients was not available. Therefore this study concerns 168 patients who underwent 179 biopsies. They found 41 cancers (PPV = .229). In these 41 patients, 32 had invasive carcinoma and 9 were in situ. Of the 30 patients who had axillary dissections, only 7 had positive nodes. None had distant metastatic disease.

They separated soft tissue lesions from calcifications in discussing their mammographic indications for surgery. The soft tissue lesions were divided into three types: mass, asymmetric density, and architectural distortion. The masses were defined as stellate, irregular, or well defined. They determined the size of the mass as the arithmetic average of two dimensions in millimeters.

The calcifications were classed by their size. Fine calcifications were those less than 0.4 mm, medium from 0.4 to 0.9 mm, and coarse greater than 0.9 mm. The calcifications were also classed by their number (less than 5, 5 to 10, or more than 10), and their distance of scatter in millimeters. Calcifications were also defined as to their shape, being regular, irregular, pleomorphic, or linear with branched castings.

Table 5-8 represents an excellent outline of the mammographic signs of malignancy and would be an excellent foundation for an information system used to develop a database of any screening mammography system or radiologic practice. By knowing which signs are most effectively reacted to in the preoperative identification of breast cancer, each radiologist may be able to improve the mammographic interpretation.

The mammographic criteria of Skinner et al revealed

Table 5-8. Mammographic criteria*

Soft tissue lesions
Type
    Mass
    Asymmetric density
    Architectural distortion
Definition (mass only)
    Stellate
    Irregular
    Well-defined
Size
    Arithmetic average of two dimensions in millimeters

Calcifications
Size
    Fine (<0.4 mm)
    Medium (0.4-0.9 mm)
    Coarse (>0.9 mm)
Number
    <5
    5-10
    >10
Distribution
    Distance of scatter in millimeters
Shape
    Regular
    Irregular
    Pleomorphic
    Linear, branched castings

From Skinner MA et al: *Ann Surg* 208(2):203-208, 1988.
*Each mammogram was reviewed by a radiologist who was blind to the final diagnosis. The radiologic soft tissue lesions and calcifications were characterized by these criteria.

that 60 patients had calcification only (34%) and of these 8 were malignant (PPV = .133). Calcification and soft tissues were found in 33 patients (18%) of which 14 were malignant (PPV = .412). A soft tissue lesion was identified in 86 of the patients (48%) in which 19 cancers were found (PPV = .221) (Table 5-9). A detailed analysis of the various mammographic features used to indicate the need for surgical biopsy included 31 patients with asymmetric density with 6 malignancies (PPV = .193), 17 patients with architectural distortion with 7 cancers (PPV = .412), 71 patients with mass not associated with architectural distortion, of which 20 had cancer (PPV = .281). There were 8 stellate masses, 34 irregularly defined masses, and 29 well-defined masses. The stellate masses revealed cancers in 6 of the 8 (PPV = .750); the irregularly defined masses revealed cancers in 12 of 34 (PPV = .353); and the well-defined masses revealed cancers in 2 of 29 (PPV = .069). The number of calcifications was correlated with the probability of cancer. These were more than 10 calcifications in 31 patients. Fourteen of these patients had malignancy (PPV = .341). If the number of calcifications was less than 10, 8 out of 52 patients were found to have malignancy (PPV = .153). Thus more than 10 calcifications significantly increased the probability of cancer. Concerning the size of the clusters, if they were less than 4 mm, 13 out of 54 patients had cancer (PPV = .235); and

if the clusters were larger than 4 mm, 9 out of 39 had cancer (PPV = .231). This size distribution had no effect on the probability of cancer. In those patients with more than 5 calcifications, they analyzed whether they were clustered or scattered. In the clustered series, cancer was found in 9 out of 46 (PPV = .196), whereas, in the scattered calcifications, cancer was found in 9 of 15 (PPV = .375). Most of the calcifications were large enough to suggest an irregular or pleomorphic shape. There were only three cases where there were many small, linear, and branching calcifications suggestive of intraluminal casting. Cancer was found in 2 of these 3 patients. The definitions of calcifications as being fine, medium, or coarse failed to uncover a subgroup more significantly associated with any particular pathologic diagnosis.

In this series, no necessary improvement in the ability to predict cancer merely due to the clustering of the calcifications was found. Malignancy was found in 20% of the lesions associated with 5 or more calcifications located within the distance of 1 cm. Overall, calcifications in 93 of the 168 patients were found either with or without associated soft tissue lesions. Skinner et al conclude that the greatest diagnostic accuracy of mammographic examination of nonpalpable breast lesions is in those lesions with no calcifications. Radiographs in this group may be more easily classed as benign or malignant. *The most reliable characteristic of the mammogram, which suggests the presence of malignancy, is the presence of architectural distortion.* This may be either frankly stellate or more subtle tethering of adjacent breast structures in association with less well-defined mass lesions. In their series, only 1 of 23 patients with well-defined masses not having calcifications was malignant.

Their indications of the mammographic features, which were most likely associated with malignancy, were: (1) curvilinear and branched calcifications, (2) changes from the previous mammogram, (3) soft tissue lesion with calcification, (4) focus with greater than 10 calcifications, and (5) architectural distortion.

Considerable attention was devoted to the analysis of the mammographic abnormalities that were to have a low likelihood of being malignant. The mammographic features more likely to be benign than malignant included well-defined masses and asymmetric densities, if there were no calcifications present; no associated soft tissue lesions; and calcifications having fewer than 10 calcifications. In this series, there were 73 biopsies performed for these mammographic abnormalities and only 4 were positive for cancer (PPV = .055). These authors suggest that it will be necessary to further understand the risk of delaying biopsy in some of these suspicious radiographic findings. How long can these lesions be safely followed? They suggest a prospective study of patients presenting with low-risk mammographic findings and evaluate the safety of following certain features. They clearly outline a reasonable

Table 5-9. Biopsy results for various mammographic features

Mammographic feature*	Malignant	Benign	PPV
Asymmetric density†	6	25	.193
Architectural distortion	7	10	.412
Mass†	20	51	.281
Mass subtotals			
Stellate	6	2	.750
Irregularly defined	12	22	.353
Well-defined	2	27	.069
Number of calcifications			
>10	14	27	.341
≤10	8	44	.153 (p = 0.07)
Size of calcifications			
≥0.4 mm	13	41	.235
<0.4 mm	9	30	.231 (p > 0.25)
Distribution of calcifications‡			
Clustered	9	37	.196
Scattered	9	15	.375 (p = 0.15)

From Skinner MA et al: *Ann Surg* 208(2):203-208, 1988.
*The radiographic features are considered independently (i.e., lesions having both a soft tissue lesion and calcifications are included twice).
†Lesions not associated with an architectural distortion.
‡Lesions having more than five calcifications.

Table 5-10. Benign mass lesions

Dominant characteristic	No. (%)
Poorly defined or irregular borders	106 (47%)
Lobulated, round, or oval	99 (44%)
Distortion of normal architecture	20 (9%)
TOTAL	225 (100%)

From Meyer JE et al: *Radiology* 150:335-337, 1984.

Table 5-11. Malignant mass lesions

Dominant characteristic	No. (%)
Spiculated	39 (55%)
Poorly defined or irregular borders	19 (26%)
Distortion of normal architecture	8 (11%)
Lobulated, round or oval	6 (8%)
TOTAL	72 (100%)

From Meyer JE et al: *Radiology* 150:335-337, 1984.

direction for further research in auditing one's practice in interpreting screening mammograms.

Inclusion of certain abnormalities decreases positive biopsy rate. Meyer et al presented the results of 500 preoperative radiographically guided localizations for occult breast carcinoma over a 5-year period.[33] Of these 500, 297 cases had a mass, asymmetry, or architectural distortion on mammograms. Seventy-two were malignant (PPV = .242). The remaining 203 cases presented with calcification without a mass, of which 45 were malignant (PPV = .234). They had a total of 117 malignancies in the 500 patients (PPV = .234). A comparison of benign and malignant mass lesions can be seen in Tables 5-10 and 5-11.

Spiculation occurred in 55% of malignant mass lesions and in none of the benign lesions. Of the 135 mass lesions with poorly defined or irregular borders, 19 were malignant (PPV = .141). There were 105 mass lesions defined as lobular, round, or oval. Six of these were malignant (PPV = .057). Twenty-eight mass lesions were classified as distorting the normal architecture and 8 were malignant (PPV = .286). To detect malignancy, special attention must be paid to spiculated masses or architectural distortion found in two thirds of the cancerous masses. None of the benign mass lesions presented with a spiculated feature.

Seventy-four patients had axillary lymph node removal. In 16 of these patients, axillary metastases were found for an incidence of 22%. The incidence of malignancy in 52 patients referred after having mammography at another institution was 13% (PPV = .134) (some of these patients had their initial mammograms interpreted at another hospital), whereas the 448 patients whose mammograms were initially interpreted at their hospital had a PPV of .246. Thus the PPV of mammograms initially interpreted elsewhere was lower than Meyer et al were able to accomplish at their hospital.

Five of the 117 "cancers" were lobular carcinoma in situ. Which features provoked the perceived need for surgical biopsy in these patients was not defined.

Meyer et al considered the appropriate ratio of benign to malignant biopsies; the surgical staff at their hospital accepted a PPV of .234 as appropriate. Moskowitz et al and others advocate a more aggressive approach to screening mammograms with an "acceptable" PPV of .100. In their original series of 180 patients, they reported a PPV of

.30.[35] In the most recent group of 320 women, this has decreased to .190. Meyer et al claim this decreasing PPV is due to an increasingly aggressive approach to mass lesions, especially asymmetric densities and small lobulated abnormalities.[33]

It seems apparent from this and other studies that radiologists' change in behavior leads to increased surgical biopsy rate in suspicious mammographic lesions. This may relate to the well-known effect of negative diagnostic experiences of radiologists when interpreting the film. When a cancer is missed on a mammogram with subtle abnormalities, the radiologist will tend to overread subsequent mammograms, leading to an increased number of benign biopsies. In this series, Meyer et al recognize that small lobulated abnormalities in asymmetric densities have a low probability of yielding positive biopsies and yet have decreased their positive biopsy rate to include these abnormalities.

FNA use may decrease "unnecessary" surgery. Hann et al used standard mammographically guided wire localization techniques to study the utility of cytology in evaluating nonpalpable breast lesions.[21] The studies were performed in women who were scheduled for biopsy of nonpalpable lesions or microcalcifications detected at mammography. They used a 19 g thin-walled needle, and two aspirates were obtained by using a 22 g needle passed through the 19 g needle. Following aspiration, the hook guide wire was positioned through the same 19 g needle. The aspirated material was placed in a 50% ethanol solution and centrifuged. The pellet was fixed; slides were prepared and stained with the Papanicolaou stain.

The cytologic samples were evaluated for cellularity, cellular arrangement, nuclear/cytoplasmic ratio, nucleoli, and nuclear characteristics. Each aspirate was classified as follows:

1. Positive, which meant unequivocally malignant cells present
2. Suspicious, which meant very abnormal cells present, that are almost certainly malignant but are too degenerate or too few for unequivocal diagnosis
3. Atypical, abnormal cells present, judged to be atypical intraductal hyperplasia or suggestive of in situ carcinoma

4. Negative, which equal benign ductal cells present consistent with normal breast, fibroadenoma, fibrocystic changes, or other benign conditions, or inadequate, which meant too few cells were seen

The mammographic lesions were graded for degree of suspicion, based on the margin characteristics of masses, or the morphology of microcalcification.

Twenty-one of the 23 cancers with adequate aspirates were correctly diagnosed by cytology (PPV = .913). Only two lesions with adequate cells and benign cytology were found to be malignant at histologic examination of a surgical biopsy specimen. One of these was an incidental focus of lobular carcinoma in situ and not in the area of suspicious microcalcifications. The second case was an infiltrating ductal carcinoma, which the authors conclude was missed due to a sampling error.

Using this technique, the aspirates from 35 of the 96 breast lesions were considered inadequate because of insufficient cellular material. The surgical biopsy revealed marked fibrosis in 16 (46%) of the breast abnormalities, which yielded inadequate cytologic samples. In the group with inadequate cytologic samples, the pathologic examination revealed 6 malignant and 29 benign histologies. Three of these cancers were DCIS.

No cancers were found in the 31 women whose mammograms were considered to have a low probability for malignancy. Of the 46 moderately suspicious mammograms, 12 cancers were identified (PPV = .261). Sixteen of the 19 highly suspicious mammograms yielded cancer at surgical biopsy (PPV = .842). These investigators demonstrate that if no biopsy had been done, based on mammograms considered having a low probability for malignancy, no cancers would have been missed, and 31 fewer biopsies would have been possible. Then the results would have been 65 biopsies yielding 28 cancers (PPV = .431). Four of these cancers were LCIS.

These authors feel that FNA results can be improved with experience. They are concerned about occasional erroneous needle placement and sampling errors. Two radiographs at 90 degree angles were obtained to identify the lesion and place a needle. They believe that the 1 mm needle–placement accuracy with stereotactic devices could significantly decrease the frequency of sampling error. However, even with this precise localization, it may be possible to sample from areas surrounding a dense scar, and thus miss the foci of a tumor.

Hann et al feel that a benign FNA sample can be of diagnostic value, if the cytologic results are closely correlated with the mammographic findings.[21] Negative cytology in a lesion with low suspicion at mammography should eliminate the need to do a surgical biopsy.

The number of inadequate aspirates may, in part, have been related to the technique of aspiration. These authors report a 36% inadequate aspirate, which they find is com-parable with the range 14% to 37% rates of inadequate samples reported for palpable masses. However, they note that it is significantly higher than the 16.6% of inadequate samples reported for FNA with stereotactic guidance by Gent et al.[15] Almost half of the inadequate samples in the Hann et al study were due to the presence of hypocellular tissue found at histology. Hann et al conclude that using standard mammographic localization for FNA, a vigorous aspiration is problematic, since it could compromise the needle position. This may not be a problem with the more accurate positioning of the stereotactic localization systems.

These authors believe that FNA, when correlated with mammographic findings, can decrease the need for "unnecessary" surgery. Biopsy may not be necessary in lesions that are moderately suspicious at mammography and have a negative FNA.

Architectural distortion has highest PPV. Rusnak et al reported a series of preoperative needle localizations to localize early breast cancer.[50] They found 48 cancers from 200 biopsies (PPV = .240). Their criteria for fine-needle localization biopsies were evidence of a mass, microcalcifications, or architectural distortions. They analyzed 192 specimens and note that the needle localization techniques missed 6 lesions (3%). Of these 6 cases, 3 returned for more tissue and the lesion was identified.

The indications for biopsy in this series were microcalcification in 55%, mass in 23%, and architectural distortion in 10%, with a combination of microcalcification and a mass in 12%.

Table 5-12 displays the surgical biopsy experience from

Table 5-12. Indications for biopsy

	Calcification	Mass	Distortion	Calcification and mass
Benign				
Fibrocytic disease	70	18	8	12
Fibroadenoma	2	12	—	2
Hyperplasia	16	—	—	2
Other benign	2	4	1	—
Other*	—	3	—	—
TOTAL	90	37	9	16
Malignant				
Invasive ductal	16	8	8	4
In-situ ductal	4	—	3	1
Invasive lobular	1	1	—	—
In-situ lobular	1	—	—	1
TOTAL	22	9	11	6
PPV	.196	.196	.550	.272

From Rusnak CH et al: *Am J Surg* 157:505-507, 1989.
*No disease was found in three patients.

Rusnack et al. These biopsies were done in 1986 to 1987 and evaluated retrospectively. In this series, the mammographic impression of architectural distortion had the highest PPV. Some 27% of these lesions were noninvasive, while all of the cancers that presented as mammographically detected masses without calcification were invasive cancers. Twenty-three percent of patients, in whom mammographic calcification led to a surgical biopsy that revealed cancer, had invasive cancer. In this series there were only 2 cases of LCIS (4%).

Increased PPV with mass and calcification combined. Gisvold and Martin presented their experience with 343 nonpalpable lesions of the breast.[16] This paper emphasizes the techniques of prebiopsy localization for nonpalpable breast cancers. They used a combination needle-hookwire technique. They encountered a substantial number of vasovagal reactions, which necessitated the presence of a cot adjacent to the procedure to accommodate the fainting patient. All patients who experienced the vasovagal reactions responded to rest in the recumbent position. In nine cases they failed to remove the located lesion by the hookwire technique. This accounts for a 3% failure rate.

Their indications for biopsy in these 343 cases were classified as a mass, calcification, and mass and calcification. Their designation of mass included any suspicious characteristic other than calcification (Table 5-13).

These authors note that when the calcification occurred with the mass, there was marked increased PPV. Of the in situ cancers, only one was an LCIS. These authors do not define the reason for biopsy in that case. The indication of calcification yielded 45% malignancy lesions, while presence of mass yielded 19%, distortion 23%, and calcification with a mass 12%.

Clusters of microcalcification indicate noninvasive and minimally invasive cancers. Marrujo et al[32] reported a surgical biopsy series with 237 breasts that contained suspicious, nonpalpable lesions in 225 women. Biopsies of these lesions revealed 64 cancers (PPV = .270). These cancers included 25 invasive, 16 minimally invasive, and 23 noninvasive lesions. They observed that the noninva-

sive and minimally invasive cancers tended to occur in younger women and almost uniformly appeared as clusters of microcalcifications (22 of 23 of the noninvasive and 14 of 16 of the minimally invasive lesions). The invasive cancers, however, affected an older population, average age of 65 years, and the mammographic appearance was that of a mass in 16 of the 25 cases.

In this series, virtually all noninvasive and minimally invasive cancers appeared as clustered microcalcifications. They consider that this mammographic finding is the most favorable indicator of early breast cancers. These authors report that in reviewing the natural history of noninvasive ductal cancer treated by biopsy alone, the risk of subsequent development of invasive cancer has been between 28% and 39%, and the average time for development of these cancers is 9.7 years after biopsy. They conclude that some one third of noninvasive cancers will eventually become invasive. Furthermore, the risk has been shown to be restricted to the ipsilateral breast, in most cases to the same quadrant as the original lesion. When consecutive autopsy cases were examined, two clinically occult noninvasive breast cancers were demonstrated for every invasive cancer that existed before death or was discovered at autopsy.[37] Marrujo et al point to the experience of Page et al, who found that biopsy demonstration of atypical epithelial lesions resulted in a four-fold to eleven-fold increase in the risk of development of invasive cancer.[32,40] This risk is equal for both breasts, and the latency period averages more than 10 years.[40]

Multicentric breast cancer. Schwartz et al. (1980) reported a series of 62 nonpalpable cancers and found unsuspected foci of cancer present in another quadrant of the breast in 39% of the patients.[53] Rosen et al published a series of 103 patients with noninvasive breast cancer who underwent mastectomy.[48] They found an independent focus of disease in 33% of the patients. In 53 patients with noninvasive ductal cancer, 3 had an unsuspected focus of invasion. Marrujo et al found a 34% incidence of multicentric cancer and a 15% incidence of atypia in their series.[32] They conclude that patients treated with lesser procedures than total mastectomy remain at high risk for the development of subsequent invasive cancer. However, Bedwani et al, who studied 323 cases of noninvasive breast cancer, found no significant difference in the 5-year cure or recurrence rate for those patients treated by radical surgery or breast-conserving surgery and radiation.[6] The 5-year cure rate and recurrence rate were 76.2% and 7.7%, respectively, for those women who underwent radical surgery, which compares with 72.89% and 8.5% for those women treated by conservative procedures. Marrujo et al argued that the treatment plan for patients with the diagnosis of nonpalpable breast lesions must address the high incidence of residual disease at the biopsy site, multicentricity, and proven capacity for invasive lesions to

Table 5-13. Reasons for biopsy in 343 cases of nonpalpable breast lesions

Reason	All lesions	All cancers	In situ cancers	PPV
Mass	185	45	2	.243
Calcification	125	26	11	.208
Mass and calcification	33	21	1	.636
TOTAL	343	92	14	

From Gisvold JJ, Martin JK Jr: *AJR* 143:477-481, 1984.

metastasize to the axillary nodes regardless of the size of the primary tumor.[32] Fisher et al published a definitive response to this concern.[13] They used data from the US National Surgical Adjuvant Breast and Bowel Project (NSABP) to establish that there is no significant difference between lumpectomy, lumpectomy plus breast irradiation, and total mastectomy in terms of disease-free survival (NSABP B-06). Breast-conserving surgery had previously been established as a replacement for radial mastectomy (NSABP B-04). In 1991, Fisher et al used 9-year follow-up data from NSABP B-06 to study the issue of ipsilateral breast tumor recurrence.[13] In contradistinction to the inference of Marrujo et al, although ipsilateral breast cancer recurrence was a powerful independent predictor of distant disease, it was a marker of risk for and not a cause of distant metastasis.[32] Fisher et al stated, "while mastectomy or breast irradiation following lumpectomy prevent expression of the marker, they do not lower the risk of distant disease. These findings further justify the use of lumpectomy."[13]

Benign versus malignant calcifications. Colbassani et al sought a mammographic and pathologic correlation of breast microcalcifications.[11] These authors reported on 55 women who participated in the Georgetown University Breast Cancer Screening Study. They had no palpable lesions. Fifteen patients had malignant disease. All had ductal carcinoma (PPV = .273). Seven were noninvasive, 3 minimally invasive, and 5 were invasive. Thus 66% of the carcinomas were noninvasive or had minimal invasion, and 93.3% had no metastases to the axillary nodes. The most frequently encountered benign lesion was some type of fibrocystic disease. The carcinomas tended to exhibit clusters of calcifications that were less dense than were the benign lesions. Calcifications associated with cancer appeared less clustered and possessed more calcifications per cluster on the average than did benign lesions. In this small series, regardless of the area covered by the cluster, in those clusters with more than 30 calcifications, carcinoma occurred in 81%. Whereas, when less than 9 calcifications were evident, no carcinoma was detected. The size of the calcification was not the distinguishing feature between benign and malignant lesions, as both had between .74 and .73 mm for their average size.

The most striking observation they found was that calcification appeared in tissue adjacent to rather than within the carcinoma in many of the cases. In 20%, the calcification was located in adjacent fibrocystic disease. In another 20%, the location was in both malignant and benign tissue. Curiously, only 15% of benign biopsies revealed calcification within the adjacent tissue that appeared normal.

These authors attempted to study the distinction between benign and malignant calcifications. They studied the size of the calcifications, the distribution of the calcification, the number of calcifications, and the proximity of adjacent calcifications within the cluster. In this small series they were unable to demonstrate a significant difference in the nature of the calcifications. This led them to the erroneous conclusion that malignant calcifications have no characteristic features. Others have effectively refuted that conclusion.[10] Colbassani et al noted that the curious feature was the high incidence of calcification in normal tissue adjacent to a malignancy.[11] They conclude this observation indirectly supports the hypothesis that calcification in disease of the breast is a result of increased cellular secretory activity and does not require the pathologic transformation of necrosis and ossification of debris within a cancer.

Mammographic findings compared with pathology. Solmer et al presented a retrospective review of patients where a specimen radiograph was performed to confirm the removal of suspicious mammographic abnormalities.[56] They studied 40 patients; 11 had cancer (PPV = .275). During this period they did a total of 340 surgical breast biopsies. Specimen mammography was used in 13% of the cases. This series, restricted to specimen mammography, is not necessarily representative of the frequency of carcinoma in all biopsies performed. Their use of specimen mammography was restricted to those cases that had three or more distinct calcifications 1 mm in size or less within 1 square cm on the mammogram. Cancer was found only in cases where there were at least 5 calcifications within 1 square cm. This criterion is used for surgical biopsy on the basis of mammographic microcalcifications. In this series a history of previous breast surgery did not correlate with a higher incidence of carcinoma.

The mammographic findings were reviewed in relation to the final pathology. Microcalcifications only occurred in 31 of the 40 patients; 8 had cancers (PPV = .258). Grouped microcalcifications associated with a mass occurred in two patients, both of which were benign. A non-calcified soft tissue density was seen in 6 patients; 3 were malignant (PPV = .500). There was one case of a soft-tissue density with microcalcification that was benign. Thirty-one of the 33 patients, who had microcalcifications as the indication for the specimen mammogram, had no associated soft-tissue mass on their mammograms. In this study, the physical examination revealed no palpable masses or other symptoms in 20 of the 40 patients and, in these, 4 were malignant (PPV = .330). In the other cases, there were 10 patients with bilateral nodularity, 5 patients with palpable mass, 3 patients with a possible mass, and 2 patients in whom palpation revealed induration. In the 10 patients with bilateral nodularity, 3 had cancer (PPV = .330). In the 5 patients with a mass palpable, 1 was malignant. In the 3 patients with a possible mass, 1 was malignant. In the 2 patients with induration, both were malignant.

The meaning of this series is difficult to evaluate, other

than it adds a dimension in reorganizing the type of breast biopsies submitted for specimen mammography and the probability of detecting cancer in such lesions. The limitation to those biopsy cases undergoing specimen mammography, and the mix of symptomatic and asymptomatic patients, makes it difficult to ascribe a contribution of this series to our understanding of how often one may expect to find a cancer when a breast is biopsied.

Staging from the TNM classification recommended. Schwartz et al sought to determine if the nonpalpable carcinomas should be staged and categorized separately from those detected in the more traditional manners.[52] They studied the 1132 biopsies obtained from 1059 women. Of these biopsies, 330 revealed cancer (PPV = .292). Histology demonstrated 190 invasive ductal carcinomas, 13 invasive lobular carcinomas, 81 in situ ductal carcinomas, 25 microinvasive ductal carcinomas, and 20 lobular carcinomas in situ. One of the 330 malignancies was a malignant carcinoid.

They pointed out that the traditional staging methods of breast cancer require the clinical indications for the diagnosis that includes, for the most part, a palpable mass. Traditional staging methods were not adequate to address the issue of nonpalpable mammographically detected breast cancers. The indications for the 1132 surgical biopsies in this series were clustered calcifications 594 (52.5%); masses 391 (34.5%); masses with associated calcification 80 (7.1%); and density distortion 67 (5.9%).

The microscopic findings in the 330 patients with malignant disease were distributed as follows. Invasive ductal carcinoma was present in 190 patients, accounting for 58% of the cancer cases and 17% of all the biopsies done. Invasive lobular carcinoma was found in 13 patients, accounting for 3.9% of the malignancies and 1.1% of the biopsies. DCIS was seen in 81 patients, accounting for 24.5%

of the cancers and 7.2% of the total biopsies. Microinvasive ductal carcinoma was seen in 25 patients, accounting for 7.6% of the malignant diseases and 2.2% of the biopsies. LCIS was found in 20 patients, accounting for 6.1% of the total malignant diseases and 1.8% of the biopsies. A similar relative number of biopsies was done for each histologic classification of cancer.

Schwartz et al compared the mammographic findings with histologic findings and observed that 56.1% of all malignant lesions were presented as clustered microcalcifications. If one considered only DCIS and the microinvasive duct carcinomas, 86.4% and 80%, respectively, were detected as clustered microcalcifications. This large series clearly points to the utility of clustered microcalcifications as an indication for surgical biopsy in the earliest of breast cancers (Table 5-14).

Of the invasive carcinomas, only 40.1% had areas of clustered microcalcification. One hundred and twenty-nine cancers presented as nonpalpable masses with or without accompanying calcifications, and in these, 85% were invasive carcinoma. When these authors found a noninvasive or microinvasive cancer in a biopsy specimen that was removed because of a nonpalpable mass, the cancer was almost always an incidental finding and the mass itself was benign. The size of mammographically detected masses was considerably less than breast cancers detected by palpation (Fig. 5-2). This requires alternative staging considerations. The presence of microcalcification or nonpalpable mass did not influence the likelihood of an axillary metastasis.

They recommend staging from the TNM classification based on the greatest diameter of the mass or area of calcification seen on the mammogram, and adding the subscript "M" to indicate that the cancer was detected only by mammography. In this series, of 167 women with invasive

Table 5-14. Roentgenographic findings

X-ray findings	No. of patients (%)	Invasive carcinoma (%)	Microinvasive carcinoma (%)	DCIS (%)	LCIS (%)	Total (%)	PPV including LCIS	PPV not including LCIS
Clustered calcifications	594(52.5)	83(40.1)	20(80.0)	70(86.4)	12(60.0)	185(56.1)	.311	.291
Masses	391(34.5)	83(40.1)	0(0.0)	1(1.2)	7(35.0)	91(28.9)	.233	.215
Mass with calcifications	80(7.1)	27(13.2)	4(16.0)	6(7.4)	1(5.0)	38(20.5)	.475	.463
Density	67(5.9)	11(5.4)	1(4.0)	4(4.9)	0(0.0)	16(4.8)	.239	.239
TOTAL	1132	204	25	81	10	330	.292	.274

From Schwartz FG, Feig SA, Patchefsky AS: *Surg Gynecol Obstet* 166(1):6-10, 1988.

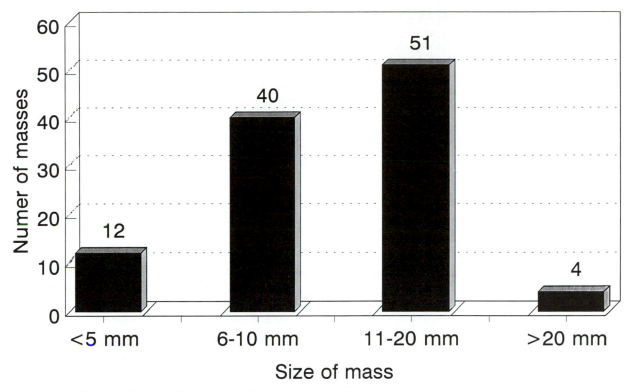

Fig. 5-2. Size of 107 mammographically detected malignant masses (From Schwartz et al: *Surg Gynecol Obstet* 166:6-10, 1988.)

cancer who had axillary dissection, 32.9% had at least one positive lymph node. Cancers, which presented as clustered calcifications in the breast, had the same chance of developing metastases as those presenting as nonpalpable masses. This challenges the term *minimal* as a description for any invasive cancer regardless of size. They acknowledge that the in situ carcinomas should continue to be called minimal or stage 0. Invasive cancers, even when detected by mammography, should be staged according to their measured size on the mammogram.

Criteria for surgical biopsy. Ciatto et al, in a classic paper, reviewed 512 consecutive cases of nonpalpable lesions detected by mammography.[10] They sought to establish reliable criteria for the surgical biopsy of nonpalpable breast lesions. Mammograms were performed as a breast cancer screening test in two separate patient populations. Some subjects were self-referred women from Florence, Italy. Whereas the other subjects were from a rural area in northern Italy, where a population-based breast cancer detection program has been operating since 1970. Subjective symptoms, other than pain, were present in 30% of the self-referred women and in 2% of the invited women.

They classed the radiographic patterns into the following 6 categories: (1) opacity with smooth, irregular borders; (2) opacity with poorly defined borders; (3) opacity with irregular, spiculated, or stellate borders; (4) parenchymal distortion without opacity; (5) moderately suspicious clustered microcalcifications; and (6) strongly suspicious clustered microcalcifications. The distinction between the moderately suspicious and the strongly suspicious microcalcification groups was based on the irregular shape, rodlike, or branching morphologic characteristics in a high spatial density for the strongly suspicious group. When microcalcifications were associated with opacity or parenchymal distortion, they were classified according to either the degree of the opacity or the parenchymal distortion pattern. All the cases were reviewed in retrospect based on the previous criteria. They correlated these mammographic observations with major outcome assessments. They evaluated the change in the PPV as they gained more experience in 1970 to 1985 (Table 5-15).

The PPV decreased as they sought to detect even earlier cancers. A decline in the PPV from .500 to .254 was associated with an increase in their cancer detection rate from 0.2 to 1.3 per 1000. A 50% decrease in PPV was associated with a 6.5-fold increase in cancer detection. The preclinical cancer detection rate was defined as the total number of preclinical cancers detected in every 1000 mammograms. Postmenopausal women had a much higher PPV (Table 5-16).

Table 5-15. Preclinical cancer DR and PPV by calendar period

Calendar period	Benign lesions (no.)	Malignant lesions (no.)	Mammograms (no.)	DR (per 1000)	B/M ratio	PPV
1970-1973	6	6	30,416	0.2	1:1	.500
1974-1977	24	24	58,219	0.4	1:1	.500
1978-1981	71	34	50,054	0.7	2.1:1	.324
1982-1985	259	88	66,592	1.3	2.9:1	.254
TOTAL 1970-1985	360	152	205,281	.07	2.4:1	.297

From Ciatto S et al: *Radiology* 165:99-102, 1987.
DR, Diagnostic rate.

Table 5-16. Preclinical cancer DR and PPV according to age group (1978-1985)

Age group (year)	Benign lesions (no.)	Malignant lesions (no.)	Mammograms (no.)	DR (per 1000)	B/M ratio	PPV
30-39	9	2	3082	0.6	4.5:1	.182
40-49	134	28	42,725	0.6	4.8:1	.172
50-59	103	45	35,956	1.2	2.3:1	.304
Over 59	75	42	24,406	1.7	1.8:1	.359

From Ciatto S et al: *Radiology* 165:99-102, 1987.
Dr, Diagnostic rate.

Table 5-17. Distribution of cases according to histologic diagnosis and radiologic pattern

Radiologic pattern	Histologic diagnosis				
	Benign	Hyperplasia	In situ cancer	Invasive cancer	PPV
Opacity with regular borders (66)	60	6	0	0	0.000
Moderately suspicious microcalcifications (157)	130	23	1	3	0.025
Parenchymal distortion (18)	11	5	0	2	0.111
Opacity with poorly defined borders (93)	49	11	2	31	0.355
Strongly suspicious microcalcifications (106)	36	11	22	37	0.556
Stellate opacity (72)	17	1	1	53	0.750
TOTAL (512)	303	57	26	126	0.300

From Ciatto S et al: *Radiology* 165:99-102, 1987.

The biopsies in 512 women yielded infiltrating cancer in 126, DCIS in 26, ductal or lobular hyperplasia in 57, and other benign lesions in 303 cases. Thus there were 152 malignant lesions identified in the 512 biopsies. The PPV of the various radiologic patterns is seen in Table 5-17.

Well-defined, smooth borders in 66 opacities had a PPV of 0. Moderately suspicious calcifications (157) had a PPV of .025. In this group 223 biopsies were performed to detect 4 cancers. Conversely, 106 strongly suspicious calcifications had a PPV of .556. This clearly demonstrates an ability to distinguish the calcifications more likely associ-ated with malignancy from benign-appearing calcifications. This refutes the contention by Colbassani et al that there are no distinguishing features of malignant microcalcifications.[11] Eighteen patients with parenchymal distortion had a PPV of .111. Mammograms showing opacities with poorly defined borders (93) had a PPV of .355. The most specific mammographic appearance of cancer was a stellate opacity. The 72 mammograms with stellate opacities had a PPV of .750.

The age-based detection rate provided data to assess the probability of a false-negative diagnosis (Table 5-16). One could correlate the detection rate to the ambient frequency of breast cancer in the screening populations and determine whether they detected as many cancers as there were known to be in the population under study. They observed a cancer detection rate of .6/1000 from 30 to 39 years of age; .6/1000 from 40 to 49 years of age; 1.2/1000 from 50 to 59 years of age; and 1.7/1000 in the over 59 years age-group. This is a slightly lower than expected incident cancer rate in older women. The PPV increased with age of the patient. The PPV went from .182 in women under the age of 40 years to .359 in women age 60 years and older. The lower PPV in the younger women is due to the fact that breast cancer becomes more easy to detect in older women. The dense breasts of younger women are more likely to mask a cancer.

Axillary dissection was carried out in 115 of the cases. Lymph node metastasis were not found in any of the 24 cases where the tumor diameter was less than 10 mm nor in 40 of 45 cases (89%) where the tumor diameter was between 1 and 2 cm. Of the tumors over 2 cm, 50% had nodal metastases.

Optimal criteria for surgical biopsy would have the highest possible PPV and cancer detection rate. A high cancer detection rate in a screening population would mean, in effect, a low false-negative rate. These authors have suggested criteria for surgical biopsy, which is among the best reviewed, if one depended entirely on the clinical profile and mammographic findings without the benefit of FNA or biopsy. These authors obtained PPV of .297 and 3.37 biopsies per cancer. Others have done slightly better, but in no other large series has there been as explicit a presentation of the implications of alternative criteria for selecting biopsy candidates.

Ciatto et al found parenchymal distortion associated with a moderate PPV of 0.11.[10] However, they believe that cases with this pattern merit a biopsy, since these lesions are relatively infrequent, and even their elimination from biopsy would not affect the overall PPV signifi-

cantly. In this case, the parenchymal distortion criterion was responsible for only 4% of the "unnecessary noncancer" biopsies (16 of 360).

They establish their basic mammographic criteria used in selecting patients for surgical biopsy from the practice audit of the involved radiologists. A PPV of each mammographic pattern is established in review of the clinical experience of each radiologist. The criteria are not drawn only from the experience of others published in the medical literature; in this case, the mammographic patterns based on their experience include parenchymal distortion, opacity with poorly defined borders, strongly suspicious microcalcifications, and stellate opacities. Using this approach they would have eliminated opacities with regular borders and moderately suspicious microcalcifications from surgical breast biopsy. These criteria would have decreased the total number of biopsies by 223 and missed only 4 cancers, one of which was LCIS.

Ciatto et al also pointed out the impact of different radiologists reading the films: "Differences in skill among radiologists are to be expected." In Table 5-18, radiologist A and radiologist F have high PPVs and cancer detection rates.[10] Radiologist D misses more cancers than his colleagues. His high false-negative rate is evident by his low rate of diagnosis when observing the same population of patients. He had the lowest true-positive mammographic interpretations per 1000 mammograms read. These data demonstrate how a practice audit can be used to determine the quality of the breast cancer detection system and decision each individual makes.[10] The difference in radiologic skill is reflected in the quality of performance. Despite the large absolute differences in the number of films read, the cancers detected, and the PPV, these numbers can be normalized through simple Z-score calculations. The Z-score is the number of standard deviations on individual's performance when compared to the normal or average performance of the entire group of observers. Z-scores are very simple to calculate.

$$Z\text{-score} = A - B/C$$

Table 5-18. Preclinical cancer DR by reporting radiologist (1978-1985)

Reporting radiologist	Benign lesions (no.)	Malignant lesions (no.)	Mammograms (no.)	DR (per 1000)	B/M ratio	PPV
A	81	33	20,025	1.6	2.4:1	.289
B	59	17	15,497	1.1	3.3:1	.224
C	101	38	39,955	0.9	2.7:1	.273
D	26	7	13,073	0.5	3.7:1	.212
E	22	3	2883	1.0	7.3:1	.120
F	41	13	6929	1.9	3.1:1	.241

From Ciatto S et al: *Radiology* 165:99-102, 1987.
DR, Diagnostic rate.

Table 5-19.   Z-score representation of the effect of reading volume on PPV

	Raw numbers			Z-score calculations			
	Mammograms	DR/1000	PPV	Mammograms	DR/1000	PPV	Sum
A	20025	1.6	0.289	0.30	0.94	1.15	2.09
B	15497	1.1	0.224	−0.03	−0.14	−0.05	−0.19
C	39955	0.9	0.273	1.98	−0.58	0.85	0.27
D	13073	0.5	0.212	−0.28	−1.45	−0.27	−1.71
E	2883	1.0	0.120	−1.13	−0.36	−1.95	−2.32
Standard	11918.28	0.46	0.055				
Average	16393.67	1.17	0.227				

From Ciatto S et al: *Radiology* 165:99-102, 1987.
DR, Diagnostic rate.

where A is an individual's performance, B is the average performance of the group, and C is the standard deviation of the group.

Z-score analysis allows for numerically equivalent determinations of the various elements of performance. Table 5-19 presents the Z-score calculations from Table 5-18. The three relevant measures of performance are the number of films read, the diagnostic rate (true positives), and the PPV. The lower the PPV, the higher the false-positive rate. Simple summarizing of the Z-scores of the diagnostic rate (DR) and PPV can be used to determine the relative quality of each radiologist's performance. Those with higher summed Z-scores are performing better than those radiologists with lower scores.

Fig. 5-3 presents graphically the data in Table 5-19. Simple visual inspection of this figure reveals the relative performance of the different radiologists. These data can be easily determined from any mammographic practice that keeps the records of individual radiologists.

For example, radiologist E read the fewest films and has the most false-positive interpretations, while maintaining only slightly less than average true-positive cancer detection rate. The summed data reveal his performance to be the worst of the group.

Radiologist F ranks 5 out of 6 in the number of films read. He has the highest true-positive rate, and a better than average false-positive rate (PPV). His summed performance ranks 2 out of 6.

Radiologist D has the most false negatives and slightly fewer than average false positives. He has read fewer than the average number of films, and his summed performance places him 5th out of 6 in overall mammographic skill.

Radiologist B read an average number of films and functions near the norm of the entire group in terms of both false-positive and false-negative interpretations.

Radiologist A functions the best of the entire group in terms of combining both the true positives and true negatives. He ranks number 1 in PPV and number 2 in cancer detection rate.

Radiologist C read the most films, but his overall performance in terms of combined false positives and false negatives is only slightly better than the group norm seen in the summed value of 0.27. While he has the second best false-positive rate, it appears that this is accomplished by a lower than normal cancer detection rate.

The optimal PPV can be determined only in relation to the cancer detection rate with which it is associated. In isolation, PPV may mean very little. Fig. 5-3 clearly depicts the issues.

This type of analysis can be done by any group of radiologists who require a firm commitment on the mammographic report and who keep accurate records of what has happened to the patients in whom a surgical biopsy is recommended. Obviously, the overall performance of the group may be improved, if those radiologists with a higher than normal false-positive or false-negative rate are aware of how their performance compares with that of their colleagues reviewing the mammograms from the same pool of patients. It is obviously important to maintain an adequate information system so that the receiver operating curves (ROC) of each radiologist can be monitored. This allows for experience-based modification of practice patterns to increase the PPV without increasing the false-negative rate. Ciatto et al signify the importance of keeping a database for each radiologist separately, and for each of the diagnostic criteria used in selecting which mammographic pattern warrants a surgical biopsy or even consideration for further presurgical diagnostic studies, such as FNA or stereotaxic biopsy.[10]

Hall et al reported on recommendations for biopsy based on the suspicion of carcinoma at mammography. They found carcinoma in 119 of 400 surgical biopsies based on mammograms (PPV = .298). These results are very similar to the experience of Ciatto et al. Both of these groups keep relevant experiential data and are concerned with equality mammography. Hall et al base their opinions on the experience derived from a large community-based clinical practice in Boston, where biweekly conferences

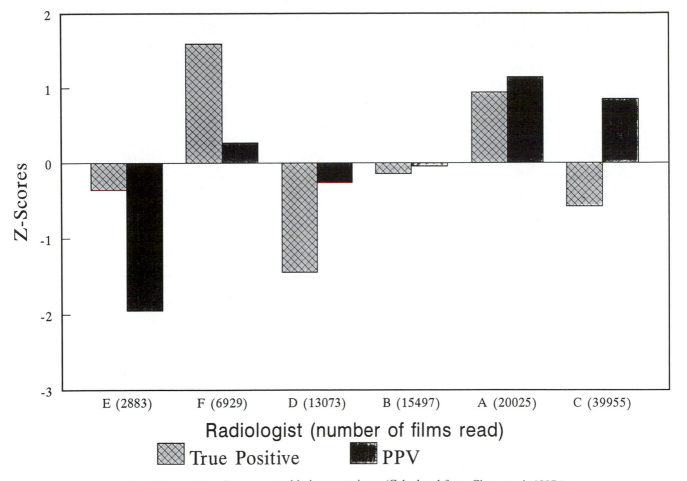

Fig. 5-3. Quality of mammographic interpretations. (Calculated from Ciatto et al: 1987.)

review recent mammograms and pathology reports including the breast biopsies.

Hall et al use a four-scale system in evaluating suspicious mammograms. The mammographic suspicions were minimal, slight, moderate, or high.[18] All poorly marginated masses were judged moderately or highly suspicious. Well-defined masses more than 2 cm in diameter were considered moderately suspicious. Sharply marginated 1 to 2 cm lesions, regardless of lobulation, were slightly suspicious. If they were less than 1 cm, they were considered minimally suspicious.

The classification of microcalcification was more difficult and more subjective than the assessment of masses. They considered three microcalcifications minimally suspicious, four slightly suspicious, and five moderately suspicious. But they emphasize the appearance of the calcifications as much as their number. If calcifications were linear or branching, suggesting an intraductal location, their suspicion was increased, whereas the larger rounded or more

sharply defined calcifications were more suggestive of a benign lesion.

They found a PPV of .298 (119 of 400) in the entire series and .371 (93 of 251) in women 50 years of age and older. This fell to .175 (26 of 149) in women less than 50 years and .158 (6 of 38) in women 40 years and younger.

The PPVs for cancers were clearly distributed along the mammographic classification criteria (Table 5-20). Minimally suspicious lesions had a PPV of .037; slightly suspicious, .13; moderately suspicious, .33; and highly suspicious, .89. In this series there were 72 invasive carcinomas, 34 DCIS, and 13 LCIS. Their accuracy in classifying calcifications was less than the accuracy in classifying masses (Fig. 5-4).

The composite ROC curves displayed in Fig. 5-4 clearly indicate the relative accuracy of mammography in diagnosis of nonpalpable breast cancer if the biopsy is performed for a high, moderate, or slight suspicion of carcinoma. Minimally suspicious calcification had a PPV of

Table 5-20. Positive predictive value of mammography in the diagnosis of nonpalpable breast cancer

	Cancer	
Mammographic suspicion	**Including LCIS (no.)**	**Excluding LCIS (no.)**
Moderate, high	.458 (104/227)	.433 (94/217)
Slight (calcifications only), moderate, high	.414 (113/273)	.387 (101/261)
Slight, moderate, high	.365 (116/318)	.340 (104/306)
Minimal, slight, moderate, high	.298 (119/400)	.274 (106/387)
Minimal, slight	.087 (15/173)	.071 (12/170)
Minimal, slight (masses only)	.047 (6/127)	.040 (5/126)
Minimal	.037 (3/82)	.025 (2/81)

From Hall FM et al: *Radiology* 167:353-358, 1988.

.061 (2/33), whereas carcinoma was found in only 1 of 49 patients with minimally suspicious masses (PPV = .020). Hall et al recommended that the biopsy criteria include only those patients with slight, moderate, or highly suspicious calcifications, and those patients with moderate or highly suspicious masses.[18] If these criteria were used alone, the PPV for cancer would have risen from .298 (119 of 400) to .414 (113 of 273). They would not have had biopsies on 6 of 127 patients with cancer. However, they "believe this trade off is acceptable in a screening program because only one of the 6 'missed' malignancies was invasive. The diagnosis of each of these carcinomas would have required 20 to 25 biopsies and an equal number of radiologic localizations and pathologic assessments."

Ciatto et al and Hall et al demonstrated excellent results when using mammography and clinical profile to select patients for surgical biopsy, although others may have had higher PPV's (Table 5-1). Ciatto et al and Hall et al were vigilant to the detail needed to improve on the use of

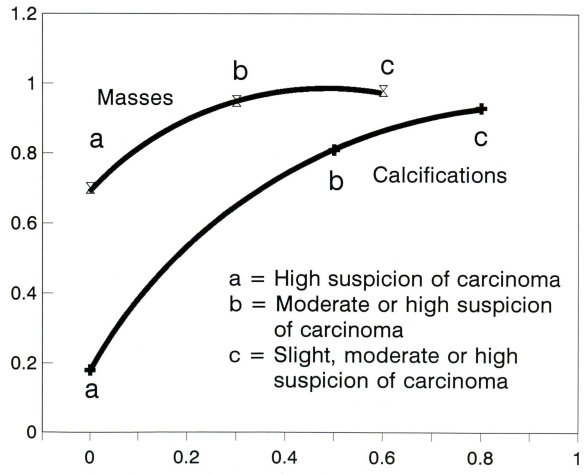

Fig. 5-4. Composite ROC curves. (From Hall, Storella, LSilverstone, Wyshak: *Radiology* 167:353-358, 1988.)

screening mammography to detect early breast cancer. All radiologists should keep accurate records of their individual experience to constantly refine their experience-based mammographic criteria for surgical biopsy. Excellent mammography can be assisted by additional presurgical information, such as that obtained by FNA cytology.

Correlation between FNA cytology and surgical biopsy. Fajardo et al undertook a study of SFNA cytology in nonpalpable breast lesions to reduce the number of surgical biopsies performed for benign disease.[12] They sought to reduce the cost and morbidity of breast cancer detection. They performed FNA cytology on 100 patients undergoing mammographically guided stereotactic localization of breast lesions before open surgical biopsy. Thirty of these patients had cancer (PPV = .300). Mammograms and FNA cytology results were classified according to a numerical code. These were based on the relative probability of malignancy (Table 5-21).

They used a prototype stereotactic device,* which has 15-degree angle views to calculate the three-dimensional lesion location. They evaluated this device and found that its accuracy was 0.5 ± 0.9 mm from the center of simulated lesions. They used a 22 g needle for aspiration. The samples were stained by the Papanicolaou method. All specimens were evaluated independently by senior cytotechnologists and cytopathologists. They evaluated cellularity, cellular arrangements, nuclear cytoplasmic ratio, and characteristics of the nuclei and nucleoli. They then classed them on a scale of 0 to 4 as indicated in Table 5-21. This series does not replicate the utility of the FNA

*LoRad Medical Systems, Inc, Danbury, CT.

as a criterion for surgical biopsy, since these patients were all scheduled for surgical biopsy on the basis of mammographic and clinical findings. The SFNA information was not used in the decision to biopsy. This undoubtedly accounts for the fact that this series with FNA biopsy has considerably more biopsies performed per cancer found than other series where the information from the stereotactic was used to select patients for surgical biopsy. However, Fajardo et al made an important contribution to the understanding of the correlation between FNA cytology and surgical biopsy.[12]

Table 5-22 displays the results of comparing surgery with mammography and FNA cytology. From these data in a mammographic diagnosis, ROC curves (ROC) can be drawn. These data are useful for every radiologist to be able to ascertain their fidelity in preoperative diagnosis of probable malignancy. Merely classifying the mammographic diagnosis as benign, probably benign, suspicious, and malignant allows for definition of probability. This is similar to the codes that have been used at the Karolinska Institute. These authors were able to demonstrate a remarkably high PPV of mammograms when they felt the lesion was malignant. Similarly, when the lesion was interpreted as benign, or probably benign, the PPV reached .887. Two of the errors were in patients who had lobular carcinomas in situ. If LCIS was eliminated from the carcinoma category and classed as benign, the PPV of the mammographic impression or probably benign reaches .919.

Even more impressive is these authors' experience with FNA. When the cytologic impression was benign, a PPV of .97 was obtained. If atypical cells were identified, the

Table 5-21. Mammographic and FNA cytology diagnosis

Diagnosis	Mammographic findings	FNA cytology
0	Not applicable	Inadequate, acellular specimen
1	Benign	Benign
	Circumscribed, low-density mass, *or*	Normal epithelial pattern of aggregates and cytologic
	Round, uniformly dense microcalcifications, few in number (<5)	features
2	Probably benign	Atypical
	Low-density mass with partial border loss, *or*	Atypical with regard to cell groupings and nuclei
	Round, uniformly dense microcalcifications (<15)	
3	Suspicious for malignancy	
	Low-density mass with architectural distortion, *or*	
	Circumscribed, high-density mass, *or*	
	Microcalcifications of irregular shapes and density	
4	Malignant	Malignant
	Circumscribed, high-density or stellate, spiculated mass with architectural distortion, *or*	Cells indicative of malignancy
	Microcalcifications of irregular shape and density with architectural distortion	

Data from Fajardo LL et al: *AJR* 155:977-981, 1990.

Table 5-22. Correlation of surgery with mammography and FNA cytology

		Surgical diagnosis					
	Benign	Infiltrating carcinoma: Ductal	Infiltrating carcinoma: Lobular	In situ carcinoma: Lobular	In situ carcinoma: Ductal lobular	Total cancers	PPV*
Mammographic diagnosis							
Benign	37	1	0	1	1	3	.925
Probably benign	18	1	0	2	1	4	.818
Suspicious	13	4	1	2	0	7	.350
Malignant	2	11	1	2	0	14	.875
FNA cytology diagnosis							
Benign	54	0	0	2	1	3	.947
Atypical	16	1	1	1	1	4	.800
Suspicious	0	4	0	1	0	4	1.000
Malignant	0	12	1	3	0	16	1.000
TOTAL	70	16	2	8	2		

Data from Fajardo et al: *AJR* 155:977-981, 1990.

*PPV is calculated as benign and probably benign mammograms predicting benign surgery, and benign and atypical FNA cytology predicting benign surgery. Suspicious and malignant PPVs are calculated as predictors of carcinoma.

PPV dropped to only .800. However, when the FNA was either suspicious or malignant, every case at surgery yielded a cancer. Thus Fajardo et al attempted to establish a predefined cut-off point for recommending biopsy based on both the FNA and the mammography appearance.[12] They found the optimal cut-off was between diagnosis code 2 (mammography probably benign, cytology atypical) and code 3 (mammography and cytology both suspicious for malignancy). At this cut-off, the FNA had a sensitivity of .77 and a specificity of 1, versus .73 sensitivity and .79 specificity for mammography. They conclude that FNA plus mammography should reduce the number of breast biopsies performed for benign lesions.

Surgical approaches to nonpalpable lesions. Papatestas et al[41] reported on surgical approaches to nonpalpable breast lesions. They reported on 475 women seen between the years of 1976 and 1988 in which 1049 biopsies showed malignant lesions (PPV = .314). Some of these cases had previously been reported by Hermann et al in their study of the accuracy of prebiopsy mammographic diagnosis.[22] Papatestas et al noted a remarkable increase in the number of breast biopsies for nonpalpable breast cancer from the years 1980 to 1988. Before 1980, only 28 such biopsies were done, whereas between 1986 and 1988, 234 were done. Over this time the PPV has decreased slightly from .400 to .300. These authors paid special attention to the mammographic indications for surgical biopsy and the age of the patients.

Table 5-23 reveals that a mammographic mass under the age of 40 years is often benign. Most often these are cystic lesions in somewhat dense breasts. This clearly points to the difficulties encountered in younger women. However, these authors were able to identify a substantial number of premenopausal breast cancers on mammography alone. These authors point out that premenopausal cancers, which presented as masses or calcification and mass, had a high likelihood of invasiveness. Table 5-24 reveals that there are a substantial number of invasive cancers when lesions other than calcification is the indication for breast biopsy. The association between invasiveness and the mammographic findings in the malignant tumors was highly significant (PPV = .001). Obviously, cancers detected by calcification alone will be less likely to be invasive. LCIS accounted for 8 (13%) of the noninvasive lesions.

These authors argued that because of the frequency with which invasive lesions are discovered at mammography and their associated axillary metastases, a low PPV is appropriate for surgical biopsies. They state that since "we accept a benign to malignant ratio of 5:1 (PPV = .200) for palpable lesions and consider that evidence of reasonable and prudent judgment." In essence, better results should not be demanded from mammographically detected lesions. Their criteria for surgical biopsy are essentially based on an external standard (i.e., their results in palpable lesions) rather than seeking to optimize within the limits of possibility as exemplified in the work of Ciatto et al and Hall et al. Paptestas et al conclude that their institution is yielding "the optimal ratio of benign to true cancers (invasive) lesions."[41]

These authors found axillary lymph nodes positive in 21% of the 57 infiltrating ductal carcinomas and 28% of

Table 5-23. Mammographic indications for surgical biopsy in nonpalpable breast cancer

	Age <40 yrs total malignant PPV			Age 40-49 yrs total malignant PPV			Age 50 yrs and older total malignant PPV			All years total malignant PPV		
Calcification	31	6	.193	69	21	.304	106	40	.377	206	67	.325
Calcification and mass	1	0	.000	8	3	.375	30	13	.433	39	16	.410
Mass	17	0	.000	50	9	.180	163	55	.337	230	64	.278
TOTAL	49	6	.020	127	33	.260	299	108	.361	475	147	.310

From Papatestas AE et al: *Arch Surg* 125:390-402, 1990.

Table 5-24. Relation between mammographic findings and invasiveness of breast cancer

	Age <40 yrs cancers invasive (%)			Age 40-49 yrs cancers invasive (%)			Age 50 yrs and older cancers invasive (%)			Total all years cancers invasive (%)		
Calcification	6	2	33	21	8	38	40	15	38	67	25	36
Calcification and mass	0	—	—	3	2	67	13	8	66	16	10	63
Mass	0	—	—	9	6	67	55	48	87	64	54	84
TOTAL	6	2	33	33	16	48	108	71	66	147	89	60

From Papatestas AE et al: *Arch Surg* 125:390-402, 1990.

their 7 lobular carcinomas. They concluded that the majority of breast cancers detected on mammography are biologically significant lesions and represent infiltrating carcinomas. The systemic disease, as seen by axillary node involvement, is more frequent in younger women before malignant lesions become palpable. Thus they conclude there is no evidence of an overdiagnosis in radiologically detected lesions. These authors advocate that rather than radiographic monitoring of any suspicious lesion in a young women, early surgical biopsy is more appropriate.

Correlation of mammography and pathology. Owing et al reported on their experiences with correlation of mammography and pathology in patients who had surgical biopsies performed for the presence of microcalcifications.[39] This report may contain some cases described in Hann et al and in Hall et al[18,21] and represents a prospective study of 157 consecutive needle localization breast biopsies that yielded 50 cancers (PPV = .318). The relationship of calcifications as seen on specimen mammography with the histologic assessment of the tissue in pathology was specifically studied. In the 50 patients with carcinoma, the calcifications were exclusively within the carcinomas in 8 cases (16%). They found calcification in both the carcinoma and adjacent benign breast tissue without atypia in 39 of the 50 patients (78%). In 3 of the 50 patients (6%) they found calcification histologically in be-

nign breast tissue without atypia. However, in 2 of these 3 cases the benign breast tissue containing the calcifications was on the same slide as the carcinoma. Thus it was immediately adjacent to the carcinoma histologically. The relationship between mammographic microcalcifications and carcinoma differed from the relationship of calcifications and atypical hyperplasia. In none of the 19 cases of atypical hyperplasia were calcifications identified exclusively within the lesion. Indeed, in 10 of the 19 cases (53%) with atypical hyperplasia, the microscopic calcifications were found exclusively in benign breast tissue without atypia.

These authors concluded that by restricting the histologic sectioning to specimen mammography, some 66% of total tissue blocks would have been eliminated. This would markedly improve the efficiency of the pathologic assessment of breast biopsy materials. The need for close correlation between specimen mammography and the mammographic appearance of the lesion is reinforced by the experience at Karolinska. Close correlation between the prebiopsy mammogram and the histologic specimens evaluated by the pathologist is an essential prerequisite to quality control.

Prorok et al had a similar experience to that published by Owings et al.[39,46] Prorok et al reviewed 62 consecutive patients with microcalcifications who presented for surgical biopsy.[46] Twenty of these patients had carcinoma (PPV

= .323). In this series 10 of the 20 had calcification limited to the carcinoma and 6 were limited to the area of benign breast disease adjacent to the carcinoma. In 4 cases, calcification was present in both the carcinoma and adjacent benign breast disease. Owings et al found a close correlation between the location of the calcifications on clinical and specimen mammography and the location of the cancer. This is especially important in considering the location of FNA sampling based on mammograms. Roses et al had a similar experience in biopsying for mammographic microcalcifications, as did Owings et al and Prorok et al.[39,46,49] These three series have remarkably close PPV based on microcalcifications alone. Roses et al studied 52 patients who were biopsied for clustered microcalcifications without any definable mass on the mammogram or physical examination.[49] Carcinoma was found in 17 patients (PPV = .327). In these patients the calcification was in the carcinoma alone in 5 of the 17 and in the carcinoma and adjacent benign disease in 8 of the 17. Calcification was found in benign disease alone but adjacent to the carcinoma in 4 of the 17 patients. These results reinforce the perception that tissue sampling in immediate proximity to calcifications will most often represent where the cancers are ultimately found. These authors were concerned that precise localization and removal of only the microcalcification without excision of a margin of surrounding tissue may exclude the adjacent carcinoma. These authors conclude that generous excisional biopsy with confirmatory specimen mammography is necessary when mammographic microcalcification is the only indication for surgical biopsy. However, it is unusual to find the calcification more than 1 cm from the cancer that caused mammographic microcalcifications.

These three series reported using characteristic microcalcifications as the only criterion for surgical biopsy. The PPV of characteristic microcalcifications is considerably higher than the overall PPV of all of the series reviewed. When one restricts the review to patients in whom the diagnosis has been based on the presence of characteristic microcalcification only, the increase in PPV is impressive. The earliest papers on microcalcification as indices for surgical biopsy by Murphy et al and Rogers and Powell (1972) had PPV of .355 and .413, respectively. These are consistent with the subsequent PPV published by Roses et al, Prorok et al, and Owings et al. In 1985, Tinnemans et al published a series of 150 consecutive female patients with nonpalpable clusters of microcalcifications seen in The Netherlands between 1975 and 1983.[58] In this series, 51 malignancies were detected. Most of these (56%) were noninvasive. Of the 29 noninvasive in situ carcinomas, 22 were DCIS and only 7 were LCIS. Thus these 150 consecutive patients, with clusters of at least 5 microcalcifications and no palpable lesion, yielded a PPV of .295. However, if one were to exclude LCIS, this PPV decreases to .287.

Tinnemans et al reviewed their experience in detecting nonpalpable breast cancers from 1975 to 1985.[57] They published the data on 359 surgical biopsies that revealed 118 carcinomas for a PPV of .329. The PPV for patients whose mammograms were derived from population screening was greater than that seen in patients who had breast complaints. In their 359 biopsy procedures performed for clinically occult lesions of the breast, the PPV for population screening was .350, whereas for individual mammograms not derived from the screening population study, the PPV was .303 (Table 5-25).

The PPV of this group's series improved markedly in the years after 1982. The PPV had been in the range of .25 to .30 from the years 1974 to 1982. In 1982 the PPV began to increase, so that by 1984 the PPV of these experienced mammographers attained .680 from mammography alone. These 359 reported cases, however, are over the entire period of time from 1975 to 1985. The authors suggest that the marked improvement in the PPV since 1982 may be due to the development of technical improvements in January, 1982. At that time a mammographic grid and microfocus of 0.09 mm began to be used routinely. All of the mammograms were seen by the same radiologists over this entire period of time. Therefore the improved ability of the radiologist alone is unlikely to explain the remarkable improvement in PPV. This observation points out the importance of film technique in improving the PPV of a system of breast cancer diagnosis.

Table 5-26 demonstrates the correlation between the mammographic criteria and surgical biopsy yield. These authors obtained similar results to others in that a stellate-shaped mass had the highest PPV and a circumscribed or nodular mass had the lowest PPV. These authors conclude that since suspicious mammograms by population and individual screening had similar PPVs, a suspicious mammogram should be considered on its own merits and not be

Table 5-25. Indications for mammography in 359 biopsy procedures performed because of clinically occult lesions of the breast

	Total (no.)	Malignant findings (no.)	PPV
Population screening	174	62	.356
Individual screening	185	56	.303
Breast complaints	99	28	.283
Control "premalignant lesions"	33	16	.485
Contralateral mastectomy	27	8	.296
Carcinophobia	9	0	.000
Positive family history	3	2	.667
Other reasons	14	2	.143

From Tinnemans JGM et al: *Surg Gynecol Obstet* 165:523-529, 1987.

Table 5-26. Correlation between mammographic criteria and biopsy

Mammography	Total (no.)	Malignant findings (no.)	PPV
Circumscribed or nodular mass	71	9	.127
Clustered microcalcifications	188	61	.324
Mass with microcalcifications	49	14	.286
Stellate-shaped mass	51	34	.667
TOTAL	359	118	.329

From Tinnemans AM et al: *Surg Gynecol Obstet* 165:523-529, 1987.

influenced by the fact that the women belong to high-risk groups. This series had an unusually high number of slow-growing tubular carcinomas. Seventeen of the 118 carcinomas were tubular (14.4%). Curiously, these were seen more often in stellate-shaped masses. Tubular carcinomas accounted for 41% of the stellate-shaped masses. This finding of slow-growing tubular carcinomas has implications on the length bias issue. The radiologist interpreting these films has obtained a PPV of .680 by mammography alone. This is remarkable; unfortunately, these authors do not report the exact criteria. A single radiologist was used to obtain this result. Perhaps this outstanding PPV is related to the criteria used to assess microcalcifications, as previously reported by Tinnemans et al.[57]

Schreer and Frischbier[51] published one of the largest series of breast cancer detected by mammography. They assess the predictive value of mammography in the early detection of breast cancer, using the histologic findings of breast biopsies that were indicated only by mammography. They studied 1385 patients, 460 of whom were shown to have cancer (PPV = .332). Of the 1385 patients, 913 (65.5% of the biopsies) were based on the presence of microcalcifications on the mammograms. Mammographically detected masses, which were indicative for surgical biopsy, were found in 333 (24.1%) of the patients. Combinations of masses, or microcalcifications, occurred in 89

patients (6.4%). The remaining 50 patients had surgical biopsies based on architectural distortion or asymmetry. The mammographic features, which correlated with histology, are seen in Table 5-27.

Schreer and Frischbier attained a PPV of .332 from mammography alone. They had a relatively high proportion of in situ carcinomas, which were diagnosed by microcalcification as the sole mammographic feature. Of the 186 in situ cancers, 127 were DCIS, 38 were LCIS, and 21 were combined DCIS and LCIS. They do not distinguish the mammographic features that occasioned the surgical biopsies for LCIS. This LCIS rate was only 2.7%. This is slightly less than the ambient frequency of LCIS expected in the population they studied.

The results attained by Schreer and Frischbier compare favorably with those of Hall et al and Ciatto et al in relating PPV to the age of the patients.[10,18,51] Ciatto et al and Hall et al had approximately a .300 PPV, and Schreer and Frischbier had a PPV of .332. The correlation between the PPV and the age of the patients is seen in Table 5-28.

All of these authors observed an increase in PPV with increasing age of the patients being screened. These series represent a large volume of quality mammography, where mammography plus clinical examination was used as the criterion for surgical biopsy without the addition of FNA.

Mass plus microcalcification gives higher PPV. Hallgrimsson et al studied 123 patients from October, 1981 to December, 1985.[20] These were derived from 12,520 patients submitted for mammography. Thus, their biopsy rate per mammogram done is 9.8/1000. They found 45 malignant lesions for a PPV of .352. They found 3.6 cancer/1000 mammograms. Since they don't define the source of their patients, it is not possible to determine a true-positive rate that can be compared with other studies. The criteria used as indications for mammographic indices for breast biopsy were similar to those of other published series. However, the results are different. These authors had the highest PPV with a mass plus microcalcification (Table 5-29).

In this instance, the criteria of microcalcifications resulted in a lower PPV than did the criteria of mass alone. They conclude that an exact analysis of the character of microcalcifications is important. Irregular microcalcifica-

Table 5-27. Correlation of mammographic features with histology

	Total (no.)	Benign	In situ cancer	Invasive cancer	Total cancer	PPV
Microcalcifications	913	614	171	128	299	.327
Masses	333	227	6	100	106	.318
Combinations	89	48	8	33	41	.461
Architectural distortion or asymmetry	50	36	1	13	14	.280
TOTAL	1385	925	186	274	460	.332

From Schreer I, Frishbier H-J: *Euro Radiol* 1:165-168, 1991.

Table 5-28. Correlation between predictive value and age of patients

Patient's age (yrs)	Ciatto et al (1970-1985)	Hall et al (1984-1987)	Schreer and Frischbier (1985-1989)
<40	0.18	0.16	0.22
40-49	0.17	0.18	0.25
50-59	0.30	0.31	0.40
>59	0.36	0.41	0.46
TOTAL	0.30	0.30	0.33

From Schreer I, Frischbier H-J: *Euro Radiol* 1:165-168, 1991.

Table 5-29. Mammographic findings in the breast correlated to the number of malignancies

Radiologic findings	Total	Malignant lesions (no.)	PPV
Mass	46	17	.370
Microcalcification	52	13	.250
Mass plus microcalcification	29	15	.517

From Hallgrimsson P et al: *Acta Radiol* 29:285-288, 1988.

Table 5-30. Radiographic appearance of nonpalpable breast lesions

Appearance	Total	Malignant	PPV
Grouped microcalcifications	46	39	.406
Small mass, <15 mm	112	30	.268
Mass and calcifications	12	8	.666
TOTAL	220	77	.350

From Hermann G et al: *Radiology* 165:323-326, 1987.

tions with differential density, and having the cast appearance of a duct, were extremely important criteria in favor of malignancy. They note that the combination of "atypical malignant (spiculated) mass" with typical malignant microcalcifications yields the highest PPV possible.

Hermann et al studied 220 women who had mammographic examinations from 1982 to 1985.[22] Some of these cases may have been included in the report of Papatestas et al.[41] Hermann et al's primary emphasis was the accuracy of preoperative mammographic diagnosis. They found malignancy in 77 cases (PPV = .350) and observed that in the radiologic appearance of nonpalpable breast lesions (Table 5-30) the highest PPV was obtained when masses were presented with calcifications.

In this instance, they had better PPV with grouped microcalcifications than with small masses. Each of the radiographs were reviewed by 3 authors independently and categorized as probably benign or probably malignant. They found no significant interobserver variation. In these 220 cases, they had a 12% false-negative retrospective interpretation of the mammograms. The malignant tumor would have been missed had the biopsy not been performed. They do not tell us what criteria they used for surgical biopsy with evidence of a "normal" mammogram and nonpalpable breast lesion. This study focused on the accuracy of prebiopsy mammographic diagnosis and nonpalpable breast lesions.

Aspiration cytology substantially decreases need for surgical biopsy. The Swedish experience, in the detection of nonpalpable breast cancer using FNA cytology as an adjunct to mammography, had been published in three separate series from three different institutions. Andersson et al published the first major clinical series in 1979, which was the result of the Malmö breast screening experience.[2] Subsequently, Arnesson et al published results of the Linkoping Program in 1986.[3] More recently, Azavedo et al presented the results of the Karolinska experience in 1989 and 1991.[4,5] These results, with the addition of FNA, markedly increased the PPV. These results are clearly distinguished from the experiences of others published in the medical literature. Other countries have also used FNA as an adjunct to screening mammography. The results of Lamb et al and Fajardo et al are representative samples of these other experiences.[12,27]

Arnesson et al presented results of surgical biopsy in nonpalpable breast lesions based on their experience at Linkoping, Sweden.[3] They screened 47,000 women twice with an interval of 2.5 years. They had an 80% attendance in the first round and 74% at the second round. Of these 47,000 women, 1284 had mammograms suggestive of malignancy. These occurred in 973 of the first-round attendees and 311 of the second round of attendees. These patients were called back for subsequent clinical examination, and 93% of them had aspiration cytology. In 314 of these 1284 patients, surgical biopsies were done for nonpalpable breast lesions. In 925 of the 1284 mammograms suggestive of malignancy, aspiration cytology was sufficient to confirm benign or malignant diagnosis. *Thus aspiration cytology eliminated 72% of the surgical biopsies that would have been performed had they been based on mammography alone without the aspiration cytology.* Of the 311 surgical biopsies performed, 129 were malignant and 185 turned out to be benign (PPV = .411). Of the 129 cancers, 40 were carcinoma in situ. The authors do not distinguish in the report how many were LCIS versus DCIS.

Table 5-31 presents the results of two serial screens, and demonstrates clearly that incidence screening 2 increased the PPV. The frequency of malignancy in the second screening was due to a change in the mammographic

Table 5-31. Results of two serial screens

	Total (no.)	Benign	Infiltrative cancer	Cancer in situ microinvasive	Cancer in situ	PPV
Prevalent screening 1	257	161	56	14	26	.374
Incidence screening 2	57	24	17	2	57	.579
TOTAL	314	185	73	16	40	.411

From Arnesson L-G et al: *Acta Chir Scand* 152:97-101, 1986.

appearance as one of the causes to initiate surgical biopsy in the second screen. Obviously, this indication was not possible on the initial prevalence screen.

Lamb et al presented the results of FNA cytology in breast screening of 397 women, of whom 173 were shown to have cancer (PPV = .436).[27] They evaluated the accuracy of FNA cytology in the preoperative diagnosis of breast cancers. Of the 562 women who had FNA cytology, 397 had subsequent surgical biopsy. This study occurred within a 6-year period that ended in December, 1985. The cytology results were used to avoid surgical biopsy in 165 women who had a suspicious lesion on a mammogram. One patient returned 2 years later with a cancer in the same breast. In this series they were able to follow all their patients. These 397 surgical biopsies represented 57% of the all surgical breast biopsies generated by the entire project during these years. These authors experienced some difficulty with those cases categorized as suspicious by the cytologist. The cytologic diagnosis of "suspicious" ranged from 3.1% to 24.4% and signified variation of reporting policy of the cytologist. The frequency of "suspicious" cytology in asymptomatic patients was double what they had found in a larger series of symptomatic patients. They feel this is due to poor representation of malignant cells in the specimen as a consequence of the size and occult nature of the lesion. Based on this experience, the Edinburgh group concludes that a combination of FNA cytology in triple assessment with physical and mammographic findings can substantially reduce the number of benign surgical biopsies. They were able to eliminate 165 surgical biopsies in 562 women who would have had surgical biopsy but for the availability of FNA cytology.

Highly accurate mammographic interpretation. In 1990, Perre et al published their experience in 101 nonpalpable suspicious breast lesions.[42] These 101 lesions occurred in 94 patients. They found 46 malignancies (PPV = .455). This series includes symptomatic women. Only 47 of the 194 patients had mammography as part of a screening program. Mammography was recommended by a physician because of patient symptoms or anxiety in 22 patients or for follow-up reasons in 25 patients. These mammographic lesions consisted of microcalcifications in 55 cases (54%) or masses in 40 (40%). Nine of the 46 cancers were carcinoma in situ. Seven were DCIS and only two were LCIS. These authors present the overall series with the highest PPV obtained using mammography alone. They do not comment on the mechanism for this highly accurate mammographic interpretation, which resulted in only 2.2 biopsies per cancer found. They also do not present any data concerning the possible false negatives in this series. There are no incidence data nor is their subsequent screening experience presented.

Remarkable rate of detection. In 1979, Andersson et al published the results of the Malmö Breast Cancer Screening Project.[2] These results are some of the most remarkable in the breast cancer detection literature. They obtained the highest breast cancer detection rate of any program before the work of Azavedo and Svane in 1991. This work was done in the 1970s, which was a time when many programs were still having difficulty maintaining adequate quality of mammography. They did a population-based randomized screening project and invited 17,447 women to attend. These women were between the ages of 50 and 69. They obtained a 73% attendance.

Fig. 5-5 presents the outline of the Malmö system of breast cancer screening. This system is quite similar to that being used at the Karolinska, where even better results have now been attained.

Table 5-32 displays the results of the Malmö breast cancer screening experience by age group. Of the 12,765 women screened, 3.2% were called back after the initial screen. This compares to 3.6% in the subsequent Karolinska series. If the patients were to have surgical biopsy on the basis of screening, as is commonly done in some other parts of the world, they would have had a PPV of .234 from the mammogram alone. In this program, the suspicion of malignancy on a screening mammogram is followed up by a call back and a complete mammographic examination. These additional views reduce the number of patients who require further diagnostic studies. Some 48% of the patients who had suspicious mammograms on the initial screen were returned to the pool of normal patients without suspicion of malignancy after the additional studies were obtained. Two-hundred and eleven patients subsequently underwent clinical examination and cytologic assessment of the lesions. Cytology eliminated 25% of these cases. The patients who ultimately had surgical biopsy represented only 39% of the patients who would have had

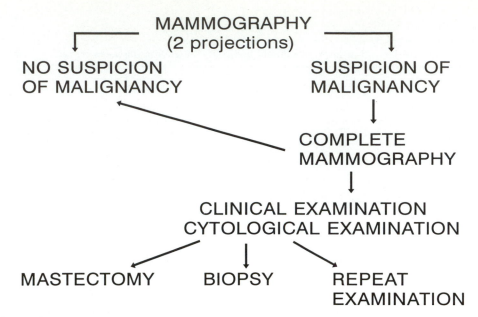

Fig. 5-5. The Malmö system of breast cancer screening. (From Andersson et al: *Radiology* 132:273-276, 1979.)

Table 5-32. Malmö breast cancer screening experience

Age	Screened (no.)	Called back after screening No.	(%)	PPV of complete mammography screening alone	Suspected after complete mammography No.	(%)	PPV of complete mammography without FNA	Surgical biopsy after FNA and clinical examination No.	(%)	Cancers found (no.)	Prevalence rate/1000 women screened	PPV of system
50-54	3455	111	(3.2)	.189	64	(1.9)	.328	46	(1.3)	21	6.1	.457
55-59	3530	88	(2.5)	.239	48	(1.4)	.438	36	(1.0)	21	6.0	.583
60-64	3103	100	(3.2)	.250	49	(1.6)	.510	41	(1.3)	25	8.1	.610
65-69	2677	106	(4.0)	.264	50	(1.9)	.560	36	(1.3)	28	10.1	.778
50-69	12,765	405	(3.2)	.234	211	(1.7)	.450	159	(1.2)	95	7.4	.603

From Andersson I et al: *Radiology* 132:273-276, 1979.

Table 5-33. Comparison of the Malmö and Karolinska breast cancer screening experience

	Screened (no.)	Called back No.	(%)	PPV of screening alone	FNA and clinical exam Suspected after complete mammography	PPV without FNA	Surgery No.	(%)	Cancer No.	(%)	Prevalence rate	PPV of the system	Biopsies/ cancer
Azavado et al (1991)	8370	302	(3.6%)	.202	219 2.6%	.279	70	(0.84%)	61	(0.73%)	7.3	.871	1.1
Andersson et al (1979)	12765	405	(3.2%)	.234	211 1.7%	.450	159	(1.2%)	95	(0.74%)	7.4	.603	1.7

surgical biopsy, if the biopsies were based on the suspicion of malignancy screening mammography alone. These authors detected cancer at a prevalence rate of 7.4/1000. The increasing prevalence with age basis is similar to what would be expected in the population being studied. This cancer detection rate suggests that very few, if any, cancers were missed with this screening program. As early as 1979 the Malmö group obtained a PPV of .603 through the combination of screening mammography and FNA cytology. Even without the FNA cytology, these authors were able to obtain a PPV of .450, which is considerably better than most any other published series of that time.

The only other group to use a system similar to the Malmö program in a large number of patients, which has been published in the refereed press, is the Karolinska Hospital in Stockholm.[4,5] The experience of the Karolinska is discussed in Chapter 1.

Malmö versus Karolinska screening experiences. Table 5-33 compares the Malmö and the Karolinska breast cancer screening experience. These studies show remarkable similarities, despite the fact that they were accomplished over a decade apart. The Karolinska call-back rate of 3.6, versus 3.2 for the Malmö experience, is indeed similar. A major difference relates to the PPV without FNA in the Malmö versus the Karolinska data. At Malmö, they were able to accomplish much greater PPV by the additional films obtained after call back. The Karolinska experience compensated for this difference with a lower surgical biopsy rate. Only 8.4 out of 1000 screening patients underwent surgical biopsy at the Karolinska, whereas 12 out of 1000 screening patients underwent surgical biopsy at Malmö. Both of these are considerably less than almost any other published series. Their low false-negative rate, accomplished by this system, is evident from the similarity between the prevalence rate of cancer and the cancer detection rate of the system. However, their subsequent interval cancer rate has caused debate on this issue. The numbers, 7.3 and 7.4, are approximately equal to the number of cancers that are anticipated in the populations being screened. Thus, if many cancers were being missed by the system, they are not apparent on the basis of the prevalence rate of cancers detected by the system.

The difference in the PPV of the two approaches is evident in the use of FNA. The FNA procedures at the Karolinska resulted in a greater reduction of cases requiring surgery than in Malmö. Of the 219 patients undergoing FNA at the Karolinska, only 70 underwent surgery (31%). They experienced an almost 70% reduction of surgical biopsies by the addition of FNA. At Malmö, 75% of patients who had FNA and clinical examinations underwent subsequent surgical biopsy, which was a reduction of only 25% by the addition of FNA. The improved fidelity of FNA over the intervening decade is due to the experience at the Karolinska. This suggests that the strategy for using FNA

could be learned and improved throughout the world. The amount of improvement depends in part on the experience of the cytopathologist involved in the procedures. Obviously, this strategy, used both at the Karolinska and at Malmö, results in the most effective and efficient diagnosis of nonpalpable breast cancer in asymptomatic women. They detect cancer at the known prevalence rate with fewest surgical biopsies. They have the highest PPV of any diagnostic system in the published literature. Therefore the role of aspiration biopsies in the diagnosis of nonpalpable breast cancer in asymptomatic women is discussed in Chapter 6.

REFERENCES

1. Albert MP, Sachsse E, Coe NP, et al: Correlation between mammography and the pathology of nonpalpable breast lesions, *J Surg Oncol* 44(1):44-46, 1990.
2. Andersson I, Andren L, Hildell J, et al: Breast cancer screening in mammography. A population-based, randomized trial with mammography as the only screening mode, *Radiology* 132:273-276, 1979.
3. Arnesson L-G, Fagerberg G, Grontoft O, Lundstrom B: Surgical biopsy of non-palpable mammary lesions, *Acta Chir Scand* 152:97-101, 1986.
4. Azavedo E, Auer G, Svane G. Stereotactic fine-needle biopsy in 2594 mammographically detected non-palpable lesions, *Lancet* 1(8646):1033-1036, 1989.
5. Azavedo E, Svane G: Radiologic aspects of breast cancers detected through a breast cancer screening program, *Eur J Radiol* 3:88-90, 1991.
6. Bedwani R, Vama J, Rosner D, et al: Management and survival of female patients with "minimal" breast cancer, *Cancer* 47:2669-2678, 1981.
7. Bigelow R, Smith R, Goodman PA, Wilson GS: Needle localization of nonpalpable breast masses, *Arch Surg* 120(5):565-569, 1985.
8. Chetty U, Kirkpatrick AE, Anderson TL, et al: Localization and excision of occult breast lesions, *Br J Surg* 70(10):607-610, 1983.
9. Choucair RJ, Holcomb MB, Mathews R, Hughes TG: Biopsy of nonpalpable breast lesions, *Am J Surg* 156(6):453-456, 1988.
10. Ciatto S, Cataliotti L, Distante V: Nonpalpable lesions detected with mammography: review of 512 consecutive cases, *Radiology* 165(1):99-102, 1987.
11. Colbassani HJ Jr, Feller WF, Cigtay OS, Chun B: Mammographic and pathologic correlation of microcalcification in disease of the breast, *Surg Gynecol Obstet* 155(5):689-696, 1982.
12. Fajardo LL, Davis JR, Wiens JL, Trego DC: Mammography-guided stereotactic fine-needle aspiration cytology of nonpalpable breast lesions: prospective comparison with surgical biopsy results, *AJR* 155:977-981, 1990.
13. Fisher B, Anderson S, Fisher ER, et al: Significance of ipsilateral beast tumour recurrence after lumpectomy, *Lancet* 338(8763):327-331, 1991.
14. Galakhoff C, Sassoon C, Vanel D, et al: Preoperative radiologic localization of nonpalpable breast lesions. Technics and value. Apropos of 33 cases, *J Radiol* 64(5):313-317, 1983.
15. Gent HJ, Sprenger E, Dowlatshahi K: Stereotaxic needle localization and cytological diagnosis of occult breast lesions, *Ann Surg* 204(5):580-584, 1986.
16. Gisvold JJ, Martin JK Jr: Pre-biopsy localization of nonpalpable breast lesions, *AJR* 143:477-481, 1984.

17. Graham NL, Bauer TL: Early detection of occult breast cancer: the York experience with 678 needle localization biopsies, *Am J Surg* 54(4):234-239, 1988.

18. Hall FM, Storella JM, Silverstone DZ, Wyshak G: Nonpalpable breast lesions: recommendations for biopsy based on suspicion of carcinoma at mammography, *Radiology* 167(2):353-358, 1988.

19. Hall WC, Aust JB, Gaskill HV, et al: Evaluation of nonpalpable breast lesions. Experience in a training institution, *Am J Surg* 151:467-469, 1986.

20. Hallgrimsson P, Karesen R, Artun K, Skjennald A: Non-palpable breast lesions. Diagnostic criteria and preoperative localization, *Acta Radiol* 29:285-288, 1988.

21. Hann L, Ducatman BS, Wang HH, et al: Nonpalpable breast lesions: evaluation by means of fine-needle aspiration cytology, *Radiology* 171(2):373-376, 1989.

22. Hermann G, Janus C, Schartz I, et al: Nonpalpable breast lesions: accuracy of prebiopsy mammographic diagnosis, *Radiology* 165:323-326, 1987.

23. Hicks MJ, Davis JR, Layton JM, Present AJ: Sensitivity of mammography and physical examination of the breast for detecting breast cancer, *JAMA* 242(19):2080-2083, 1979.

24. Hoehn JL, Hardacre JM, Swanson MK, Williams GH: Localization of occult breast lesions, *Cancer* 49(6):1142-1144, 1982.

25. Kessler HB, Rimer BK, Devine PJ, et al: Corporate-sponsored breast cancer screening at the work site: results of a statewide program, *Radiology* 179:107-110, 1991.

26. Knaus JV, Dolan JR, Isaacs JH: Detection of localized breast cancer by prospective mammographic screening criteria, *Am J Obstet Gynecol* 158(1):147-149, 1988.

27. Lamb J, Anderson TJ, Dixon MJ, Levack PA: Role of fine needle aspiration cytology in breast cancer screening, *J Clin Pathol* 40:705-709, 1987.

28. Landercasper J, Gundersen SB Jr, Gundersen AL, et al: Needle localization and biopsy of nonpalpable lesions of the breast, *Surg Gynecol Obstet* 164(5):399-403, 1987.

29. Landstrom J, Osgood G, Young SC: Needle localization in occult breast lesions, *J Surg Oncol* 40(1):1-3, 1989.

30. Lang NP, Talbert GE, Shewmake KB, et al: The current evaluation of nonpalpable breast lesions, *Arch Surg* 122(12):1389-1391, 1987.

31. Lefor AT, Numann PJ, Levinsohn EM: Needle localization of occult breast lesions, *Am J Surg* 148(2):270-274, 1984.

32. Marrujo G, Jolly PC, Hall MH: Nonpalpable breast cancer: needle-localized biopsy for diagnosis and considerations for treatment, *Am J Surg* 151(5):599-602, 1986.

33. Meyer JE, Kopans DB, Stomper PC, Lindfors KK: Occult breast abnormalities: percutaneous preoperative needle localization, *Radiology* 150(2):335-337, 1984.

34. Molloy M, Azarow K, Garcia VF, Daniel JR: Enhanced detection of preinvasive breast cancer: combined role of mammography and needle localization biopsy, *J Surg Oncol* 40(3):152-154, 1983.

35. Moskowitz M: The predictive value of certain mammographic signs in screening for breast cancer, *Cancer* 51(6):1007-1011, 1983.

36. Murphy WA, DeSchryver-Kecskemeti K: Isolated clustered microcalcifications in the breast: radiologic-pathologic correlation, *Radiology* 127:335-341, 1978.

37. Nielsen M, Jensen J, Anderson J: Percutaneous and cancerous breast lesions during lifetime and at autopsy: a study of 83 women, *Cancer* 54:612-615, 1984.

38. Ostrow LB, DuBois JJ, Hoefer RA Jr, Brant WE: Needle-localized biopsy of occult breast lesions, *So Med J* 80(1):29-32, 1987.

39. Owings DV, Hann L, Schnitt SJ: How thoroughly should needle localization breast biopsies be sampled for microscopic examination? *Am J Surg Pathol* 14(6):578-583, 1990.

40. Page DL, Dupont WD, Rogers LW, et al: Atypical hyperplastic lesions of the female breast: a long-term follow-up study, *Cancer* 55:2698-2708, 1985.

41. Papatestas AE, Hermann D, Hermann G: Surgery for nonpalpable breast lesions, *Arch Surg* 125:399-402, 1990.

42. Perre I, Hoynck Van Papendrecht AAGM, Sierinkk HD, Muller JW: The non-palpable, radiographically suspicious breast lesion: an analysis of 101 cases, The Netherlands, *J Surg* 42(3):69-71, 1990.

43. Petrovich JA, Ross DS, Sullivan JW, Lake TP: Mammographic wire localization in diagnosis and treatment of occult carcinoma of breast, *Surg Gynecol Obstet* 168(3):239-243, 1989.

44. Poole GV Jr, Choplin RH, Sterchi JM, et al: Occult lesions of the breast, *Surg Gynecol Obstet* 163(2):107-110, 1986.

45. Powell RW, McSweeney MB, Wilson CE: X-ray calcifications as the only basis for breast biopsy, *Ann Surg* 197(5):555-559, 1983.

46. Prorok JJ, Trostle DR, Scarlato M, Rachman R: Excisional breast biopsy and roentgenographic examination for mammographically detected microcalcification, *Am J Surg* 145:684-686, 1983.

47. Rogers JV, Powell RM: Mammographic indications for biopsy of clinically normal breast: correlation with pathologic findings in 72 cases, *AJR* 115:794-800, 1972.

48. Rosen PP, Senier R, Schottenfeld J, et al: Non-invasive breast carcinoma: frequency of unsuspected invasion and implications for treatment, *Ann Surg* 189:377-383, 1979.

49. Roses DF, Harris MN, Gorstein F, Gumport SL: Biopsy for microcalcification detected by mammography, *Surgery* 87(3):248-252, 1980.

50. Rusnak CH, Pengelly DB, Hosie RT, Rusnak CN: Preoperative needle localization to detect early breast cancer, *Am J Surg* 157(5):505-507, 1989.

51. Schreer I, Frischbier H-J: Predictive value of mammography in early detection of breast cancer: analysis of histological findings in breast biopsies indicated only by mammography, *Euro Radiol* 1:165-168, 1991.

52. Schwartz GF, Feig SA, Patchefsky AS: Significance and staging of nonpalpable carcinomas of the breast, *Surg Gynecol Obstet* 166(1):6-10, 1988.

53. Schwartz GF, Patchefsky AS, Feig SA: Clinically occult breast cancers: multicentricity and implications for treatment, *Ann Surg* 191:8-12, 1980.

54. Silverstein MJ, Gamagami P, Colburn WJ, et al: Nonpalpable breast lesions: diagnosis with slightly overpenetrated screen-film mammography and hook wire-directed biopsy in 1,014 cases, *Radiology* 171(3):633-638, 1989.

55. Skinner MA, Swain M, Simmons R, et al: Nonpalpable breast lesions at biopsy. A detailed analysis of radiographic features, *Ann Surg* 208(2):203-208, 1988.

56. Solmer R, Goodstein J, Agliozzo C: Nonpalpable breast lesions discovered by mammography, *Arch Surg* 115:1067-1069, 1980.

57. Tinnemans AM, Wobbes T, Holland R, et al: Mammographic and histopathologic correlation of nonpalpable lesions of the breast and the reliability of frozen section diagnosis, *Surg Gynecol Obstet* 165:523-529, 1987.

58. Tinnemans ERG, Wobbes T, Lubbers E-J, et al: The significance of microcalcifications without palpable mass in the diagnosis of breast cancer, *Surgery* 99:652-657, 1986.

Chapter 6

INVESTIGATION OF BREAST ABNORMALITIES

In the premammographic era, breast cancer was diagnosed on the basis of symptomatology. Most often it presented as a palpable mass. Other clinical symptoms such as pain, skin thickening, retraction, or nipple discharge were occasionally present. Mammography has allowed for the detection of breast cancer before it has clinical symptoms. Screening for breast cancer in presumed asymptomatic women has usually included mammography and clinical palpation. Thus, some palpable lesions are detected in asymptomatic women who otherwise have not identified the palpable abnormality through breast self-examination. On a screening examination a mass may be felt or a mammographic abnormality detected, both of which will require further diagnostic steps. Before the advent of fine-needle aspiration cytology or needle-directed histology, the standard approach to further diagnosis of either a palpable lesion or a mammographic abnormality was the use of open surgical biopsy.

As can be seen in the preceding chapter, the use of fine needle aspiration has markedly diminished the need for open surgical biopsy of lesions that ultimately turn out to be benign. This chapter will attempt to place in perspective the various diagnostic modalities. To do so, it will be necessary to discuss some aspects in the diagnosis of both palpable and nonpalpable breast cancer. We seek to further define and characterize the various approaches to cytologic or histologic tissue sampling prior to surgical biopsy. In addition, it is necessary to define further the marking techniques that are required for surgical biopsy of a mammographically detected occult breast lesion.

PALPABLE BREAST ABNORMALITIES
Clinical examination

Physical examination is the simplest and cheapest way to detect palpable lesions in the breast. It does not involve any equipment and can be performed regularly by the woman herself or by her doctor. It may result in detection of breast cancers at an early stage. An annual physical examination performed by a physician, without any self-examination in between, may detect tumors of larger size than if self-examinations are regularly performed, since the interval between the examinations is much longer. Many breast cancer screening programs encourage women to perform breast self-examination between screening examinations. Although this is intuitively logical, there is as yet no large series similar to the HIP data on mammography that establishes a decrease in breast cancer mortality due to the practice of breast self-examinations.

Palpable breast lesions of various types are a common finding during physical examination of women with different kinds of breast symptoms. When a woman has detected a lump in her breast, an experienced physician must examine and evaluate the lesion. It can be clinically difficult, however, even, for an experienced physician, to differentiate a malignant tumor from a benign one. Hardness and movability of the lump, skin retraction, position of the lump in the breast, and palpable enlarged lymph nodes in the ipsilateral axilla are all helpful diagnostic signs in evaluating palpable tumors.

Role of mammography in detecting palpable breast lesions

Mammography was initially used to aid the clinical investigation of patients with breast symptoms and to improve diagnostic accuracy. In most cases it can discriminate benign lesions from malignant tumors. Erickson et al.[22] reported that 102 of 214 women referred over an 8-year period for abnormal mammograms could be spared surgical biopsy. The patients, who were followed closely, had benign lesions by clinical and mammographic criteria. However, it should be recalled, a "normal" mammogram does not always exclude the presence of cancer in a patient with dense breasts and a newly palpable lump but can be frequently false-negative in such situations.

Kopans and Swann[47] noted that benign and malignant lesions can have similar morphology. Benign lesions more commonly have smooth well-defined margins, but cancers may be sharply outlined as well. Swann et al.[80] emphasized that the translucent zone around the edge of a tumor, the so-called halo sign, does not exclude malignant changes. A newly palpable mass in a patient with dense breasts or a circumscribed mammographic lesion will usually require further studies.

Fine-needle aspiration in palpable breast lesions

Fine-needle aspiration cytology (FNA) has been used for seven decades in diagnosing tumors of different origin. Only a few items are needed: needles, syringe, syringe holder, glass slides. Changes in cells from various organs and in tumors anywhere in the body can be interpreted by this technique. The technique yields hundreds, even thousands, of cells for microscopic evaluation.

Martin and Ellis,[56] who have been performing aspiration needle biopsies from tumors of different origin since 1926, reported on 65 cases in which they used an ordinary 18-gauge needle attached to a syringe. When the needle entered the tumor, the piston of the syringe was partly withdrawn to produce a vacuum. They found that the vacuum and a moving needle were necessary for adequate sampling of cellular material. In most cases aspiration with the needle at rest was not adequate to draw sufficient tissue into the needle. These authors placed a small fragment of the sampled material on a slide for smearing and left the remainder in a specimen bottle for fixation and staining. Tissue was successfully sampled in 80% of the cases. The failures occurred in harder fibrous tumors, but they were able to distinguish benign from malignant tumors in all cases in which adequate tissue was aspirated. Although they did not perform aspiration from abdominal tumors, they successfully sampled diagnostic material from lung tumors, tumors and lymph nodes in the neck, intraoral and nasal antral tumors, breast tumors, sarcomas of bone, and miscellaneous tumors. Their indications for the procedure were tumor masses that lay below the surface of normal tissue when surgical exposure was deemed contraindicated. Their contraindications included danger or the "dissemination of disease or fungation of tumor tissue through the operative wound; the interference with subsequent therapeutic surgical procedures; [and] the surgical risk and lack of justification for any procedure involving physical or mental discomfort or expense to the patient, where the information gained [might] be of doubtful value to the patient or of academic interest only." They found that in most cases the information from the smear was sufficient to discriminate between benign and malignant tumors and the procedure was well accepted by the patients.

The technique has spread rapidly throughout the world, and FNAs are now widely used. The clinical advantages, presented by Linsk and Franzen,[53] are as follows:

1. Efficiency in obtaining a specific diagnosis of a mass before irreversible surgery, radiotherapy, or chemotherapy
2. Staging accuracy
3. Ease of obtaining material, which invariably means an earlier diagnosis and thus better diagnostic and therapeutic planning
4. The psychologic advantage of relieving anxiety and convincing the patient of the need for immediate treatment

It also has substantial economic advantages[53]:

1. Rapid accurate diagnosis reduces the need for hospitalization
2. Preoperative diagnosis may eliminate the need for some surgical procedures.
3. Particularly in rural or undeveloped areas, submission of slides to regional cytopathologic laboratories may allow diagnosis without the need for more sophisticated diagnostic equipment.

This method has been used in many breast centers for years to further improve the diagnostic reliability of clinical examination and mammography. FNA has made it possible to get a cytomorphologic diagnosis of both benign lesions and cancers preoperatively. It has proved in many studies to have a diagnostic accuracy around 90%.

Franzen and Zajicek[26] did a critical review of 3479 consecutive aspiration biopsies of palpable breast lesions in 3023 women between 1955 and 1966 at Radiumhemmet, Karolinska Hospital. Eighty-six cases were excluded because the aspiration was performed after surgery/radiotherapy or because surgery was delayed until 6 months or more after the aspiration. Surgery was performed on 1713 breast lesions in 1686 women. Cytologic and clinical findings were compared for the rest of the women. A syringe with a special handle that permitted single-hand gripping was used, and a 0.6 mm needle. A larger needle was sometimes used when the first aspiration indicated the presence of dense fibrotic tissue. Only the first FNA was considered in presenting the result, even if more than one aspiration was performed. The cytology reported cancer in 75.8% and suspicious for cancer in another 13.4% of the histologically proved cases. There was only one false-positive cytologic report.

Zajdela et al[86] presented results from FNAs in 2401 consecutive cases. All underwent histopathologic examination. There were 1745 malignant tumors, and 656 benign. The cytologic diagnosis of cancer was confirmed in 996 cases out of 1000 (PPV, 0.996) but was missed in 3.6% (PPV = 0.964).

Many authors have emphasized that the experience of

the individual who performs the procedure is of utmost importance to the result. Linsk and Franzen[53] reported that the percentage of false-negative results varied in several large series from 7.4% to 26.7%. They suggested that a reduction of false-negatives must come from increased experience rather than from "any conscious effort," since the latter may cause too many false-positive readings.

Barrows et al.[7] assessed FNA biopsies on 689 women with breast cancer. The clinical factors relating to success of the aspiration were evaluated. Although the size of the lesion was important, the physician who did the aspiration was the most significant factor. With an experienced physician doing the aspiration, positive results were obtained in more than 80% of the breast malignancies.

Cohen et al.[15] showed that training and experience of the cytopathologist are important in interpreting breast fine-needle aspiration biopsies (FNABs). Fifty specimens were reviewed by five observers. All cases had histopathologic follow-ups. Two reviewers were experienced, three relatively inexperienced. The experienced observers had significantly better sensitivity and specificity.

Gautenbein et al.[28] evaluated FNABs from 1768 cases. A palpable mass was the indication in 92.1%, and a radiologic finding in 2.7%. The other aspirations were for various reasons (e.g., skin changes and unilateral enlargement of the breast). The aspirations were performed by either cytopathologists or other physicians. The two groups with different experience were compared. The specificity was 100% for both. A nonrepresentative diagnosis was obtained in 5% of the histologically proved cancers in the experienced group, compared to 19.2% in the other group. The authors concluded that the experience of the doctor performing the biopsy is of greatest importance to the diagnostic results.

Aardal et al.[1] reported on 3743 FNAs in 3188 patients. Histologic examination was performed in 798 patients, and cancer histologically verified in 421. There were no false-positive and only 13 false-negative cytologic diagnoses. Specificity was 100%, and sensitivity 77.9% or 96.4% depending upon the criteria used. Twenty-three doctors performed the aspirates, which they suggested caused a high proportion of inadequate smears. Inadequate smears were only 4% to 7% when experienced doctors did the procedure.

FNA provides many advantages in evaluating palpable breast lesions. One advantage is that, when it is positive, a single surgery can be planned as a curative measure rather than a diagnostic surgical biopsy followed by a second curative surgery. The patient with such a tumor can thus be informed preoperatively that she has a cancer, which may be psychologically important to her. The surgeon can explain the different possibilities of curative treatment available, and together they can tailor the treatment to her particular situation. If mammography suggests an invasive component, sampling of lymph nodes in the axilla can also be performed at the same time as the surgical treatment. Another advantage is that surgery can be avoided if benign cells are aspirated and the benign cytologic diagnosis is consistent with the clinical examination and mammography.

Many articles have presented the experiences with FNA of palpable breast lesions.

Furnival et al.[27] studying FNA in 237 patients with a palpable breast tumor, showed a diagnostic accuracy of 95.5% in both benign and malignant lesions. They found that FNA improved the management of breast lesions by giving an accurate preoperative diagnosis.

Rimsten et al.[71] evaluated clinical examination and FNA in 1244 women with breast symptoms, performing FNA on 984 lesions. Histologic examination showed cancer in 115 of 411 cases (28%)—in 92.5% of the patients when palpation suggested "definite cancer" and in 50% when there was a clinically "strong suspicion of cancer." All cytologic diagnoses of cancer were verified histologically. In patients with grave atypia on cytology, 87.5% had cancer at histologic examination. Cytology was false-negative in 4% of the malignant tumors but found cancer in 6 and 12 cases, respectively, when palpation showed no cancer or only a slight suspicion of cancer. None of the histopathologically proved cancers evaluated both clinically and cytologically were benign. The authors suggested that the number of "unnecessary" surgical biopsies could be reduced by combining palpation and cytology.

Kiovuniemi[43] presented a comparison of FNA and histology in 503 cases. Cancer was histologically proved in 192 tumors. FNA originally showed 137 (71.4%) of these to be malignant and, after review of the specimen, in an additional 24 (12.5%). Strongly suspicious findings were originally reported in 19 (9.9%) and, after review, in an additional 6 (3.1%). Fourteen (7.3%) were reported as moderately suspicious. Four of the negative cases (2.1%) were due to inadequate specimens. Of the 311 histologically benign lesions a strong suspicion of malignancy was reported in 5 (1.4%) and a moderate suspicion in 22 (7.1%). No strongly suspicious findings were left after review, and only 9 (2.9%) cases were moderately suspicious. There were no false-positive reports.

Deschenes et al.[19] reported on 2050 FNAs of breast lesions. Cytology diagnosed 92 (78%) of 118 histologically proved cancers. In another 13 (11%) malignancy was cytologically suspected; only 9 (7.6%) were false-negative. In the 287 histologically confirmed benign lesions, cytology reports were correct in 237 (83%). There were no false-positive reports. FNA was found to be a safe, simple, and quick method, well accepted by the patient, and to have a positive predictive value of 100%. However, if cancer is suspected clinically, cytology reports that are negative should be disregarded.

Kline et al.[44] studied 3545 aspirates performed over 8 years. The material included solid and cystic masses. Abnormal cells were found in 90% of the 368 malignant tumors. FNA proved to be rapid and accurate, without significant complications.

Salter et al.[73] reported the accuracy of 2334 breast biopsies performed during a 9-year period. They concluded that with FNA the number of surgical biopsies could be reduced, increasing the efficiency of hospital resources, and diminishing patient anxiety. Bell et al.[10] reviewed 1680 FNA biopsies in 1410 patients. The cytologic diagnoses were malignant in 131, suspicious for malignancy in 102, atypical in 198, benign in 1019, and unsatisfactory in 230 cases. No false-positive results were obtained. Seventeen percent of the cytologically atypical cases had malignant tumors, and 4% of the cytologically benign cases. Ninety-three percent of the cancers were detected by the combination of clinical, mammographic, and cytologic examinations. Clinical examination and cytology detected 87%, and clinical examination and mammography 79%, of the cancers. The authors found that a two-stage surgical procedure could be avoided if FNA had demonstrated cancer preoperatively.

Wanebo et al.[84] performed FNA on 398 patients and found 136 to be cancers. One hundred of these (74%) could be diagnosed preoperatively by cytology. Seventy-one patients underwent mastectomy without frozen section. Thirteen had had an excisional biopsy previous to the mastectomy. There were no false-positive diagnoses. Thirty-one patients had tumors that were cytologically diagnosed as suspicious for malignancy and open biopsy was suggested. Twenty-two of these had cancer histologically, and one a metastatic cancer. One hundred three patients had negative cytology and open biopsy. One hundred two were negative by histopathology, but one had cancer. Insufficient material was obtained in 38 patients, and 12 of those had cancer. The authors found FNA to be a safe, atraumatic, and rapid method, obviating the need for frozen section and reducing anesthesia and operative time. "FNA is highly accurate in the diagnosis of breast cancer."

Wollenberg et al.[85] evaluated FNA in all patients who received that procedure between 1973 and 1982. Correlations were made between cytologic and histologic diagnoses when the patients were operated upon and between mammography results and clinical evaluation when surgery was not performed. Their results for sensitivity, specificity, and predictive value of a positive and negative diagnosis were respectively 65%, 100%, and 89.6%. They felt that their use of FNA permitted early diagnosis, treatment, and management of breast cancer.

Somers et al.[76] described their results in 369 FNA specimens. Sensitivity was 78%, specificity and positive predictive value both 100%, and negative predictive value 78%. They found that a negative FNA report did not exclude malignancy in a clinically suspicious lesion but suggested that FNA showing malignancy could be the basis for planning and performing a definitive surgical procedure when it confirmed a clinical and mammographic impression of cancer.

Grant et al.[30] examined 100 women with aspiration cytology before surgical excision of a palpable mass. Their false-negative rate was 6%, and their accuracy 94%. They stated that FNA may add confidence in diagnosis of benign lesions, prevent misdiagnosis of cancers, and reduce costs of managing both primary and recurrent breast cancer.

Lamb et al.[50] used FNA in a 6-year program screening for breast cancer. Healthy women were invited to participate. Aspiration cytology was performed in 562, and surgical biopsy in 397. One hundred seventy-three cancers were confirmed by histology. The main causes of false-negative results were the small size of the cancers and the occult nature of mammographically detected lesions. The authors opined that the triple diagnosis with FNA, mammography, and physical examination meant that the number of benign biopsies could be reduced considerably.

Patel et al.[69] presented results of a study of 1458 patients with breast masses who underwent aspiration cytology. Fifty percent (731 patients) had histopathologic diagnoses. The sensitivity was 64% for patients having one aspiration, but 91% for those having three. The specificity was 56%, which was due to inadequate or unsatisfactory cytologic preparations. Invasive lobular carcinoma was more difficult to cytologically diagnose than invasive ductal carcinoma. Fibroadenoma yielded a higher rate of correct diagnosis than fibroadenosis. The size of the mass was important for the ductal invasive cancers and fibroadenomas, but not for invasive lobular cancer or fibroadenosis. Thirty of 32 false-negative results were caused by the needle missing the mass, and the remaining two were due to misinterpretation. The authors concluded that aspiration cytology was accurate and should be used as a preoperative diagnostic procedure for breast masses but that negative aspirates should be regarded as nonresults if there was mammographic or clinical suspicion of malignancy.

Carlson et al.[14] reported on needle aspirations in 86 patients with solid breast masses. Cancers were histopathologically found in 27 patients, and 59 had benign lesions. The authors reported no false-positive findings and five (11.9%) false-negatives. Sensitivity was 73.7%, and specificity 100%.

Kwok et al.[48] found that aspiration cytology was useful in allowing a better psychologic preparation of patients before surgery. They used preoperative aspiration cytology in a group of patients with breast lumps and compared the diagnosis with the histopathologic diagnosis of the excised specimen. Aspiration cytology correctly diagnosed 89% of malignant lesions and 92.6% of benign lesions based upon histologic diagnosis. Cytologic diagnosis of benign disease had a false-negative rate of 6%, whereas that of malignant disease had a 2.7% false-positive rate. Inadequate diagnosis was reported in only 3.5%. The authors suggested that a palpable lesion that can be cytologically proved to consist of normal breast tissue or benign changes of the breast tissue may be left in the breast without any surgical treatment if the clinical evaluation is consistent with the cytologic diagnosis.

Painter et al.[67] reviewed 245 FNAs of solid breast masses and found that 178 aspirations revealed benign lesions, 7 intermediate, and 53 malignant. In seven cases the aspirations were unsatisfactory. Fifty-two of these masses were histopathologically diagnosed as cancers. One hundred one patients with negative findings were followed, and in none did cancer develop. The authors found that aspiration biopsy gave additional information and allowed greater diagnostic accuracy that could result in the elimination of many breast biopsies.

Rangwala et al.[70] studied cytologically 131 fine-needle aspirations and 85 discharge smears from the nipple and correlated the cytology with histology. They found cytologic examination accurate and useful.

Langmuir et al.[51] presented results from 257 palpable breast masses in 200 patients. FNA was found to have a sensitivity of 96% and a specificity of 94%. No false-positive diagnoses were reported. The authors reported that FNA improved the diagnoses of benign lesions and decreased the risk of missing cancers.

Gelabert et al.,[29] who performed 107 FNABs in 98 patients with palpable solid breast masses, found that 84 tumors showed malignancy. Eighty patients were treated by mastectomy without open biopsy or frozen section. The sensitivity was 95%, and the specificity 100%, for diagnosis of breast cancer. The authors stated that it is a simple and reliable method that also proves to be cost-effective.

Triple diagnosis

As early as 1975 Johnsen[42] showed that almost all palpable breast lesions could be correctly diagnosed by using combined physical examination (inspection as well as palpation), mammography, and FNA, the so-called "triple diagnosis." Butler et al.[13] also evaluated the efficacy of a combined physical, mammographic, and FNA examination. One hundred thirteen women were prospectively evaluated. Eighty-six patients underwent all three studies. The authors concluded that the combination was highly accurate in diagnosing breast masses. Patients in whom all three examination results were benign could be safely observed without the need of open biopsy.

Lamarque and Rodiere[49] reported that 95% to 98% of breast cancers can be correctly diagnosed by a combination of clinical examination, mammography, and cytology.

The use of FNA to diagnose palpable breast masses has thus been firmly established as an effective means of facilitating the early diagnosis of breast cancer and diminishing the need for surgical biopsy of benign lesions.

Surgical biopsy

A surgical diagnostic biopsy is recommended if any of the three procedures (physical examination, mammography, and FNA) show findings suspicious of malignancy. Frozen section diagnosis during surgery can be performed if no conclusive cytomorphologic diagnosis is available preoperatively. When that is necessary, the patient cannot be prepared psychologically for the whole treatment and, in addition, a correct diagnosis may be difficult to obtain from frozen section, especially if the tumor is extremely small.

Fessia et al.,[24] studying 4436 consecutive breast biopsies, compared frozen section diagnosis (FSD) with the final pathology report. In 96.57% (4284 cases) there was no difference. There were no false-positive FSDs, although in 1.66% (74 cases) false-negative reports did occur. The main source of false-negatives was minimal breast cancer and in situ cancers. In minimal cancers the FSD was correct in 80.21%, compared to 99.42% in the nonminimal cancers; and in minimal cancers the false-negative results were 8.79%. In carcinomas in situ the false-negative FSDs were 76.82%.

NONPALPABLE BREAST LESIONS

Because of the expanding use of mammography both in the clinical examination of patients with breast symptoms and as a screening modality, nonpapable breast lesions are increasingly being detected. Palpable breast lesions detected by physical examination can be further investigated by mammography and FNA. A surgical excision must be performed, however, if any of these modalities arouses the suspicion of malignancy. Surgical diagnostic biopsies can be avoided if the triple diagnostic procedure reveals a benign lesion. What alternatives are there for further investigation of a nonpalpable breast lesion detected by mammography? Clinical examination does not help since these tumors are nonpalpable despite physical examination performed by an experienced clinician. Perhaps regularly scheduled follow-up mammograms would be an alternative, to avoid too many surgical biopsies for benign lesions; but is it desirable to diagnose cancers by letting them grow? The diagnostic accuracy of investigating nonpalpable lesions can be increased by adding cytomorphologic examinations.

Follow-up mammograms

An abnormality detected by mammography is always to be worked up as well as possible with additional views. For example, rolled views and/or coned down views with or without magnification may clarify the diagnosis (see Chapters 3 and 4). These have to be done before any definite report is given. Is it a real lesion or just a superimposition of structures? Worked-up mammograms may show the area to be normal without need of further investigation or follow-up mammograms. However, a real lesion that cannot be evaluated as truly benign must be further investigated in some way. The report to the clinician should include a recommendation of further diagnostic steps. Regular follow-up mammography may be preferred; but then there are questions: how many months shall we wait before the next examination? how often should mammography be repeated and for how long? how do we know that the same size, shape, and appearance on a subsequent 6-month mammogram all mean that the lesion is benign? when can we stop the follow-up mammograms? does a minimal increase in size mean that the lesion is malignant, or can it still be benign?

It is sometimes difficult to exactly measure the diameter of a tumor, especially in a dense breast. Although the rapid change in size and shape helps decide in favor of a surgical biopsy, the possibility of curing a patient with a malignancy may be missed by the delay in diagnosis. Even a tumor of 5 mm diameter can metastasize during the follow-up period. It may still be localized to the breast and axillary nodes only, but it could also be a generalized illness that will affect the prospect for survival.

Rosen and Kimmel[72] evaluated 48 patients with nonpalpable breast tumors who presented with metastatic adenocarcinoma in the axilla. Tumor size ranged from 0.1 to 6.5 cm (median 1.5 and mean 1.9 cm). One to 65 lymph nodes were involved. Only 20 cases had fewer than four positive lymph nodes. During follow-up, which ranged from 5 to 267 months (median 60 months), 60% remained alive and free of recurrence. Only 25% died of breast cancer. These patients were compared with a matched series of equivalent stage II patients, who presented with palpable tumors. The patients with palpable tumors had a less favorable overall prognosis than the patients with occult breast tumors, but the differences were not statistically significant.

Regular follow-ups may mean problems for radiologists and patients. What do we recommend to the patient? Is it possible to explain to the patient without worrying her? A lesion of unknown nature, which needs such follow-up to be clarified, undoubtedly induces anxiety in the patient. She may have many sleepless nights. When shall we stop the follow-up mammograms? When are we to recommend surgical biopsy? A decrease in density of the surrounding breast tissue because of ongoing fatty involution may simulate the increased density of a lesion. A suspicion may arise that the lesion is malignant despite the fact that no changes have in reality occurred. An "unnecessary" surgical excision may be suggested. There are other possibilities than follow-up mammograms to investigate nonpalpable lesions and to more rapidly and precisely determine the nature of the lesion.

Ultrasound

In differentiating cystic from solid lesions, ultrasound can be added to mammography. Surgery on purely cystic lesions may be avoided. However, the sonographic appearance of malignant tumors varies and may overlap the characteristics of benign solid lesions. The value of ultrasound in differentiating malignant nonpalpable solid lesions from benign solid ones is limited.

Surgical biopsy

When a questionable lesion has been detected mammographically, surgical biopsy is an alternative to regular follow-up mammograms; but the number of excisional biopsies of benign lesions will also increase as mammography is used more widely. If we are to provide accessible breast cancer detection at a cost that society can afford, this increase in excisional biopsies must be controlled by improved mammographic interpretation and further preoperative diagnostic steps. The costs for such health services will definitely increase if unwarranted surgery is performed too often.

Moskovic et al.,[60] in discussing the economic consequences of too many benign biopsies, calculated the costs for 14,000 such procedures in England to be over 10,000,000 £. These figures are important to the already financially constrained health care systems in many countries. A well worked-up mammography study can discriminate to a high degree between benign lesions and cancers, but there are always lesions in the borderline area for which optimal mammographic differentiation is not possible. The experience of the radiologist who evaluates the mammograms is important in decreasing the number of such lesions selected for surgical biopsy. Moskovic et al.[60] emphasized the need for the most experienced radiologist available to be involved in deciding which of the nonpalpable lesions require surgical biopsy. They did a retrospective study of 69 surgically occult lesions biopsied within a period of 1 year: 17 were cancers, 3 were lobular carcinomas in situ (LCIS), and 49 were histopathologically benign lesions (PPV = 0.258). The three LCIS were not included in the malignancies, since they were considered as incidental findings without specific radiologic features. The evaluations of mammograms performed by one group of radiologists (two consultants and eight junior staff at different stages of radiologic training) were compared with those performed by a single experienced mammographic radiologist. Calcifications were present in 80% of the cases. The lesions were graded as benign, suspicious, and malignant. The experienced radiologist graded all cancers as suspicious or malignant, but the group of general radiologists graded two as benign. The experienced radiologist evaluated only 14 of 69 lesions (20%) as suspicious compared to 36 of 69 (56%) by the general radiologists. The general radiologists were thus less specific in their diagnoses. Moskovic et al.[60] emphasized that the decision whether a lesion should be biopsied must be made by an experienced radiologist. If that were the case in this series, then these authors would have decreased the number of biopsies by half.

Meyer et al.[59] compared the PPVs for two groups of radiologists, classifying as true-positive all women whose mammographic abnormalities were considered "suspicious, biopsy recommended," and who had pathologically proved cancer. Twelve hundred sixty-one breast abnormalities were submitted to surgical biopsy: 280 of these had been detected on mammograms performed at the referral hospital, and the remaining 981 were detected at other radiology departments but referred for surgical consultation to the referral hospital. Cancer was histopathologically proved in 237 cases (18.8%). The PPV for the radiologists at the referral hospital was 26.1% compared to 16.7% at the others. The authors concluded that the figures supported the recommendation of a second opinion on the mammograms of patients with abnormalities at least in the borderline region.

Thompson et al.[81] stated that the ratio of benign to malignant lesions surgically removed could be acceptable if all mammograms were preoperatively reviewed by a limited number of experienced radiologists. A PPV of 0.240 was achieved in their series of 548 nonpalpable mammographically detected lesions. Those presenting as clustered microcalcifications had a PPV of 0.196, those with irregular soft tissue densities a PPV of 0.238; but when both these features were present, the PPV increased to 0.545. This review procedure excluded from surgery a large number of patients who were recommended for surgical excision by other radiologists in the community.

The surgical excision of a benign lesion can be difficult to perform without removing too much of the surrounding normal tissue. Some patients regard the cosmetic and psychologic results as undesirable and may refrain from further mammograms because of a fear of "unnecessary" surgery. Jackson and Bassett[41] suggested that some physicians do not recommend screening mammography to their patients because of the large number of unnecessary biopsies that result from false-positive mammograms. Future mammograms may also become more difficult to interpret because of parenchymal distortion by surgery.

Preoperative morphologic diagnosis

Can cytomorphologic diagnosis further improve the evaluation of nonpalpable lesions? Would it be possible to reduce the number of benign lesions recommended for surgical diagnostic biopsies by adding cytologic information preoperatively, or does the small size of the nonpalpable lesions impair a reliable morphologic diagnosis? Fessia et al[24] and Lamb et al.[50] reported that FNA of palpable breast lesions resulted in a higher percentage of false-negative reports from minimal cancers than from larger cancers. However, if representativity of the sampled cells can

be guaranteed, cytomorphologic diagnosis of nonpalpable lesions should have the same advantages as that of palpable lesions.

Nonstereotactic biopsy technique

Aspiration needle biopsies from nonpalpable lesions require mammographic guidance. The nonstereotactic approach gives correct cytologic results in less than 50% of the histologically proved malignant tumors. In most cases we are dealing with tumors of less than 10 mm size, often less than 5 mm. FNA is less accurate for small palpable lesions. Freehand, nonstereotactic FNA can never give the same diagnostic accuracy for nonpalpable lesions as for palpable ones. The prospects of sampling representative cells are too uncertain without mammographic guidance.

Better precision is achieved if a two-dimensional determination of the position of the lesion in the compressed breast is used to guide FNA. The patient is examined in an ordinary mammography unit. The regular compression plate above the breast is exchanged for another with holes or coordinate systems around an aperture. No extra equipment is required except the compression plate, which makes this technique inexpensive. One such approach was presented by Muhlow,[61] who used a perforated Plexiglas window in the compression plate above the breast and a Plexiglas screen upon which the breast was placed above the film slit. The film cassette could thus be exchanged without disturbing the compression. Novak[65] exchanged the original compression plate for one with a rectangular aperture that had engraved letters and figures along its length and breadth. The standard radiographic cone was equipped with an optic system consisting of two light indicators adjustable to the desired coordinate point so the biopsy could be achieved at the intersecting light beams. A controlled exposure with the needle in place revealed the representativity of cell sampling in two dimensions. However, the depth of needle penetration could not be controlled or calculated by either method.

Martin and Ellis,[56] reporting on needle puncture and aspiration of palpable breast tumors and tumors of other origin, found that some tumors can be felt as the needle enters the tumor. Whereas the resistance to the needle may be different within the lesion from that within the surrounding tissue, the feel by the needle will occasionally reveal even nonpalpable breast lesions. However, dense tissue surrounding the lesion, lesions of but a few millimeters' diameter, and lesions presenting as microcalcifications only without increased surrounding density can hardly be felt by this technique. Clusters of microcalcifications or areas of parenchymal distortion usually show no specific difference in needle resistance compared to normal surrounding breast tissue. The same may hold true for small areas of increased density in breasts with large amounts of dense tissue. There will be no change in feeling with the needle during this procedure and, thus, no help in determining of the correct depth of the lesion.

Stereotactic fine-needle biopsy (SFNB) technique

If truly representative cells from nonpalpable lesions of minimal size are to be sampled, equipment that permits cell sampling with very high precision is essential. A three-dimensional calculation of lesion position is necessary for the precise cell sampling that is possible with the stereotactic technique. Most of today's mammography units have attachable stereotactic devices. There are, however, some imaging devices that have been specially designed to do SFNB. The very first stereotactic device, presented by Bolmgren et al.,[12] consisted of an x-ray tube mounted on a hinged arm, a patient table, a pivoting stand, a compression device with film holder, a biopsy device, and a calculator. The equipment was used for cell sampling and preoperative marking, and its precision was ±1 mm. A further improvement in equipment was presented by Nordenström et al.[63]

All the SFNB devices have a movable compression plate with a window in front of the breast. Corresponding to that window are radiopaque coordinate systems, or reference markers, engraved in the fixed compression plate behind the breast. The breast can be compressed and examined as with any ordinary mammography views (i.e., craniocaudal, lateromedial or mediolateral, and mediolateral-oblique). Even lesions that are seen in only one projection can be biopsied by the SFNB technique. All modern equipment has a high precision of around ±1 mm. The principle is that the exact three-dimensional position of the lesion can be calculated from a pair of stereoradiographs exposed over the appropriate area of the compressed breast. By reading the coordinates of the lesion from the stereoradiographs, all three true coordinates, including the coordinate for the depth, can be calculated. Some of these systems allow for automatic calculations from the stereoradiographs whereas with others the coordinates have to be read from the stereoradiographs and fed manually into a calculator, which is used to compute the exact true coordinates. These coordinates are set on the biopsy instrument to establish the direction of the needle in all three dimensions for cell sampling. The biopsy devices are constructed differently for the different systems. Most use Cartesian coordinates. The equipment presented by Nordenström et al.[63] translates the Cartesian coordinates to polar coordinates, resulting in an angulation of the needle direction relative to the breast. One advantage is that this allows more space for the examiner between the breast and the instrument. Another is that it makes a biopsy possible from lesions placed within the corners of the compression plate aperture and from lesions situated close to or partly outside the edge of the aperture.

STEREOTACTIC BIOPSY TECHNIQUE
History of the methodology

A stereotactic device was developed in 1975 at the Karolinska Hospital to provide cell sampling with very high precision from nonpalpable breast lesions. We sought to evaluate whether fine needle biopsy would give additional information to mammography in those lesions. This equipment was described by Bolmgren et al.[12]

The same year Nordenström and Zajicek[64] presented the first results, wherein cytologic and histopathologic diagnoses were compared after surgical excision of a lesion that had been biopsied using this stereotactically guided fine-needle device. They compared the cytologic report from the SFNB and the histologic diagnosis in 23 nonpalpable lesions. Cancer was cytologically reported in 5 cases, and could be confirmed in all five by histology. The cytology report was benign for the other 18. The histologic diagnosis was benign mastopathia, usually with fibrosis, in 17 of those cases. One lesion was histologically proved to be a fibroadenoma. There were no false-negatives. These results were so promising that the equipment was further modified to improve patient acceptance and ease of use without impairing its high precision (±1 mm). The combined evaluation of the lesions by mammography and SFNB decreased the number of surgical diagnostic biopsies of benign lesions.

The first very promising results were confirmed by Svane and Silfverswärd,[79] who reported the mammographic, cytologic, and histopathologic findings from 120 nonpalpable breast lesions that had been stereotactically examined and surgically treated during the period of further development of the equipment and technique. Those patients were referred for surgical biopsy using the combined evaluation of mammography and SFNB examinations. The malignant/benign ratio for the surgically treated nonpalpable lesions was 1:1 (PPV, 0.52). This was a remarkable improvement over the results of surgical biopsies that did not use the stereotactic system for FNA. Inadequate specimens were obtained in only 7.5% of the cases.

Svane[78] presented the results of a clinical/radiologic follow-up of the other 323 patients (332 nonpalpable lesions) who had undergone stereotactic FNAB during the same period but had not been surgically biopsied immediately. Follow-up was 4 to 53 months. Four of those 332 lesions were subsequently proved to be cancers. In two surgery was recommended, irrespective of benign cytology reports, because of a strong mammographic suspicion of malignancy. The patients refused surgery until 3 and 7 months later. The other two cancers showed cytologically atypical cells but were not excised until 15 and 18 months later, also because of patient reluctance. These results showed that the combined evaluation of nonpalpable lesions by mammography and SFNB can produce a high malignant/benign ratio among surgically treated lesions and avoid surgical biopsies of benign lesions without a resulting increase in false-negatives or a loss of diagnostic accuracy.

Needles (cytology or histology)

The SFNB technique can provide a cytologic or histopathologic diagnosis of nonpalpable lesions. Fine-needle biopsies for cytology can be performed by aspiration or by Rotex needle.

In 1977 Nordenström[62] designed and presented the Rotex needle, an 0.8 mm cannula (21 gauge) with an indwelling 0.55 mm screw (25 gauge). The screw is rotated into the lesion and cells are retained within the grooves of the screw when covered with the cannula. This avoids seeding of cells along the needle tract, which can reduce the amount of material for diagnosis. Cells are "rolled off" the 17 mm grooved tip of the needle by rotating it counterclockwise against a glass slide. These smears are prepared and stained as for any ordinary aspiration technique. The dimension of the aspiration needle can be as small as 0.5 mm (25 gauge) and still provide abundant cell material, although a larger diameter (0.7 mm, 22 gauge) will usually be necessary if the lesion is partly cystic with very thick fluid. All needles must be long enough for control stereo-radiographs to demonstrate the position of their tip within the lesion. Most systems use needles that are 6 or 7 cm long.

Mammographically guided breast biopsies can also be performed by a different type of needle for histopathologic diagnosis. A core specimen for histology is obtained by numerous different automated biopsy devices that are available for percutaneous biopsies not only from breast tumors but from tumors in different locations of the body as well. Some biopsy guns are intended for a special organ, but many can be used for different organs. The best known is the Biopty gun, developed in the early 1980s.

The diameters of the needles vary from one biopsy device to another, but many go from 14 up to 20 gauge. Some needle types are available for different biopsy depths, which may be important since the lesions are nonpalpable with, in most cases, a diameter of less than 1 cm. It may not be relevant to sample tissue at a depth of 2 to 4 cm. There are biopsy devices that harvest tissue at 0.7, 0.9, or 1.2 cm, and these are more suitable for nonpalpable breast lesions.

Fine-needle aspirations with a 22- or 25-gauge needle do not generally require anesthesia. Most patients assert that the discomfort with a routine compression mammography is greater than with a simple fine-needle penetration of the breast. However, if larger needle devices are used, local anesthesia is usually required. In addition, Parker et al.[68] claim that the technique of large needle core biopsies

works better if there has been a surgical "nick" of the skin. These large needle histologic sampling techniques fall somewhere between the more noninvasive fine-needle methods and a true open surgical biopsy. The large-bore techniques do not deform the breast or subject the patient to the degree of discomfort, cost, or potential risk that an open surgical biopsy does; but they are considerably more invasive and tissue destructive than the fine-needle biopsy methods are. In addition, very small lesions may be macerated by the large-bore 14-gauge needle.

The choice between fine-needle cytologic assessment and large-core histologic assessment has been heavily influenced by the availability of pathologists who feel comfortable with breast cytology techniques. It has become standard practice in the United States for surgeons and other physicians to perform fine-needle aspirations of palpable breast lesions. When we attempt to do similar techniques with nonpalpable lesions, the amount of tissue sample is occasionally considered insufficient by American cytologists. In Europe, and particularly in Scandinavia and Sweden, cytology has become a more prominent clinical practice than in the United States. Thus, American pathologists who have trained with the Swedish cytologic techniques seem able to replicate the Swedish data even with nonpalpable lesions. However, until American pathologists feel sufficiently comfortable with the cytologic assessment, it seems apparent that initially the American techniques will be more dependent on histology than cytology. In certain instances the histologic assessment is an essential prerequisite to therapy. This is especially true for certain national breast cancer protocols, which are attempting to assess the role of hormonal therapy in ductal carcinoma in situ (DCIS). The diagnosis of DCIS cannot be made on cytology alone. If a nonsurgical approach is to be used therefore, the only choice is a large-bore histologic sample.

Although we advocate fine-needle aspiration as being less invasive than and equivalently diagnostic to large-bore techniques, it is apparent that many institutions (particularly in the United States) will continue to use large-bore methodologies. Either method is a distinct advantage, however, over the more commonly used open surgical biopsy as the initial response to newly palpated lesions or mammographically detected nonpalpable breast lesions.

Amount of sample

In most cases one pass with the needle is not enough to sample sufficient material. Even if the first cell sampling is calculated to be from the center of the lesion, cells should be obtained also from the periphery. Some tumors will have fibrous or necrotic tissue in the center, with neoplastic cells more in the periphery. Representative cells can thus be sampled only from the periphery. We recommend changing the position of the needle 1 to 4 mm from the first calculation, depending upon the size of the mammographic lesions, to assure that representative cells are sampled. Usually, three needle passes will give adequate material. Tumors presenting as clusters of calcifications sometimes need four or five passes from different parts. The calcifications may represent an in situ tumor, which may be situated within fat tissue, especially if there is no increased density or parenchymal distortion. If only two or three passes are performed, epithelial cells may be difficult to sample in sufficient number from a DCIS. This is especially important to consider if the calcifications are within only one duct, where the total length of the calcified part may be 1 to 3 cm and the diameter of the duct is less than a millimeter.

Cell preparation and stains

The sampled cells are smeared onto glass slides. Stains applied to wet-fixed material as well as those applied after air drying of the cells may be used. The method of fixation and the stains employed will depend upon the collaborating cytopathologist. Air-dried smears may be easier to handle, and the fixation is reported to be more constant. May-Grunwald-Giemsa (MGG) is satisfactory for air-dried specimens, but quick stains can also be used and will allow evaluation of the material (at least quantity of cells) before the patient leaves. In addition, more cells can be obtained if the samples are not adequate. Spraying with fixatives or immersing in 95% ethanol is done before Papanicolaou staining, used especially for membranes, nucleoli, and nuclear chromatic material. Many pathologists prefer Papanicolaou instead of MGG, but problems with loss of cells in the fixation medium have been reported when stains are applied to wet-fixed material.

Role of the preoperative morphologic diagnosis with nonpalpable lesions

The main advantages of cytomorphologic diagnosis of nonpalpable lesions are the same as for palpable ones. In many cases it is a reliable and cost-effective alternative to diagnostic surgical biopsy, thereby lowering the number of surgical biopsies of benign lesions.

Kopans[45] discussed problems caused by the increased number of open biopsies of benign lesions following the extended use of screening mammography. For both economic reasons and the negative physical and psychologic effects on the woman, we strive to reduce unnecessary surgical biopsies. Fine needle biopsy can accomplish this objective; but several requirements must be met: Extremely accurate needle placement, appropriate aspiration technique, and an experienced cytopathologist are needed if we are to replace open surgical biopsies for benign lesions with stereotactically derived cytology or histology specimens. One advantage when mammography and cytology suggest malignancy is that surgery can be performed as a therapeutic measure instead of a diagnostic one.

Masood et al.[58] reported results from 20 women prospectively evaluated with FNAB under mammographic guidance. Surgery was performed in all 20 patients. Successful localization and aspiration was achieved in 18 (90%). There was agreement between the cytologic and histologic diagnoses in 17 patients (94%). The authors suggested that mammographically guided fine-needle aspiration offers a safe, reliable, and cost-effective alternative to open biopsy of nonpalpable breast lesions.

Dent et al.[18] performed stereotactic aspiration cytology on 50 patients with 52 nonpalpable breast lesions. All underwent subsequent surgical biopsy. The aspiration did not give sufficient material in 23% of the lesions (which were small or poorly cellular, causing the inadequacy of the sample). The limitations were due to the sampling of cells rather than to tumor localization. Fifteen of the other 40 patients had benign lesions, and 10 had malignant tumors by mammography and cytology. These patients could have been spared diagnostic surgery or had definitive surgery at the first stop. Only one patient with a mammographically "probably benign" and cytologically "benign" lesion had a malignancy. It was an invasive lobular cancer with a dominant in-situ component, that was discussed as an incidental finding.

Hann et al.[32] performed a prospective study of nonpalpable breast lesions using FNA. The lesions presented as mammographic masses or microcalcifications. Ninety-six were examined with FNA at the time of presurgery wire localization. All lesions with malignant or suspicious cytologic findings were verified histologically as cancer. Five of 12 with atypical cytologic findings were malignant at surgical biopsy. Two of 33 cytologically evaluated as benign were malignant. Adequate cell sampling was obtained from 23. A cytologically correct diagnosis of cancer was achieved from 21 of these. Insufficient cellular material was obtained from 35 of the 96; 16 showed marked fibrosis at histology. The authors concluded that FNA can aid in establishing a diagnosis of mammographically detected nonpalpable lesions.

Azavedo et al.[4] presented their experiences using stereotactic FNA in 2594 nonpalpable breast lesions examined with mammography and SFNB between 1983 and 1987. On the basis of this combined evaluation, 2005 (77.3%) were diagnosed as benign without need of surgery or further periodic controls. Only one of those turned out to be a cancer (14 months later). Follow-up was 1 to 6 years. These results hold true today, when the minimum follow-up is 4 years. Twenty-two patients were mammographically and cytologically diagnosed as having cancers but were not operated upon because of reasons other than their breast lesion. Surgery was performed in 567 patients. Breast cancers were histopathologically proved in 429 (PPV, 0.757). The ratio between benign and malignant tumors was 1:3. Many patients with nonpalpable tumors could thus be spared surgery by the combined evaluation of mammography and SFNB.

Jackson and Bassett[41] suggested that stereotactic fine-needle biopsy could make a cost-effective contribution to the management of nonpalpable breast lesions by reducing excisional biopsies for benign lesions. They saw the prospect for only one, instead of two, operations for definitely malignant tumors and noted that most investigators had reported an insufficient specimen rate of less than 25% when using stereotactic FNA.

Masood et al.[57] evaluated 100 mammographically detected lesions in 100 patients. All lesions were surgically removed after mammographically guided FNAB. Sufficient cellular material for cytologic evaluation was obtained in 91% of the cases. There were no false-positive diagnoses. Seventeen of the 20 malignant tumors were cytologically diagnosed preoperatively. Cytology alone had a PPV of 0.850. Thus, sensitivity was 85% and specificity 100%. The authors concluded that mammographically guided FNAB is a safe, reliable, and cost-effective alternative to open biopsy of nonpalpable breast lesions.

Helvie et al.[33] reported results from radiographically guided FNAB in 215 nonpalpable lesions. They used a coordinate grid localization system. Seventy-four lesions were operated upon. Forty-one were malignant (PPV, 0.554) The aspirates were categorized into four cytologic groups or as simple cysts. Based on the most stringent cytologic criteria, sensitivity for detection of cancer was 97% and specificity 94%, but only 46% of the aspirates were representative. The sensitivity and specificity were 68% and 97% when based on less stringent criteria. These authors emphasized that mammographic findings and cytologic results must be integrated when the decision is made how to manage a nonpalpable lesion.

Lofgren et al.[54] examined 219 nonpalpable breast lesions submitted to SFNB. Their therapeutic decisions were made after correlation of the mammographic and cytologic findings. Representative cytologic samples were obtained in 74% of the lesions. The sensitivity was 93%, and the specificity 97% when only cases with representative cytologic yields were considered.

Fajardo et al.,[23] evaluating FNA in 100 women who had undergone surgical excisional biopsy after stereotactic FNA, found 70 lesions benign and 30 malignant. The sensitivity of fine-needle aspiration cytology in their series was 77%, and the specificity 100%. For mammography they were 73% and 79%. The authors suggested that stereotactic mammography–guided FNA could reduce the number of breast biopsies performed for benign lesions.

Parker et al.[68] did stereotactic breast biopsies with 18-, 16-, and 14-gauge cutting needles and a biopsy gun in 103 patients. Surgery was performed after the stereotactic biopsy. There was agreement between the cytologic and histologic results in 89 cases (87%), including 14 of 16 cancers (PPV, 0.875). These authors found that large-gauge automated percutaneous biopsy was an acceptable alternative to surgical biopsy.

Dowlatshahi et al.[20] described results from a prospective study of double diagnosis of nonpalpable breast lesions. Mammography and SFNB were combined when adequate tissue was aspirated for cytologic examination. Mammography was performed on 264 occult lesions preoperatively. Both mammographic appearance and stereotactic FNA results were given scores on a scale of 0 (benign) to 5 (malignant). Histologically, 53 proved to be cancer. There were 97 benign lesions. If the total threshold score for open biopsy had been set to 2, 14% of the lesions would have proved histologically benign (PPV, 0.860). There would have been no false-negative results. If the threshold score had been raised to 4, 40% of the operated lesions would have been benign, with two false-negatives in cases that had cancer in situ. Adequate cytologic tissue was obtained from 150 lesions. The authors reported that it was possible to identify many of the benign lesions without surgery and spare these women an open surgical biopsy (with its attendant cost, morbidity, and resultant breast deformity in some patients).

TISSUE CHARACTERISTICS TO ATTAIN THE MAXIMUM INFORMATION FROM SFNB

With 17 years' experience at the Karolinska Hospital we have learned some unusual aspects of the stereotactic fine-needle biopsy procedure. We will now share this knowledge, gained from this experience, with the readers of this book.

Every single true mammographic finding has a histologic explanation as to why it looks the way it does. Therefore a radiologist can confirm an opinion on most mammographic abnormalities by noting resistance offered (the feel of the needle as it goes into the lesion) before the cytology specimen is analyzed. This is very important to the proper interpretation of an SFNB procedure.

The findings of concern on a mammogram are (1) densities and (2) calcifications without or with an accompanying density. Calcifications can appear within fat or nonfat.

Density of lesions

Densities on a mammogram represent many things. Lobules with glands, ducts, fibrous/sclerotic tissue, blood vessels, cysts, tumor, etc. appear as densities.

Does this mean that not every density is likely to yield epithelial cells on a cytology smear? The answer must be a qualified "yes." In cases with many lobules the mammogram will show dense breasts and a needle inserted will always get abundant epithelial cells. It is the resistance offered by the area at the tip of the needle that is "normal" as compared to other lesions.

If a density represents a cyst, then the resistance at the tip of the needle will immediately decrease as the needle goes through the capsule into the fluid-filled lumen and the aspirate will contain protein-rich fluid, often with groups of apocrine-type cells. On the other hand, if a density represents fibrous/sclerotic tissue with or without fibroblasts, then the resistance will often be greater than in so-called "normal" tissue consisting of only lobules.

We all know that malignancies are harder than normal tissue; but they seldom feel as hard as fibrotic or sclerotic tissues when penetrated by a needle. Malignancies often give a special type of resistance on FNA, comparable to that felt when a needle is inserted into a ripe pear. The resistance of a fibrous lesion, on the other hand, resembles more that of an unripe pear or a rubber eraser. Moreover, the fibrous lesion will not yield many cells by aspiration because it has much collagen, which is very difficult to aspirate. The less cellular a fibrous tissue is, the less chance there will be of obtaining any diagnostic material by aspiration alone. In such cases the Rotex needle is of great value. It can be slowly twisted back and forth into the lesion, drilling its way into the tough substance and collecting stromal fragments in its grooves.

A well-circumscribed lesion of moderate to moderately high density is usually due to one of four common findings: (1) a cyst, (2) a fibroadenoma, (3) a mucinous cancer, or (4) a papillary tumor. From these four differential diagnostic alternatives, a qualified assumption can be made based on the feel of the inserting needle. A vast experience has taught us to differentiate these lesions by their characteristic resistance upon needle penetration. In the case of a *cyst,* resistance will immediately decrease as the needle enters the fluid-filled lumen. In the case of a *fibroadenoma,* resistance will be more than that of the preceding breast tissue, so that a slight increase in toughness is felt as the needle enters the lesion. The cellular yield may or may not be very rich depending upon the stroma of the lesion: the more sclerotic, the less the cellular yield. However, the Rotex needle will gather at least stromal fragments, with or without epithelial cells, and this finding incorporated into the mammographic image of a well-circumscribed lesion means fibroadenoma—even if the cytopathologist does not have all the morphologic criteria (e.g., myoepithelial cells and myxoid stroma). In the case of a *mucinous carcinoma,* the sample material will always be enough (because of colloid and epithelial cells) to make this diagnosis. A *papillary tumor* is a special entity that almost always will result in blood smears (bloody aspirates), which increases the suspicion of malignancy even

before the cytology specimen has been stained. In such cases we do the preoperative marking by injecting a carbon suspension directly after sampling enough material for cytologic assessment. This means that the patient is ready for subsequent surgery even before the cytomorphologic diagnosis. She does not have to return to the radiologist for a localization procedure on the day of the operation.

These are some of the ways that information from an SFNB procedure and cytomorphology can be incorporated into the mammographic assessment of a nonpalpable finding. In addition to correlation with mammography and the tactile sensation of needle penetration, the SFNB procedure itself acts as an independent separate parameter in the total assessment of a lesion.

Calcifications without accompanying density

Microcalcifications alone, without an accompanying density, may be within small ducts or lobules, but also may be scattered in fatty tissue. In such cases the abnormal mammogram should be very clear. When the background is only fat, the cellular yield may be only fat cells. In addition, the needle will not encounter any "toughness" while being inserted. If the calcifications are within ducts or lobules and these ducts or lobules are so small that they do not produce a density on the mammogram, the number of cells may be very limited. In other words, lack of resistance at the tip of the needle with a cytology specimen of just fat and blood cells is consistent with the mammographic pattern and anatomy of the area when calcifications are of benign appearance and situated in fatty tissue.

Calcifications with accompanying density

These lesions have the same characteristic tactile findings as for densities alone. The presence of calcification within a density does not alter its resistance to a needle puncture.

USE OF THE SFNB MATERIAL

The stereotactic fine needle biopsy technique is not limited to gathering cell material for cytomorphologic diagnosis and preoperative marking. It can also be used to collect cell material for further analyses of a tumor.

Azavedo et al.[6] demonstrated reproducibility in the composition of cellular material from multiple fine-needle aspirates in human malignant tumors. Several tumors were aspirated five times each with different needles and syringes and separate smears were produced. The smears were analyzed with single cell cytospectrophotometry to measure the DNA distribution patterns, which proved to be identical in the different samples. These observations were confirmed by measuring aliquots with flow DNA cytometry. This research provides the background needed to use the SFNB samples to obtain biologic information of a nonpalpable breast tumor prior to surgery. The information is useful to planning adequate therapy. Mammographically detected tumors can be extremely small, and there may not be enough material to perform important biologic analyses postoperatively. Thus, preoperative biologic analysis of the stereotactically derived cells may help design tumor specific therapy and establish the prognosis, even of small lesions.[3] We use this technique to provide clinicians with not only diagnostic but also prognostic information (DNA-ploidy) and information that can offer a patient specific therapies (estrogen receptor status, ER). Azavedo et al.[5] showed that both DNA and ER analysis can be done on smears obtained from nonpalpable tumors. Today immunocytochemistry is widely used to provide more biologic information, and molecular biology has opened the frontier to new techniques such as in situ hybridization studies on cytologic smears. Cells collected through SFNB have multiple purposes; SFNB is a multipurpose technique.

PREOPERATIVE LOCALIZATION TECHNIQUES

Mammography was introduced to improve the evaluation of patients with palpable breast lesions and other breast symptoms. Nonpalpable lesions, however, were also increasingly detected. Many of these demanded surgery, but it was difficult for the surgeon to find and excise them. Thus it became obvious that they would have to be radiologically localized preoperatively to guide surgery and minimize the loss of breast tissue. Different marking methods were invented in response to this need.

Noninvasive methods of localization

Noninvasive methods include measuring on the mammogram the distance from the lesion to the nipple and the nipple to the lesion in an effort to transform the mammographic lesional position to the operating room situation with the breast noncompressed and in a supine position. The calculated site of the lesion is marked on the skin or expressed as time on a dial or as intersections on a coordinate presentation of the breast. These noninvasive marking methods convey the approximate location of the lesion and may be used if the lesion is just beneath the skin, but they will result in an unnecessarily large excision of breast tissue if the lesion is situated deeper and/or the breast is large. The less reliable the marking of the lesion position, the more extensive the surgical excision has to be and the greater the risk of both nonradical excision of tumor and disfigurement of the breast (along with a poor cosmetic result).

Invasive methods of localization

Straight needles. For years the tip of a straight needle has been used to mark the site of a lesion. Threatt et al.[82] presented their technique for preoperatively localizing

clusters of microcalcifications by passing a long 25-gauge needle, usually to its hub, through the skin without anesthesia. Craniocaudal and lateromedial mammograms verified its position. It was then taped in place. The procedure was performed immediately prior to surgery or the afternoon before. No complications were reported. Libshitz et al.[52] reported inserting a straight needle after orthogonal mammographic localization. They verified its position by further mammograms and taped it to the skin. Sometimes two needles were used. Bigongiari et al.,[11] who also used a straight needle, presented their results in 90 cases. They taped the hub of the needle to the skin before the breast was radiographed in two planes, and reported that the lesion itself was often palpable through the incision. Histologic identification of calcifications after localization by specimen radiography or exact correlation between slide and image were the criteria used to establish the accuracy of location. Their success rate was approximately 90%, with only seven documented failures. They felt that poor communication between the surgeon and radiologist and inadequate mutual understanding of the localization procedure were the major causes of the failures. Becker[9] described a method whereby a needle was placed in the breast after measurements were transferred from the craniocaudal and mediolateral mammographic views to the breast. The depth of the lesions determined the length of the needle. He used 21- to 23-gauge needles, verifying needle position by craniocaudal and mediolateral projections. The technique was evaluated in more than 100 cases, and the lesions found to be usually within 1 cm of the needle tip. When the needle was more than 1 cm outside the lesion, a second needle was inserted with the first used as a guide. The first needle was then removed.

To prevent its pulling out of the breast, a straight needle must be carefully fixed to the skin and long enough to pass through and beyond the lesion. The surgeon can palpate its course, which may help in finding the lesion, although the needle can migrate before the scheduled surgery. To prevent dislodgement, Sitzman[75] designed a needle that could be secured with a skin suture. He reported his success (10 instances) in nine patients. The needle was fashioned from the stylet of a 3.5-inch 20-gauge spinal needle with the hub removed. The cut end of the needle was bent into a tight 3 mm loop. Three lengths of the needle were used depending on the depth of the lesion. After insertion of the needle to its full length, it was taped to the skin and two views were exposed to control its position. Then it was secured to the skin with a single 3-0 silk suture.

Straight needles have been used to mark the lesion in only two dimensions. Muhlow[61] presented a device that he developed for better marking precision that consists of a compression plate with holes and a film holder under the breast. This permits the film to be removed without releasing the compression. The needle is inserted through the hole closest to the lesion. He suggested that two marker needles be introduced from different angles and their intersection be used to guide the surgeon. Novak[65] directed the needle by means of an optical system with two light indicators adjusted to a coordinate system on the upper mammogram compression plate. This allowed for precise positioning of the needle.

Hookwire systems. Hooked markers were invented to prevent shifting between the localization procedure and the operation. Frank et al.[25] reported their experience with a commercially available device that consisted of a needle with an inner barbed wire stylet. Hoehn et al.[34] presented their updated results using this wire in 62 patients (66 needle localizations). The age of the patients was 39 to 80 years (mean 58.3), and the wire was found to be an effective flexible guide that resisted migration.

Many authors have noted the main disadvantage with a hookwire protruding from the tip of the introducing needle is that once the hook is set it cannot be repositioned. If the first position of the hook is not precise enough, either its erroneous relation to the lesion must be carefully established to guide the surgeon or an additional marker must be placed and both markers removed at the time of surgery. However, Hall and Frank[31] reported that a poorly situated guide can be extracted during localization or surgery by steady traction on its protruding end, with only some minor tissue damage. Their series included 40 patients who underwent breast wire localization during a 3-year period. In 28 cases the lesion remained nonpalpable during surgery. In 24 of these the suspicious area was completely or almost completely removed with the first biopsy. In two the area was excised on a second or third biopsy, and in two it was not removed during the initial operation. In one third (9 patients) a second wire had to be placed. Homer[38] presented results from 16 cases in which the Frank breast biopsy guide was used. This device consists of a 25-gauge 9.5 cm long wire with its distal 4 mm bent like a hook. The wire is contained in a 9 cm 25-gauge needle. All excisions were verified by specimen radiography, and all lesions successfully excised. In three patients a second wire was inserted because the first was farther than 1.5 cm from the lesion. In two of these, the wire migrated into the breast and was totally retracted.

Loh et al.[55] used a 22-gauge spinal needle with a stylet for localization. The proximal end of the stylet was cut, and the distal 5 mm bent backward like a hook. The hook protruded from the needle but was flattened against the sheath. If the position of the hook was not close enough to the lesion, a second stylet was introduced without removing the first one. Olesen and Blichert-Toft,[66] using a combination of the Muhlow localization system and the Frank needle, reported further improvement of the technique by ensuring a perpendicular introduction of the needle through the hole in the compression plate. They used a device consisting of a cut cannula melted vertically through and fused to a small plate of Plexiglas. The device was placed over the appropriate hole of the compression plate and the needle was thus steered to pass perpendicularly through the tumor. A modified hooked needle technique was presented by Kopans and De Luca,[46] who bent a wire into a spring hook that could be contained within the needle lumen and be reformed to hook into the breast tissue upon its release from the needle tip. The needle could thus be repositioned accurately prior to releasing the hook.

J- or X-shaped wires in combination with straight needles have been used to improve the anchorage of marker needles. Homer[36] (1979) has reported his experience with a curved-end retractable wire. The system consists of a 20-gauge needle, a wire with a distal end assuming a J configuration, and a plastic stabilizer. Both the needle and the wire remain in the breast until surgery. The guide is not transectable and can be palpated by the surgeon. Homer and Pile-Spellman[39] reported on a series of 100 consecutive occult lesions localized with a curved-end retractable wire system. The failure rate for initial excision was 4%. Arnesson et al.[2] presented their results from surgical biopsies of 314 nonpalpable breast lesions detected in a mammography screening program. Cancer was histopathologically proved in 129 cases. Novak's equipment[65] was used to direct the needle. A metal thread with a hook on the tip was put through the needle when the tip of the needle was correctly placed. Satisfactory results were achieved in 95% of the initial biopsies. The authors found that the failures were mostly due to the surgeon's lack of familiarity with the method. Only one failure was caused by an incorrect location. Urrutia et al.[83] presented a system with a retractable barb. They used a 20-gauge needle with a separate fenestration 1.5 cm from the tip. The hookwire projects out through the hole from the side of the needle when the position of the needle is correct. This type of needle can be repositioned. Another advantage is that it gives stiffness with great holding power. The authors found that the needle system eliminates failure caused by dislodgement or transection of the localizing wire.

Some problems with wire localization techniques have been reported. Homer[37] described transection of the wire. Previously, Hall and Frank[31] pointed out the importance of using a long guide and not cutting off excess wire outside the breast before mammography or biopsy. A short guide may retract completely into the breast because of change in body position or movements of the arm. This is especially a problem if the guide is introduced into the pectoralis musculature when a deep situated lesion is localized. Homer[36] also reported the migration of wire despite securing its external end with tape or a "bulldog" clamp. This complication was eliminated when a screw clamp was used to secure the end. Davis et al.[17] has also reported on migration of the wire.

Kopans and Swann[47] discussed different marking techniques. They suggested that if a simple needle technique is used the needle must be longer than the distance to the lesion, since the tip must be placed beyond the lesion to remain along the needle shaft despite the different positions of the breast at localization and at surgery. The authors found a stiff needle to be advantageous but that the technique provides only two-dimensional accuracy. They therefore used wires to give an accurate three-dimensional localization. If a hookwire system is used, they suggested that the tip of the needle be placed at the same level as the hook. For the springhook wire system the lesion should be located along the thickened distal segment of the wire; and the wire must be long enough, or it may disappear into the breast as the breast reexpands following the release of compressions.

Other types of metal markers. Barth et al.[8] presented a localization technique utilizing metal pellets were inserted to mark the nonpalpable lesion. The same year (1977) Nordenström and Zajicek[64] introduced a technique wherein hooked stainless steel suture threads were inserted to the edge of the lesion. They did not leave any marking out to the skin. Thus, even if the marking of lesions in the breast was accurate, this technique proved to be of little help to the surgeon and was therefore abandoned.

Dyes. Preoperative markings with dyes was attempted as early as 1965 by Hollender and Gros.[35] Dyes and combinations of dye with radiographic contrast medium have subsequently been used. Kopans and Swann[47] concluded that radiographic contrast may make it more difficult to evaluate specimen radiographs despite the use of very small amounts. The patient may have an adverse (though small) reaction to the contrast medium.

Methylene blue or Evans blue dye. Methylene blue or Evans blue has been used as a preoperative marking medium by many authors. Simon et al.[74] injected a mixture of less than 0.1 ml of Ethiodol and 0.1 ml Evans blue through a 20-gauge needle inserted into the breast tissue as close to the lesion as possible after orthogonal localization. The tissue was, thereby, colored. Horns and Arndt[40] described their experience with injection of 0.1 ml of equal parts of Evans or Sky blue and radiopaque contrast medium through a satisfactorily positioned needle. A small amount of air was flushed through the needle before withdrawal to expel the contents. They suggested that surgery follow within 4 hours of injection because of dye diffusion. No complications were found in more than 70 successful localizations. Loh et al.[55] reported that even small amounts of methylene blue injected immediately before surgery sometimes resulted in diffusion of the dye into a large volume of breast tissue. Svane[77] used methylene blue alone or in combination with water-soluble radiographic contrast medium but abandoned them because of indistinct marking resulting from rapid diffusion into surrounding

tissue. Dufrane et al.[21] suggested that this method be given up or reserved just for immediate preoperative localization because of the rapid diffusion into surrounding tissue and the disappearance of dye within a few hours.

Toluidine blue dye. Toluidine blue has the same disadvantages as methylene blue. Czarnecki et al.[16] presented their experiences with preoperative localization using toluidine blue in 20 cases. They found no difference in distance of diffusion or color intensity between toluidine blue and methylene blue. The most important disadvantage of toluidine was its rapid disappearance (a few hours).

Carbon suspension. Carbon as a marking medium was introduced in 1978 to solve the problem of rapid diffusion and, thereby, the necessity of marking close to the time of surgery. Svane[78] discussed her experiences with it in 56 nonpalpable lesions. The lesion was marked with a 4% aqueous suspension of carbon injected through a needle from the lesion out to the skin while the needle was being withdrawn. Inert medical-grade carbon suspended in water leaves a black tract of carbon particles in the breast. A black point of carbon less than 1 mm marks the site of injection in the skin, like a tattoo. Thirty-one of the 56 lesions were excised at other hospitals. In most cases surgery was performed on the same day as localization, but in one case 57 days elapsed between marking and surgery and there was no diffusion of the carbon trail. Nor were any complications reported. Since 1979 the procedure has been the only marking method used at Karolinska Hospital, and we now have experience using carbon to mark more than 1800 nonpalpable lesions. Stereotactic technique has been used to determine the relation of the lesion to the needle tip, with no complications reported.

The main advantages of the carbon suspension technique are that it:

- Is accurate, easy, and rapid to perform
- Gives a distinct marking without diffusion into surrounding tissue
- Can be performed days or even weeks in advance of surgery
- Can be done at a time convenient for both the surgeon and the patient, independent of the localization
- Is well accepted by the patient (no skin incision and no anesthesia necessary)
- Is inert and thus does not interfere with the determination of biologic parameters (e.g., estrogen and progesterone receptors, DNA measurements)
- Is not radiopaque and thus disturbs neither radiography of the specimen nor the histopathologic examination (Indeed, carbon may help the pathologist find the exact area of concern, especially if the tumor has presented radiologically as microcalcifications only when there is no visible tumor to the naked eye.)

Dufrane et al.,[21] evaluating different marking techniques, found the carbon suspension to be a promising tracer because of its high patient tolerance, efficiency, and effectiveness and its low costs.

ADVANTAGES OF THE SFNB TECHNIQUE

Stereotactic fine-needle biopsies with the Rotex needle, or aspirations with a 22-gauge or 25-gauge needle, can make a substantial contribution to the diagnosis of breast cancer. Until more experience is gained with them in the United States, interim stage large-bore stereotactic biopsies of nonpalpable lesions seem a reasonable recourse. Either of these techniques offers considerable advantages over the prior approach of direct surgical biopsy in patients with newly palpated lesions, or nonpalpable lesions detected on screening mammography. Asymptomatic patients with prospective breast lesions will usually benefit from either cytologic or histologic materials gathered prior to, or in lieu of, an open surgical biopsy.

The preoperative diagnosis of breast cancer makes it considerably easier to manage a case adequately. When the cytology or histology reveals a benign lesion, or if the combination of cytology and mammography suggests benignity, unnecessary diagnostic surgery may well be avoided. This addition to the diagnostic armamentarium will substantially diminish the need for open surgical biopsy. Thus the cost, discomfort, and anxiety induced by the frequent use of open surgical biopsy for what turns out to be a benign lesion can be largely avoided by the incorporation of either cytologic or histologic data obtained through stereotactic techniques.

In addition to the utility of a preoperative diagnosis, SFNB allows for the preoperative localization of a lesion without hook wires or other more traumatic approaches to marking a suspected breast lesion. Carbon localization with stereotactic techniques is an accurate means of identifying exquisitely small breast lesions disclosed by mammography and should permit considerably less normal breast tissue to be removed at surgical biopsy.

Finally, the addition of SFNB or histology techniques allows for characterization of the biologic aspects of a breast lesion without surgery. Cytology can yield sufficient cells for the identification of DNA-ploidy, estrogen receptors, and other cell markers relevant to the clinical therapy and prognosis of a breast lesion. In addition, it can provide information prior to surgery on the exact nature of the lesion under consideration, and thus help in managing inoperable patients. Cytologic assessment with SFNB is a way to get fresh tumor material from microscopically unidentified nonpalpable tumors for biologic analysis.

Thus, the combination of properly performed and interpreted screening mammography with clinical breast examination and stereotactically guided biopsy can markedly improve on our ability to provide humane, accurate, and cost effective diagnosis of early breast cancer in asymptomatic women.

REFERENCES

1. Aardal NP, Skaarland E, Myking AO, et al: Fine needle aspiration cytology of the breast. A simple method? *Tidsskr Nor Laegeforen* 109(23):2284-2286, 1989.
2. Arnesson L-G, Fagerberg G, Grontoft O, Lundstrom B: Surgical biopsy of non-palpable mammary lesions, *Acta Chir Scand* 152:97-101, 1986.
3. Azavedo E, Fallenius A, Svane G, Auer G: Nuclear DNA content, histological grade, and clinical course in patients with nonpalpable mammographically detected breast adenocarcinomas, *Am J Clin Oncol* 13(1):23-27, 1990.
4. Azavedo E, Svane G, Auer G: Stereotactic fine-needle aspiration biopsy in 2594 mammographically detected nonpalpable lesions, *Lancet* 1:1033-1036, 1989.
5. Azavedo E, Svane G, Skoog L: Preoperative immunocytochemical analysis of the estradiol receptor in non-palpable human breast tumors, *Oncology* 8:318-321, 1990.
6. Azavedo E, Tribukait B, Konaka C, Auer G: Reproducibility of the cellular DNA distribution patterns in multiple fine needle aspirates from human malignant tumors, *Acta Pathol Microbiol Immunol Scand Sect A* 90:79-83, 1982.
7. Barrows GH, Anderson TJ, Lamb JL, Dixon JM: Fine-needle aspiration of breast cancer. Relationship of clinical factors to cytology results in 689 primary malignancies, *Cancer* 58(7):1493-1498, 1986.
8. Barth V, Behrends W, Haase W: Methode zur präoperativen Lokalisation nicht palpabler suspekter Mikroverkalkungen im Brustdrüsenkörper, *Radiologie* 17:219, 1977.
9. Becker W: Stereotactic localization of breast lesions, *Radiology* 133:238, 1979.
10. Bell DA, Hajdu SI, Urban J, Gaston JP: Role of aspiration cytology in the diagnosis and management of mammary lesions in office practice, *Cancer* 51(7):1182-1189, 1983.
11. Bigongiari LR, Fidler W, Skerker LB, Comstock C: Percutaneous needle localization of breast lesions prior to biopsy. Analysis of failure, *Clin Radiol* 28:419, 1977.
12. Bolmgren J, Jacobson B, Nordenström B: Stereotaxic instrument for needle biopsy of the mamma, *Am J Roentgenol* 129:121-125, 1977.
13. Butler JA, Vargas HI, Worthen N, Wilson SE: Accuracy of combined clinical-mammographic-cytologic diagnosis of dominant breast masses. A prospective study, *Arch Surg* 125:893-896, 1990.
14. Carlson GW, Ferguson CM: Needle aspiration cytology of breast masses, *American Surgeon* 53(4):235-237, 1987.
15. Cohen MB, Rodgers RP, Hales MS, et al: Influence of training and experience in fine-needle aspiration biopsy of breast. Receiver operation characteristics curve analysis, *Arch Pathol Lab Med* 111(6):518-520, 1987.
16. Czarnecki DJ, Feider HK, Splittgerber GF: Toluidine blue dye as a breast localization marker, *AJR* 153:261-263, 1989.
17. Davis PS, Wechsler RJ, Feig SA, March DE: Migration of breast biopsy localization wire, *AJR* 150:787-788, 1988.
18. Dent DM, Kirkpatrick AE, McGoogan E, et al: Stereotaxic localization and aspiration cytology of impalpable breast lesions, *Clin Radiol* 40:380-382, 1989.
19. Deschenes L, Fabia J, Meisels A, et al: Fine needle aspiration biopsy in the management of palpable breast lesions, *Can J Surg* 21(5):417-419, 1978.
20. Dowlatshahi K, Jokich PM, Kluskens LF, et al: A prospective study of double diagnosis of nonpalpable lesions of the breast, *Surg Gynecol Obstet* 172:121-124, 1991.
21. Dufrane P, Mazy G, Vanhaudenaerde C: Prebiopsy localization of nonpalpable breast cancer, *JBR-BTR* 73:401-404, 1990.
22. Erickson EJ, McGreevy JM, Muskett A: Selective nonoperative management of patients referred with abnormal mammograms, *Am J Surg* 160:659-664, 1990.
23. Fajardo LL, Davis JR, Wiens JL, Trego DC: Mammography-guided

stereotactic fine-needle aspiration cytology of nonpalpable lesions: prospective comparison with surgical biopsy results, *AJR* 155:977-981, 1990.

24. Fessia L, Ghiringhello B, Arisio R, et al: Accuracy of frozen section diagnosis in breast cancer detection. A review of 4436 biopsies and comparison with cytodiagnosis, *Pathol Res Pract* 179(1):61-66, 1984.

25. Frank HA, Hall FM, Steer ML: Preoperative localization of nonpalpable breast lesions demonstrated by mammography, *N Engl J Med* 295:259, 1976.

26. Franzen S, Zajicek J: Aspiration biopsy in diagnosis of palpable lesions of the breast. Critical review of 3479 consecutive biopsies, *Acta Radiol* 7(4):241-261, 1968.

27. Furnival CM, Hocking MA, Hughes HE, et al: Aspiration cytology in breast cancer. Its relevance to diagnosis, *Lancet* 2(7932):446-449, 1975.

28. Gautenbein H, Spieler P: Fine-needle aspiration biopsy of the breast. Frequency, indication, and accuracy studied on material from the Cytological Laboratory of the Pathology Institute, St. Gallen Canton Hospital, 1981-1984, *J Suisse Med* 116(44):1513-1518, 1987.

29. Gelabert JA, Hsiu JG, Mullen JT, et al: Prospective evaluation of the role of fine-needle aspiration biopsy in the diagnosis and management of patients with palpable solid breast lesions, *Am Surg* 56(4):263-267, 1990.

30. Grant CS, Goellner JR, Welch JS, Martin JK: Fine-needle aspiration of the breast, *Mayo Clin Proc* 61(5):377-381, 1986.

31. Hall FM, Frank HA: Preoperative localization of nonpalpable breast lesions, *AJR* 132:101-105, 1979.

32. Hann L, Ducatman BS, Wang HH, et al: Nonpalpable breast lesions: evaluation by means of fine needle aspiration cytology, *Radiology* 171(2):373-376, 1989.

33. Helvie MA, Baker DE, Adler DD, et al: Radiographically guided fine-needle aspiration of nonpalpable breast lesions, *Radiology* 174:657-661, 1990.

34. Hoehn JL, Hardacre JM, Swanson MK, Williams GH: Localization of occult breast lesions, *Cancer* 49:1142-1144, 1982.

35. Hollender LF, Gros CHM: Röntgenuntersuchung der klinisch nicht tastbaren Mammacarcinome, *Langenbeck Arch Klin Chir* 313:380-384, 1965.

36. Homer MJ: Percutaneous localization of breast lesions: experience with the Frank breast biopsy guide, *J Can Assoc Radiol* 30:238-241, 1979.

37. Homer MJ: Transection of the localization hooked wire during breast biopsy, *AJR* 141:929-930, 1983.

38. Homer MJ: Preoperative needle localization of nonpalpable breast lesions, *Hospimedica*, pp 42-47, Oct/Nov 1989.

39. Homer MJ, Pile-Spellman ER: Needle localization of occult breast lesions with a curved-end retractable wire: technique and pitfalls, *Radiology* 161:547-548, 1986.

40. Horns JW, Arndt RD: Percutaneous spot localization of nonpalpable breast lesions, *AJR* 127:253, 1976.

41. Jackson VP, Bassett LW: Stereotaxic fine-needle aspiration biopsy for nonpalpable breast lesions, *AJR* 154:1196-1197, 1990.

42. Johnsén C: Breast disease. A clinical study with special reference to diagnostic procedures, *Acta Chir Scand Suppl* 454:1-108, 1975.

43. Kiovuniemi AP: Fine-needle aspiration biopsy of the breast, *Ann Clin Res* 8(4):272-283, 1976.

44. Kline TS, Joshi LP, Neal HS: Fine needle aspiration of the breast: diagnoses and pitfalls. A review of 3545 cases, *Cancer* 44(4):1458-1464, 1979.

45. Kopans D: Fine-needle aspiration of clinically occult breast lesions, *Radiology* 170:313-314, 1989.

46. Kopans DB, DeLuca SA: A modified needle-hookwire technique to simplify preoperative localization of occult breast lesions, *Radiology* 145:211-212, 1980.

47. Kopans DB, Swann CA: Preoperative imaging-guided needle placements and localization of clinically occult breast lesions, *AJR* 152:1-9, 1989.

48. Kwok D, Chan M, Gwi E, Law D: Aspiration cytology in the management of breast lesions, *Aust NZ J Surg* 58:295-299, 1988.

49. Lamarque JL, Rodiere MJ: Breast biopsy. In Dondelinger RF, Rossi P, Kurdziel JD, Wallace S, editors: *Interventional radiology*, New York, 1990, Georg Thieme Verlag, pp 27-32.

50. Lamb J, Anderson TJ, Dixon MJ, Levack PA: Role of fine needle aspiration cytology in breast cancer screening, *J Clin Pathol* 40(7):705-709, 1987.

51. Langmuir VK, Cramer SF, Hood ME: Fine needle aspiration cytology in the management of palpable benign and malignant breast disease. Correlation with clinical and mammographic findings, *Acta Cytol* 33(1):93-98, 1989.

52. Libshitz HJ, Feig SA, Fetouch S: Needle localization of non-palpable breast lesions, *Radiology* 121:557, 1976.

53. Linsk J, Franzen S: Breast aspiration. In Linsk J, Franzen S, editors: *Clinical aspiration cytology,* Philadelphia, 1983, JB Lippincott, pp 105-138.

54. Löfgren M, Andersson I, Lindholm K. Stereotaxic fine-needle aspiration for cytologic diagnosis of nonpalpable breast lesions, *AJR* 154:1191-1195, 1990.

55. Loh CK, Perlman H, Harris JH, et al: An improved method for localization of nonpalpable breast lesions, *Radiology* 130:244-245, 1979.

56. Martin HE, Ellis EB: Biopsy by needle puncture and aspiration, *Ann Surg* 92:169-181, 1930.

57. Masood S, Frykberg ER, McLellan GL, et al: Prospective evaluation of radiologically directed fine-needle aspiration biopsy of nonpalpable breast lesions, *Cancer* 66:1480-1497, 1990.

58. Masood S, Frykberg ER, Mitchum D, et al: The potential value of mammographically guided fine-needle aspiration biopsy of nonpalpable breast lesions, *Am Surg* 55:226-231, 1989.

59. Meyer JE, Eberlein TJ, Stomper PC, Sonnenfeld MR: Biopsy of occult breast lesions. Analysis of 1261 abnormalities, *JAMA* 262:2341-2343, 1990.

60. Moskovic E, Sinnett HD, Parsons CA: The accuracy of mammographic diagnosis in surgically occult breast lesions, *Clin Radiol* 41:344-346, 1990.

61. Mühlow A: A device for precision needle biopsy of the breast at mammography, *AJR* 121:843-845, 1974.

62. Nordenström B: Stereotaxic screw needle biopsy of non-palpable breast lesions. In Logan MW, editor: *Breast carcinoma: the radiologist's expanded role,* New York, 1977, John Wiley, pp 313-318.

63. Nordenström B, Rydén H, Svane G: Breast. In Zornoza J, editor: *Percutaneous needle biopsy,* Baltimore, 1981, Wiliams & Wilkins, pp 43-55.

64. Nordenström B, Zajicek J: Stereotaxic needle biopsy and preoperative indication of non-palpable mammary lesions, *Acta Cytol* 21:350-351, 1977.

65. Novak R: Position-controlled needle aspiration biopsy at mammography, *Fortschr Geb Röntgenstr* 131:659-661, 1979.

66. Olesen KP, Blichert-Toft M: Preoperative needle-marking of nonpalpable breast lesions, *Fortschr Geb Röntgenstr* 131(3):331-332, 1979.

67. Painter RW, Clark WE, Deckers PJ: Negative findings on fine-needle aspiration biopsy of solid breast masses: patient management, *Am J Surg* 155(3):387-390, 1988.

68. Parker SH, Lovin JD, Jobe WE, et al: Stereotactic breast biopsy with a biopsy gun, *Radiology* 176:741-747, 1990.

69. Patel JJ, Gartell PC, Smallwood JA, et al: Fine needle aspiration cytology of breast masses: an evaluation of its accuracy and reasons for diagnostic failure, *Ann R Coll Surg Engl* 69(4):156-159, 1987.

70. Rangwala AF, Perez-Blanco M, Reilly J: Cytological diagnosis of breast cancer, *NJ Med* 86(11):859-865, 1989.

71. Rimsten A, Stenkvist B, Johanson H, Lindgren A: The diagnostic accuracy of palpation and fine-needle biopsy and an evaluation of their combined use in the diagnosis of breast lesions: report on a prospective study in 1244 women with symptoms, *Ann Surg* 182(1):1-8, 1975.

72. Rosen PP, Kimmel M: Occult breast carcinoma presenting with axillary lymph node metastases: a follow-up study of 48 patients, *Hum Pathol* 21:518-523, 1990.

73. Salter DR, Bassett AA: Role of needle aspiration in reducing the number of unnecessary breast biopsies, *Can J Surg* 24(3):311-313, 1981.

74. Simon N, Lesnick GJ, Lerer WN, Bachman AL: Roentgenographic localization of small lesions of the breast by the spot method, *Surg Gynecol Obstet* 134:572, 1972.

75. Sitzman SB: A new needle for pre-operative localization of non-palpable breast lesions, *Radiology* 131:533, 1979.

76. Somers RG, Young GP, Kaplan MJ, et al: Fine-needle aspiration biopsy in the management of solid breast tumors, *Arch Surg* 120(6):673-677, 1985.

77. Svane G: A stereotaxic technique for preoperative marking of nonpalpable breast lesions, *Acta Radiol [Diagn]* 24:145-151, 1983.

78. Svane G: Stereotaxic needle biopsy of non-palpable breast lesions. A clinic-radiologic follow-up, *Acta Radiol [Diagn]* 24:385-390, 1983.

79. Svane G, Silfverswärd C: Stereotaxic needle biopsy of non-palpable breast lesions. Cytologic and histologic findings, *Acta Radiol [Diagn]* 24:283-288, 1983.

80. Swann CA, Kopans DB, Koerned FC, et al: The halo sign and malignant breast lesions, *AJR* 149:1145-1147, 1987.

81. Thompson WR, Bowen JR, Dorman BA, et al: Mammographic localization and biopsy of nonpalpable breast lesions, *Arch Surg* 126:730-734, 1991.

82. Threatt B, Appelman H, Dow R, O'Rourke T: Percutaneous needle localization of clustered mammary microcalcifications prior to biopsy, *AJR* 121:839-842, 1974.

83. Urrutia EJ, Hawkins MC, Steinbach BG, et al: Retractable-barb needle for breast lesion localization: use in 60 cases, *Radiology* 169:845-847, 1988.

84. Wanebo HJ, Feldman PS, Wilhelm MC, et al: Fine needle aspiration cytology in lieu of open biopsy in management of primary breast cancer, *Ann Surg* 199(5):569-579, 1984.

85. Wollenberg NJ, Caya JG, Clowry LJ: Fine needle aspiration cytology of the breast. A review of 321 cases with statistical evaluation, *Acta Cytol* 29(3):425-429, 1985.

86. Zajdela A, Pilleron JP, Ennuyer A, Bataini P: Cytological examination. Solid breast tumors examined by means of fine-needle puncture, *J Gynecol Obstet Biol Reprod* 4(2):59-66, 1975.

ATLAS OF MAMMOGRAMS OF NONPALPABLE LESIONS

Mammography is one of the most demanding areas of radiology. Enormous responsibility is assumed in dealing with both screening and diagnostic examinations.

This atlas is designed to provide an opportunity to help you examine your current skills in detecting both subtle and more obvious breast lesions. The images in this atlas are comprised of mammography screening studies. Only routine mediolateral oblique and craniocaudal projections were initially available for interpretation. Each of the atlas studies became a diagnostic examination, requiring additional radiographic workup and stereotaxic fine-needle biopsy evaluation.

To simulate the situation faced in routine screening mammography interpretation, the reader is encouraged to review initial images before moving to any additional associated films. Each separate section of the atlas is devoted to a specific mammographic pattern. Line drawings accompany many case images to assist in locating both subtle lesions and studies with multiple abnormal radiographic patterns. The photographic range employed in reproducing original mammographic images is extremely variable (Chapter 3). Every effort has been made to reproduce the atlas images exactly to the original image. In some instances, it was necessary to sacrifice the breast silhouette in order to best demonstrate the areas of pathology. We encourage use of a magnifying glass to review the images, the same way one would perform routine interpretation of mammograms.

When promulgated and perpetuated by leading medical professionals, ideas, facts, and a few fallacies about mammography carry a weight of scientific truth. The more we learn about mammography, however, the more complex it becomes. Some of what we believed yesterday we find inappropriate today. Some of what we believe we know about mammography today we may believe is wrong tomorrow.

Applying traditional techniques while developing new ones requires open minds. Each new method contributes to improved breast cancer detection. Our increasing knowledge and skill will promote early cancer detection and thereby decrease deaths from breast cancer.

BIBLIOGRAPHY

Andersen JA, Carter D, Linell F: A symposium on sclerosing duct lesions of the breast, *Pathol Annu* 21(Pt 2):145-179, 1987.

Andersen JA, Gram JB: Radial scar in the female breast: a long-term follow-up study of 32 cases, *Cancer* 53:2557-2560, 1984.

Anderson TJ, Battersby S: Radial scars of benign and malignant breasts: comparative features and significance, *J Pathol* 147:23-32, 1985.

Bassett LW, Jahanshahi R, Gold RH, Fu YS: *Film screen mammography: an atlas of instructional cases,* New York, 1991, Raven.

Cahill CJ, Boulter PS, Gibbs NM, Price JL: Features of mammographically negative breast tumors, *Br J Surg* 68(12):882-884, 1981.

Dahnert W: *Radiology review manual: differential diagnosis of breast disease,* Baltimore, 1991, Williams & Wilkins.

Dutt PL, Page DL: Multicentricity of in situ and invasive carcinoma. In Bland KI, Copeland EM, eds: *The breast: comprehensive management of benign and malignant diseases,* Philadelphia, 1991, Saunders.

Gershon-Cohen J, Ingleby H: Roentgenography of fibroadenoma of the breast, *Radiology* 59:77-87, 1952.

Gormly L, Bassett L, Gold R: Positioning in film-screen mammography, *Appl Radiol,* July 1988.

Haus AG, Feig SA, Ehrlich SM, et al: Mammography screening: technology, radiation dose and risk, quality control, and benefits to society, *Radiology* 174:627-656, 1990.

Leis H: Prognostic parameters for breast cancer. In Bland KI, Copeland EM, eds: *The breast: comprehensive management of benign and malignant diseases,* Philadelphia, 1991, Saunders.

Lesser ML, Rosen PP, Kinne DW: Multicentricity and bilaterality in invasive breast carcinoma, *Surgery* 91:234-240, 1982.

Linell F, Ljungberg O, Anderson I: Breast carcinoma: aspects of early stages, progression and related problems, *Acta Pathol Microbiol Scand* A272(Suppl):1, 1980.

Miller AB: Screening and detection. In Bland KI, Copeland EM, eds: *The breast: comprehensive management of benign and malignant diseases,* Philadelphia, 1991, Saunders.

Page DL, Anderson TJ: *Diagnostic histopathology of the breast,* New York, 1987, Churchill Livingstone.

Peeters PH, Verbeek AL, Zielhuis GA, et al: Breast cancer screening in women over age 50: a critical appraisal (review), *Acta Radiol* 31(3):225-231, 1990.

Pierson KK, Wilkinson EJ: Malignant neoplasia of the breast: infiltrating carcinomas. In Bland KI, Copeland EM, eds: *The breast: comprehensive management of benign and malignant diseases,* Philadelphia, 1991, Saunders.

Roebuck EJ: *Clinical radiology of the breast,* Oxford, 1990, Heinemann.

Shehi LJ, Pierson KK: Benign and malignant epithelial neoplasms and dermatological disorders. In Bland KI, Copeland EM, eds: *The breast: comprehensive management of benign and malignant diseases,* Philadelphia, 1991, Saunders.

Sickles EA: Further experience with microfocal spot magnification mammography in the assessment of clustered breast microcalcifications, *Radiology* 137(Pt 1):9-14, 1980.

Sickles EA: Mammographic detectability of breast microcalcifications, *Am J Roentgenol* 139(5):913-918, 1982.

Souba WW: Evaluation and treatment of benign breast disorders. In Bland KI, Copeland EM, eds: *The breast: comprehensive management of benign and malignant diseases,* Philadelphia, 1991, Saunders.

Strax P: Detection of breast cancer, *Cancer* 66(Suppl):1336-1340, 1990.

Tabar L, Dean PB: *Teaching atlas of mammography,* ed 2, New York, 1985, Thieme-Stratton.

Chapter 7

BENIGN LESIONS

PATIENT 1

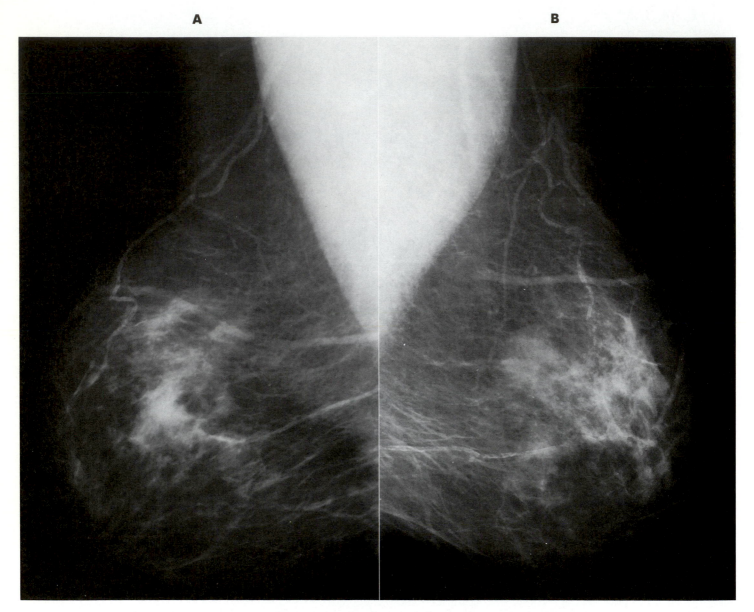

Fig. 7-1. A, Right MLO. **B,** Left MLO.

These images (Figs. 7-1 and 7-2) are from a screening mammogram of a 67-year-old asymptomatic woman with moderately lucent breasts. Do you see a worrisome mammographic appearance? Would you request additional workup for final mammographic interpretation of this screening examination?

A   B

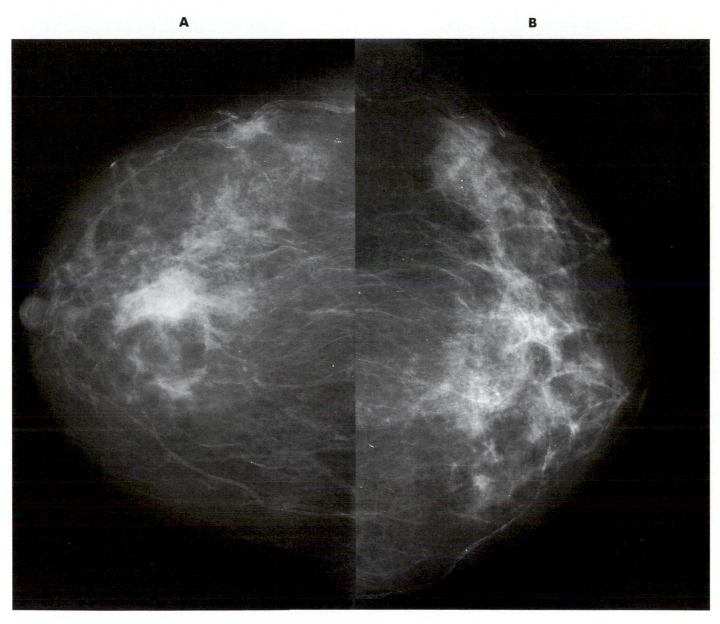

Fig. 7-2. A, Right CC. **B,** Left CC.

A   B

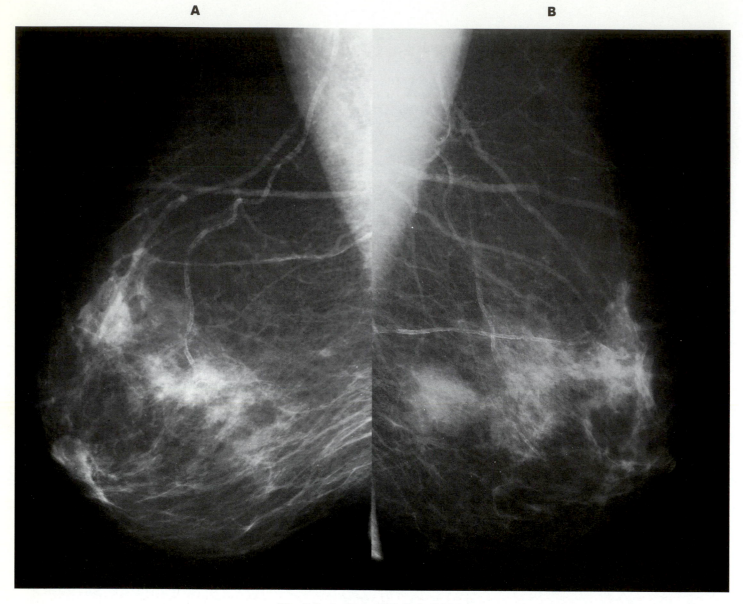

Fig. 7-3. A, Right LM. **B,** Left LM.

This woman's standard mammographic projections reveal a centrally located asymmetric density in her right breast, most clearly seen in Fig. 7-2, *A*. The area appears to be of medium density yet not greater than the density of surrounding glandular tissue. While this mammographic appearance is suggestive of a benign process, coned compression or magnified projection is recommended.

Margins of any breast density must be carefully evaluated. The coned, mediolateral oblique projection reveals minimal border irregularity but does not demonstrate distinct spiculated breast distortion typically associated with malignant lesions. Also on the coned projection, mixed densities in the center of the lesion disclose radiolucent areas indicative of fatty replacement of breast stroma (Fig. 7-4).

Stereotaxic fine-needle biopsy (SFNB) evaluation can confirm benignancy of a worrisome mammographic appearance; as in this case, the results of the stereotaxic procedure confirmed the density to be benign and surgical biopsy was unnecessary (Fig. 7-5). Supportively, no microcalcifications or other signs of malignancy are observed.

Instead of immediately performing open surgical biopsy on suspicious-looking areas in the breast, the SFNB procedure offers an initial practical alternative to evaluate benign- or malignant-appearing breast lesions. SFNB will produce the additional information to permit definitive breast diagnosis.

Code 3

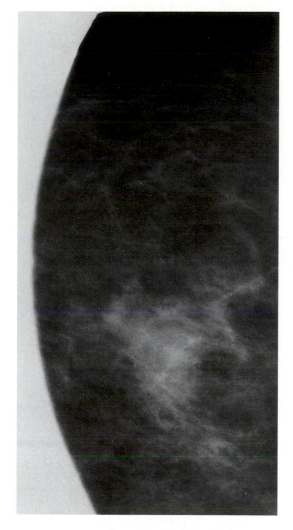

Fig. 7-4. Coned right MLO.

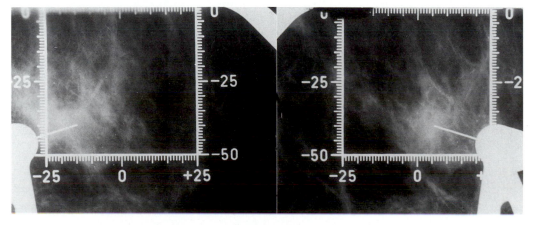

Fig. 7-5. SFNB.

PATIENT 2

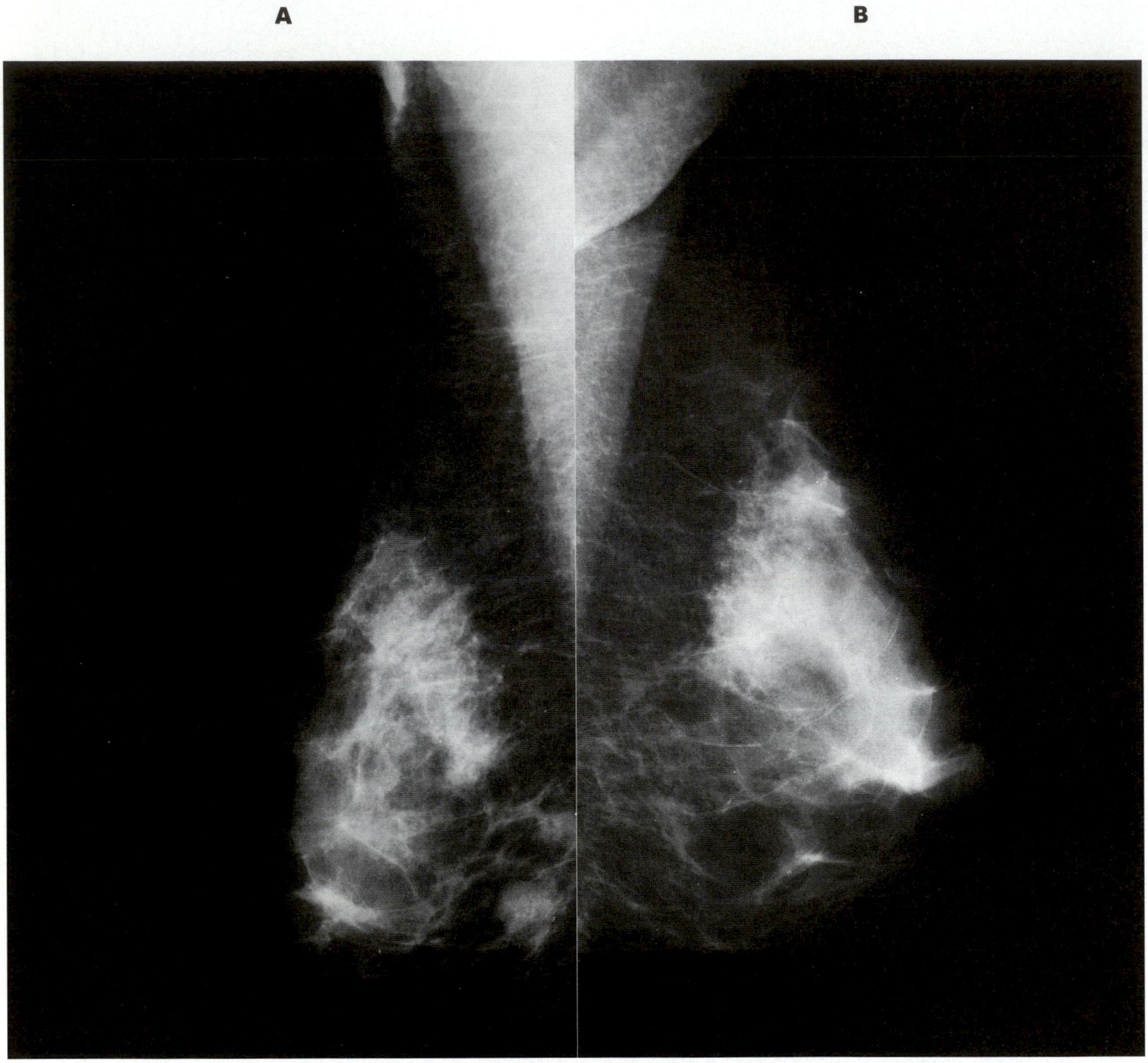

Fig. 7-6. A, Right MLO. **B,** Left MLO.

A 60-year-old asymptomatic physician with dense breasts underwent routine mammographic screening evaluation (Figs. 7-6 and 7-7).

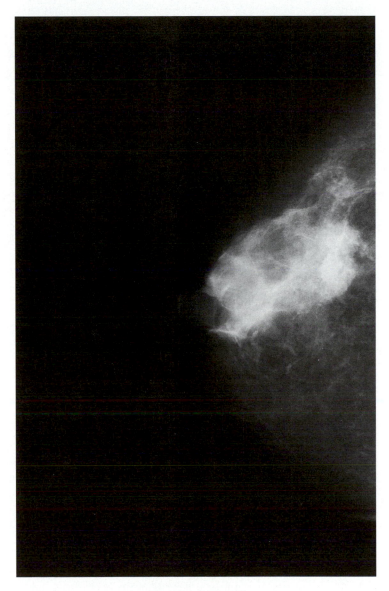

Fig. 7-7. Right CC.

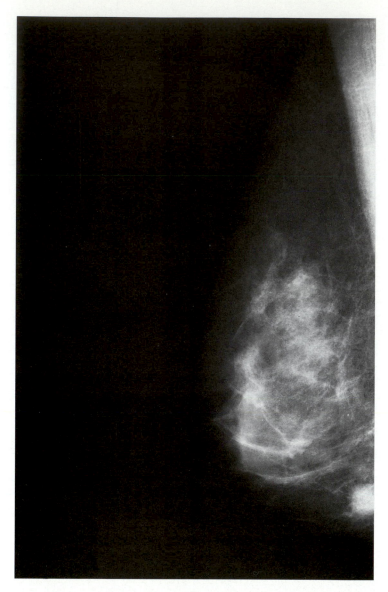

Fig. 7-8. Right LM.

A rounded density can be seen in the upper outer quadrant of the right breast (Fig. 7-7). The mammographic appearance of this density suggests a fibroadenoma. The fibroadenoma is the most common benign, solid breast lesion and is usually seen in younger women. However, fibroadenomas are not uncommon in the elderly. Often they undergo atrophy and calcify.[1] Unfortunately, its appearance often prompts surgery. The well-defined margins and the lesion's medium density, demonstrated on the coned mediolateral oblique projection, favor a benign diagnosis (Fig. 7-9).

In this woman, SFNB was performed and cytology proved negative for malignancy. Although fibroadenomas have no malignant potential and surgery was, in fact, unnecessary, in this case surgery was requested by the patient. Histology further substantiated a fibroadenoma (Fig. 7-10).

Code 3

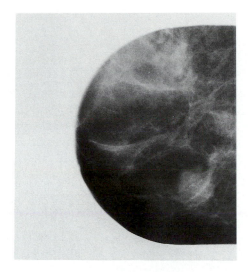

Fig. 7-9. Coned right MLO.

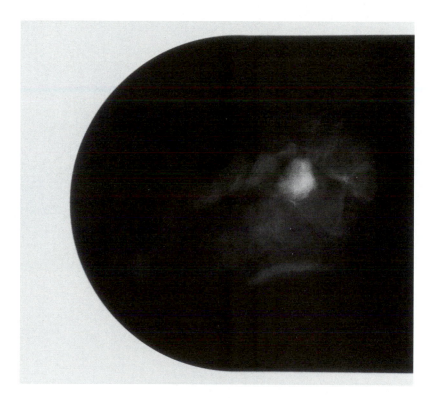

Fig. 7-10. Biopsy specimen.

PATIENT 3

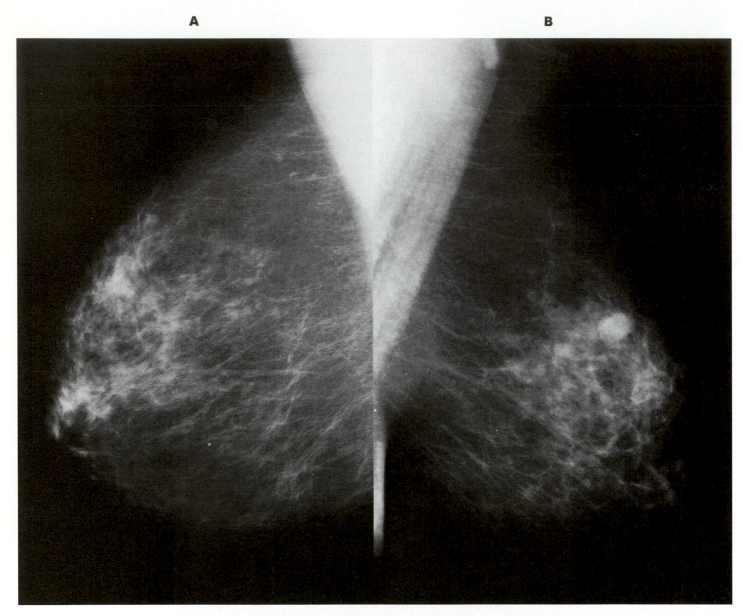

Fig. 7-11. A, Right MLO. **B,** Left MLO.

These images (Figs. 7-11 and 7-12) from a screening mammogram of a 68-year-old asymptomatic woman reveal a normal amount of breast parenchyma for her age.

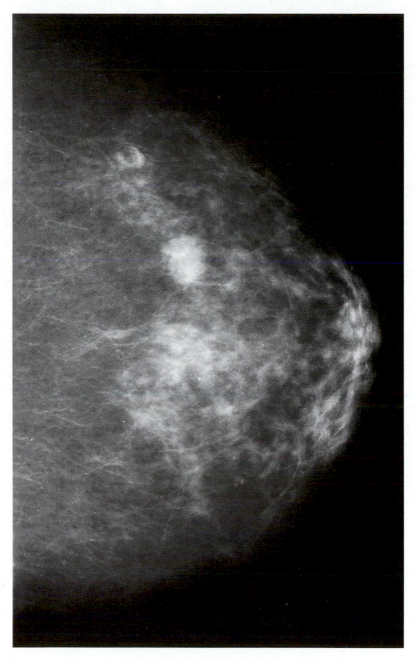

Fig. 7-12. Left CC.

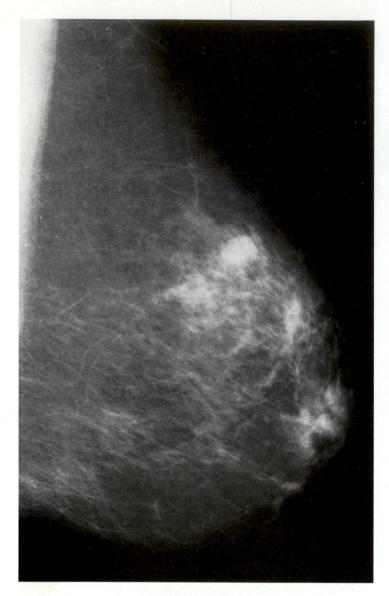

Fig. 7-13. Left LM.

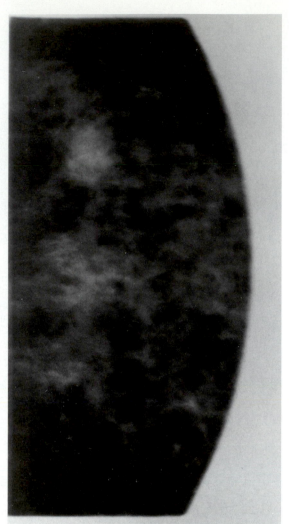

Fig. 7-14. Coned left CC.

In the upper outer quadrant of the left breast mammogram, a nonpalpable, circumscribed density with unsharp borders is identified (Fig. 7-11, *B*). The density does not exhibit clearly malignant features, and the mammographic appearance is initially suggestive of a fibroadenoma.[2]

Look carefully at the margins of this lesion (Fig. 7-13). It would be inappropriate to immediately rate this density as highly suspicious for malignancy because of some margin unsharpness. It is equally inappropriate, however, to consider this mammogram normal and the density benign. Additional coned compression views revealed persistent unsharp margins, warranting further investigation (Fig. 7-14).

SFNB evaluation was recommended and performed (Fig. 7-15). Cytology of the lesion showed benign epithelial cells. Surgical excision was still recommended in this case. Circumscribed lesions with persistently unsharp borders, whether malignant or benign, often have a similar mammographic appearance. Histology confirmed the diagnosis of fibroadenoma.

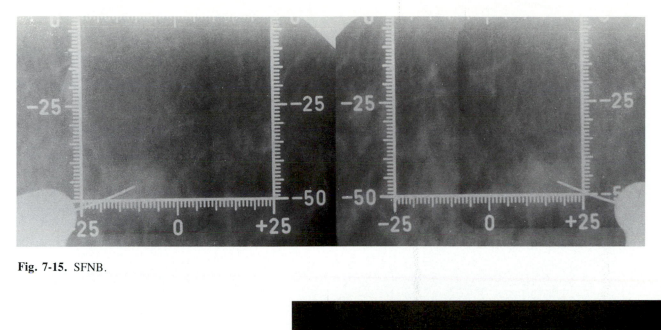

Fig. 7-15. SFNB.

It is important that each mammogram study be evaluated on its own merit and be correlated with individual mammographic features, clinical evaluation, and risk factors of the woman.

Code 3

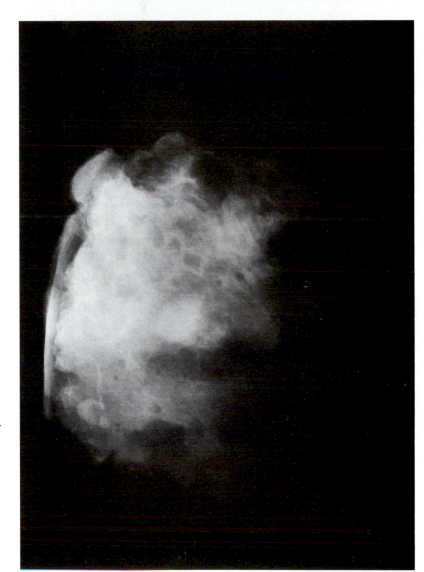

Fig. 7-16. Biopsy specimen.

PATIENT 4

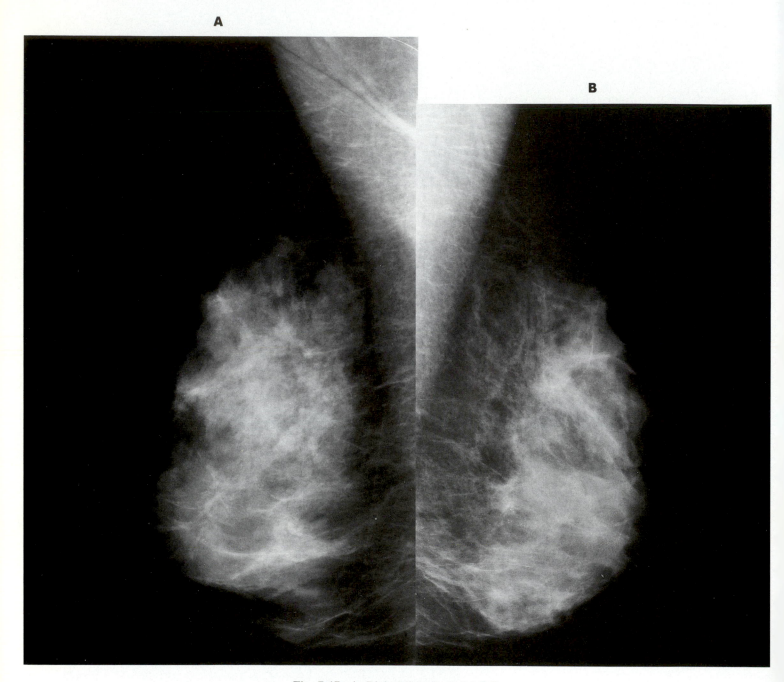

Fig. 7-17. A, Right MLO. **B,** Left MLO.

These images (Figs. 7-17 and 7-18) are from a screening mammogram of an asymptomatic 57-year-old woman with dense breasts.

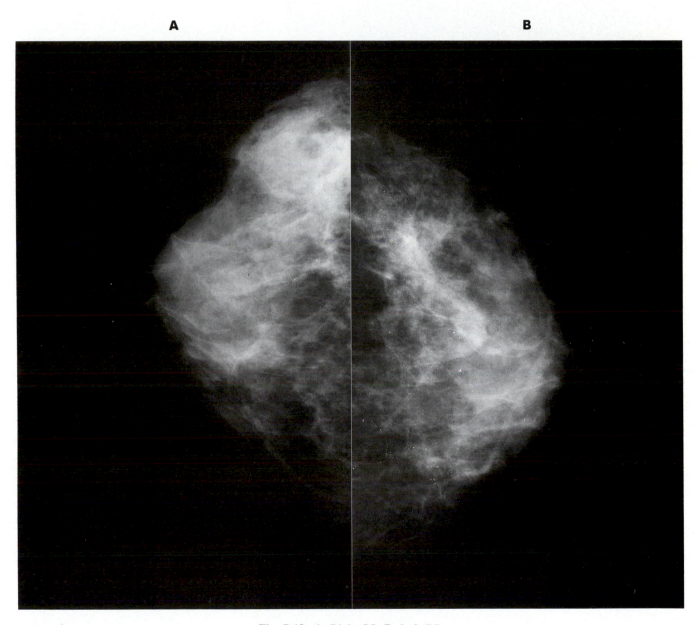

Fig. 7-18. A, Right CC. **B,** Left CC.

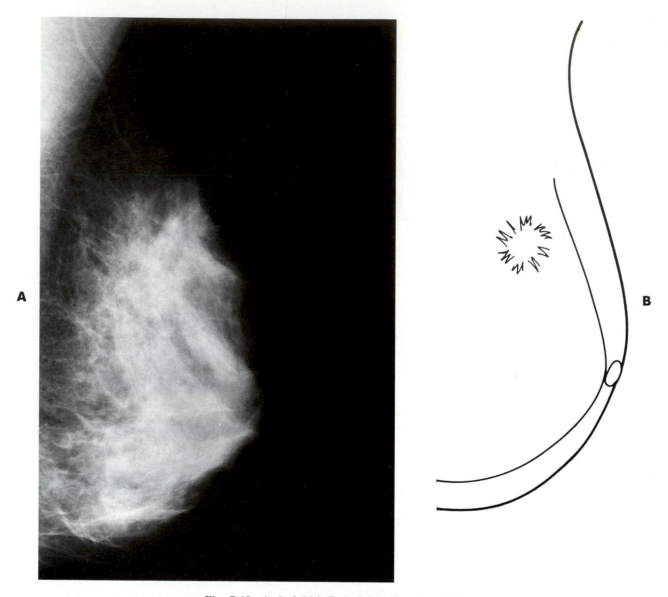

Fig. 7-19. A, Left LM. **B,** Left LM (line drawing).

This woman's screening films identified a parenchymal distortion in the left medio-lateral oblique projection and left craniocaudal projection in the upper outer quadrant (Figs. 7-17, *B*, and 7-18, *B*). This type of radiographic finding requires additional mammographic projections to complement the standard two-view mammographic examination.

Additional views of the left breast were acquired in the lateromedial projection by rotating the breast tissue in two different positions (Fig. 7-19, *A*). Additional coned mediolateral oblique and craniocaudal projections were also obtained (Figs. 7-20 and 7-21). The additional projections do not eliminate or diminish the demonstration of breast parenchymal distortion. While there are no clear and dominant mammographic malignant features, the distorted parenchyma continues to reveal increased density of the breast tissue, with some suggestion of mild spiculation. Such areas of dense parenchymal distortion can represent carcinoma.

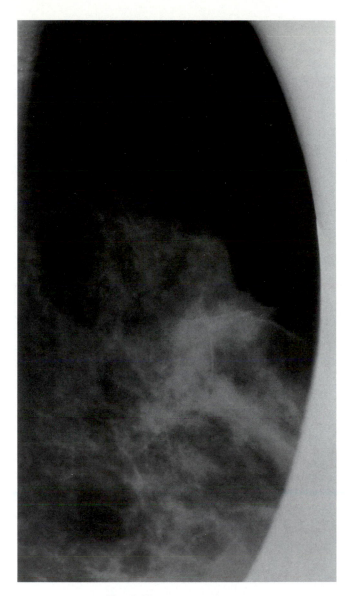

Fig. 7-20. Coned left MLO.

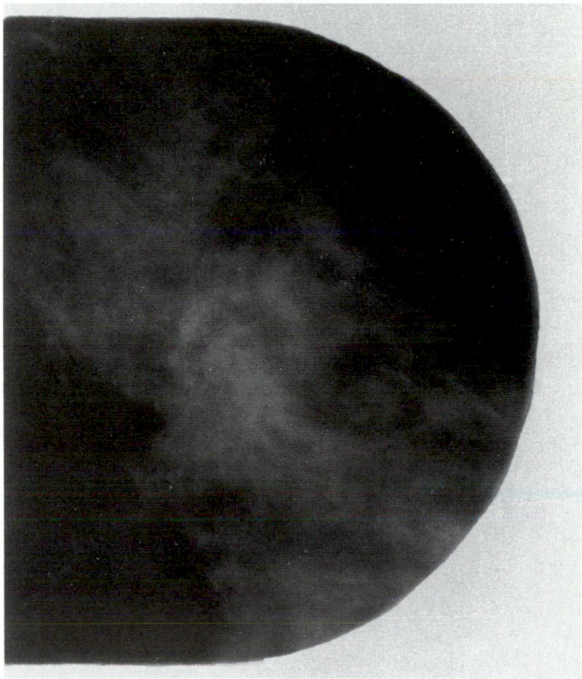

Fig. 7-21. Coned left CC.

SFNB was performed and cytologic evaluation proved negative for malignancy. Nonetheless, in this patient's case, while there were no clinical findings, surgery was carried out to exclude the possibility of a diffusely growing lobular carcinoma. Histology of this breast density confirmed benign fibrocystic changes without atypia.

Code 3

PATIENT 5

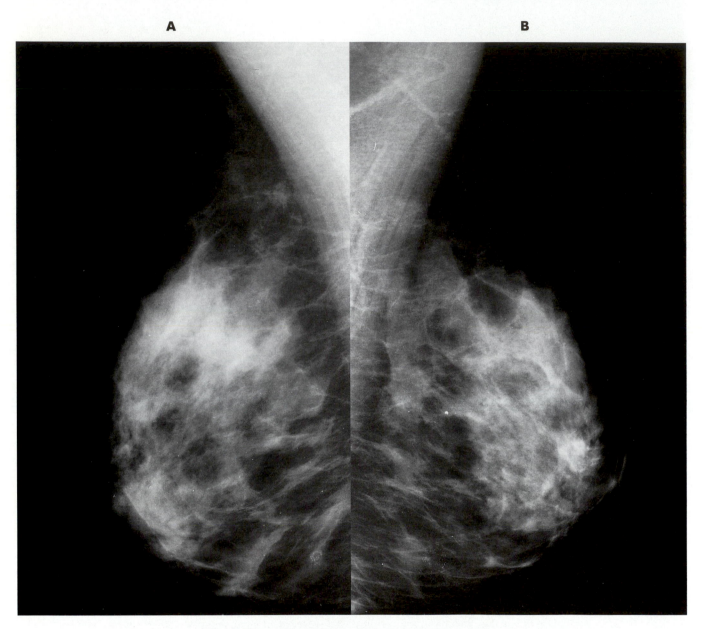

Fig. 7-22. A, Right MLO—1989. **B,** Left MLO—1989.

These images (Figs. 7-22 and 7-23) from a 54-year-old asymptomatic woman's mammogram revealed two groups of calcifications in her right breast.

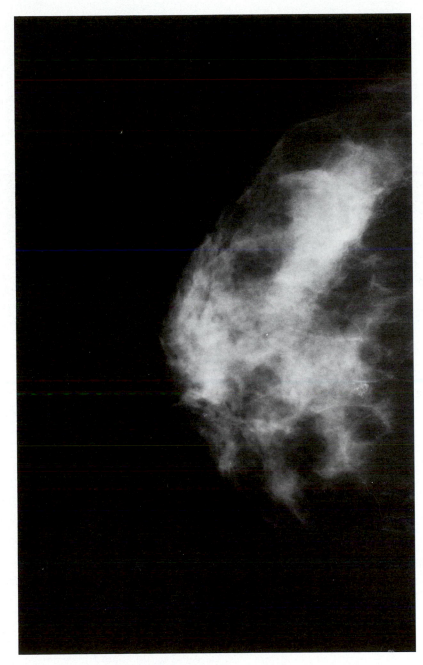

Fig. 7-23. Right CC—1989.

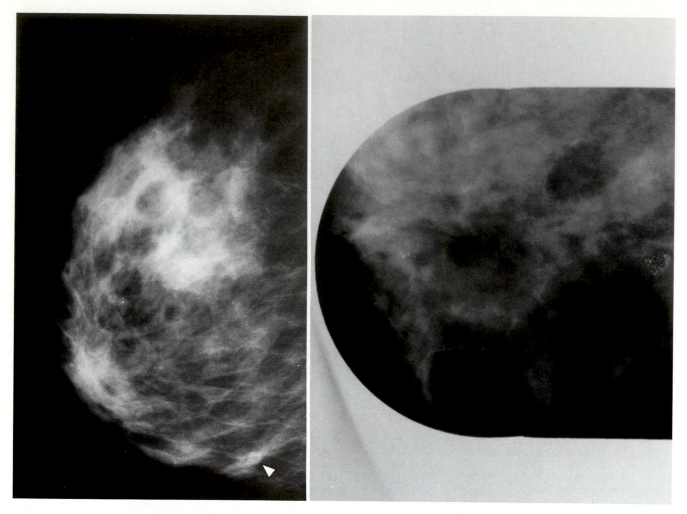

Fig. 7-24. Right LM—1989.   **Fig. 7-25.** Coned magnification, right CC—1989.

The anterior group of calcifications in the right breast near the nipple represents what are characerically categorized as benign-appearing calcifications (Figs. 7-22 to 7-24) (see also Chapter 12). The second group of calcifications in the lower quadrant of the breast demands additional radiographic workup to better understand the pathology underlying this calcific finding.

Magnification views of the right breast (Fig. 7-25), while not conclusive, do suggest that the calcifications represent benign changes. The perception of benignancy can be confirmed by SFNB. In such calcific clusters cell sampling should be obtained, not only from the center of the lesion but also from the periphery of the cluster. The SFNB illustration (Fig. 7-26) represents only one of four needle placements used to evaluate these calcifications.

In this case, SFNB cytology results revealed scattered and small groups of benign epithelial cells from both the aspirate samples and the multiple Rotex needle biopsies (see Chapter 4). This type of cytology report, when carefully integrated with a lesion's mammographic appearance, should be sufficient evidence of benignancy to avoid open surgical biopsy.

Routine screening mammogram evaluation 2 years following the stereotaxic procedure shows no change in the group of SFNB-evaluated calcifications (Figs. 7-27 and 7-28).

Code 3

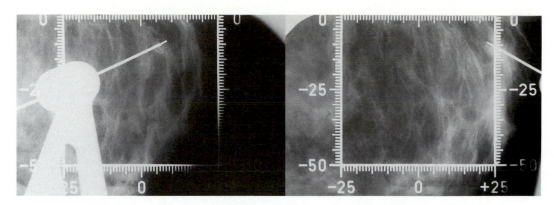

Fig. 7-26. Right SFNB—1989.

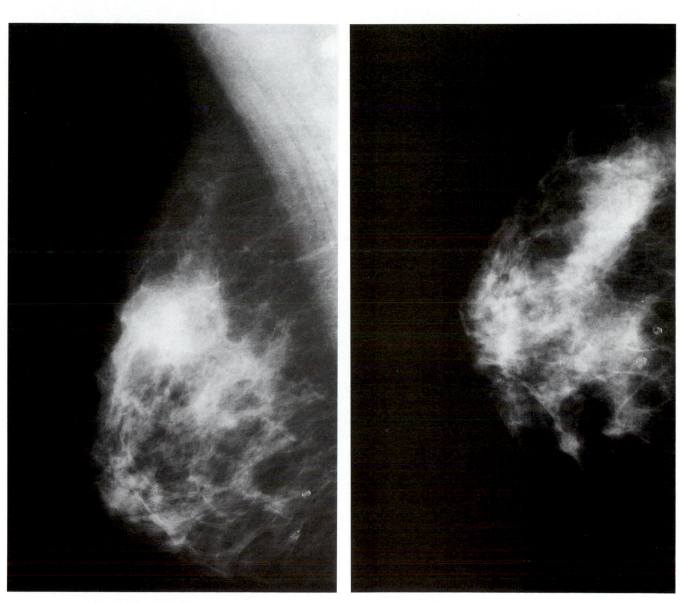

Fig. 7-27. Right MLO—1991.

Fig. 7-28. Right CC—1991.

PATIENT 6

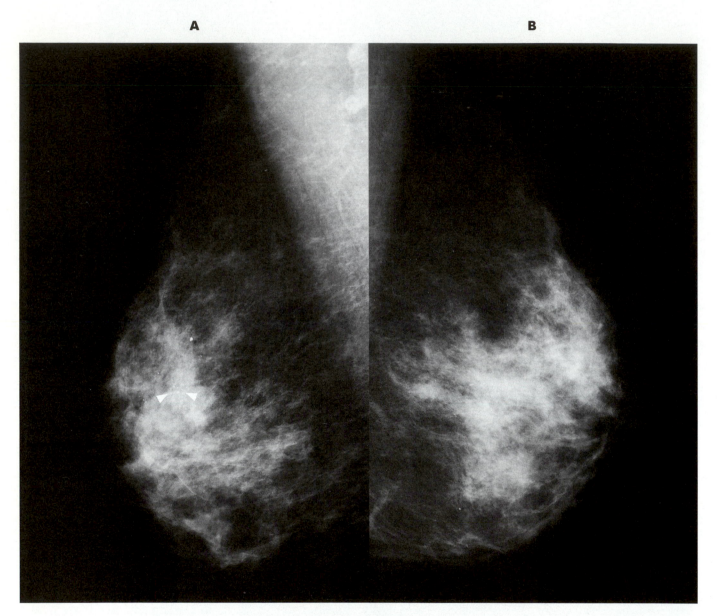

Fig. 7-29. A, Right MLO. **B,** Left MLO.

These images (Figs. 7-29 and 7-30) from a screening mammogram of a 60-year-old asymptomatic woman show bilateral dense breasts.

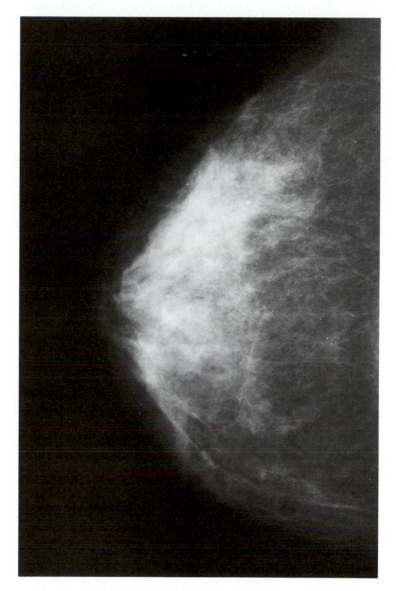

Fig. 7-30. Right CC.

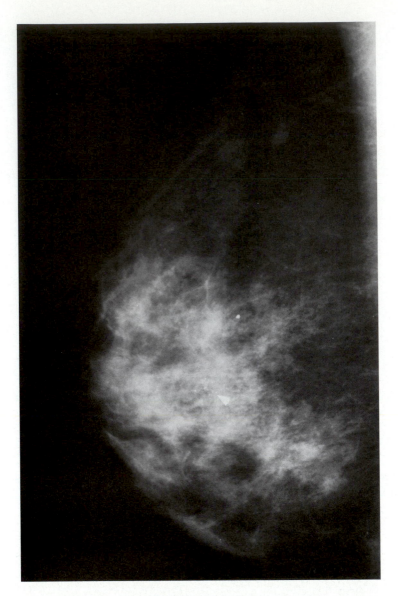

Fig. 7-31. Right LM.

Multiple clusters of irregular calcifications are seen throughout the right breast. The various shapes of calcifications show both lunar and semilunar configurations, suggesting a benign process (Fig. 7-29). On the lateral side of the right breast the calcifications are of a mixed type (Fig. 7-31). Several of the mixed type do show benign lunar and semilunar features, while others appear to have varying intensity and are arranged in linear and crushed formations. This appearance is suggestive of pathologic changes consistent with, but not necessarily, cancer. Calcific patterns such as this demand further investigation (Figs. 7-32 and 7-33).

Stereotaxic procedure was recommended and performed. Regardless of a resultant benign cytology report, surgery was still recommended for this patient because of the irregularity of the multiple clusters of microcalcifications.

Histology showed proliferative epithelium and papillomatosis with only slight atypia.

Page and Anderson point out that the terms "epitheliosis" and "papillomatosis" "have been blurred" by pathologists including too many cellular changes within the broader confines of the definitions. They propose applying the term "hyperplasia" and to specify their observations as mild, moderate, florid, or atypical.[3]

Code 3

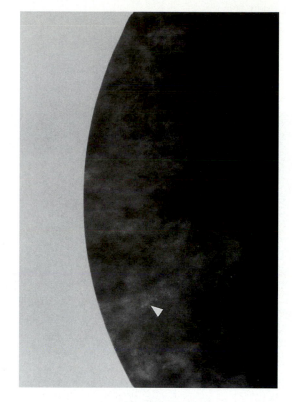

Fig. 7-32. Right coned.

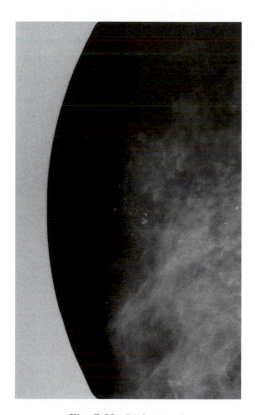

Fig. 7-33. Right coned.

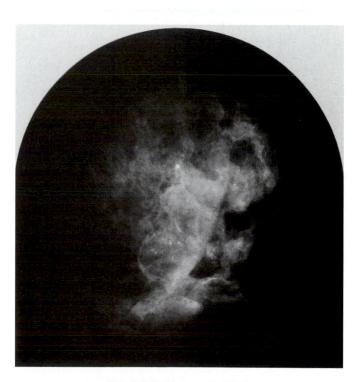

Fig. 7-34. Biopsy specimen.

PATIENT 7

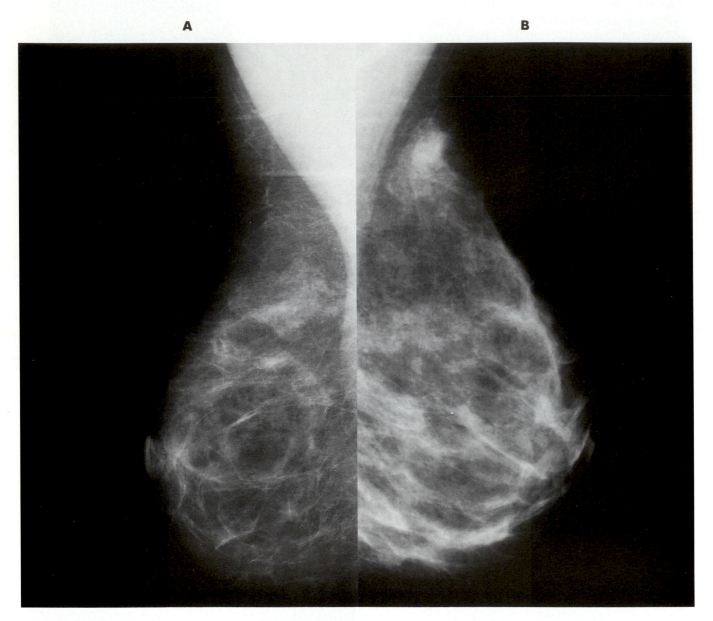

Fig. 7-35. A, Right MLO. **B,** Left MLO.

These images (Figs. 7-35 and 7-36) from a 51-year-old asymptomatic woman show mammographically lucent-appearing breasts.

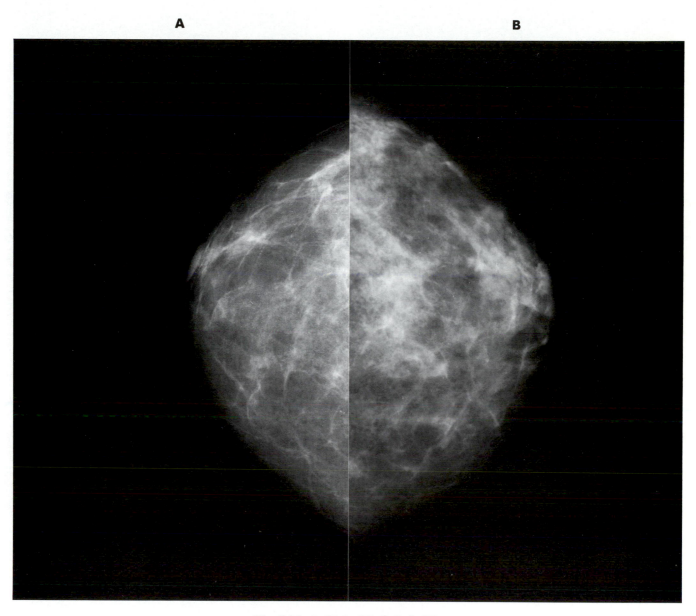

Fig. 7-36. A, Right CC. **B,** Left CC.

A   B

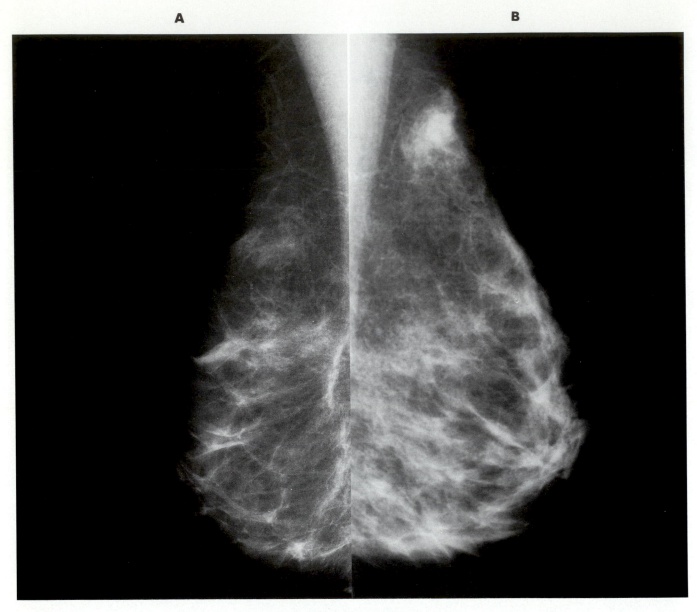

Fig. 7-37. A, Right LM. **B,** Left LM.

Asymmetry is present in this woman's entire left breast, with a single area of more dense parenchyma located in the left outer quadrant (Fig. 7-35). The same dense area is not specifically identified on the craniocaudal projection (Fig. 7-36, *B*). While the parenchymal density is identified in the left breast in both the mediolateral and the lateromedial projections, no such density is seen in the right breast in the corresponding area. Coned views of this left breast density further confirm its presence, and while this density has a normal-appearing structure, we believe focal distortion must always be approached by careful analysis (Fig. 7-38).

In addition to mammographic workup, stereotaxic procedure was recommended and confirmed a benign lesion. Cytology revealed benign epithelial cells and normal stromal breast fragments.

Code 3

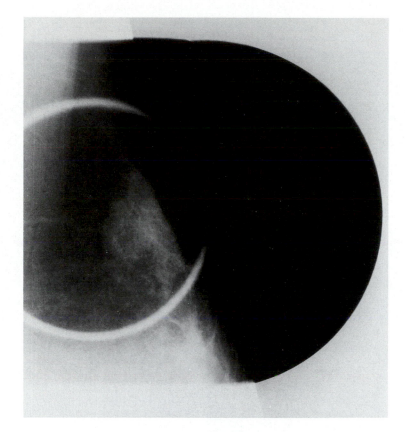

Fig. 7-38. Coned left breast.

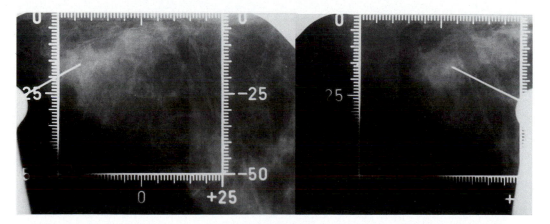

Fig. 7-39. SFNB.

PATIENT 8

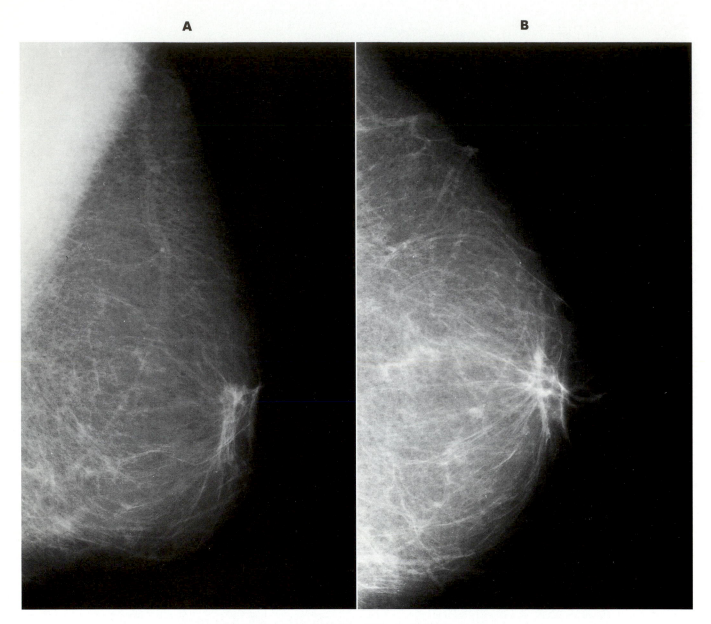

Fig. 7-40. A, Left MLO—1991. **B,** Left CC—1991.

A 52-year-old asymptomatic woman had routine mammography screening evaluation. Mammographically, her breasts are relatively lucent. The woman had undergone breast reduction surgery 15 years earlier. Compare the mediolateral (Figs. 7-40, *A,* and 7-41, *A*) and craniocaudal (Figs. 7-40, *B,* and 7-41, *B*) mammography projections, performed 10 years apart.

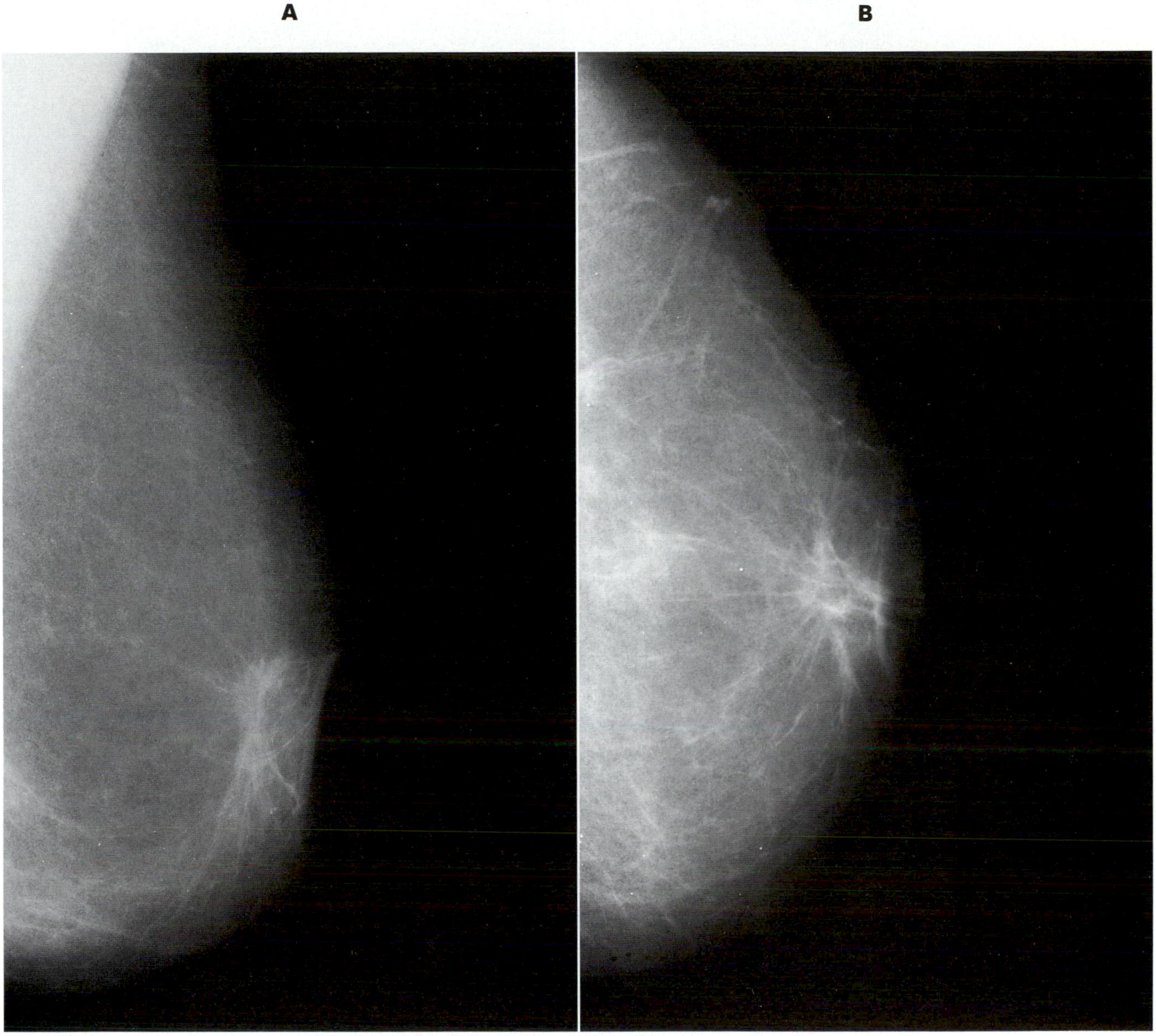

Fig. 7-41. Left MLO—1981. **B,** Left CC—1981.

A

B

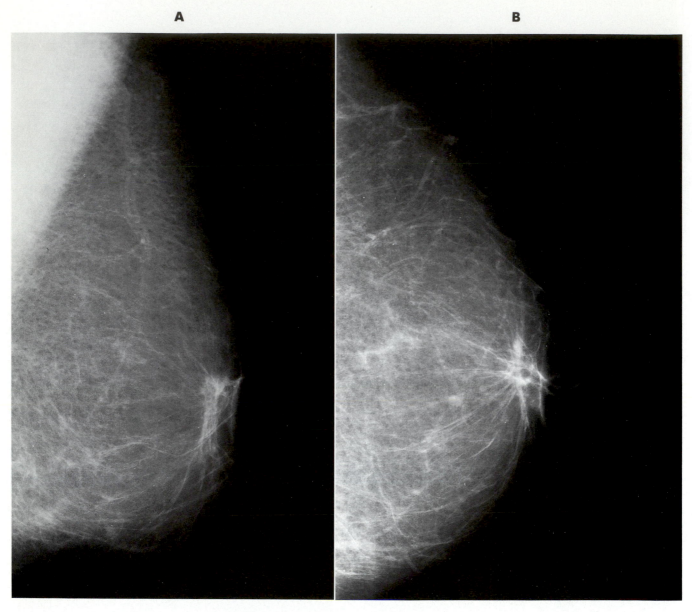

Fig. 7-42. A, Left MLO—1991. **B,** Left CC—1991.

In this woman's 1991 screening mammogram, an irregular density is detected near the nipple of the left breast. This left breast density was, in fact, mammographically present on this patient's 1981 mammogram. Examination comparison in this case detects and confirms that only minimal change has occurred in 10 years. Improved mammography techniques allow for better visualization of gross and subtle breast densities. This type of mammographic density mimics a possible malignant-type lesion, and weighing the possibility of breast skin retraction should be considered. In this case it actually represents an ordinary surgical scar.

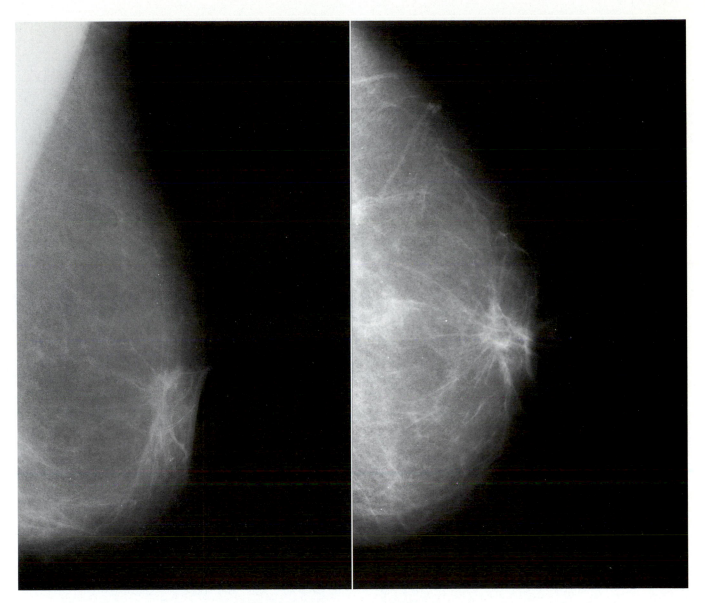

Fig. 7-43. A, Left MLO—1981. **B,** Left CC—1981.

This study reinforces the extreme importance of taking a thorough patient history and of securing all existing previous mammograms to assist in definitive diagnosis and to help eliminate unnecessary invasive diagnostic procedures.

Code 3

PATIENT 9

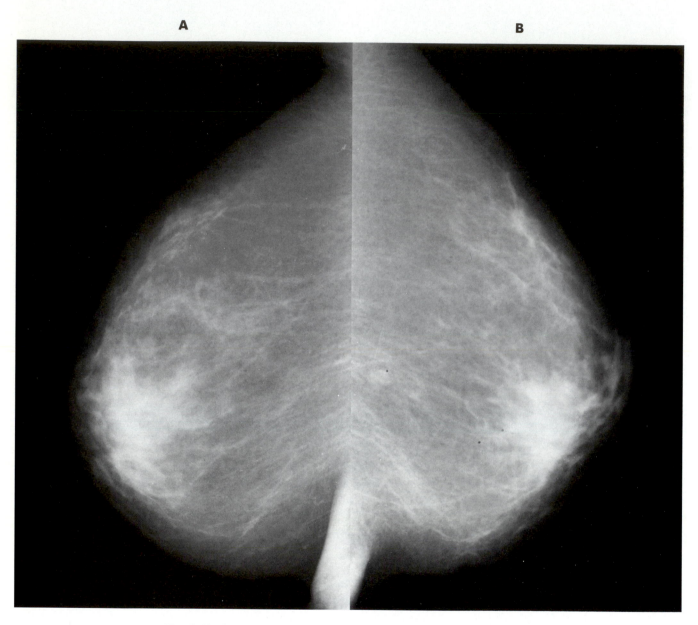

Fig. 7-44. A, Right MLO—March, 1990. **B,** Left MLO—March, 1990.

A hypertensive 74-year-old asymptomatic woman reported for routine mammography screening (Figs. 7-44 and 7-45). Her lucent breast pattern allows easy detection of even small areas of concern.

A

B

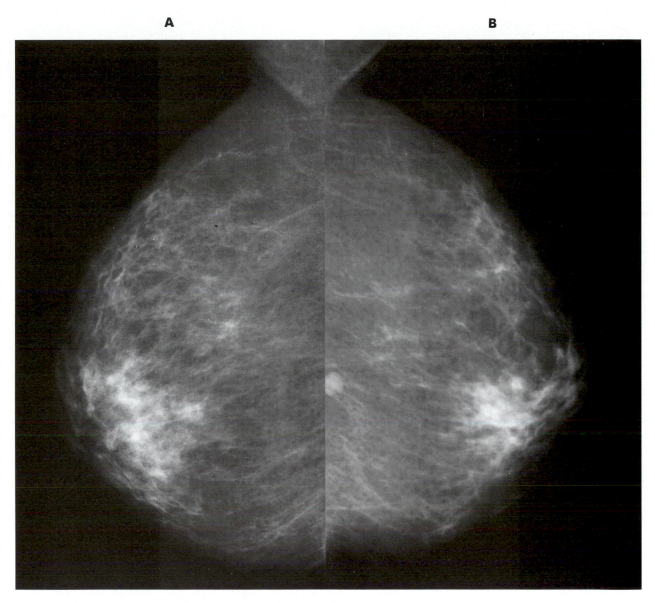

Fig. 7-45. A, Right MLO—May, 1991. **B,** Left MLO—May, 1991.

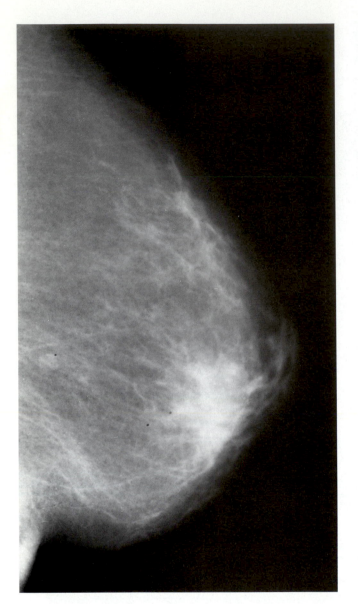

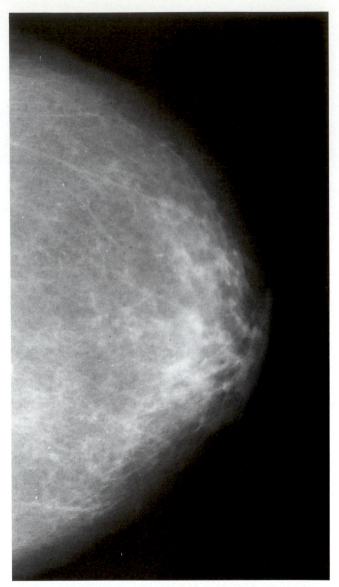

Fig. 7-46. Left MLO—March, 1990.

Fig. 7-47. Left CC—March, 1990.

A 4 mm rounded density is seen in the midposterior portion of the left breast (Figs. 7-44, *B,* and 7-45, *B*). This density was detected on her March 1990 mammography examination (Fig. 7-47). In comparing her serial examinations of March 1990 and May 1991, the density has increased to 7 mm.

The borders of the lesion appear smooth and its size is not remarkable. This finding would not ordinarily raise high suspicion for malignancy and could be presumed a cystic process. In this case, however, several factors make evaluation of the density essential: (1) the woman's age, (2) a 3 mm increase in the size of the lesion within 1 year, and (3) the most posterior orientation of the lesion in an otherwise lucent breast.

Ultrasound may be a technique of choice to evaluate this density. If ultrasound confirms a simple cyst and does not demonstrate a solid mass, biopsy of the lesion may be avoided. If mammography reveals a suspicious border and evaluation by ultrasound

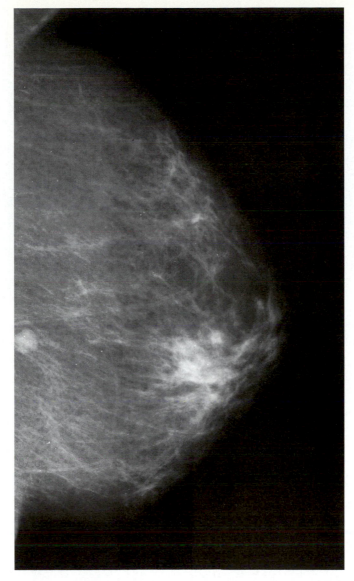

Fig. 7-48. Left MLO—May, 1991.

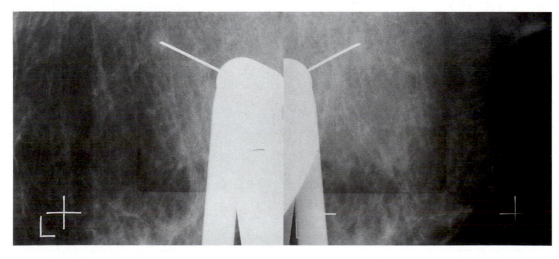

Fig. 7-49. SFNB.

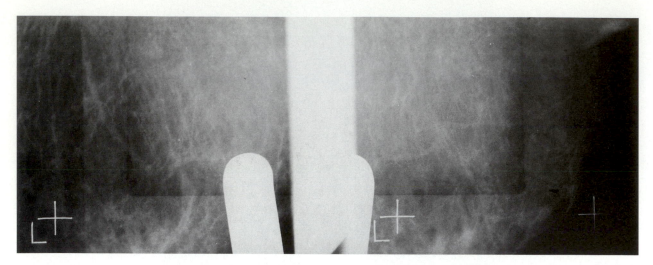

Fig. 7-50. Post–SFNB aspiration.

demonstrates internal changes, then biopsy may be necessary. In this case, the woman's family believed that cytologic evaluation of the lesion, using the SFNB technique, would immediately confirm its cellular makeup.

SFNB was recommended and performed. Cytology of the lesion produced cystic fluid, demonstrating benign ductal epithelial cells with no evidence of malignancy. The postaspiration image revealed no residual breast tissue mass (Fig. 7-50).

Ordinarily, this woman might have had to undergo surgical evaluation of the lesion. The SFNB procedure eliminated performing surgery in this hypertensive 74-year-old woman and gave complete assurance of a benign process.

Code 3

REFERENCES

1. Bassett LW, Jahanshahi R, Gold RH, Fu YS: *Film screen mammography: an atlas of instructional cases,* New York, 1991, Raven.
2. Gershon-Cohen J, Ingleby H: Roentgenography of fibroadenoma of the breast, *Radiology* 59:77-87, 1952.
3. Page DL, Anderson TJ: *Diagnostic histopathology of the breast,* New York, 1987, Churchill Livingstone.

CIRCUMSCRIBED LESIONS

PATIENT 1

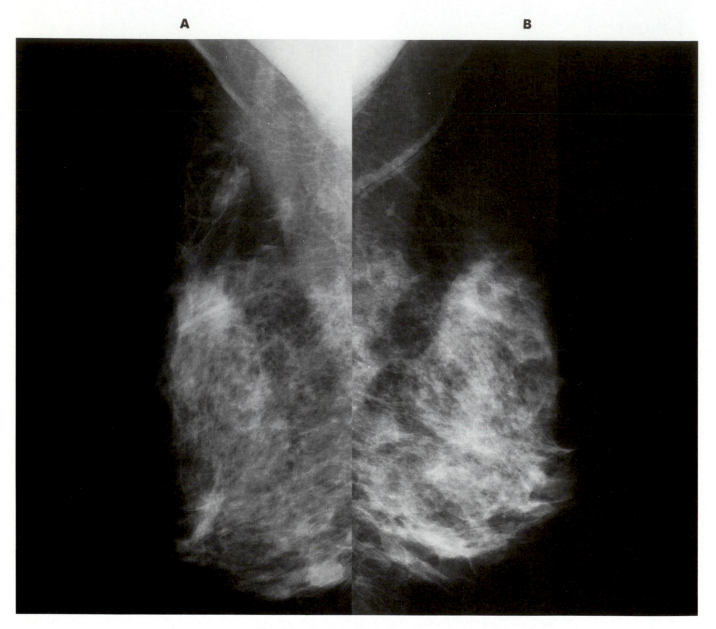

Fig. 8-1. A, Right MLO. **B,** Left MLO.

These images (Figs. 8-1 and 8-2) are from a screening mammogram of a 58-year-old asymptomatic woman.

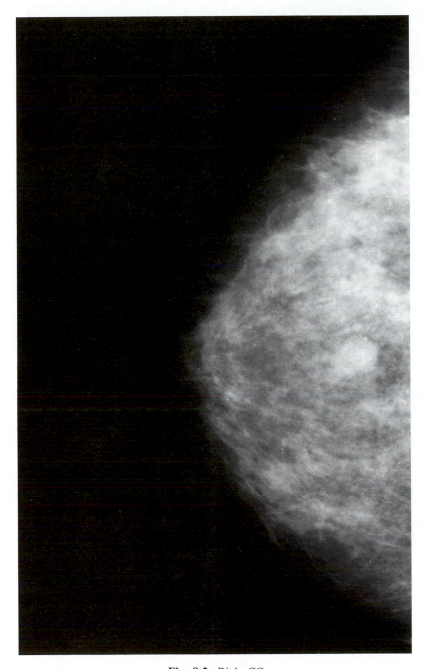

Fig. 8-2. Right CC.

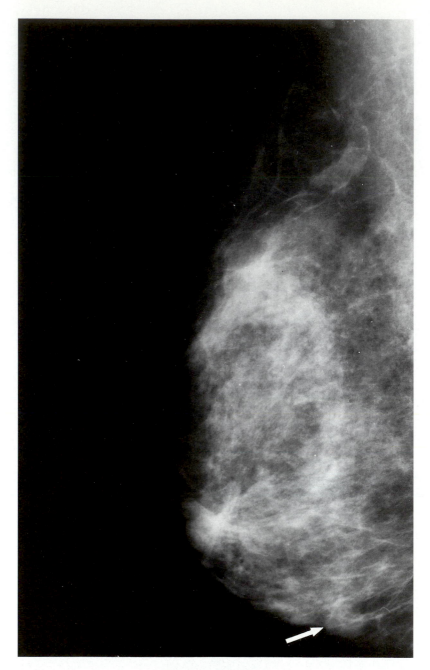

Fig. 8-3. Right LM.

Bilateral variation in the breast parenchyma is within normal limits. Mammographic appearance, however, of a right breast density raises suspicion. Study the margin of the circumscribed density located below the right nipple (Fig. 8-1, *A*). In the lateromedial projection the density is less obvious, while in the craniocaudal projection the density is readily detected in the midportion of the breast (Figs. 8-2 and 8-3). The coned compression film demonstrates unsharp portions in the margin of the density, delineating discrete border lobulation (Fig. 8-4).

Stereotaxic evaluation of this circumscribed density, with cytologic and histologic correlation, confirmed a highly differentiated ductal carcinoma with some mucinous areas. Mucinous cancers are not usually fast growing; consequently, when they are detected and immediately treated, prognosis is good.

Code 3

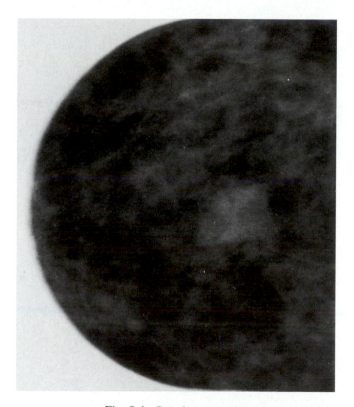

Fig. 8-4. Coned compression.

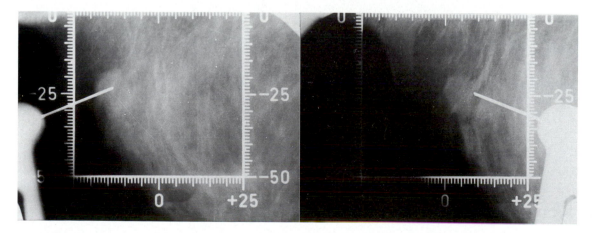

Fig. 8-5. SFNB.

PATIENT 2

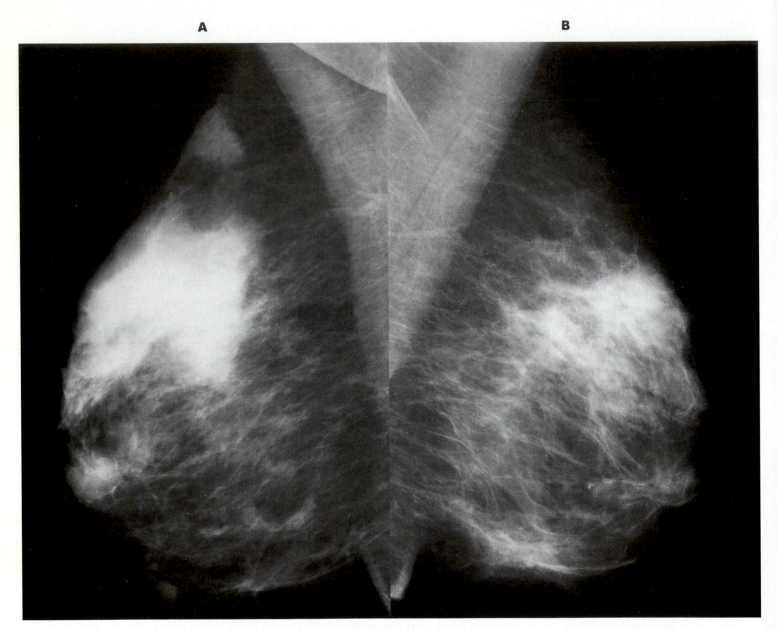

Fig. 8-6. A, Right MLO. **B,** Left MLO.

These images (Figs. 8-6 and 8-7) represent a screening mammogram of a 52-year-old asymptomatic woman with moderately dense breasts.

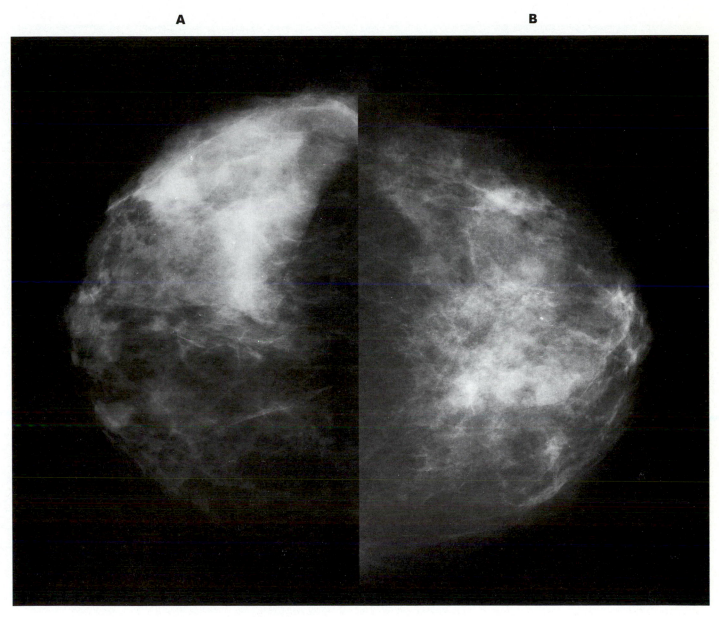

Fig. 8-7. A, Right CC. **B,** Left CC.

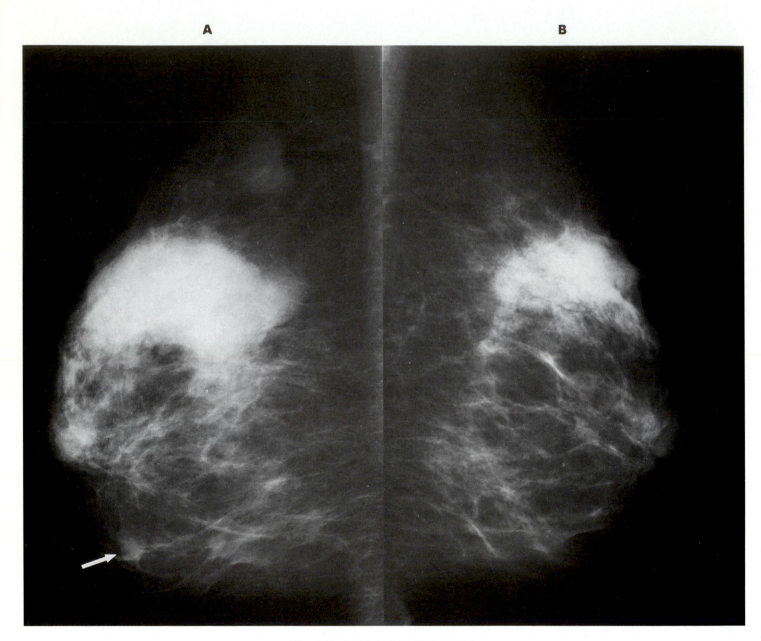

Fig. 8-8. A, Right LM. **B,** Left LM.

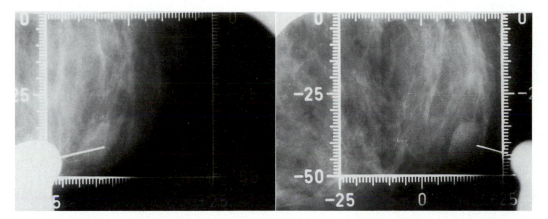

Fig. 8-9. SFNB.

This woman's right breast is considerably more dense than her left. In addition, an asymmetric density is seen in the upper portion of the right breast (Fig. 8-6, *A*). Performing clinical breast examination and securing an accurate medical history are essential but can be particularly helpful when evaluating dense asymmetric breasts. Clinical breast examination of this patient revealed no palpable masses.

A discrete nonpalpable density is visualized in the right lower inner quadrant of the breasts (Figs. 8-6, *A*, and 8-8, *A*). The mammographic appearance is typical of fibroadenoma. Eighty percent of all common or "typical" fibroadenomas reach a diameter of between 1 and 3 cm.[7]

SFNB was performed and cytology showed only stromal fragments. Key to cytologically classifying fibroadenomas is to demonstrate fibrous stroma with minimal cellularity and without cytologic atypia.[7] In this case, surgery was avoided based on correlation of the mammographic appearance of the density with the resultant cytology of the lesion.

At the Karolinska Institute and Michigan State University, when mammography, cytology, and clinical evaluation confirm these findings, removal of a fibroadenoma is not recommended.

Code 2

PATIENT 3

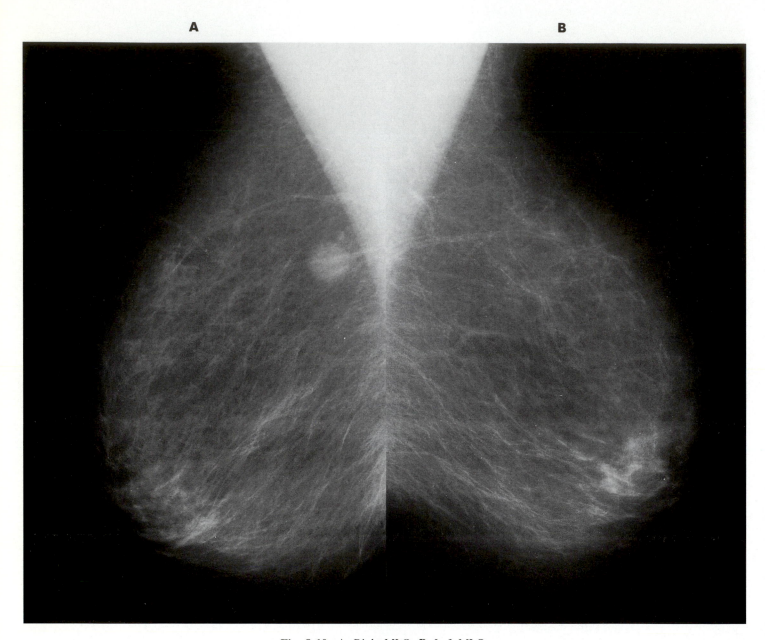

Fig. 8-10. A, Right MLO. **B,** Left MLO.

This 57-year-old woman had a *palpable* mass and was referred for a diagnostic mammogram (Figs. 8-10 and 8-11). This case illustrates how certain types of benign lesions can mimic malignant-appearing lesions. (This is the single atlas example of a case with a known *palpable* mass.)

A   B

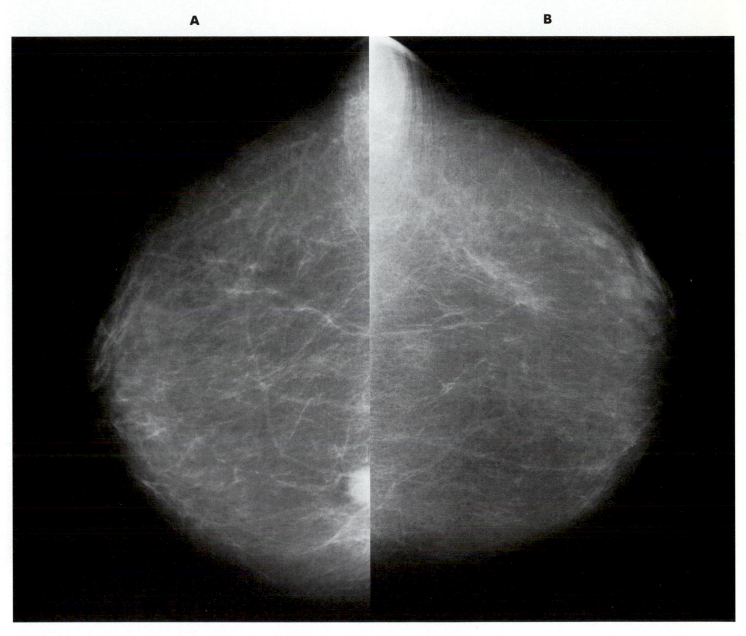

Fig. 8-11. **A,** Right CC. **B,** Left CC.

A   B

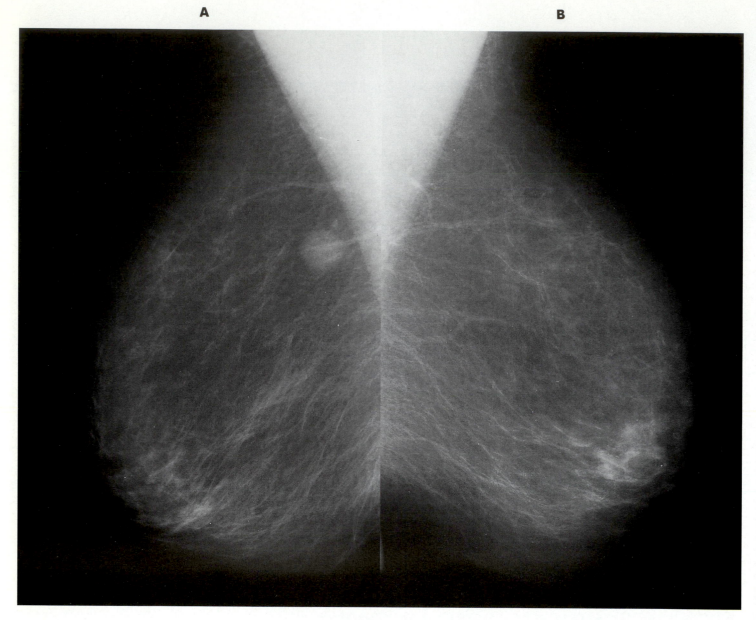

Fig. 8-12. A, Right MLO. **B,** Left MLO.

The circumscribed lesion in the upper inner quadrant of the right breast is of moderate density. This woman's clinical evaluation included breast skin inspection and palpation of a firm, elevated breast lesion revealing an epidermal cyst. Surgical incision of the lesion emptied squamous debris. Routinely, epidermal cysts occur on the face, neck, and trunk, but occasionally they appear on breast skin. This case illustrates how certain lesions mammographically mimic cancer.[6]

Code 2

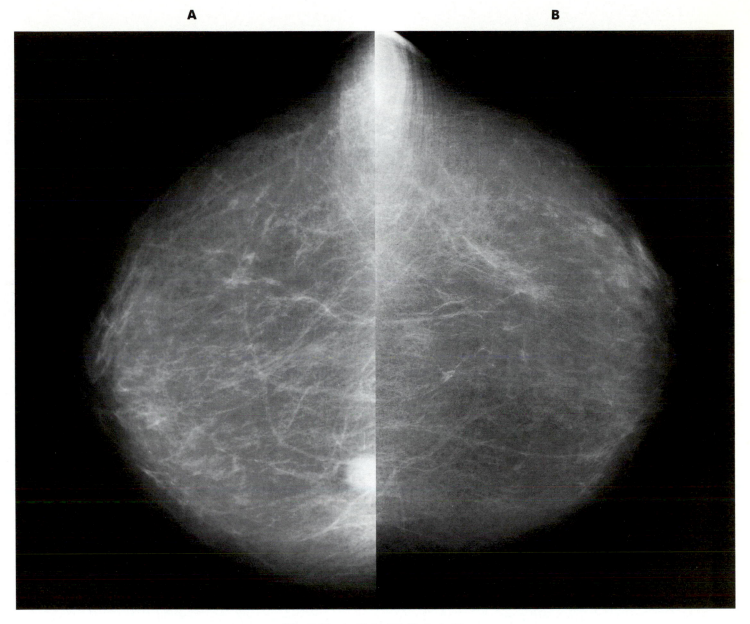

Fig. 8-13. A, Right CC. **B,** Left CC.

PATIENT 4

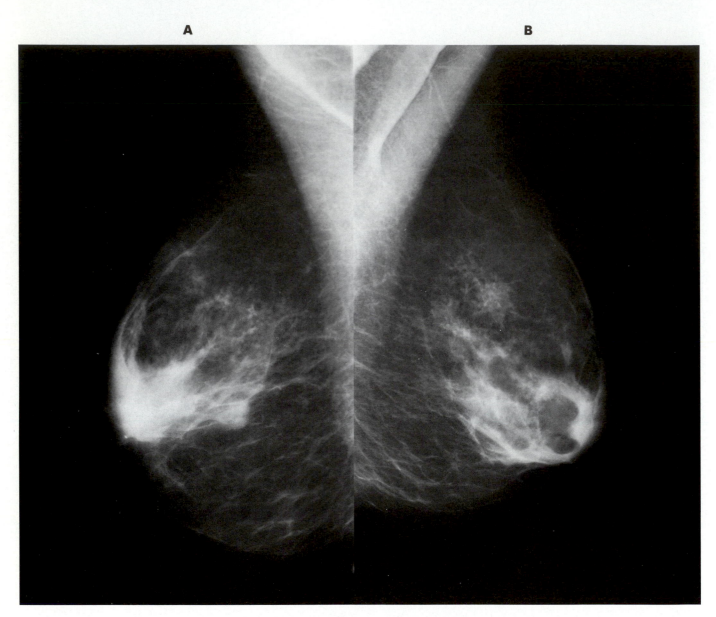

Fig. 8-14. A, Right MLO. **B,** Left MLO.

These images (Figs. 8-14 and 8-15) are from a screening mammogram of a 60-year-old asymptomatic nurse.

A

B

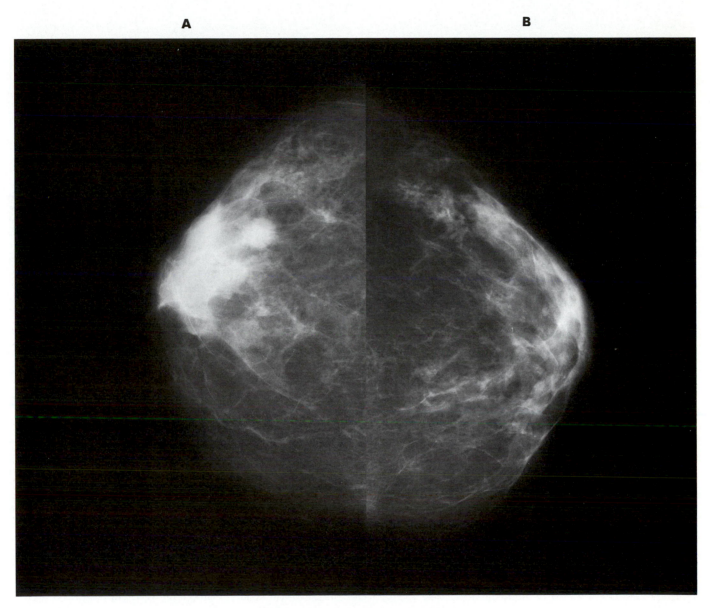

Fig. 8-15. A, Right CC. **B,** Left CC.

A   **B**

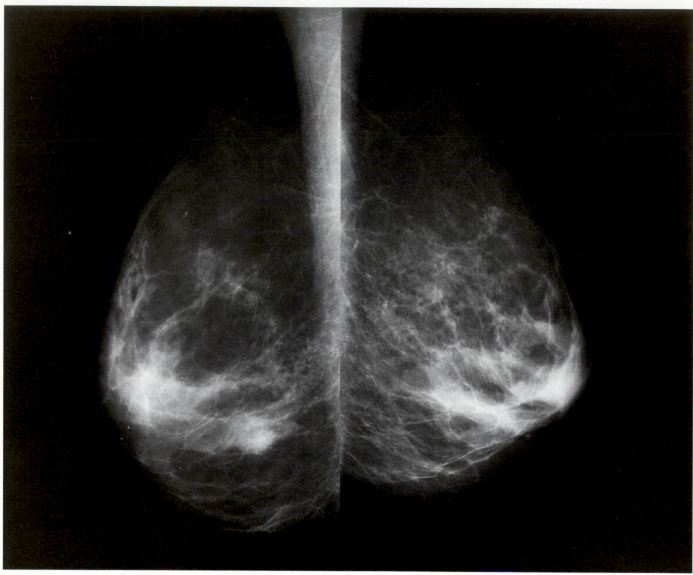

Fig. 8-16. A, Right LM. **B,** Left LM.

A 12 mm, circumscribed, dense lesion in the lower outer quadrant of the right breast is easily identified (Figs. 8-14, *A,* and 8-15, *A*). Bilateral comparison of the mediolateral oblique, craniocaudal, and lateromedial breast projections confirms its presence (Figs. 8-14, *A,* 8-15, *A,* and 8-16, *A*). The unsharp margins of the lesion are especially appreciated on the right coned compression view (Fig. 8-17). This woman's clinical breast examination, performed by an oncologist and a surgeon, failed to reveal a palpable mass.

SFNB was performed and cytology was positive for malignancy. Following carbon localization of the lesion, the biopsy specimen confirmed histology of colloid carcinoma.

Colloid tumors (mucinous) occur in approximately 2% of breast carcinomas.[4] While these tumors are generally palpable and are thought to occur in women in their sixth or seventh decade, a more recent discovery is the occurrence of colloid tumors in younger

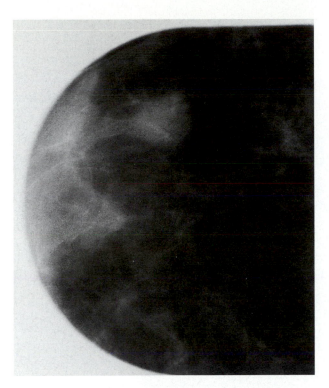

Fig. 8-17. Coned compression of right breast.

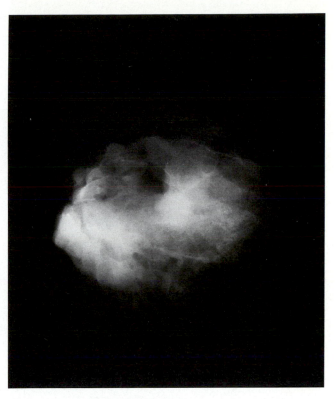

Fig. 8-18. Biopsy specimen.

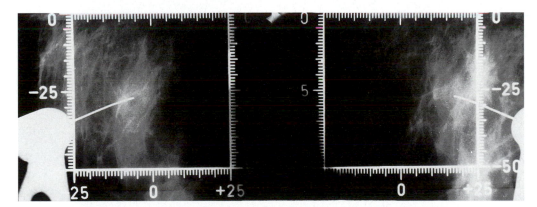

Fig. 8-19. SFNB.

women. These tumors are smaller and nonpalpable when detected in younger women, questioning "the belief that bulky, mucinous tumors are largely confined to the older patient."[5]

If we correlate mammographic features, SFNB, and histology results we may learn to specify breast pathology better from the mammographic pattern. Eventually we may even be able to distinguish tumor types.

Code 4

PATIENT 5

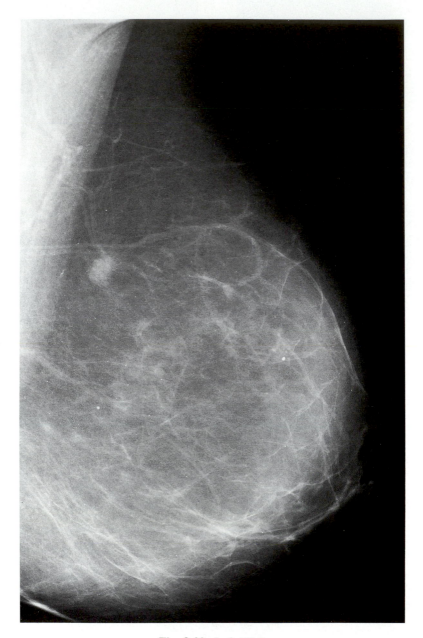

Fig. 8-20. Left MLO.

These films (Figs. 8-20 and 8-21) represent a screening mammogram in a 49-year-old asymptomatic woman.

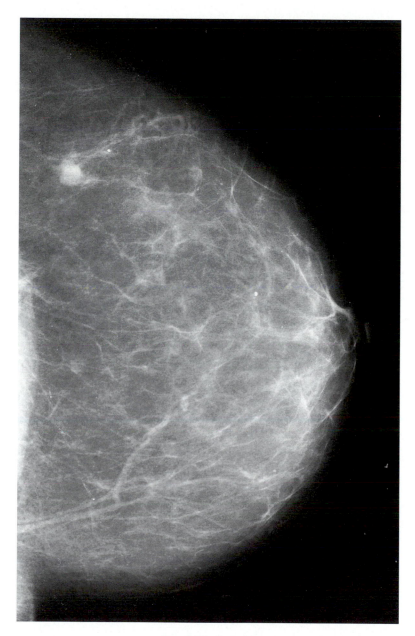

Fig. 8-21. Left CC.

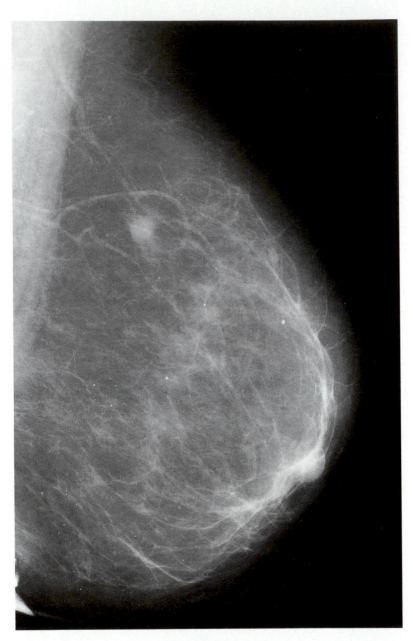

Fig. 8-22. Left LM.

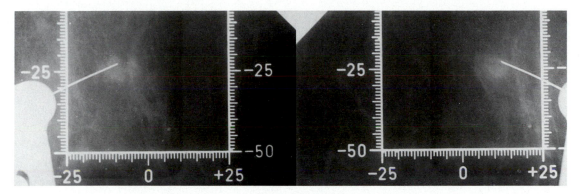

Fig. 8-23. SFNB.

An ill-defined circumscribed density is seen in the left upper outer quadrant in a fatty breast (Fig. 8-21). This single circumscribed lesion has somewhat unsharp margins (Fig. 8-20). These same characteristics can, in fact, be representative of malignant tumor types such as ductal or medullary cancer. It appears "soft" and rather "bulky" in nature, which mammographically is typical of a medullary cancer (Fig. 8-22).

To determine the nature of the lesion, we recommended and performed SFNB (Fig. 8-23). Cytology revealed cancer cells. Histology of the biopsied lesion confirmed medullary carcinoma.

Medullary carcinoma is mainly composed of epithelial elements and very little dense, fibrous stroma. Medullary carcinoma accounts for 5% to 7% of all breast cancers, with 11% of diagnosed medullary cancers occurring in women less than 35 years of age.[1,2] This type of cancer is shown to have one of the lowest rates of multicentricity. Histologically, medullary cancer is highly cellular. Despite this tumor's high degree of cellular pleomorphism and mitosis, prognosis is good.[2,3]

Code 4

REFERENCES

1. Dahnert W: *Radiology review manual: differential diagnosis of breast disease,* Baltimore, 1991, Williams & Wilkins.
2. Leis H: Prognostic parameters for breast cancer. In Bland KI, Copeland EM, eds: *The breast: comprehensive management of benign and malignant diseases,* Philadelphia, 1991, Saunders.
3. Lesser ML, Rosen PP, Kinne DW: Multicentricity and bilaterality in invasive breast carcinoma, *Surgery* 91:234-240, 1982.
4. Page DL, Anderson TJ: *Diagnostic histopathology of the breast,* New York, 1987, Churchill Livingstone.
5. Pierson KK, Wilkinson EJ: Malignant neoplasia of the breast: infiltrating carcinomas. In Bland KI, Copeland EM, eds: *The breast: comprehensive management of benign and malignant diseases,* Philadelphia, 1991, Saunders.
6. Shehi LJ, Pierson KK: Benign and malignant epithelial neoplasms and dermatological disorders. In Bland KI, Copeland EM, eds: *The breast: comprehensive management of benign and malignant diseases,* Philadelphia, 1991, Saunders.
7. Souba WW: Evaluation and treatment of benign breast disorders. In Bland KI, Copeland EM, eds: *The breast: comprehensive management of benign and malignant diseases,* Philadelphia, 1991, Saunders.

Chapter 9

ASYMMETRIC DENSITY

PATIENT 1

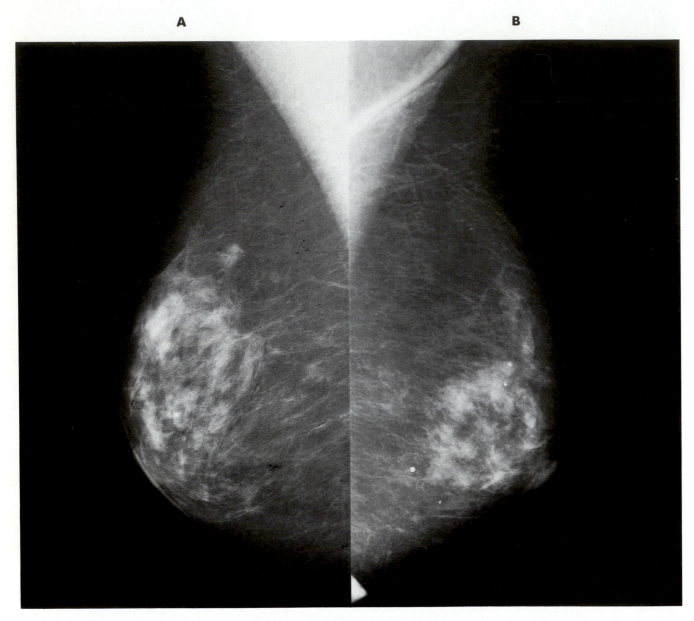

Fig. 9-1. A, Right MLO; **B,** left MLO.

These films (Figs. 9-1 and 9-2) represent a screening mammogram of a 69-year-old asymptomatic woman.

A

B

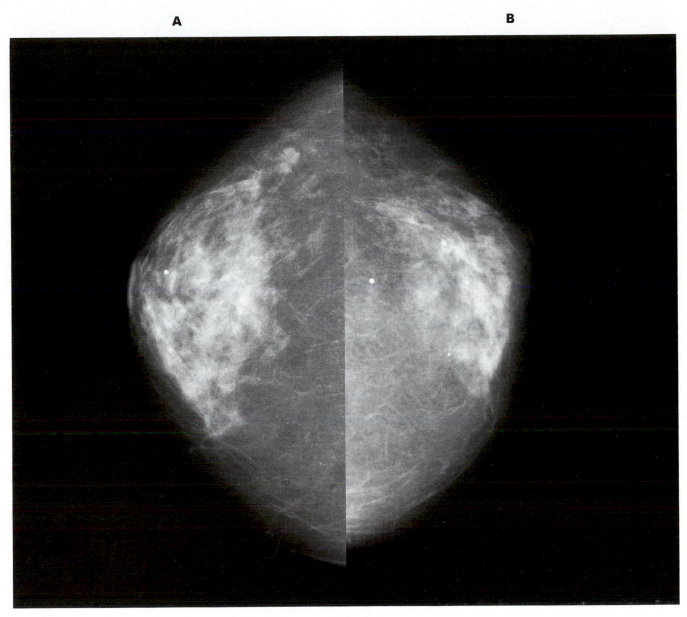

Fig. 9-2. A, Right CC; **B,** left CC.

A   B

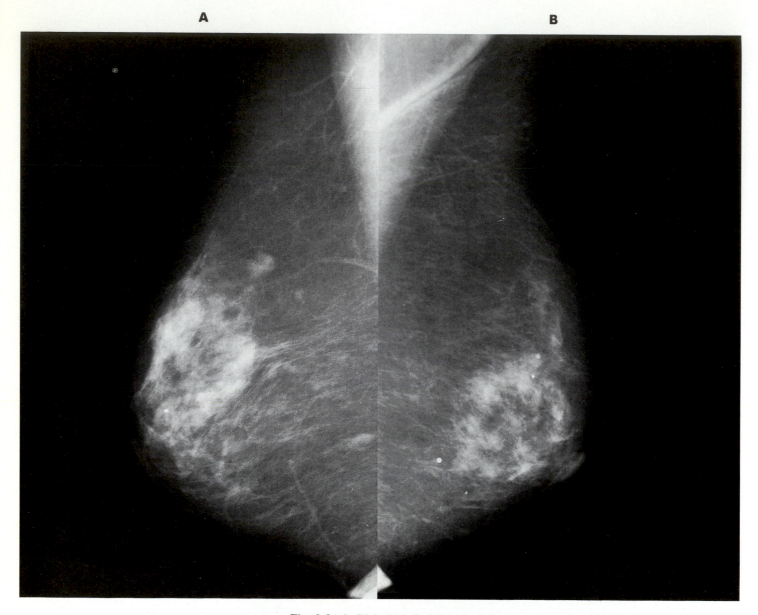

Fig. 9-3. **A,** Right LM; **B,** left LM.

Over 20 years before this screening mammogram, this woman had bilateral breast surgery. Palpable lesions were discovered in the upper outer quadrants of her breasts. At that time, both surgically removed lesions were proved benign. The woman did well postsurgically and, since she was otherwise healthy, she saw little benefit in reporting for routine breast check-ups. Subsequent to her breast surgery, mammography was not nearly as popular or routinely ordered. As mammography improved and campaigns were designed to educate women about early cancer detection, she decided to participate in a screening evaluation.

Her present screening mammography examination reveals an asymmetric density in the upper outer quadrant of the right breast. The density has somewhat unsharp margins with a suggestion of spiculated features on the lower medial side of the lesion (Fig. 9-1, *A*). Coned projections delineate the asymmetric area, and it remains particularly persis-

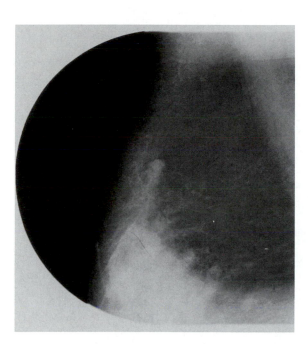

Fig. 9-4. Coned right MLO.

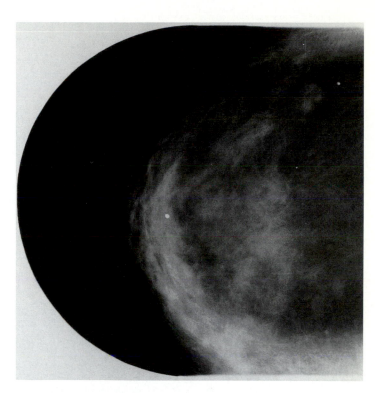

Fig. 9-5. Coned right CC.

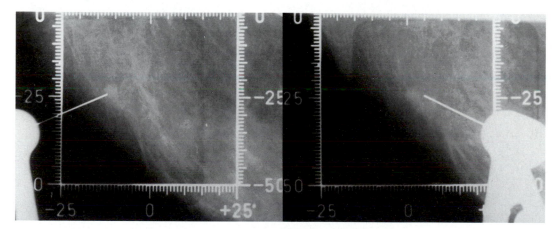

Fig. 9-6. SFNB.

tent in the coned mediolateral oblique projection (Figs. 9-4 and 9-5). This mammographic pattern is suspicious for malignancy. Stereotaxic fine-needle biopsy (SFNB) was performed and demonstrated cytology positive for cancer (Fig. 9-6). Histology confirmed poorly differentiated invasive ductal carcinoma.

Vigilance in requesting mammograms is incumbent on women themselves and on their physicians. The implications for continuing cancer education are obvious. We do not yet know what causes breast cancer or how to prevent it. We must, however, include mammography to assist in early diagnosis of breast disease.[6]

While advocacy of breast screening is not shared by all, detection of the "minimal" breast lesion and decreasing unnecessary biopsies are preferred by most. As Peeters suggests, well-trained screening teams can accomplish both and, in doing so, assist to minimize interval breast cancers.[3]

Code 4

PATIENT 2

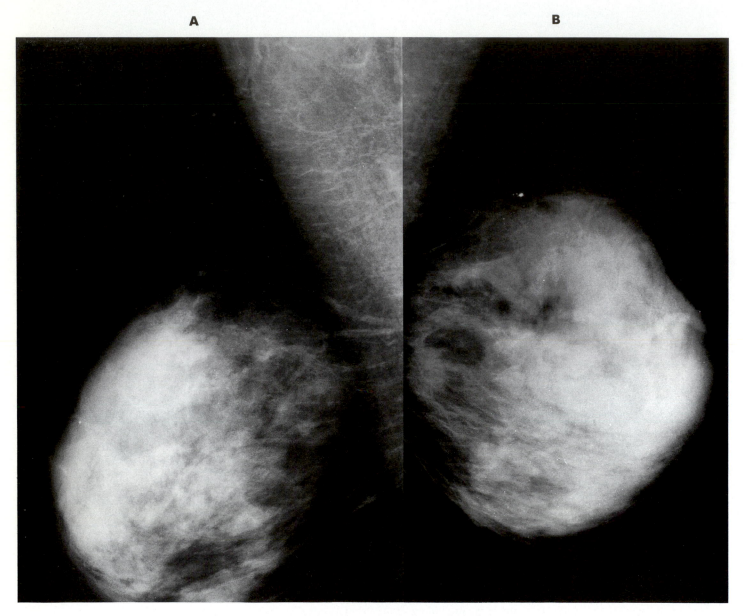

Fig. 9-7. A, Right MLO; **B,** left MLO.

These images (Figs. 9-7 and 9-8) are from a screening mammogram of a 50-year-old asymptomatic woman with dense breasts.

A

B

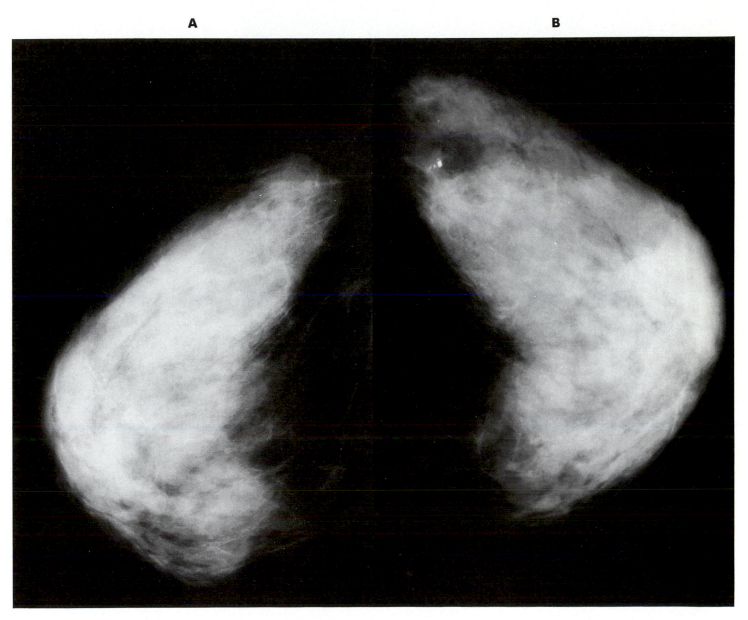

Fig. 9-8. A, Right CC; **B,** left CC.

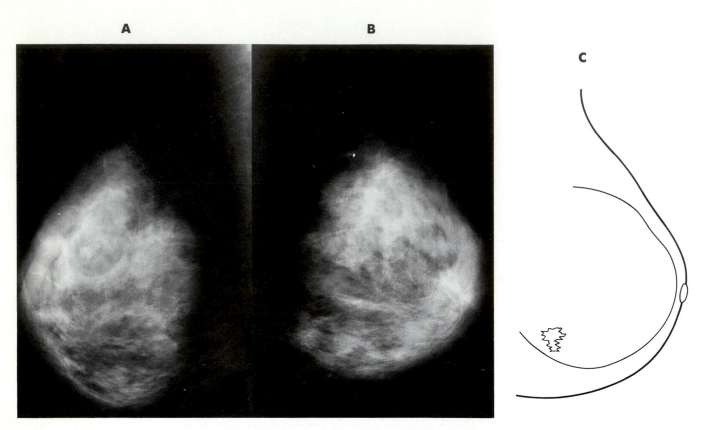

Fig. 9-9. A, Right LM; **B,** left LM; **C,** left LM (line drawing).

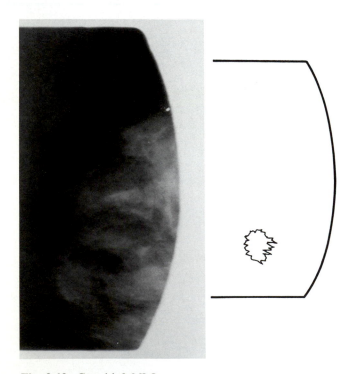

Fig. 9-10. Coned left MLO.

This woman's dense breast parenchyma makes it particularly difficult to identify existing breast pathology (Figs. 9-7 and 9-8). An asymmetric density is identified in the upper outer quadrant of the left breast (Fig. 9-8, *B*). An area of benign-appearing calcification is seen in the mediolateral oblique projection. Careful evaluation of the left magnification projection further demonstrates a stellate-patterned type of lesion that is not otherwise well appreciated (Fig. 9-11, *A*). Study of the density reveals spiculation within the dense breast tissue. Mammographically, this represents cancer.

SFNB demonstrated malignant epithelial cells. Histology of the lesion confirmed poorly differentiated invasive ductal carcinoma.

Despite mammography's high sensitivity and specificity in diagnosing breast problems, diagnostic difficulties, including the misinterpretation of carcinoma as benign, were found to be a main cause of error in dense breasts.[1] Methods of systematic evaluation for viewing all mammography examinations should be established. One way to assist in detecting subtle breast asymmetry is to compare corresponding breast parenchyma using the Tabar masking

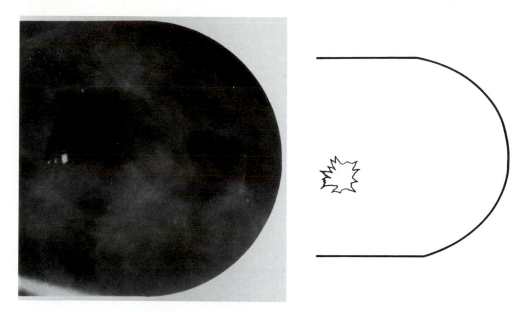

Fig. 9-11. Coned magnification left CC.

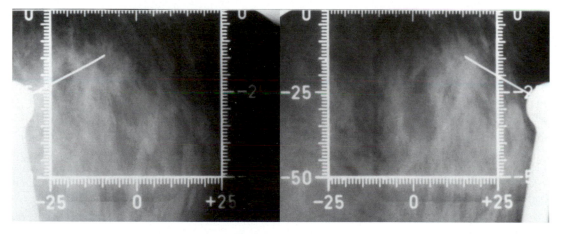

Fig. 9-12. SFBN.

method.[7] In any case, implementing a consistent pattern of analysis is important to first detect breast normality or abnormality. Interpretation of any "finding" and subsequent recommendation for further evaluation can only be a consequence of its initial detection.

Code 5

PATIENT 3

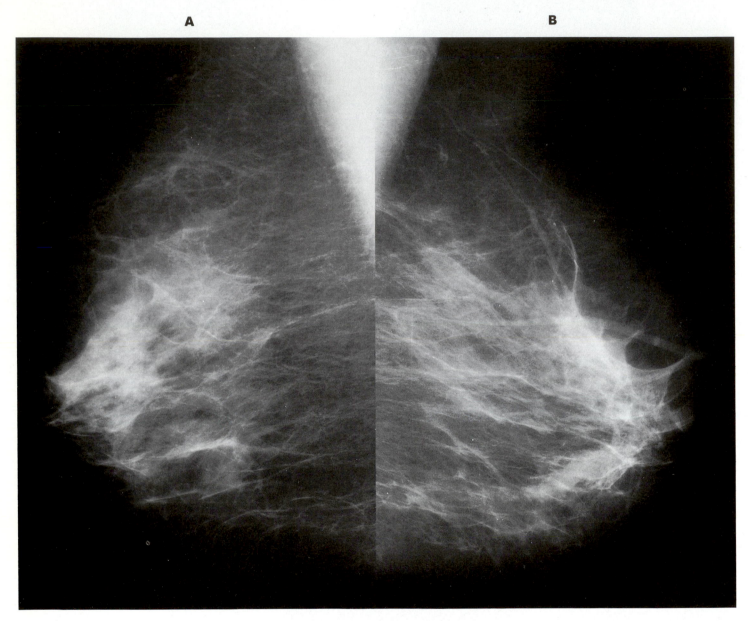

Fig. 9-13. A, Right MLO; **B,** left MLO.

These images (Figs. 9-13 and 9-14) are from a screening mammogram of a 58-year-old asymptomatic woman with a moderate amount of breast parenchyma.

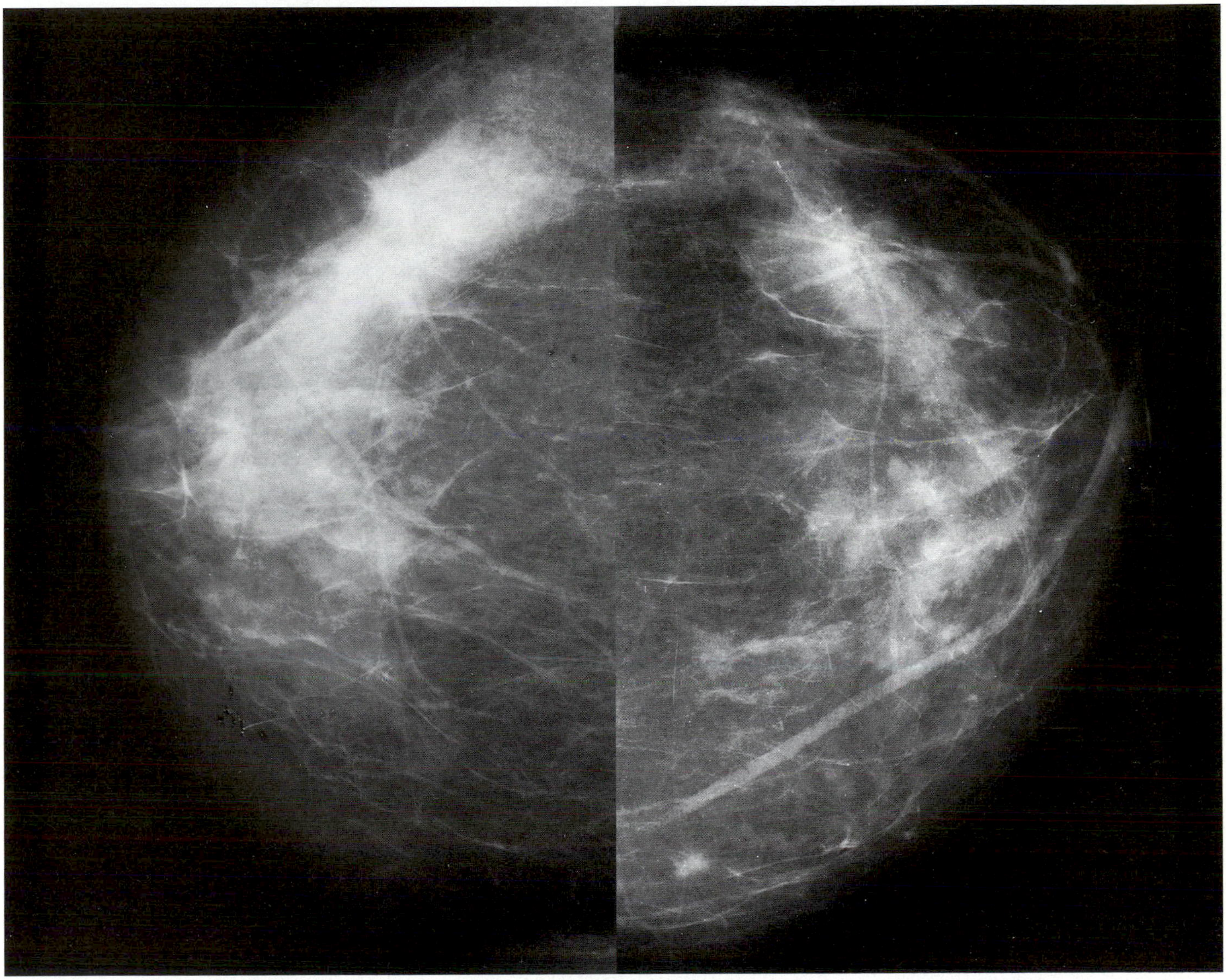

Fig. 9-14. A, Right CC; **B,** left CC.

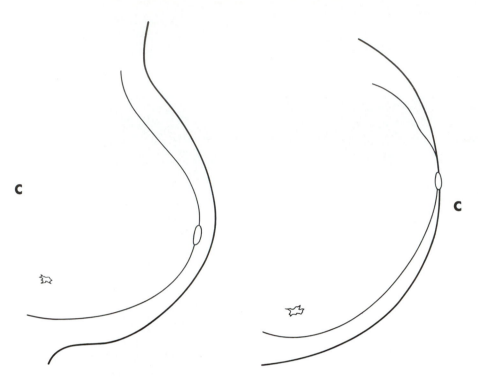

Fig. 9-13, cont'd. C, Left MLO (line drawing).

Fig. 9-14, cont'd. C, Left CC (line drawing).

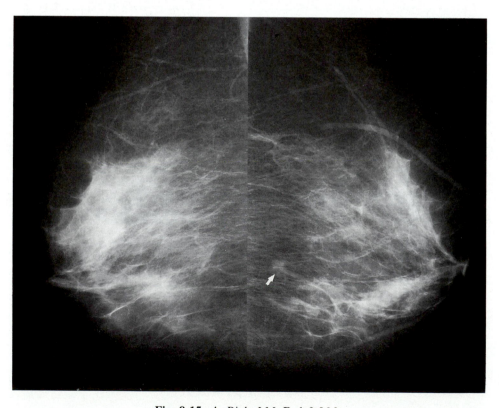

Fig. 9-15. A, Right LM; **B,** left LM.

In comparing the right and left breast, an overall asymmetric parenchymal distribution is noted on the left (Figs. 9-13 and 9-14). On the medial side of the left breast, approximately 12 cm from the nipple, a small asymmetric density, with suspicion of suggested spiculation, is observed (Fig. 9-14, *B*). In the coned projection of this small area of dense tissue, a few discrete microcalcifications are also seen within the lesion (Fig. 9-16). This lesion, best appreciated in the craniocaudal projection, is mammographically suggestive of a malignancy.

SFNB was performed and cytology revealed cancer cells (Fig. 9-17). Following carbon localization and surgery, the diagnosis of highly differentiated invasive ductal carcinoma was histologically confirmed.

Code 5

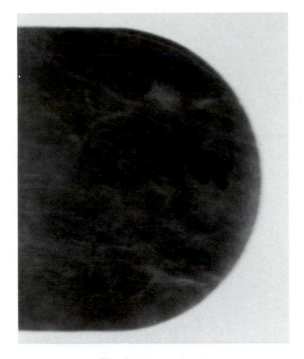

Fig. 9-16. Coned left CC.

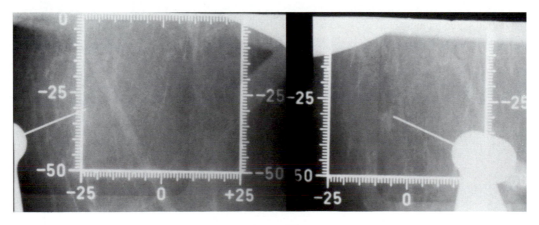

Fig. 9-17. SFNB.

PATIENT 4

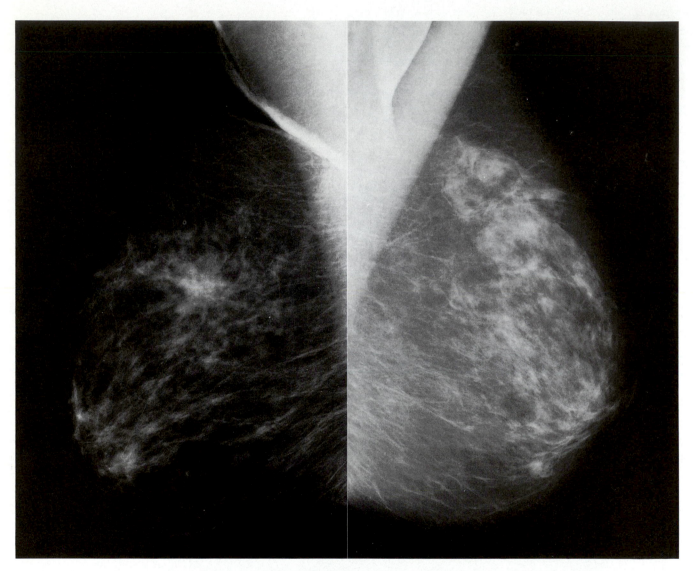

Fig. 9-18. A, Right MLO; **B,** left MLO.

These images (Figs. 9-18 and 9-19) represent a screening mammogram of a 67-year-old asymptomatic woman with lucent breasts.

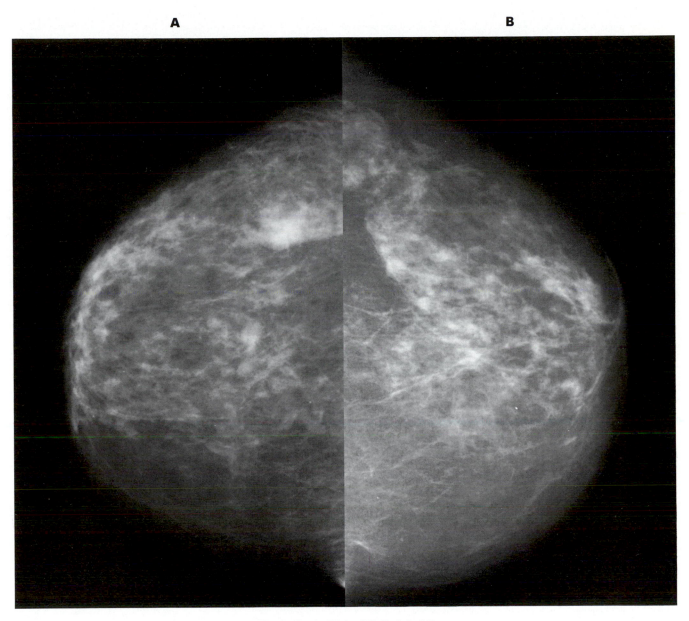

Fig. 9-19. A, Right CC; **B,** left CC.

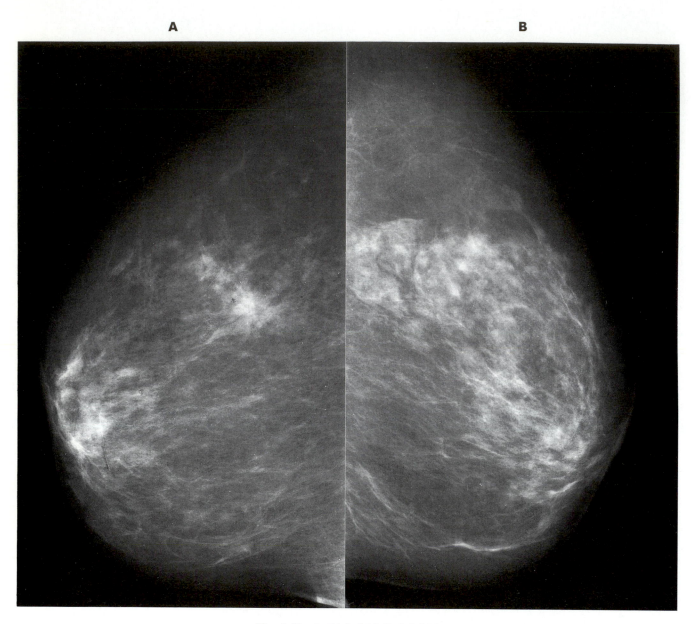

Fig. 9-20. A, Right LM; **B,** left LM.

There is radiographic evidence of bilateral asymmetric distribution of breast parenchyma. In the mediolateral oblique projection, initial comparison of the breasts may lead some to concentrate on the asymmetric pattern in the left breast, at the expense of ignoring the density in the upper outer quadrant on the right (Fig. 9-18). However, the craniocaudal projection demonstrates the dense right breast area and diminishes concern for a potential worrisome asymmetric pattern on the left.

As evidenced in this case, the depiction of significant or less significant areas of concern depends on both routine and special mammographic views (Fig. 9-19). Both the lateromedial projection and the coned compression film revealed the lesion's asymmetric and stellate-like qualities (Figs. 9-20 and 9-21).

Mammographically, this lesion is classified as a code 4 with a high probability of neoplasm. SFNB confirmed malignant epithelial cells, and histologic evaluation of the lesion confirmed invasive lobular carcinoma (Fig. 9-22).

Code 4

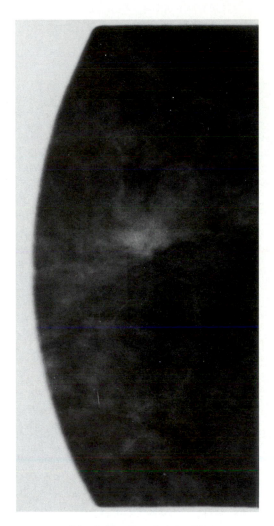

Fig. 9-21. Coned right CC.

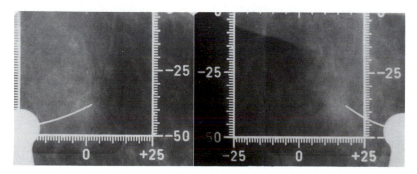

Fig. 9-22. SFNB.

PATIENT 5

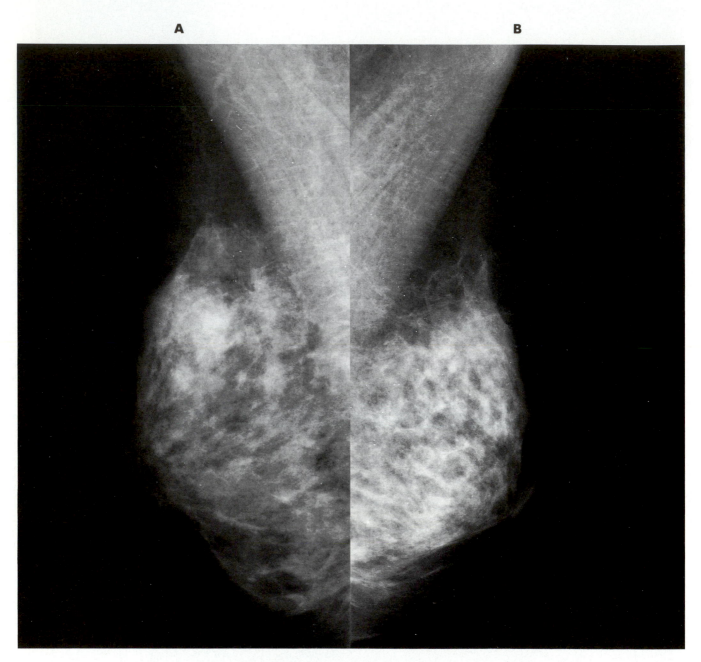

Fig. 9-23. A, Right MLO; **B,** left MLO.

These images (Figs. 9-23 and 9-24) are from a screening mammogram of a 67-year-old asymptomatic woman with dense breast parenchyma.

A   B

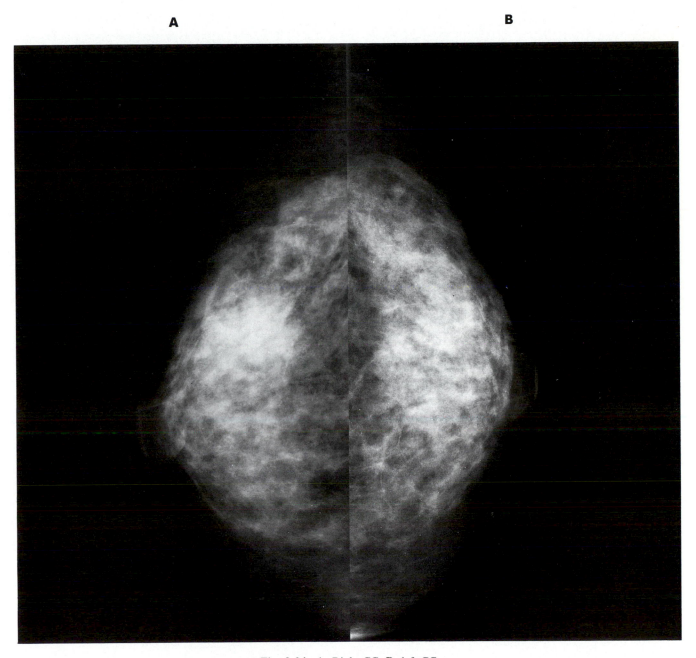

Fig. 9-24. A, Right CC; **B,** left CC.

In the standard mediolateral and craniocaudal projections, an asymmetric density is seen in the upper outer quadrant of the right breast (Figs. 9-23, *A,* and 9-24, *A*). The value of coned mammography projections has been previously discussed.[5]

It is noteworthy that in this woman's case the coned craniocaudal projection does not help to reliably distinguish the presence of a lesion (Fig. 9-25). In contrast, however, in positioning this woman for a mediolateral oblique projection and applying coned compression, a very worrisome-appearing lesion is identified with certainty (Fig. 9-26). The value of combining coned compression projections and varying the breast's position to confirm a suspected lesion is again appreciated.

SFNB and cytology of the density proved it to be carcinoma. Following carbon marking of the lesion and its surgical removal, histology reconfirmed the cancer diagnosis of invasive lobular carcinoma.

Code 5

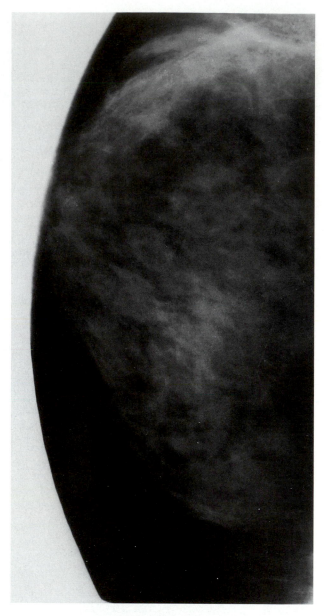

Fig. 9-25. Coned right CC.

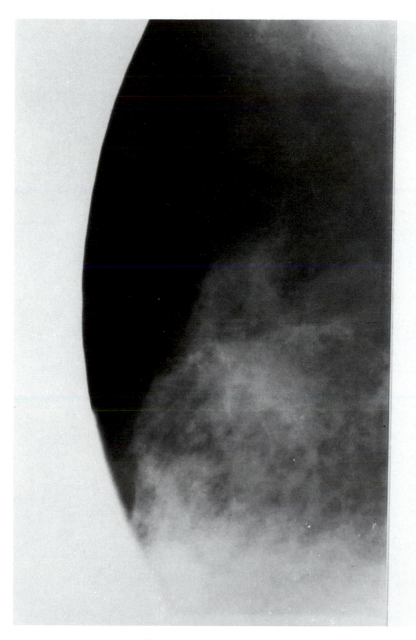

Fig. 9-26. Coned right MLO.

PATIENT 6

A   B

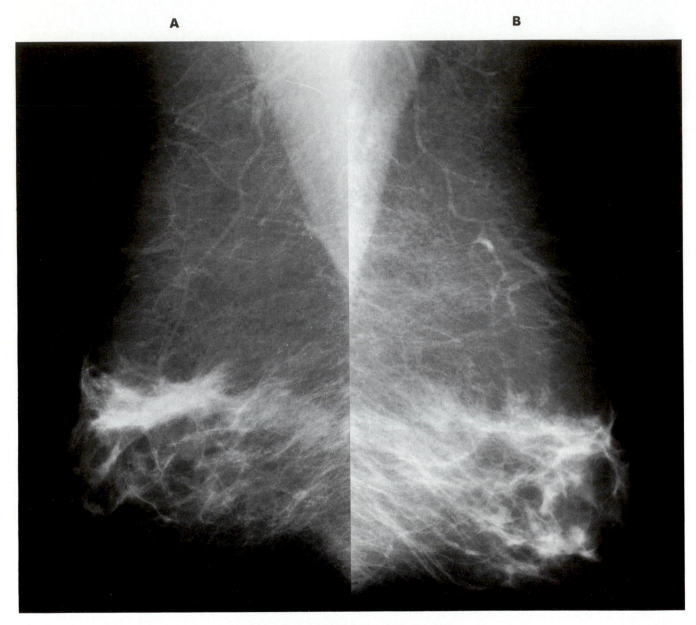

Fig. 9-27. A, Right MLO. **B,** left MLO.

These images (Figs. 9-27 and 9-28) are from a screening mammogram of a 56-year-old asymptomatic woman.

A

B

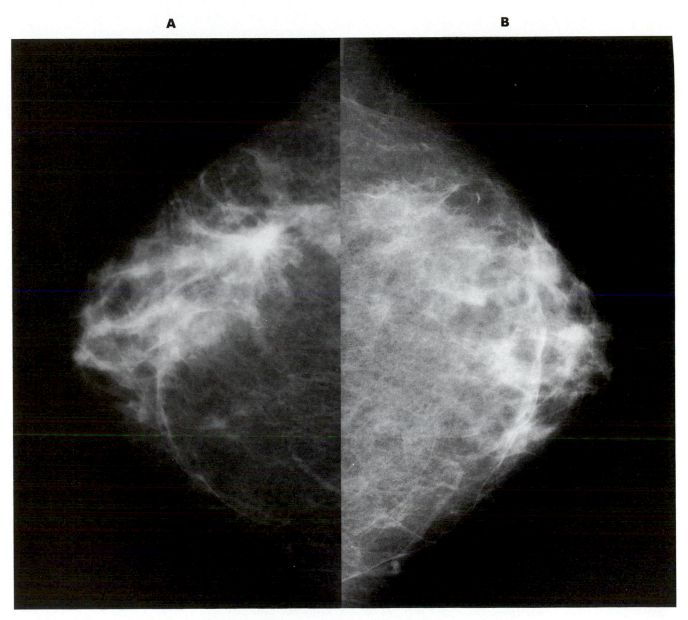

Fig. 9-28. A, Right CC; **B,** left CC.

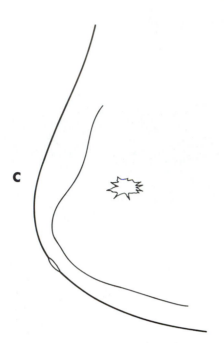

Fourteen years before this screening evaluation, this woman had undergone bilateral breast reduction. This woman had not been vigilant about continuing breast examination and neglected mammography follow-up.

If one had access to only the mediolateral projections, considering her history of previous surgery, an initial radiology perception of "postsurgical changes" would be a feasible consideration. However, in viewing both the routine craniocaudal mammography projection and the coned compression projections of the right breast, a pattern of mammographic cancer is soon revealed (Fig. 9-28 and 9-30). Mild parenchymal asymmetry with denser breast tissue is noted in the right breast (Fig. 9-27, *A*). Evalua-

Fig. 9-27, cont'd. **C,** Right MLO (line drawing).

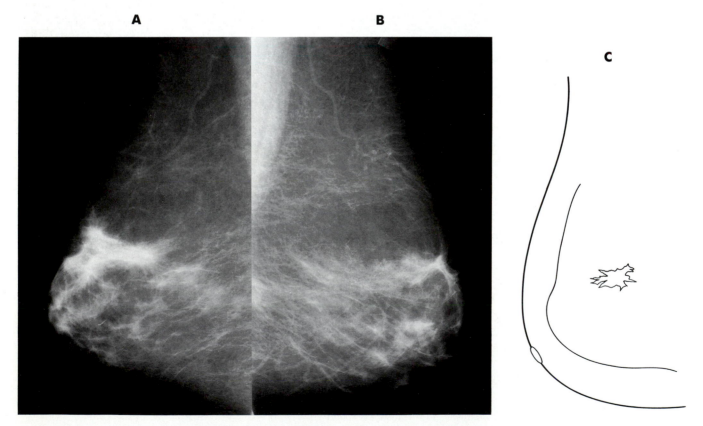

Fig. 9-29. **A,** Right LM; **B,** left LM; **C,** right LM (line drawing).

tion of the right upper outer quadrant in both the craniocaudal and the lateromedial projections immediately reveals that the dense breast area also consists of spiculate
borders (Figs. 9-28, *A,* and 9-29, *A*). Further confirmation
of this pattern is evidenced on the coned magnification
projection (Fig. 9-30). This now easily distinguishable
mammographic pattern is automatically assigned a code 5
classification.

SFNB and carbon localization were performed. Cytology of the lesion revealed gross atypia and enlarged nuclei
representing cancer (Fig. 9-31). Histology of the lesion
confirmed moderately differentiated invasive ductal carcinoma.

Code 5

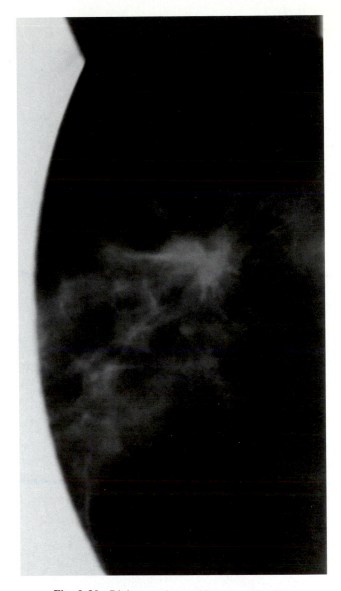

Fig. 9-30. Right coned magnification projection.

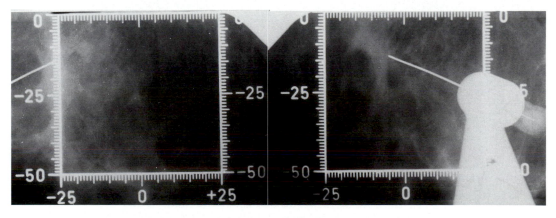

Fig. 9-31. Right SFNB.

PATIENT 7

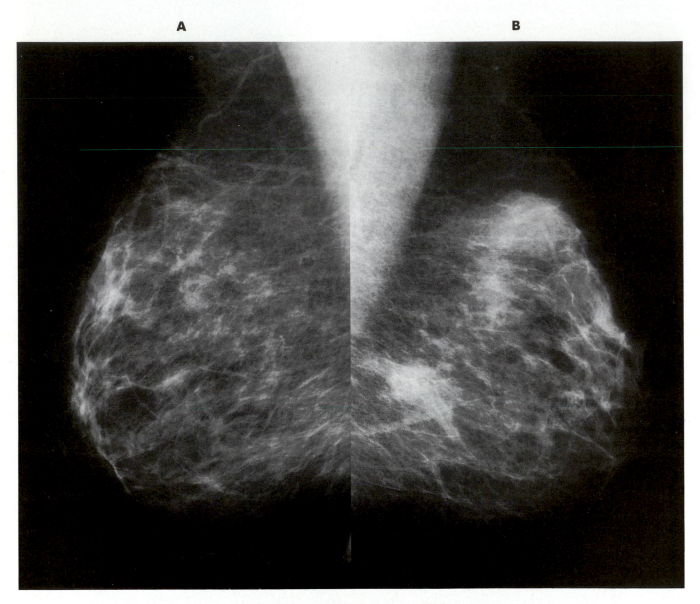

Fig. 9-32. A, Right MLO; **B,** left MLO.

These images (Figs. 9-32 and 9-33) represent a screening mammogram of a 68-year-old asymptomatic woman.

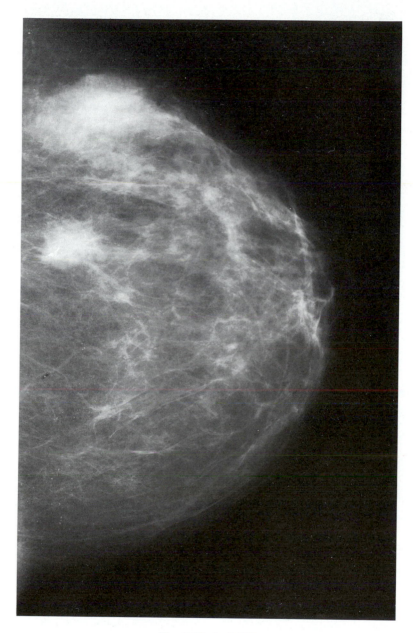

Fig. 9-33. Left CC.

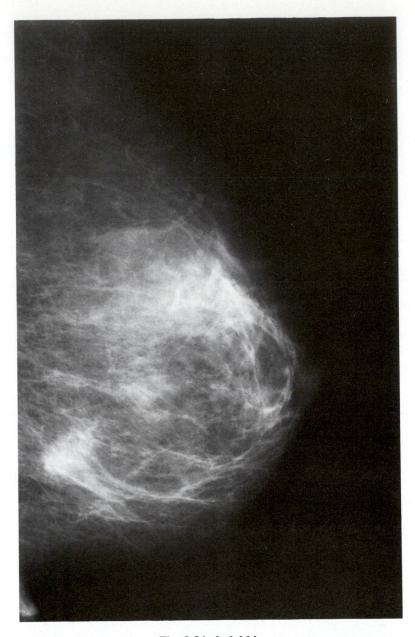

Fig. 9-34. Left LM.

There is obvious asymmetry of the left breast. Most notable is the asymmetric density in the outer quadrant on the left. This rather ill-defined lesion is void of typical spicula. However, microcalcifications are apparent both within the density and within the surrounding breast stroma (Fig. 9-35). Despite the 2 cm diameter of this asymmetric lesion, the density was not palpable at clinical breast examination because of its central location within the breast tissue.

SFNB was recommended, and cytology confirmed malignant epithelial cells (Fig. 9-36). Histology of the lesion confirmed poorly differentiated invasive ductal carcinoma.

Code 5

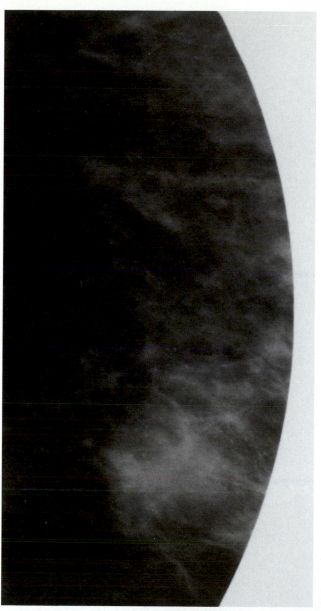

Fig. 9-35. Coned left LM.

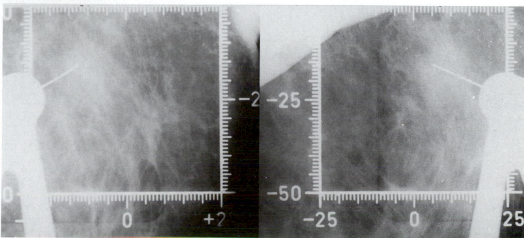

Fig. 9-36. SFNB.

PATIENT 8

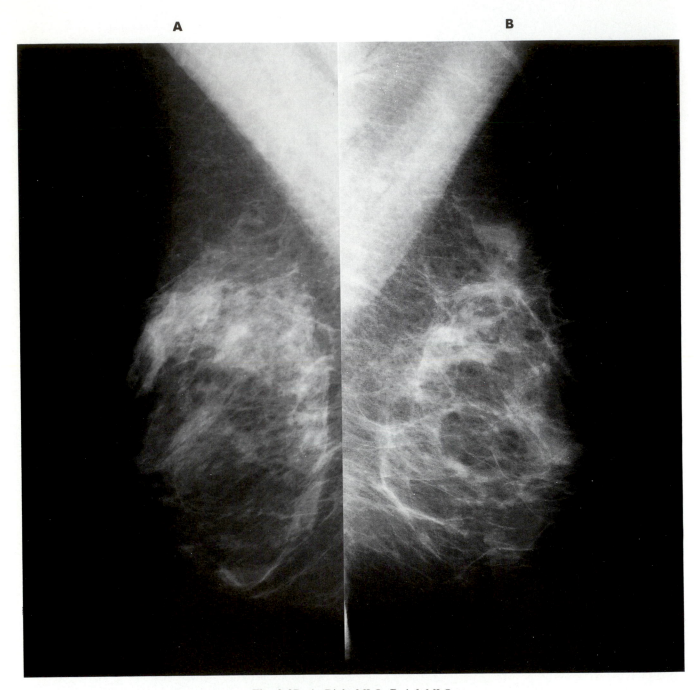

Fig. 9-37. A, Right MLO; **B,** left MLO.

These images (Figs. 9-37 and 9-38) represent a screening mammogram of a 60-year-old asymptomatic woman with moderately dense breasts.

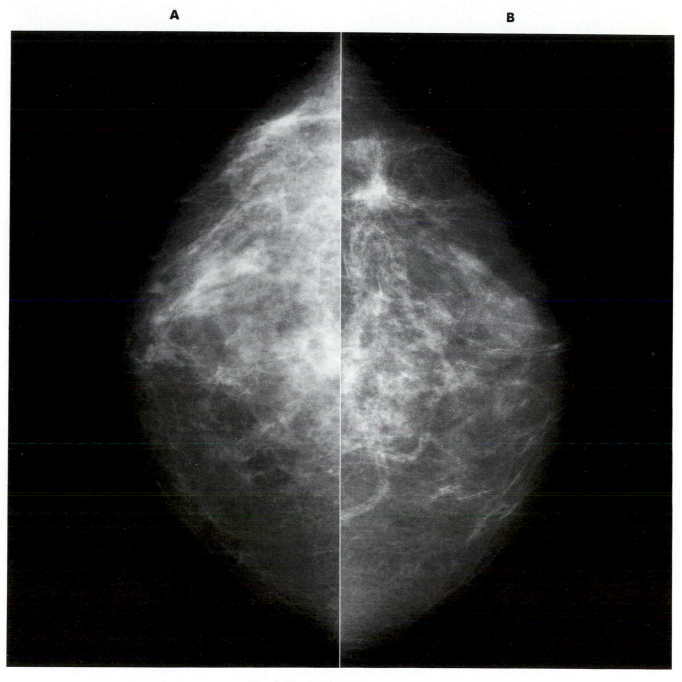

Fig. 9-38. A, Right CC; **B,** left CC.

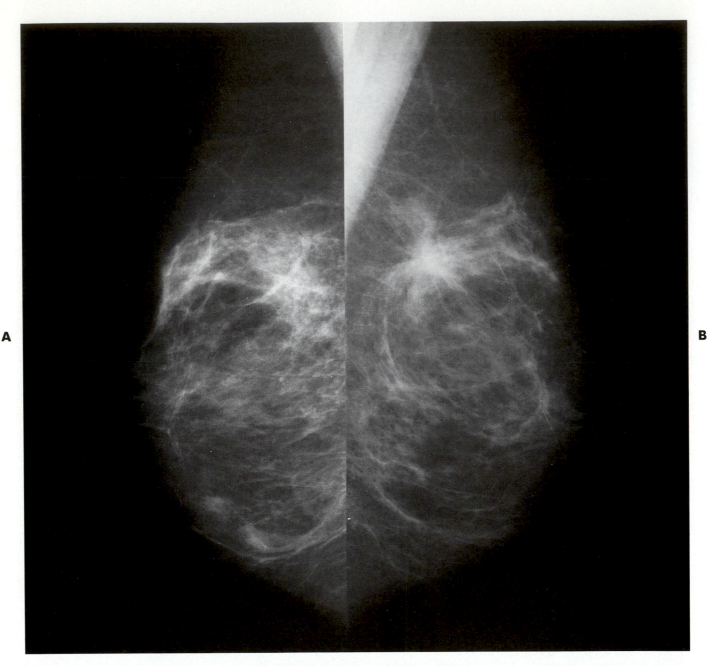

Fig. 9-39. A, Right LM; **B,** left LM.

At initial breast screening evaluation, an asymmetric density with minimal paren-chymal distortion is detected in the upper outer quadrant of the left breast (Fig. 9-37, *B*). The lesion is not readily apparent on the mediolateral oblique projection but is easily detected on the craniocaudal projection (Fig. 9-38, *B*). Further mammographic workup of this highly suspicious area is warranted. Both the lateromedial and the coned projec-tions obviously reconfirm the mammographic finding of an asymmetric mass, which mammographically represents a malignant lesion (Figs. 9-39, *B,* and 9-40).

SFNB and carbon marking of the lesion were performed. Cytology revealed malig-nant epithelial cells (Fig. 9-41). Histology proved the lesion to be a moderately well-differentiated invasive ductal carcinoma (Fig. 9-42).

Code 5

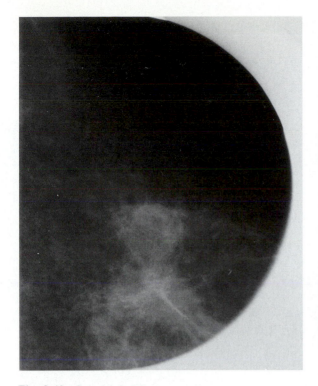

Fig. 9-40. Coned left CC.

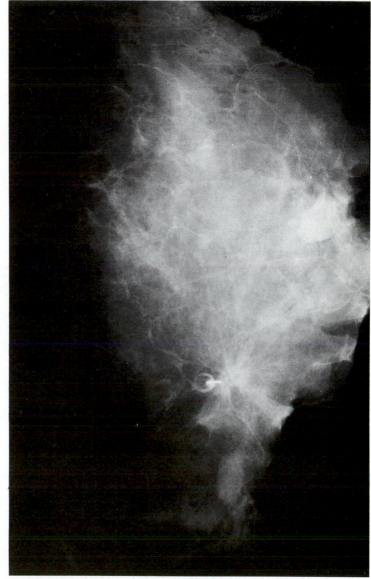

Fig. 9-42. Biopsy specimen.

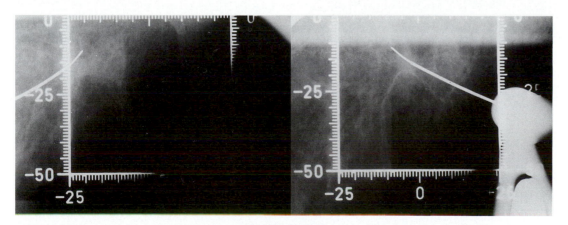

Fig. 9-41. SFNB.

PATIENT 9

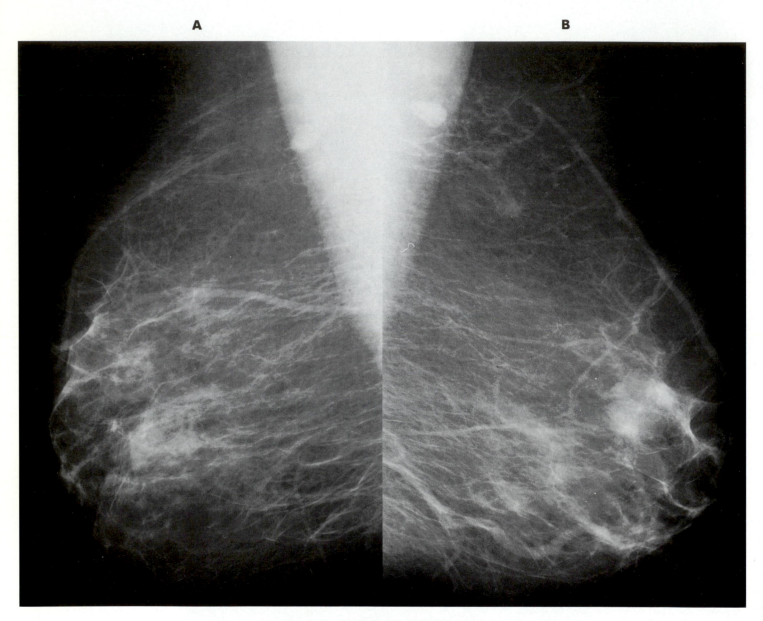

Fig. 9-43. A, Right MLO; **B,** left MLO.

These images (Figs. 9-43 and 9-44) are from a screening mammogram of a 65-year-old asymptomatic woman with moderately lucent breasts.

A

B

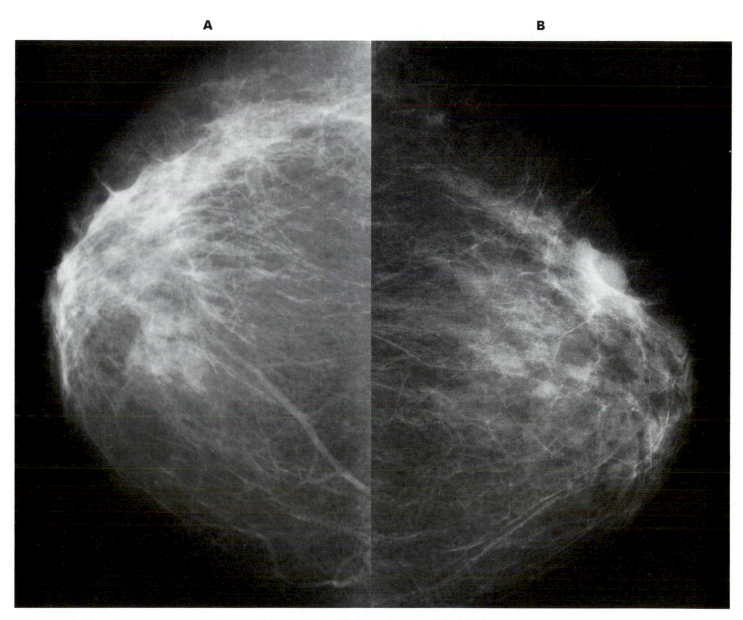

Fig. 9-44. A, Right CC; **B,** left CC.

Parenchymal asymmetry of the breast is seen near the left nipple (Fig. 9-43, *B*). Careful evaluation of this area helps to conclude that the breast changes are most likely within normal limits. There is, however, a small, solitary asymmetric density in the left upper outer quadrant that warrants further evaluation (Figs. 9-43, *B,* and 9-45, *B*). Coned compression projections were taken of both areas in question. When compressed, the dense tissue area near the nipple was relieved and offered normal breast texture. The coned projection of the solitary asymmetric density, however, reveals subtle spiculations surrounding the lesion (Fig. 9-46). Once this spiculated pattern is mammographically evident, it represents carcinoma until proved otherwise.

SFNB was performed on the lesion in the upper outer quadrant and cytology revealed malignant cells (Fig. 9-47). Histology of the lesion confirmed moderately differentiated invasive ductal carcinoma.

Code 5

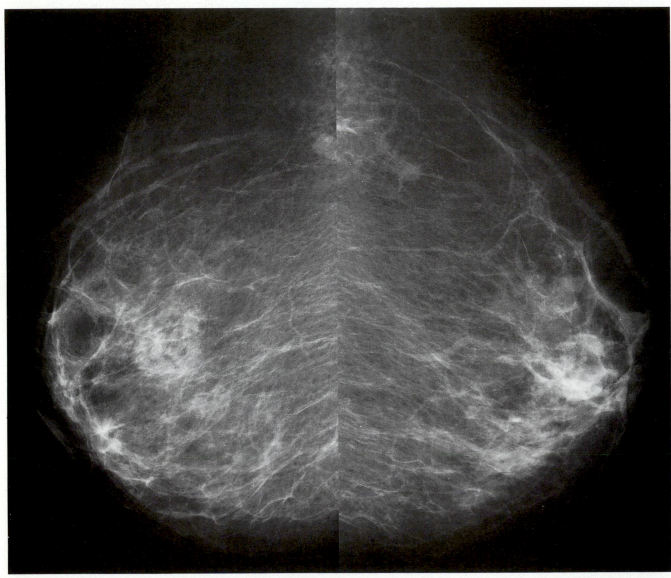

Fig. 9-45. A, Right LM; **B,** left LM.

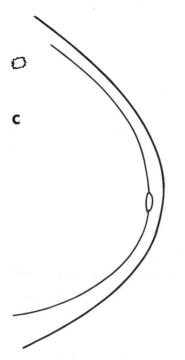

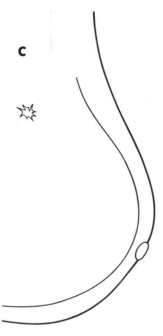

Fig. 9-44, cont'd. C, Left CC (line drawing).

Fig. 9-45, cont'd. C, Left LM (line drawing).

Fig. 9-46. Coned left LM.

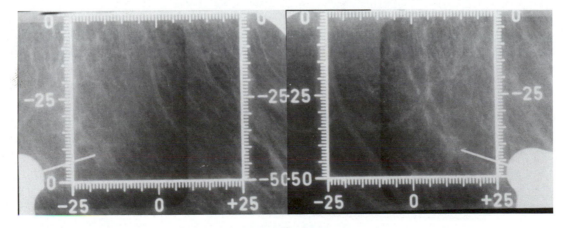

Fig. 9-47. SFNB.

PATIENT 10

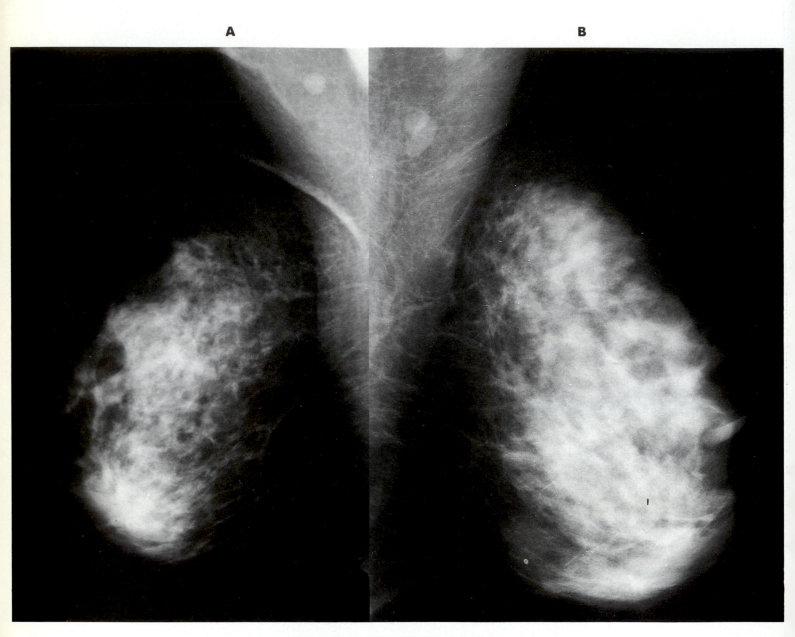

Fig. 9-48. A, Right MLO; **B,** left MLO.

These images (Figs. 9-48 and 9-49) are from a screening mammogram of a 50-year-old woman with dense breasts.

A   B

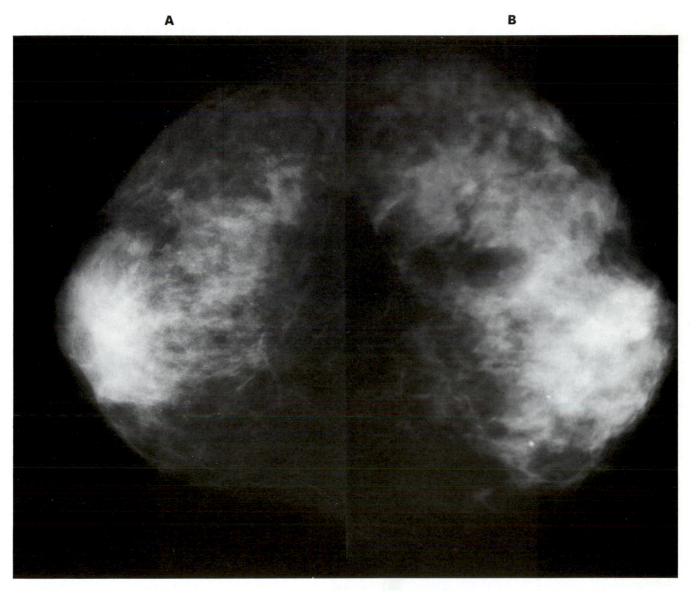

Fig. 9-49. A, Right CC; **B,** left CC.

C

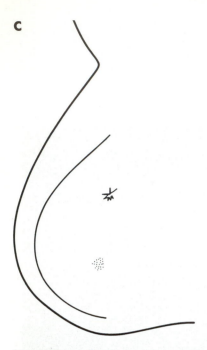

Two findings are present in the right breast. An asymmetric density is seen in the right upper inner quadrant. This mammographic finding is suggestive of malignancy (Fig. 9-48, *A*). A second finding is a group of benign-appearing calcifications also located in the inner quadrant of the breast and inferior to the asymmetric pattern (Figs. 9-48, *A*, and 9-49 *A*). While the calcifications appear dense and rounded, they are nonetheless mammographically nonspecific and require further evaluation.[2]

C

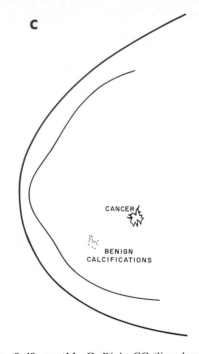

Fig. 9-48, cont'd. C, Right MLO (line drawing).

Fig. 9-49, cont'd. C, Right CC (line drawing).

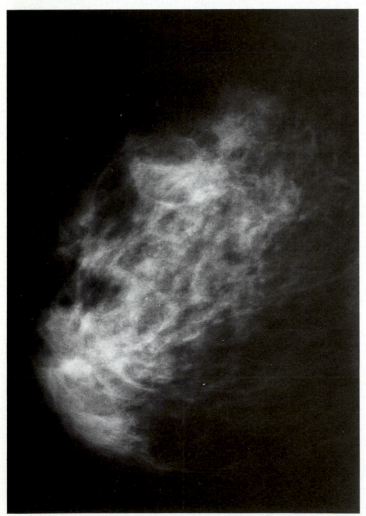

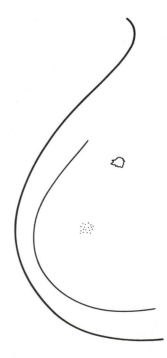

Fig. 9-50. A, Right LM; **B,** right LM (line drawing).

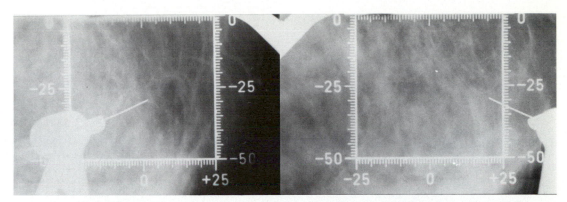

Fig. 9-51. SFNB, benign calcifications.

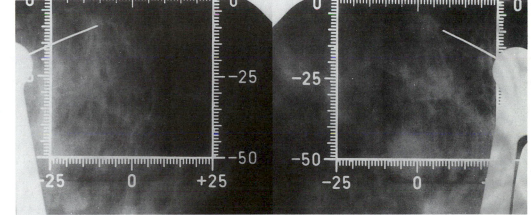

Fig. 9-52. SFNB, cancer.

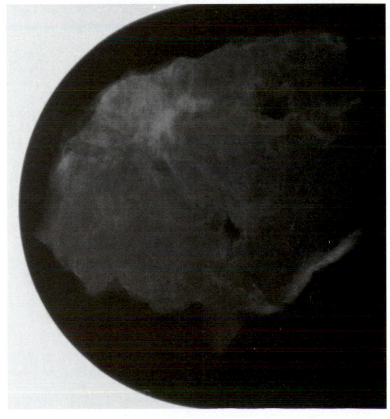

SFNB was performed at both sites. The mammographic interpretations of benignancy in the area of calcifications and of malignancy in the stellate-like asymmetric breast tissue were cytologically confirmed (Figs. 9-51 and 9-52). Removal of only the cancerous lesion was required. Histology of the asymmetric lesion confirmed a moderately well-differentiated invasive ductal carcinoma (Fig. 9-53).

Code 2—benign calcifications
Code 4—asymmetric density with spicula (probable cancer)

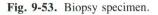

Fig. 9-53. Biopsy specimen.

PATIENT 11

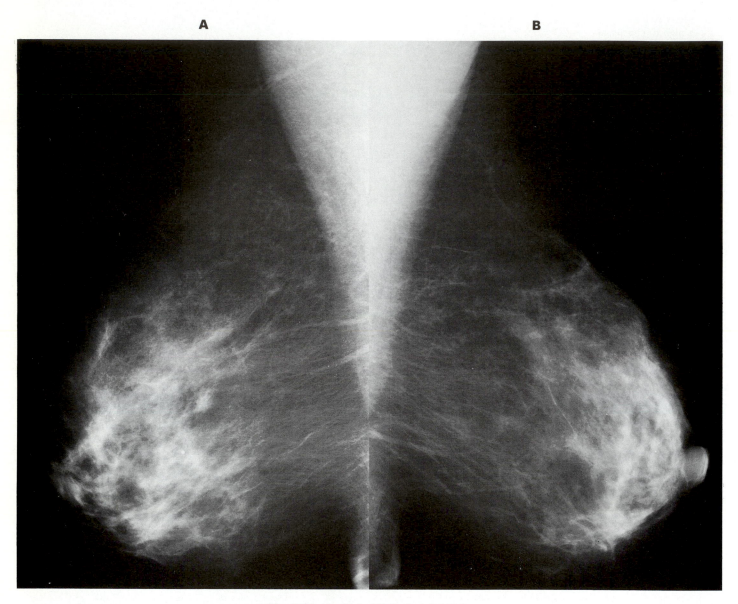

Fig. 9-54. A, Right MLO; **B,** left MLO.

These images (Figs. 9-54 and 9-55) represent a screening mammogram of a 58-year-old asymptomatic woman with dense breasts.

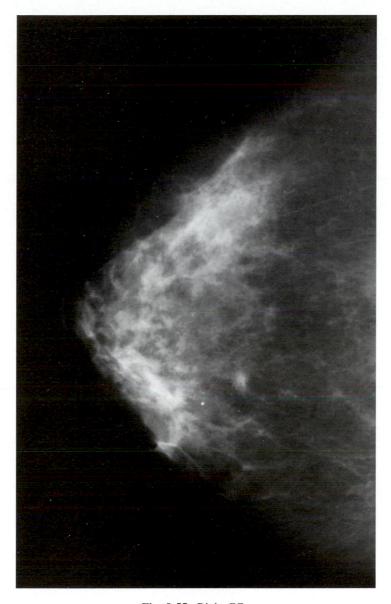

Fig. 9-55. Right CC.

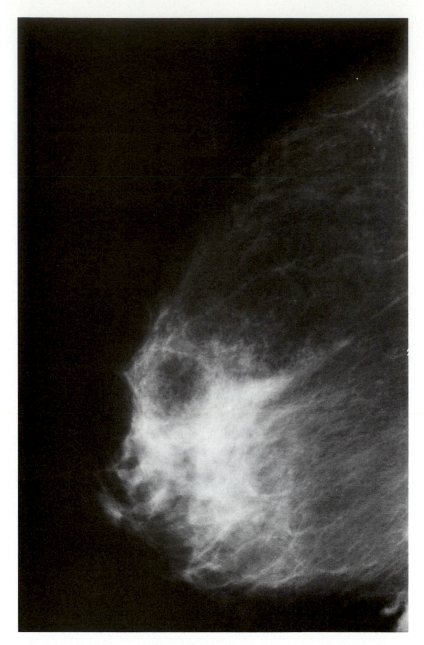

Fig. 9-56. Right LM.

An asymmetric density is observed on the medial side of the right nipple. Several discrete microcalcifications and a dense, benign-appearing calcification are also seen within surrounding breast tissue (Figs. 9-55 and 9-56). Coned compression views of the lesion confirm its presence, but again appearance of the lesion is more persistent on the standard mediolateral oblique and craniocaudal projections (Fig. 9-57). Various combinations of mammography views either elevate or diminish our concern and help achieve a definitive diagnosis (Patients 4 and 5). This density is mammographically suspicious for malignancy.

SFNB was performed and cytology demonstrated cancer cells (Fig. 9-58). Histology of the density confirmed well-differentiated invasive ductal carcinoma.

While involution changes do not occur equally in each breast quadrant, it is recognized that glandular density usually diminishes initially in the lower inner quadrant of the breast. Mammographic involution patterns assist in the detection of previously obscured dense breast lesions against the more lucent background of postinvolutional breast tissue.[4]

Code 4

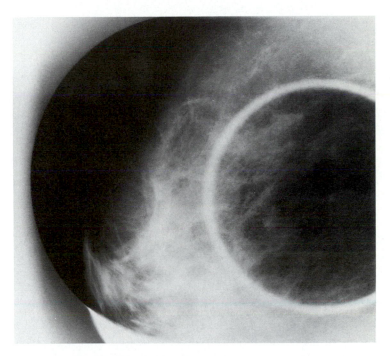

Fig. 9-57. Coned right breast.

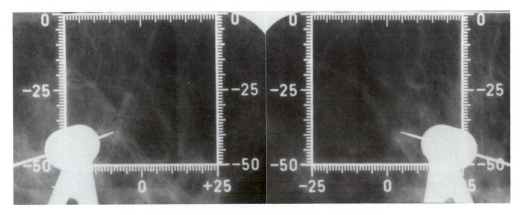

Fig. 9-58. SFNB.

PATIENT 12

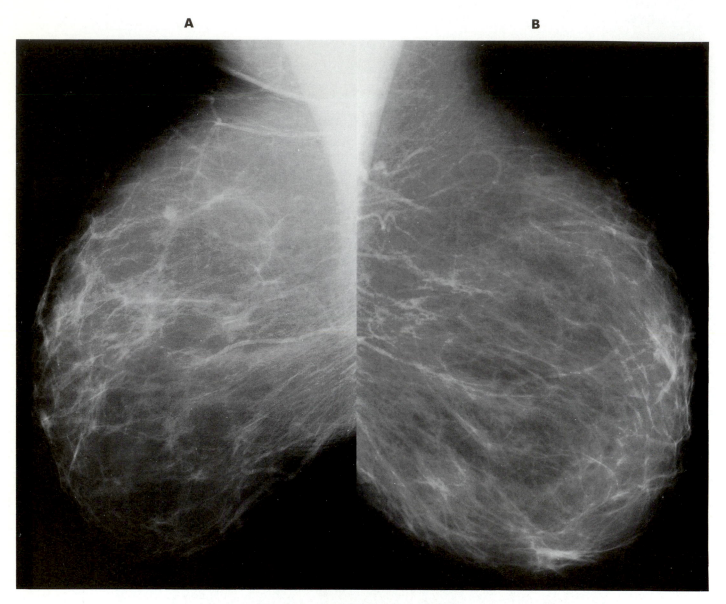

Fig. 9-59. A, Right MLO; **B,** left MLO.

These images (Figs. 9-59 and 9-60) are from a screening mammogram of a 66-year-old asymptomatic woman with large, lucent breasts.

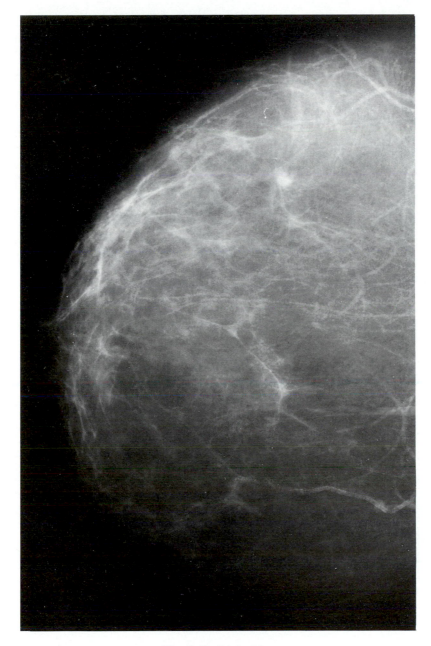

Fig. 9-60. Right CC.

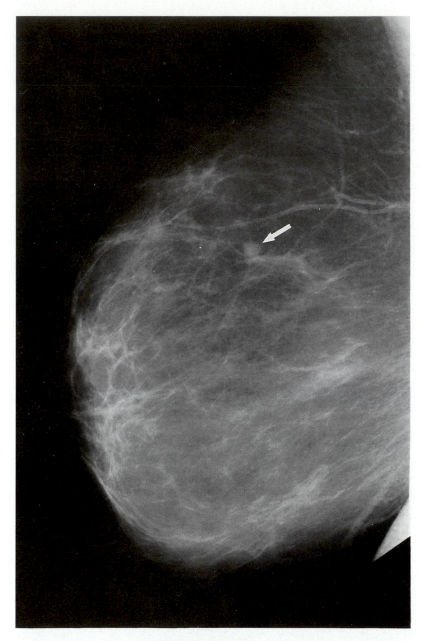

Fig. 9-61. Right LM.

An asymmetric density is seen in the upper outer quadrant of the right breast (Fig. 9-59, *A*). This screening-detected abnormality, while small, is readily evident because of the rather lucent nature of this woman's breasts.

Lack of homogeneity, usually seen in larger lesions, is not usually present in smaller lesions. However, this lesion appears to have had enough time to begin developing secondary signs of asymmetry, suggesting a slightly stellate pattern (Fig. 9-60). Mammographically, this lesion is very suspicious for malignancy.

On the basis of this mammographic finding, SFNB of the lesion was performed. Cytology revealed cancer cells. Histology of the lesion confirmed poorly differentiated invasive ductal carcinoma.

Code 5

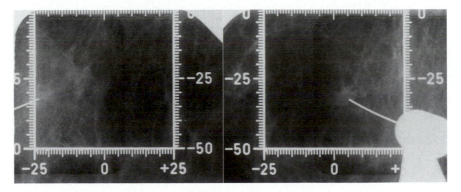

Fig. 9-62. SFNB.

PATIENT 13

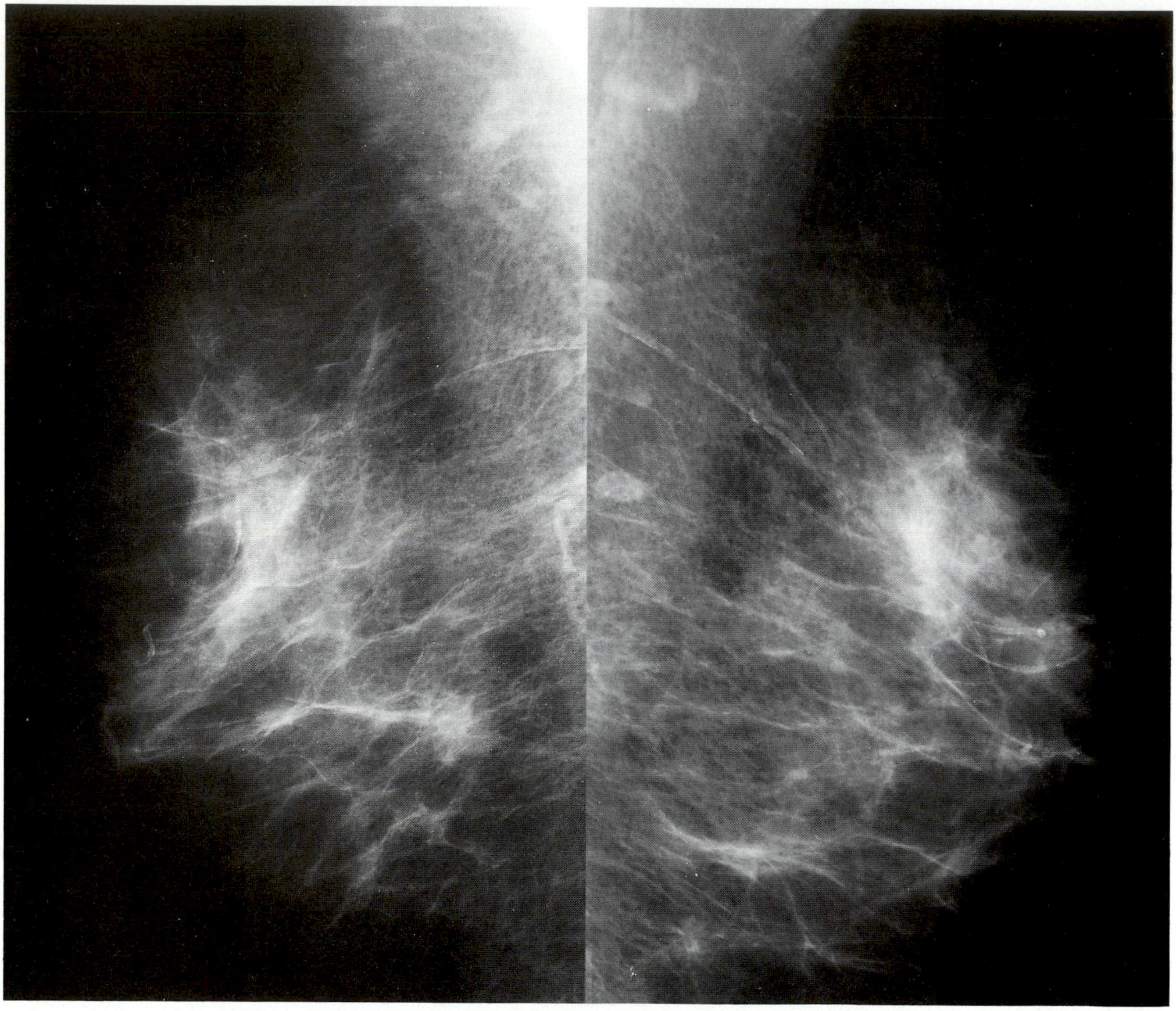

Fig. 9-63. A, Right MLO; **B,** left MLO.

These images (Figs. 9-63 and 9-64) represent a screening mammogram of a 59-year-old asymptomatic woman.

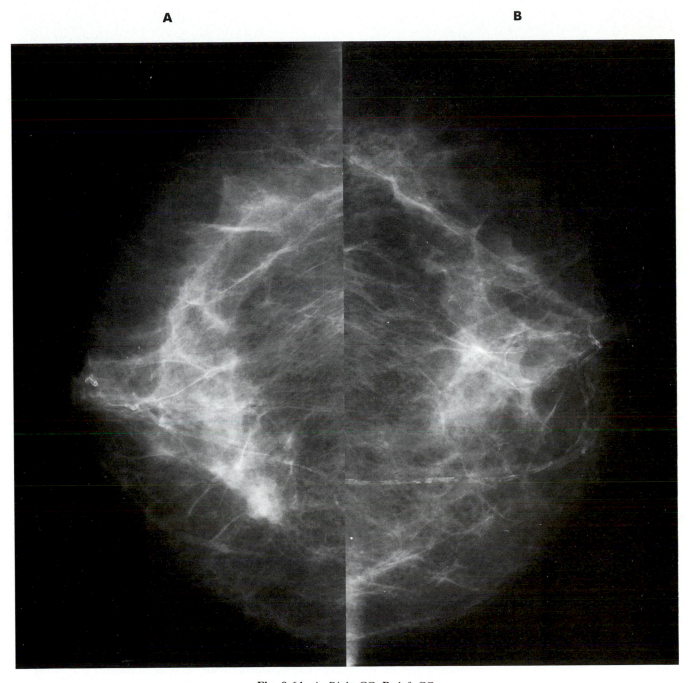

Fig. 9-64. A, Right CC; **B,** left CC.

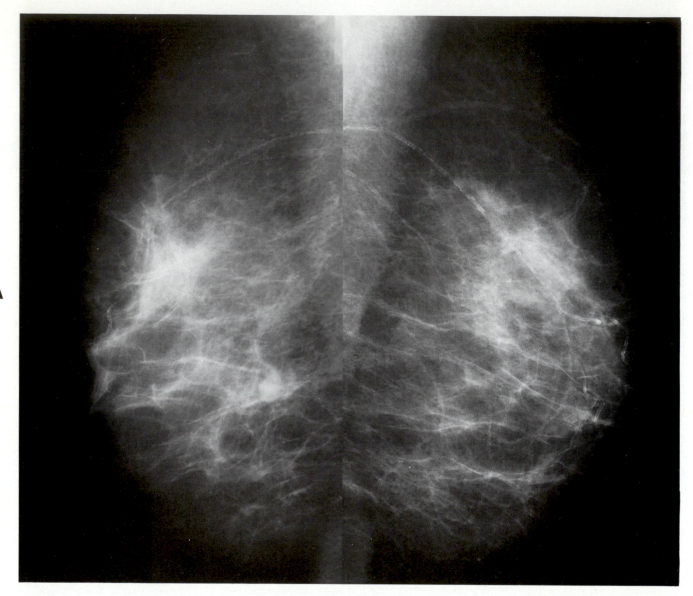

Fig. 9-65. **A,** Right LM; **B,** left LM.

While this woman's mammogram reveals a moderate amount of breast parenchyma bilaterally, an asymmetric density is observed on the medial side of the nipple in the right breast, requiring further work-up (Fig. 9-63, *A*).

This asymmetric density initially appears somewhat circumscript in nature on the lateromedial projection (Fig. 9-65, *A*). A closer look at the craniocaudal projection confirms one's aroused suspicion for an increase in fibroglandular tissue with associated spiculation (Fig. 9-64, *A*). The right coned projection confirms the density and its unsharp margins. This projection also lends further evidence of the spiculated nature of involved breast tissue (Fig. 9-66). Mammographically, this suggests cancer, and the density is immediately designated as a code 5 lesion.

SFNB was performed and carbon localization was accomplished. Cytology confirmed malignant cells, and histology of the lesion confirmed moderately differentiated invasive ductal carcinoma and several areas with ductal carcinoma in situ. The radial spiculated pattern of the lesion is easily recognized in the biopsy specimen (Fig. 9-68).

Code 5

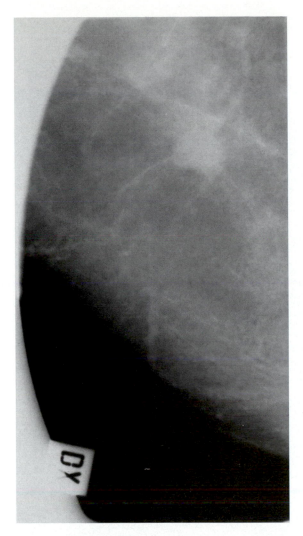

Fig. 9-66. Right coned projection.

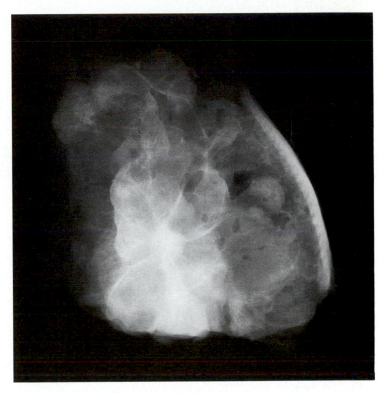

Fig. 9-68. Biopsy specimen.

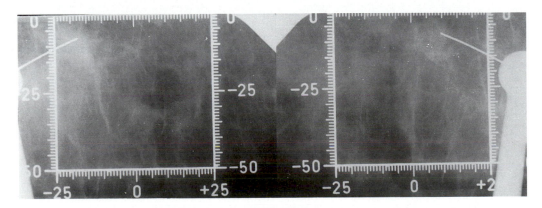

Fig. 9-67. SFNB.

PATIENT 14

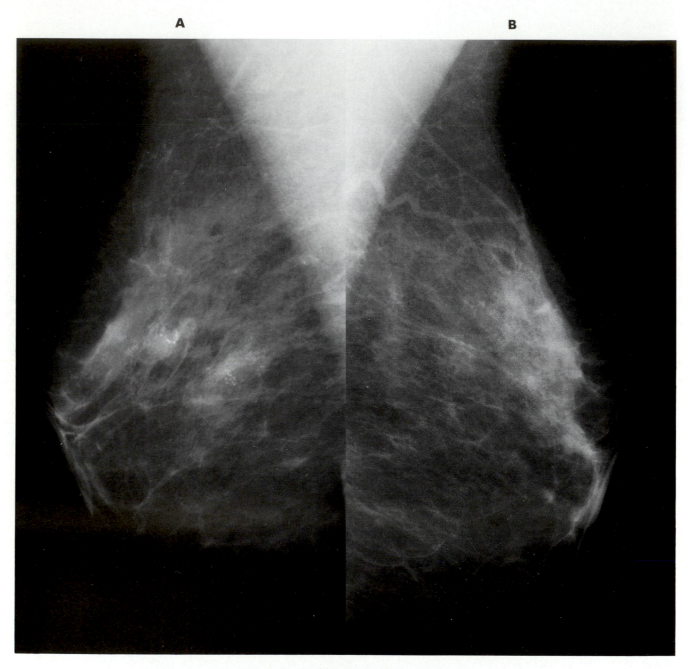

Fig. 9-69. A, Right MLO; **B,** left MLO.

These images (Figs. 9-69 and 9-70) represent a screening mammogram of a 50-year-old asymptomatic woman with a moderate amount of breast parenchyma.

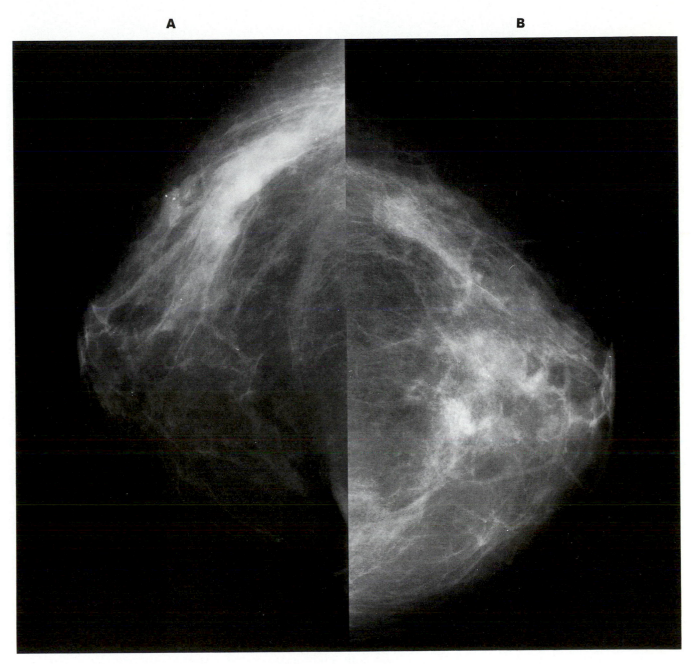

Fig. 9-70. A, Right CC; **B,** left CC.

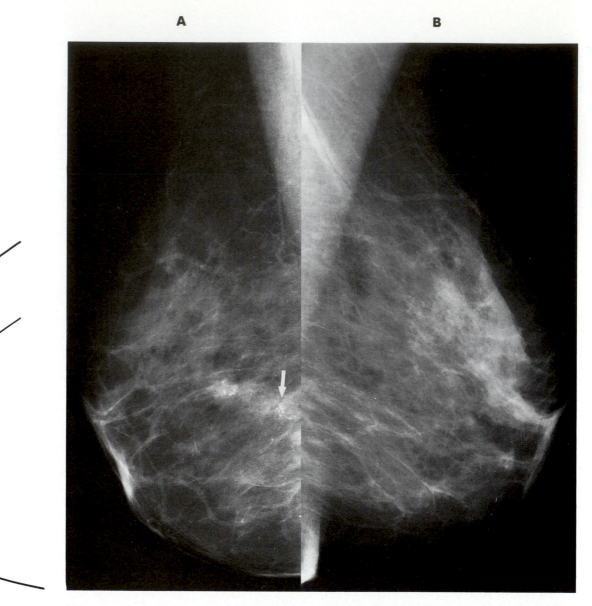

Fig. 9-70, cont'd. C, Right CC (line drawing).

Fig. 9-71. A, Right LM; **B,** left LM.

There is a combination of findings in this woman's breast screening evaluation. Groups of irregular calcifications and increased density of the breast tissue are seen in both the right mediolateral oblique and the right craniocaudal breast projections. In the medial aspect of the left breast, there is a more subtle asymmetric density, best seen in the craniocaudal projection (Fig. 9-70, *B*). Both lesions are mammographically suspicious for malignancy, with a slightly higher index of suspicion for neoplasm in the right breast lesion.

Unfortunately, this woman had no previous mammograms to compare with these current findings. Further radiographic work-up employing coned compression views, especially of the left breast, demonstrate not only the persistent increase in breast density but also associated calcifications within the lesion (Fig. 9-72).

SFNB was performed on both suspicious areas, with cytology revealing malignant cells in both lesions (Figs. 9-73 and 9-74). Histology confirmed bilateral ductal carcinoma in situ and a bilateral mastectomy procedure was performed in this case.

NOTE: See Chapter 4 for an explanation of the coding system and the importance of code 3.

Code 4—right breast
Code 3—left breast

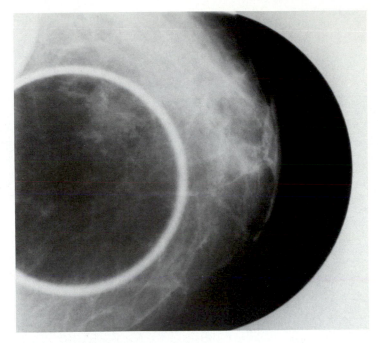

Fig. 9-72. Coned left CC.

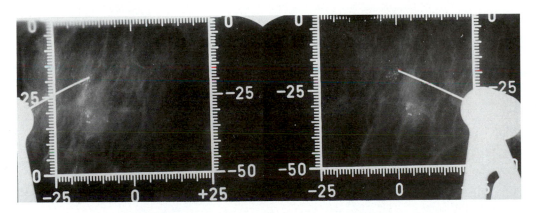

Fig. 9-73. Right SFNB.

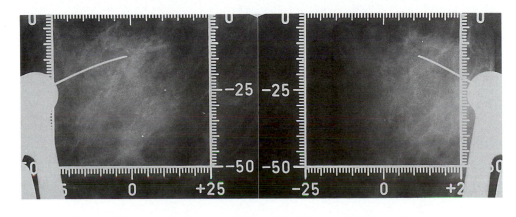

Fig. 9-74. Left SFNB.

PATIENT 15

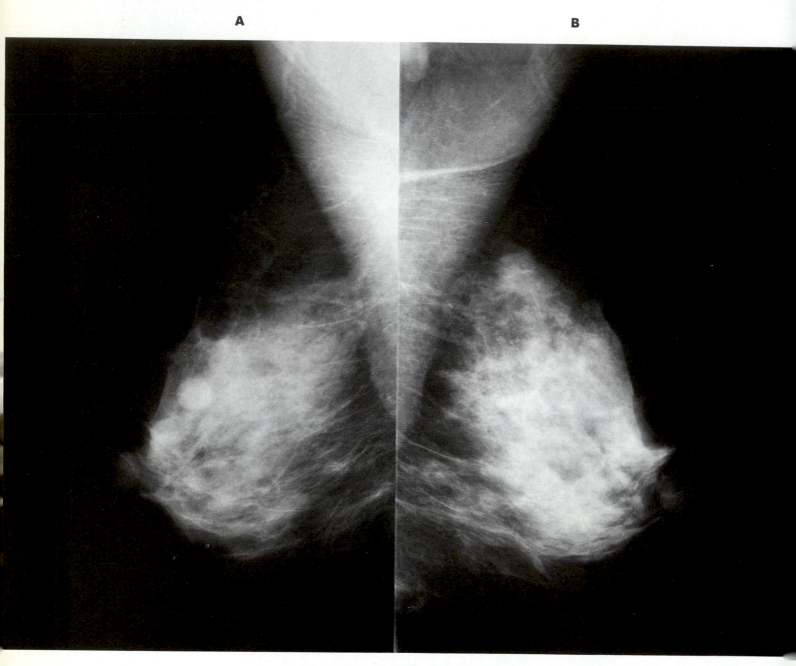

Fig. 9-75. A, Right MLO; **B,** left MLO.

These images (Figs. 9-75 and 9-76) represent a screening mammogram of a 51-year-old asymptomatic woman with very dense breasts.

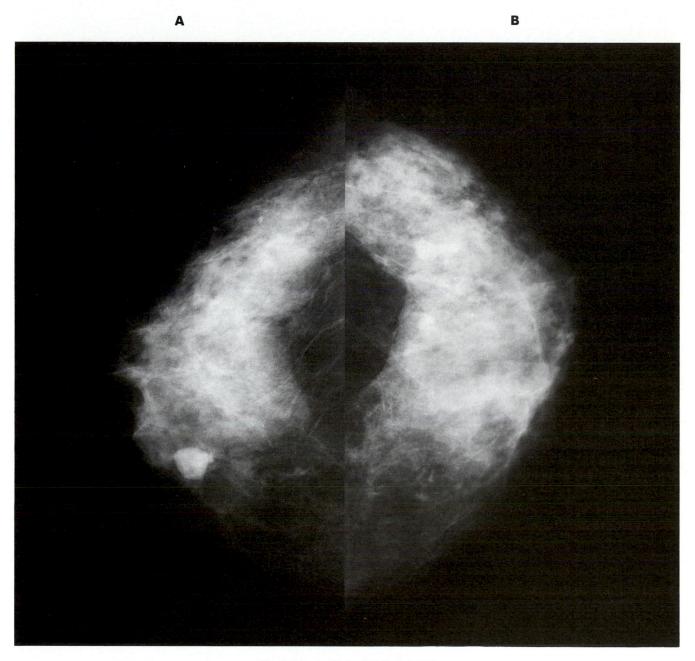

Fig. 9-76. A, Right CC; **B,** left CC.

A B

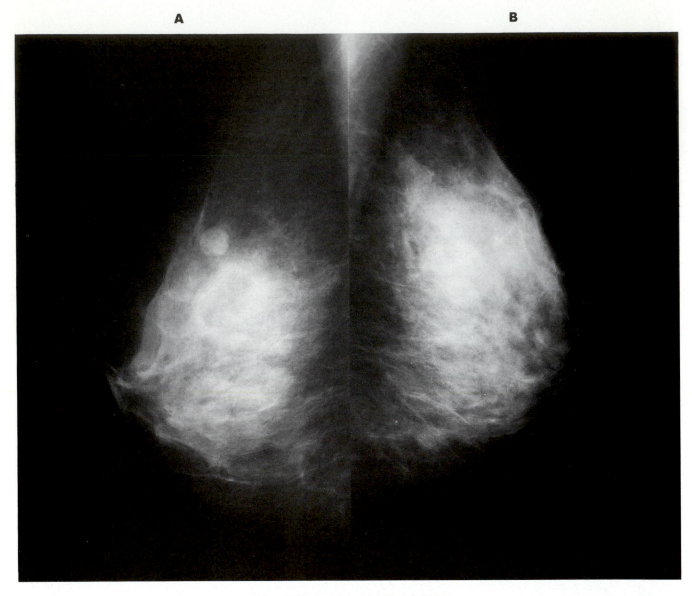

Fig. 9-77. A, Right LM; **B,** left LM.

This woman clearly demonstrated bilateral breast lesions. In the upper inner quadrant of the right breast, there is a well-defined density (Figs. 9-75, *A* and 9-76, *A*). The lesion is very well circumscribed and the margin of the lesion is well defined. This pattern is significant, particularly when detected in younger women. Mammographically, this lesion is suggestive of a fibroadenoma.

SFNB of the right breast was performed. Cytology revealed benign epithelial cells and stromal fragments. No further diagnostic evaluation or surgical intervention of the right breast was necessary.

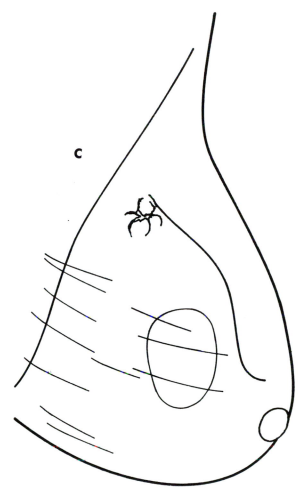

Fig. 9-75, cont'd. C, Left MLO (line drawing).

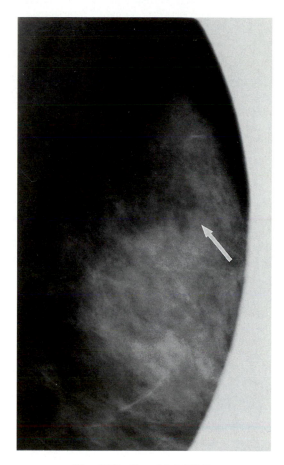

Fig. 9-78. Coned left MLO.

In the mediolateral oblique projection, an asymmetric density in the upper outer quadrant of the left breast can also be appreciated with certainty. This density, unlike the right breast lesion, has unsharp margins (Fig. 9-77). Mammographically this lesion is very suspicious for malignancy.

SFNB of the left breast lesion revealed cytology of cell atypia suspicious for cancer. Histology of the left breast lesion confirmed poorly differentiated invasive ductal carcinoma.

Code 2—right breast
Code 4—left breast

REFERENCES

1. Cahill CJ, Boulter PS, Gibbs NM, Price JL: Features of mammographically negative breast tumors, *Br J Surg* 68(12):882-884, 1981.
2. Lanyi M: *Diagnosis and differential diagnosis of breast calcifications,* Berlin, 1986, Springer-Verlag.
3. Peeters PH, Verbeek AL, Zielhuis GA, et al: Breast cancer screening in women over age 50: a critical appraisal (review), *Acta Radiol* 31(3):225-231, 1990.
4. Roebuck EJ: *Clinical radiology of the breast,* Oxford, 1990, Heinemann Professional Publishing.
5. Sickles EA: Further experience with microfocal spot magnification mammography in the assessment of clustered breast microcalcifications, *Radiology* 137(1):9-14, 1980.
6. Strax P: Detection of breast cancer, *Cancer* 66(Suppl):1336-1340, 1990.
7. Tabar L, Dean PB: *Teaching atlas of mammography,* ed 2, New York, 1985, Thieme-Stratton.

Chapter 10

RADIAL SCAR

PATIENT 1

A

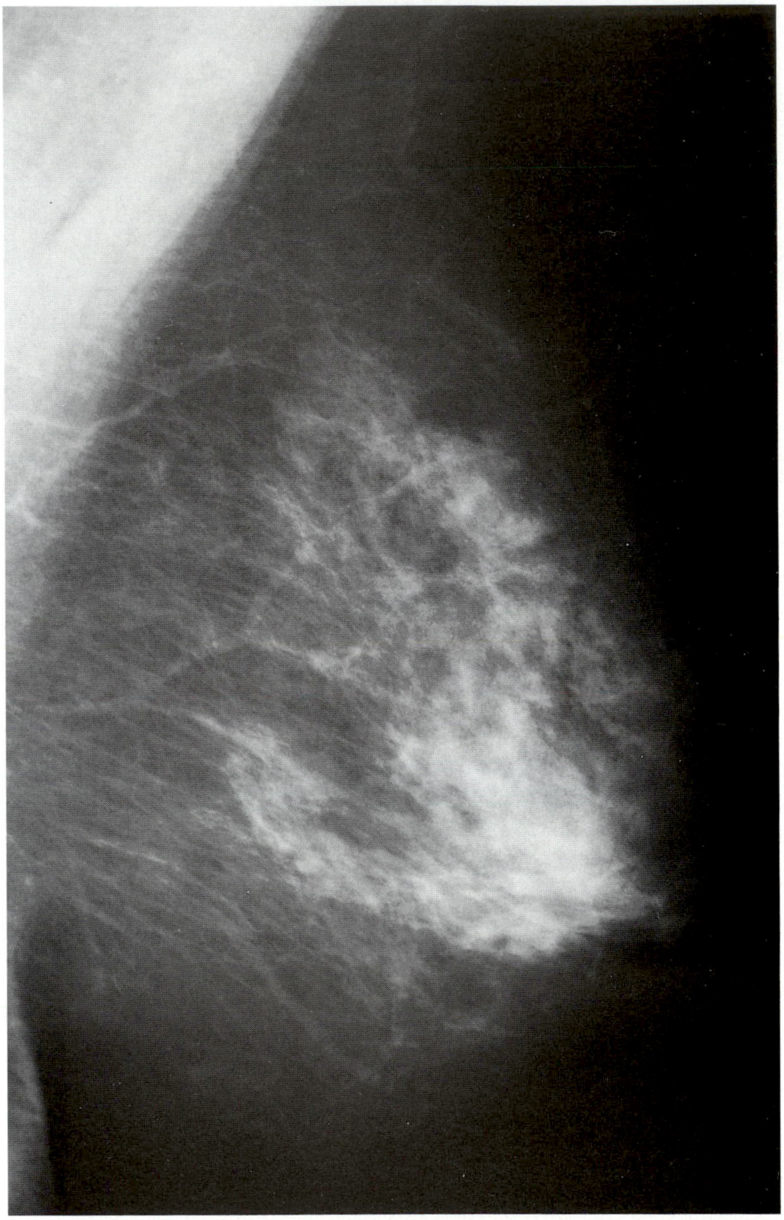

Fig. 10-1. A, Left MLO.

These images (Figs. 10-1, *A*, and 10-2) represent a routine screening mammogram of a 67-year-old woman with moderately dense breast parenchyma.

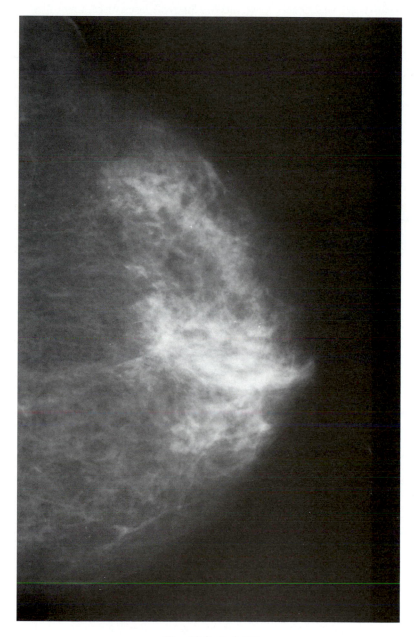

Fig. 10-2. Left CC.

A spiculated density is evident in the craniocaudal view of the left breast (Fig. 10-2). Additional lateromedial and coned magnification projections of the density confirm its stellate-pattern configuration and irregular spiculations (Figs. 10-3, *A,* 10-4, and 10-5).

Stereotaxic fine-needle biopsy (SFNB) was performed in this case and cytology proved negative for malignancy (Fig. 10-6). Surgical biopsy specimen also confirmed the lesion to represent radial scar.

Radial scar lesions have an irregular stellate pattern but are benign and routinely small. This breast lesion is frequently confused with cancer because its mammographic traits are similar to malignant breast conditions.[1] Consequently, with no reliable mammographic characteristic to specifically differentiate benign from malignant, biopsy of this breast lesion is routinely endorsed.

While performing surgery is never deliberately delayed, the SFNB procedure that reveals positive cytology allows for immediate carbon localization and also allows more options of freedom to schedule definitive surgery of the lesion. The stereotaxic procedure, detecting malignant cells, provides the surgeon an opportunity to discuss surgical management and postsurgical treatment plans with the patient.

Code 3

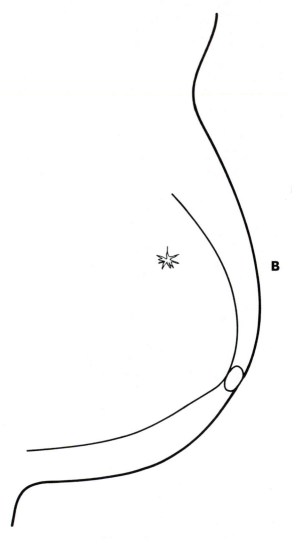

Fig. 10-1, cont'd. B, Left MLO (line drawing).

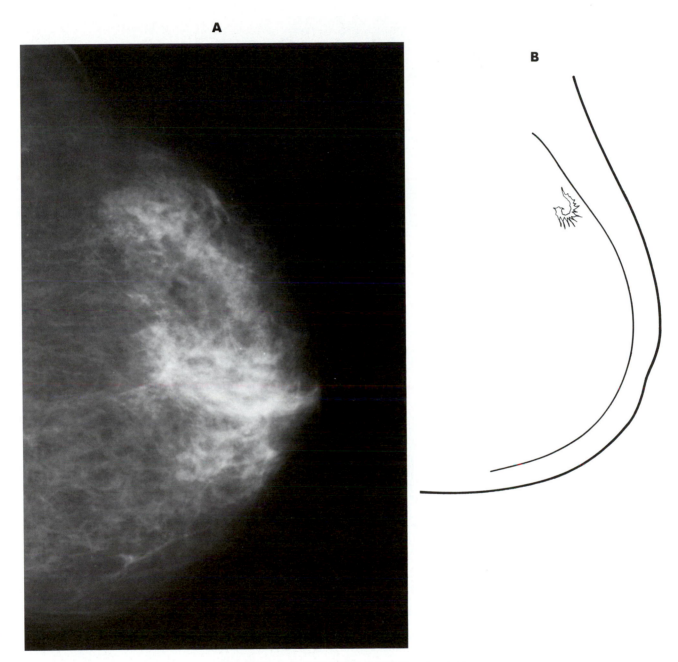

Fig. 10-3. A, Left LM; **B,** left LM (line drawing).

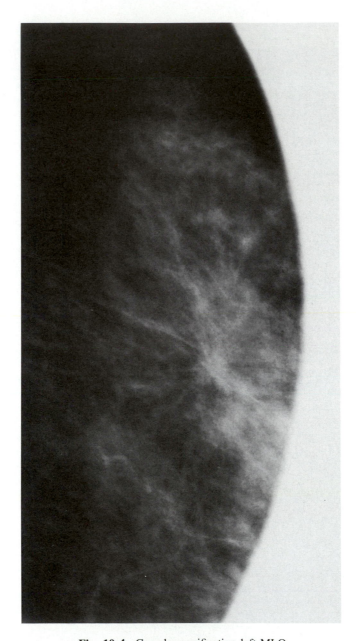

Fig. 10-4. Coned magnification left MLO.

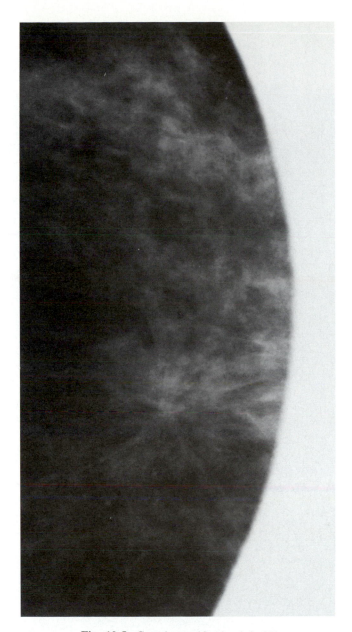

Fig. 10-5. Coned magnification left CC.

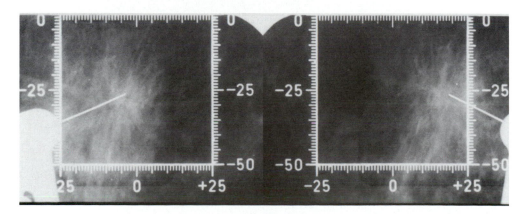

Fig. 10-6. SFNB.

PATIENT 2

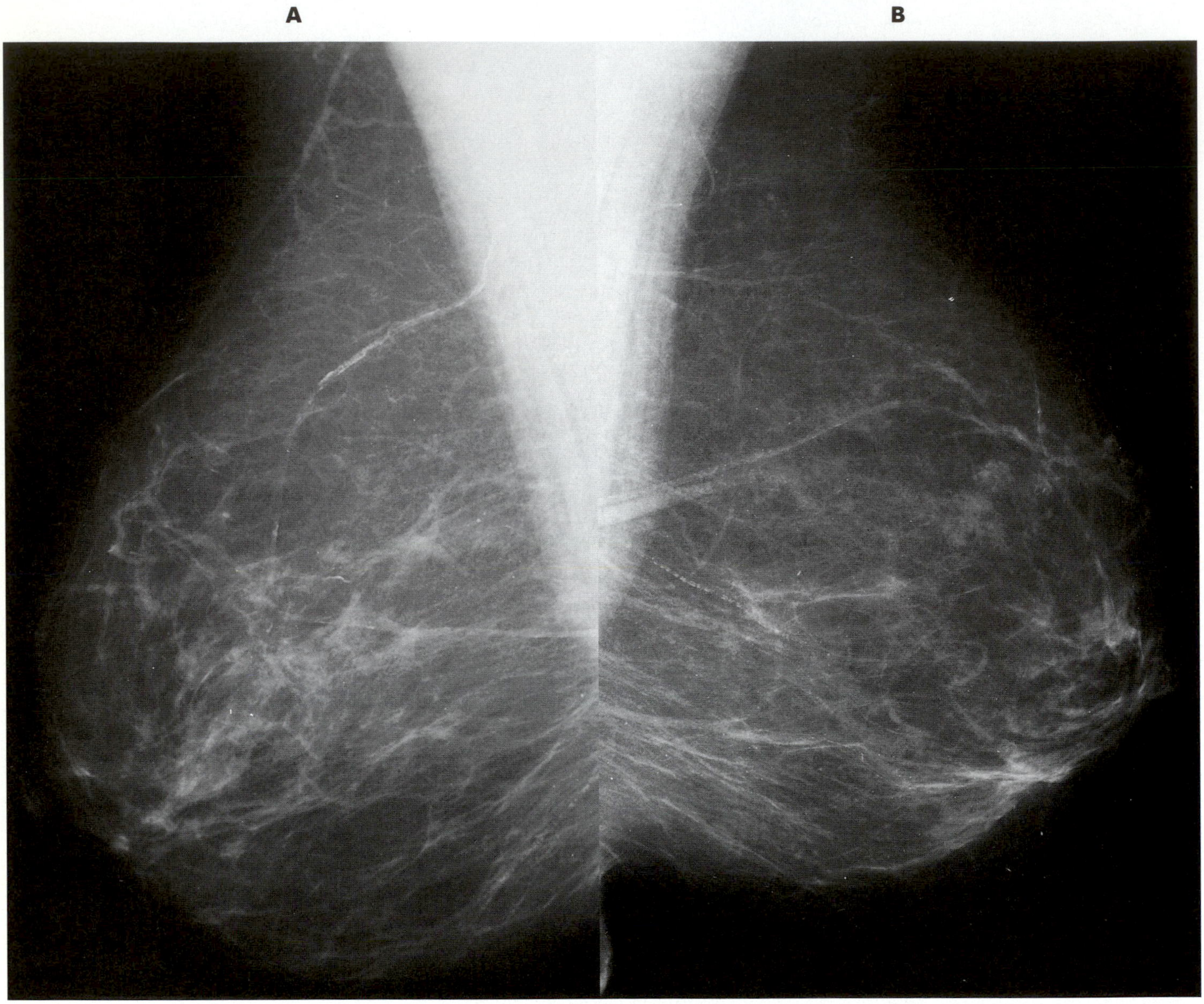

Fig. 10-7. A, Right MLO; **B,** left MLO.

These images (Figs. 10-7 and 10-8) represent a screening mammogram of a 53-year-old asymptomatic woman with moderately lucent breasts.

A

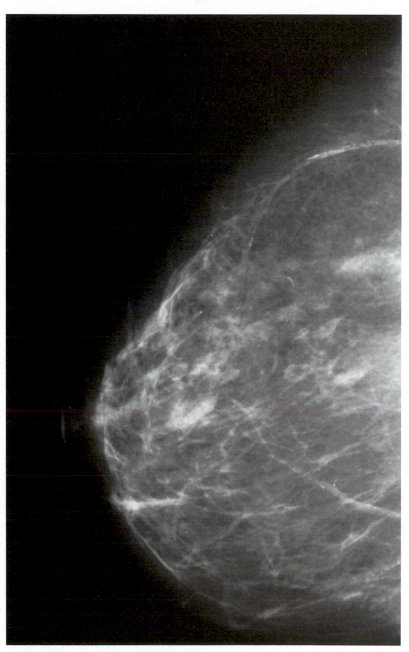

Fig. 10-8. A, Right CC.

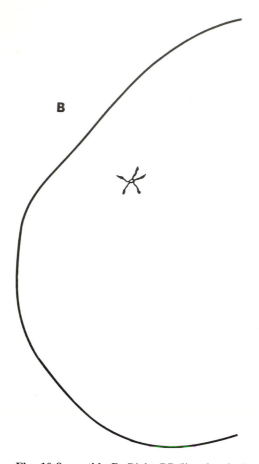

Fig. 10-8, cont'd. B, Right CC (line drawing).

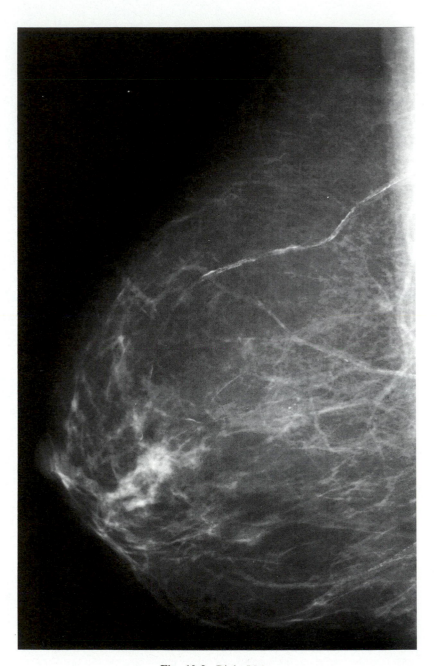

Fig. 10-9. Right LM.

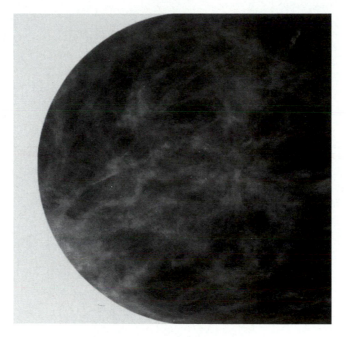

Fig. 10-10. Coned magnification right MLO.

In the mediolateral projection, a coarse, stellate-pattern lesion is seen on the lateral side of the right nipple (Fig. 10-7, *A*). The lesion, also evident on the craniocaudal and lateromedial projections, is most clearly seen on the coned magnification image (Figs. 10-8 to 10-10).

SFNB was performed and cytology confirmed the mammographic appearance of radial scar. Examined histology tissue sections of the lesion further confirmed the benign diagnosis, showing sclerosing adenosis with a scleroelastic and atrophic center.

Characteristic of radial scar is a central density with radiolucent areas and spiculations. The range of size and structure—that is, radiality and elastosis in these lesions—contributes to variations in their mammographic appearance in response to variations of mammographic projections that are obtained (Figs. 10-7, *A;* 10-8, *A;* 10-9; and 10-10).[3,4]

Code 3

PATIENT 3

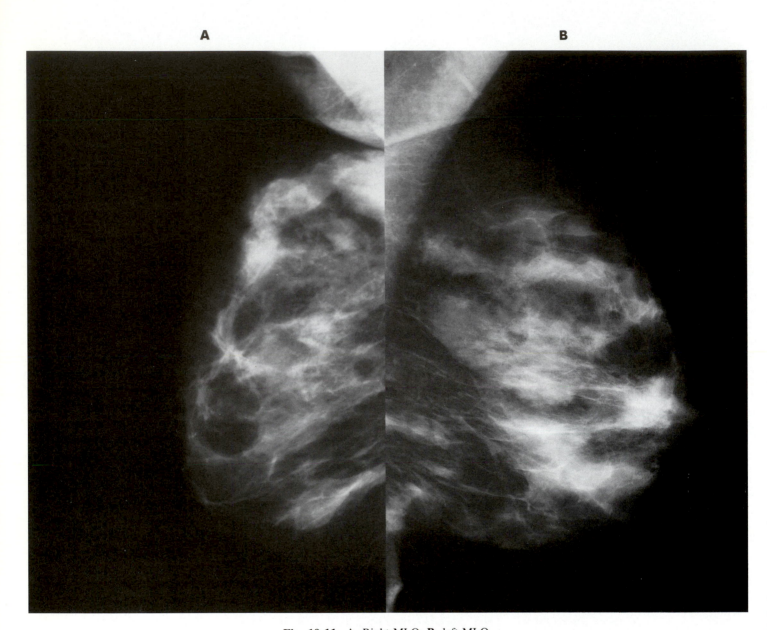

Fig. 10-11. A, Right MLO; **B,** left MLO.

These images (Figs. 10-11 and 10-12) are a screening mammogram of a 50-year-old asymptomatic woman with a moderate amount of breast parenchyma. This woman was difficult to position for mammography because of her previous right-sided thoracic surgery, which explains the difference in the mammographic appearance between the right and left breasts. Routine inclusion of the axillary tail on the right was precluded. Right breast nipple retraction is a postsurgical result.

A

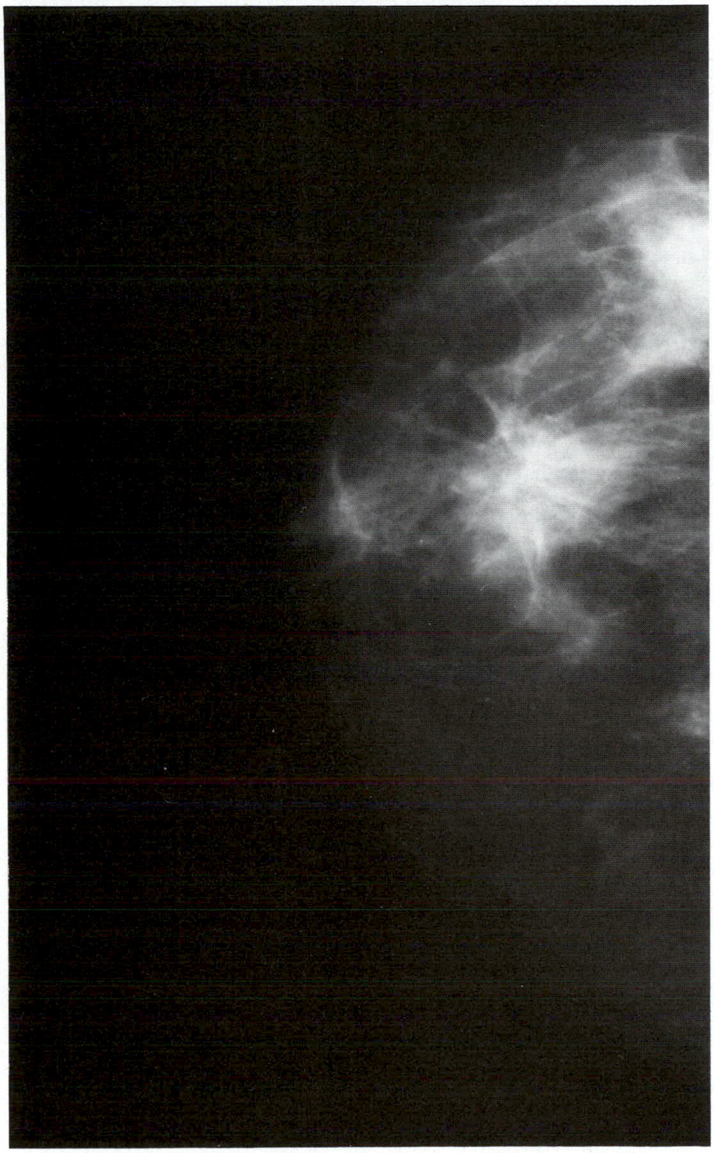

Fig. 10-12. A, Right CC.

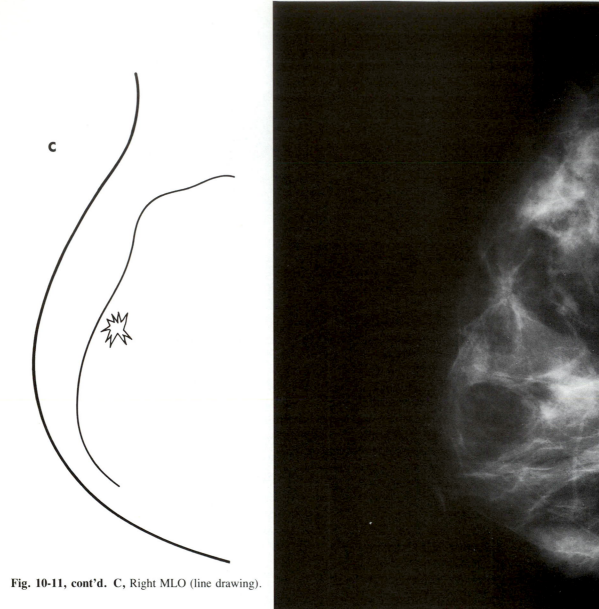

Fig. 10-11, cont'd. C, Right MLO (line drawing).

Fig. 10-13. Right LM.

Distortion of the breast parenchyma is observed approximately 5 cm above the right nipple (Fig. 10-11, *A*). As previously discussed, and depending on the mammographic projection, this distorted area also shows variations in lesion density and radial configuration (Fig. 10-12, *A*) (patient 2).

SFNB of this stellate-appearing lesion yielded stromal fragments and benign epithelial cells. Histology of the lesion also confirmed a radial scar (Figs. 10-14, *A*, and 10-15). As demonstrated in Fig. 10-14, *B*, the breast was placed in the craniocaudal position with the center of the lesion optimally located to perform SFNB evaluation.

Histologic degrees of fibroelastic distortion of a lesion itself may contribute to variations in mammographic appearance. Such fibroelastic distortion is one of the classic

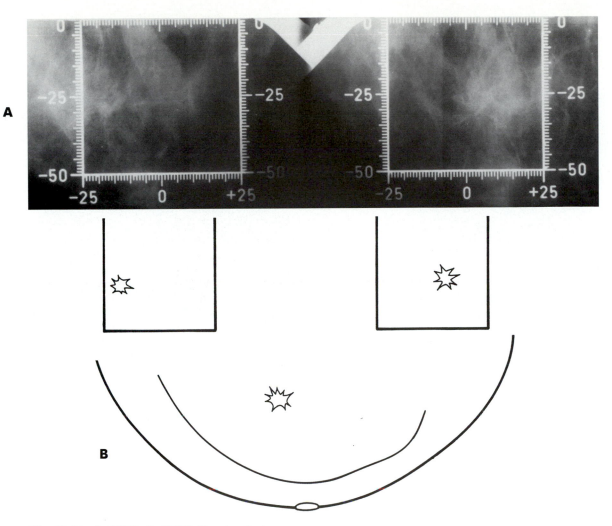

Fig. 10-14. **A,** SFNB; **B,** SFNB (line drawing).

features of radial scar lesions.[3] These confounding variations of mammographic observation cannot, however, be casually followed.

It has been demonstrated that radial scars are often multiple, and even on local excision of one, others may be left in the breast.[2,6] This supports the perception that many radial scars remain dormant and there is simply not enough information as to how often or which radial scar develops into cancer.[5]

Code 3

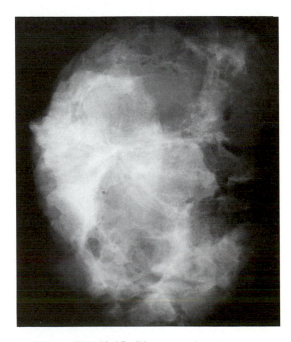

Fig. 10-15. Biopsy specimen.

PATIENT 4

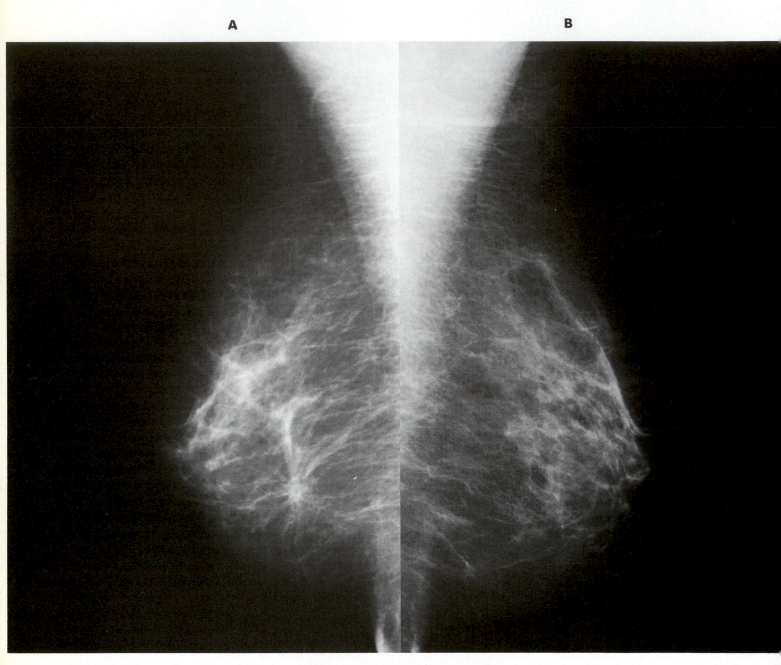

Fig. 10-16. A, Right MLO; **B,** left MLO.

These images (Figs. 10-16 and 10-17) represent a screening mammogram of a 51-year-old asymptomatic woman with lucent breasts.

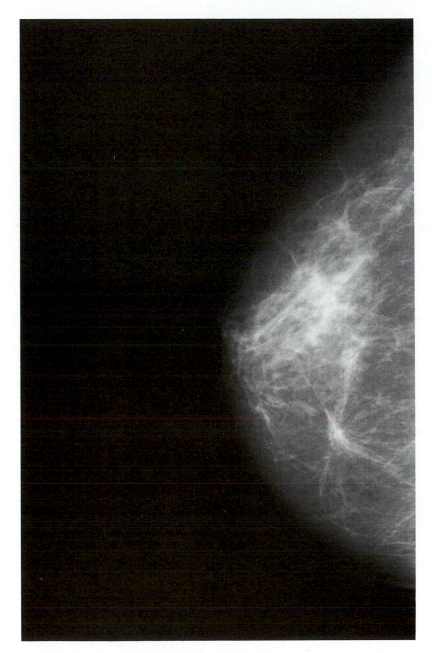

Fig. 10-17. Right CC.

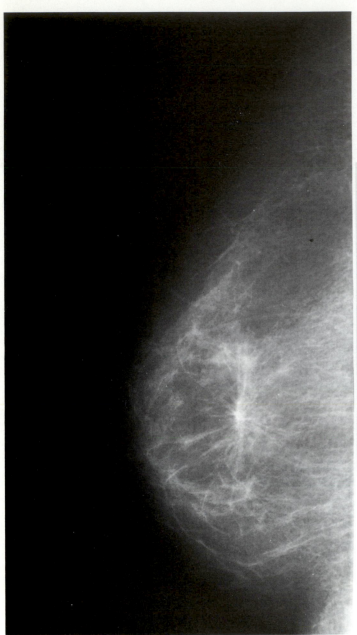

Fig. 10-18. Right LM.

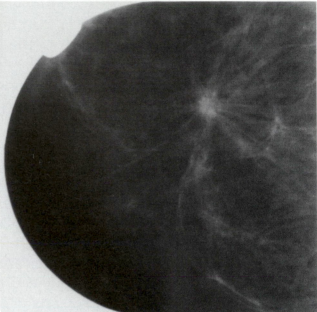

Fig. 10-19. Coned magnification right.

The obvious stellate lesion has broad, extended spiculations on the medial side of the right nipple (Fig. 10-16, *A*). The center of the lesion, especially well visualized in the mediolateral oblique projection, is not totally dense, suggestive of nonmalignant change (Fig. 10-19). This lesion, well demonstrated in all mammographic projections, shows that the center of the lesion remains radiolucent. The mammographic report indicated a radial scar and SFNB was recommended.

The SFNB projection, shown prior to needle placement for cytologic evaluation, further illustrates the radiolucent center, an expected feature of radial scar (Fig. 10-20). Stereotaxic procedure was performed and cytology confirmed benign epithelial cells (Fig. 10-21). Histology of the surgical specimen further proved the lesion to be radial scar (Fig. 10-22).

Code 4

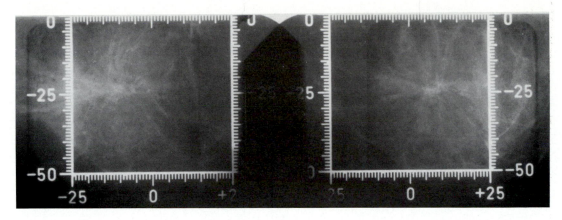

Fig. 10-20. SFNB scout film.

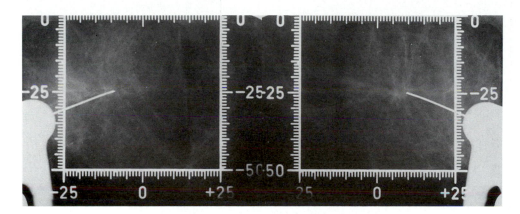

Fig. 10-21. SFNB; right LM.

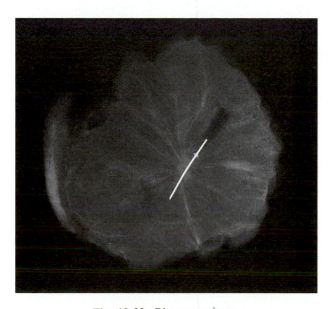

Fig. 10-22. Biopsy specimen.

PATIENT 5

A B

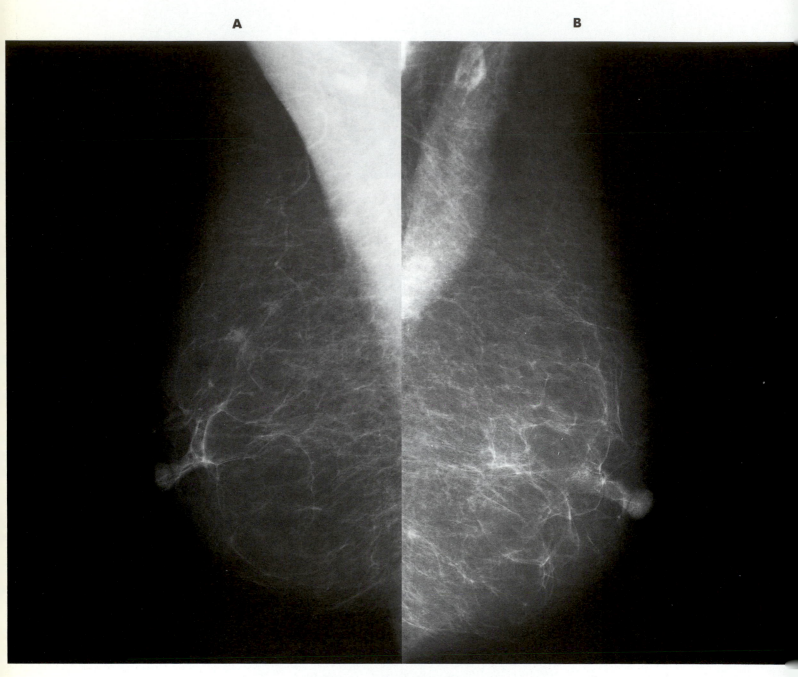

Fig. 10-23. A, Right MLO; **B,** left MLO.

These films (Figs. 10-23 and 10-24) are from a screening mammogram of a 63-year-old asymptomatic woman with lucent breasts.

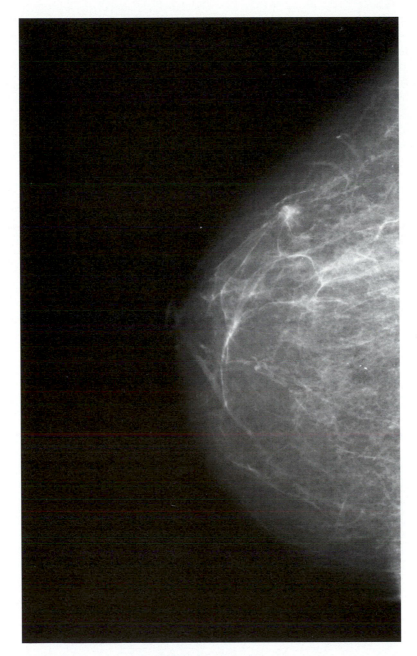

Fig. 10-24. Right CC.

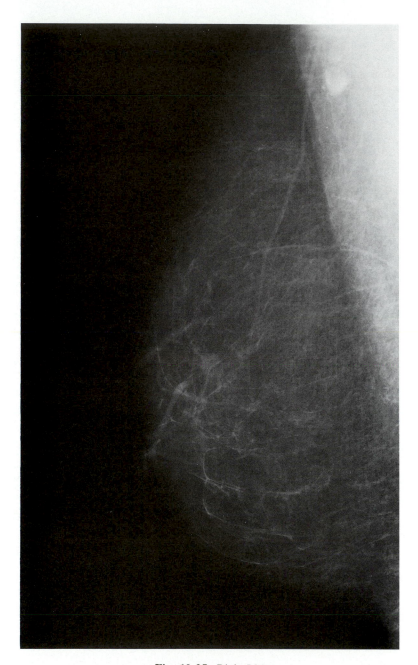

Fig. 10-25. Right LM.

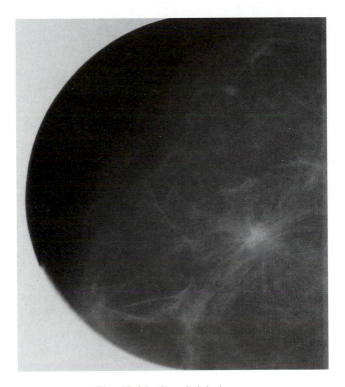

Fig. 10-26. Coned right breast.

A discrete spiculated lesion is seen in the upper outer quadrant of the right breast (Fig. 10-23, *A*). The density of the center of this lesion also changes depending on the mammographic projection (Patient 2) (Figs. 10-23, *A;* 10-24; and 10-25). The coned projection shows long and somewhat broad spicula coursing through the lesion (Fig. 10-26). This lesion is mammographically suggestive of radial scar.

SFNB and histology of the lesion confirmed benign cells and the diagnosis of radial scar.

While pathogenesis of radial scars remains unknown, Andersen et al.[1] hypothesize that they may begin as a result of unknown injury. These authors suggest fibrotic changes and elastosis may heal as focal areas, with central contraction involving ductal and lobular elements that together form a radial pattern.

Code 4

REFERENCES

1. Andersen JA, Carter D, Linell F: A symposium on sclerosing duct lesions of the breast, *Pathol Annu* 21;(Pt 2):145–179, 1987.
2. Andersen JA, Gram JB: Radial scar in the female breast: a long-term follow-up study of 32 cases, *Cancer* 53:2557-2560, 1984.
3. Anderson TJ, Battersby S: Radial scars of benign and malignant breasts: comparative features and significance, *J Pathol* 147:23-32, 1985.
4. Dahnert W: *Radiology review manual: differential diagnosis of breast disease,* Baltimore, 1991, Williams & Wilkins.
5. Linell F, Ljungberg O, Anderson I: Breast carcinoma: aspects of early stages, progression and related problems, *Acta Pathol Microbiol Scand* (Sect A) 272(Suppl):1, 1980.
6. Nielson J, Jensen J, Andersen JA: An autopsy study of radial scar in the female breast, *Histopathology* 9:287, 1985.

Chapter 11

STELLATE LESIONS

PATIENT 1

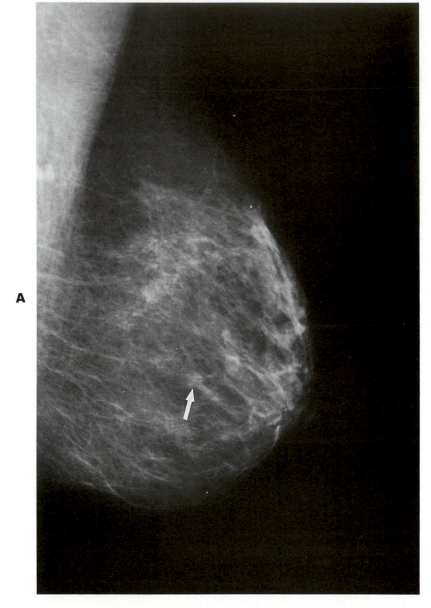

A

Fig. 11-1. A, Left MLO.

These images (Figs. 11-1, *A*, and 11-2) of the left breast are from a screening mammogram in a 53-year-old asymptomatic woman.

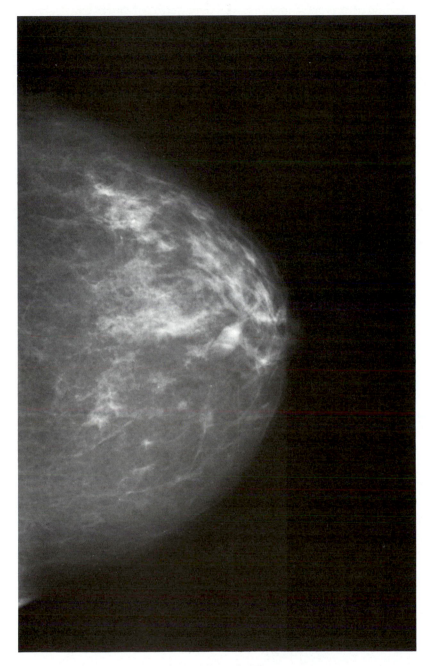

Fig. 11-2. Left CC.

Interpretation of the ratio of isolated areas of dense breast parenchyma and adipose tissue of this mammogram presents something of a challenge. Initial observation of the breast in the craniocaudal projection reveals a subtle yet suspicious dense area with spiculated "tails" that requires additional mammographic work-up (Fig. 11-2).

A left lateromedial projection does provide more obvious confirmation of the lesion. Coned images in both the craniocaudal and the mediolateral projections are required to isolate and confirm the 4 to 6 mm stellate pattern of the lesion located in the left lower inner quadrant of the breast (Figs. 11-4 and 11-5). Stereotaxic fine-needle biopsy (SFNB) was performed and cytology demonstrated malignant cells (Fig. 11-6). Histology confirmed well-differentiated invasive ductal carcinoma.

Arthur et al. found that epithelial parenchymal structures were highly variable, with diversity in fibrous tissue and intralobular stroma not necessarily associated with epithelial parenchymal structure.[1] Mammographic patterns and their associated risk for cancer, while inexact, do significantly contribute to warranted levels for suspicion of malignancy. When detected, the stellate-pattern configuration, whether subtle or obvious, warrants immediate and further investigation.

Code 5

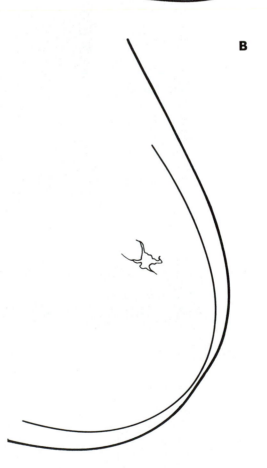

Fig. 11-1, cont'd. B, Left MLO (line drawing).

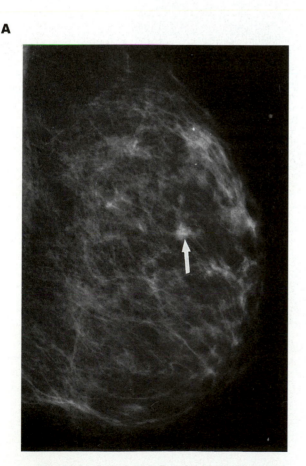

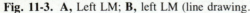

Fig. 11-3. A, Left LM; **B,** left LM (line drawing.

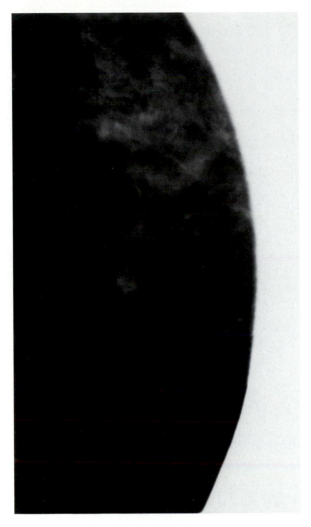

Fig. 11-4. Coned Left CC.

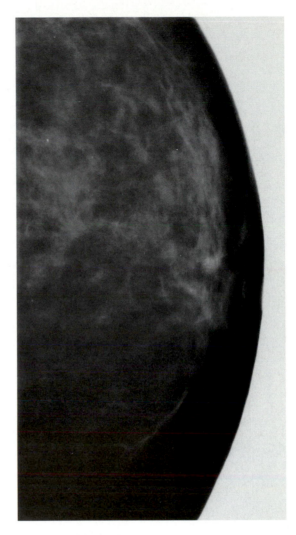

Fig. 11-5. Coned Left MLO.

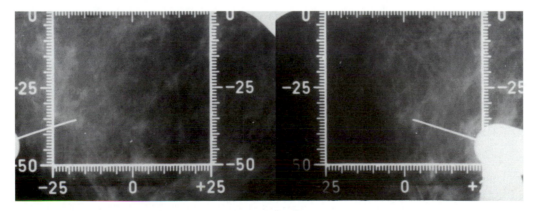

Fig. 11-6. SFNB.

PATIENT 2

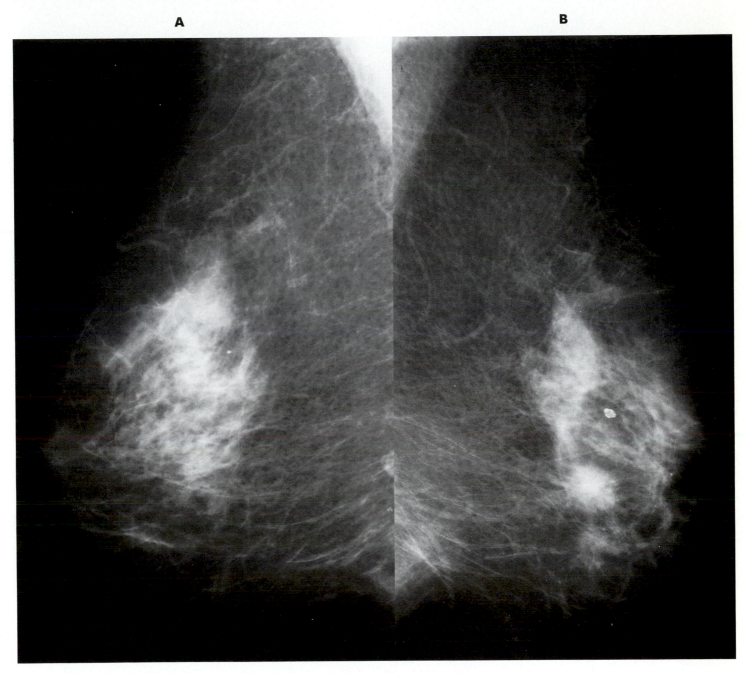

Fig. 11-7. A, Right MLO; **B,** left MLO.

These images (Fig. 11-7) represent a screening mammogram in a 60-year-old asymptomatic woman with a moderate amount of breast parenchyma.

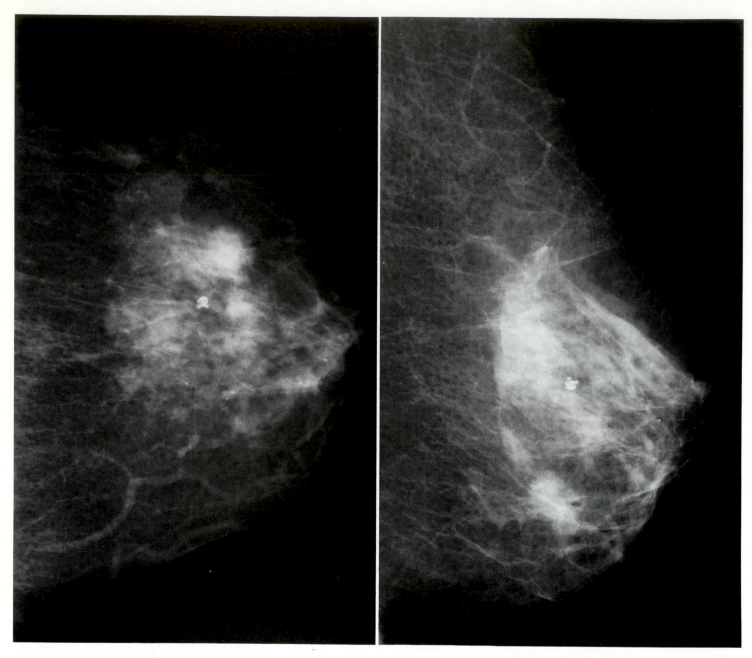

Fig. 11-8. Left CC.   **Fig. 11-9.** Left LM.

This woman's right breast is unremarkable. In the left breast is one large, obvious benign-appearing calcification. In addition, two suspicious densities are detected in the left lower outer quadrant (Fig. 11-7, *B*).

The first lesion is more obvious and more dense, with a stellate configuration. The second suspicious area, while not as dense, is located approximately 1 cm inferior to the stellate lesion.

The stellate lesion is a classic mammographic cancer with a code 5 designation. The second density, while not as classically characteristic of cancer, is nonetheless too sus-

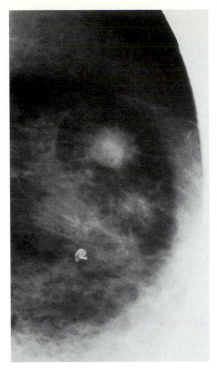

Fig. 11-10. Coned left CC.

picious for malignancy to be designated a code 3. The mere presence and configuration of the code 5 lesion also increase the index of suspicion of the second finding. Consequently, the second lesion is given a code 4 designation.

SFNB was therefore performed at both suspicious areas. Cytology indicated malignant cells on both lesions. Histology of the lesions confirmed invasive lobular carcinoma.

Code 5 — lesion 1
Code 4 — lesion 2

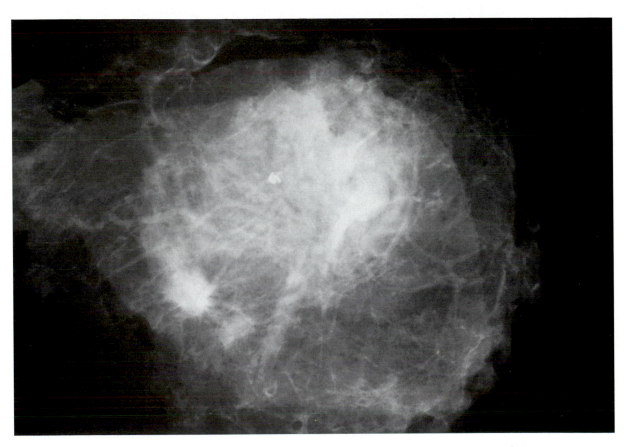

Fig. 11-11. Biopsy specimen.

PATIENT 3

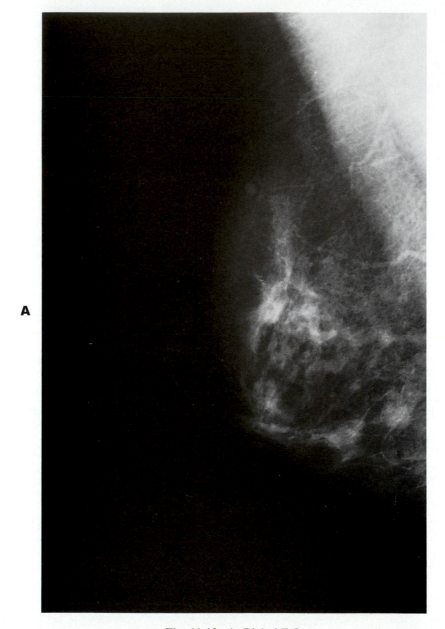

Fig. 11-12. A, Right MLO.

These images (Figs. 11-12, *A*, and 11-13) of the right breast are from a screening mammogram of a 64-year-old asymptomatic woman.

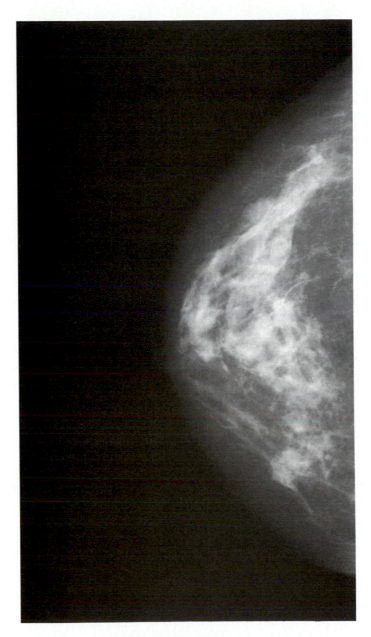

Fig. 11-13. Right CC.

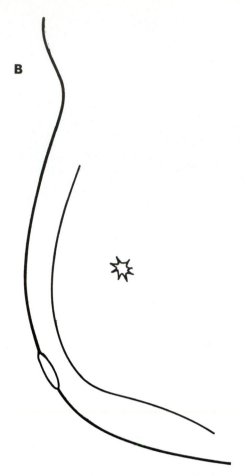

Fig. 11-12, cont'd. B, Right MLO (line drawing).

The craniocaudal projection of the right breast reveals a rather dense parenchymal pattern in this 64-year-old woman (Fig. 11-13). In addition, the mediolateral oblique projection reveals a small stellate-patterned lesion. While only approximately 4 mm in size, this mammographic pattern should always arouse concern (Fig. 11-12, *A*). A lateromedial projection further verifies the stellate pattern and spiculated changes of the affected right breast parenchyma (Fig. 11-14, *A*).

SFNB demonstrated gross cellular atypia with enlarged nuclei consistent with malignancy. After surgical removal, histology confirmed infiltrating highly differentiated ductal carcinoma (Fig. 11-15).

This nonpalpable area, initially evident only on the mediolateral oblique projection, points to the importance of multiple images to confirm the presence of a suspected lesion. A diagnostic examination must be tailored to the specific breast problem.[2]

Code 5

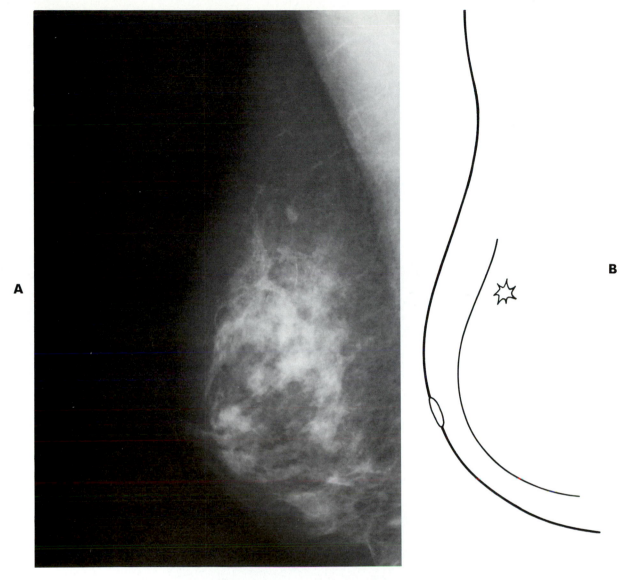

Fig. 11-14. A, Right LM; **B,** right LM (line drawing).

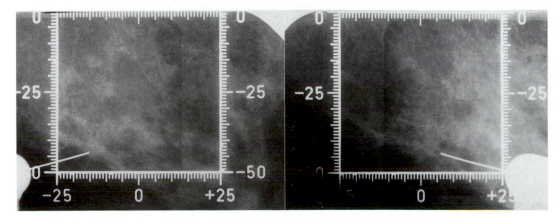

Fig. 11-15. SFNB.

PATIENT 4

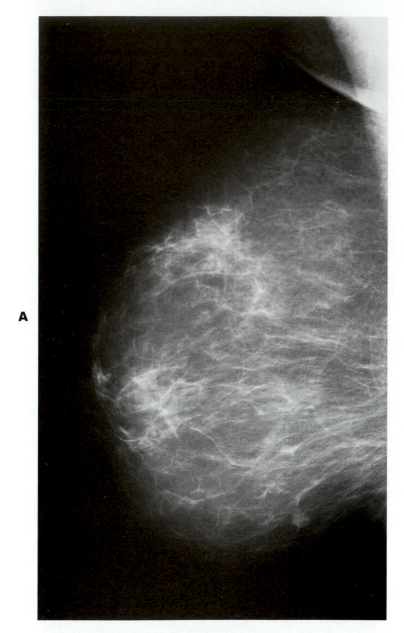

Fig. 11-16. A, Right MLO.

These images (Figs. 11-16, *A,* and 11-17) of the right breast are from a screening mammogram of a 52-year-old asymptomatic woman.

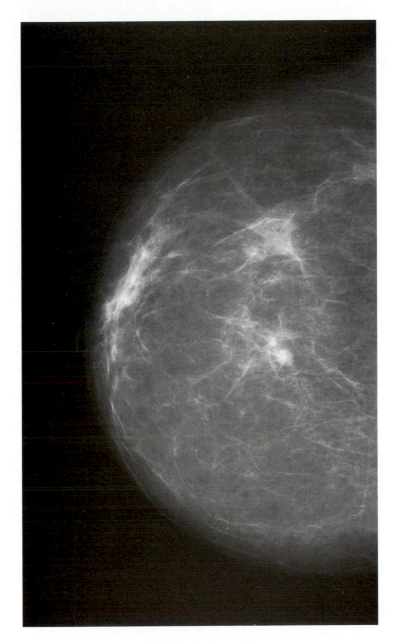

Fig. 11-17. Right CC.

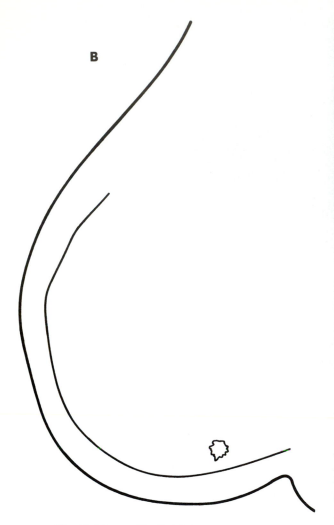

Fig. 11-16, cont'd. B, Right MLO (line drawing).

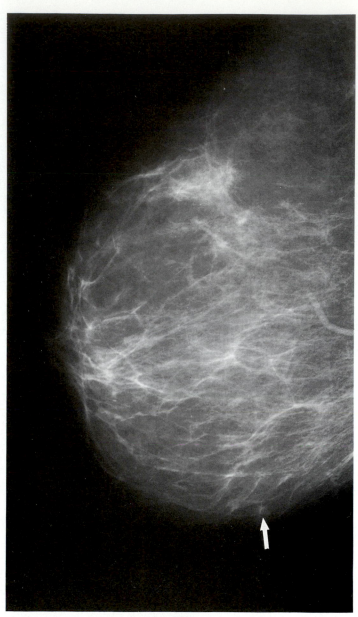

Fig. 11-18. Right LM.

Involutional changes are seen in the upper outer portion of this woman's fatty breast (Fig. 11-16, *A*). Without the benefit of the craniocaudal projection, one may dismiss the 5 mm stellate density located posteriorly below the right nipple in the mediolateral oblique projection (Fig. 11-17).

Mammography work-up confirmed the presence of the density. A coned compression projection reconfirmed its location. The lateromedial projection depicts the lesion, but only as subtly as the mediolateral oblique. The biopsy specimen demonstrates, as did the coned compression view, the exact dense and stellate nature of this cancerous lesion (Fig. 11-20).

SFNB was performed, and cytology demonstrated malignant epithelial cells. Histology confirmed invasive well-differentiated ductal carcinoma.

Code 5

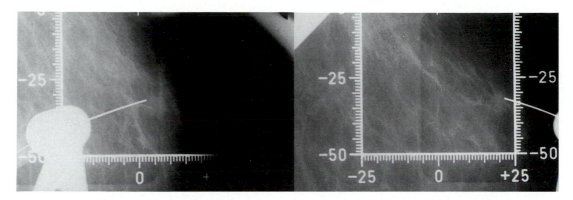

Fig. 11-19. Right SFNB.

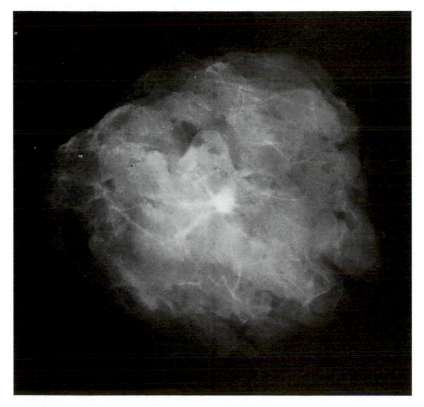

Fig. 11-20. Biopsy specimen.

PATIENT 5

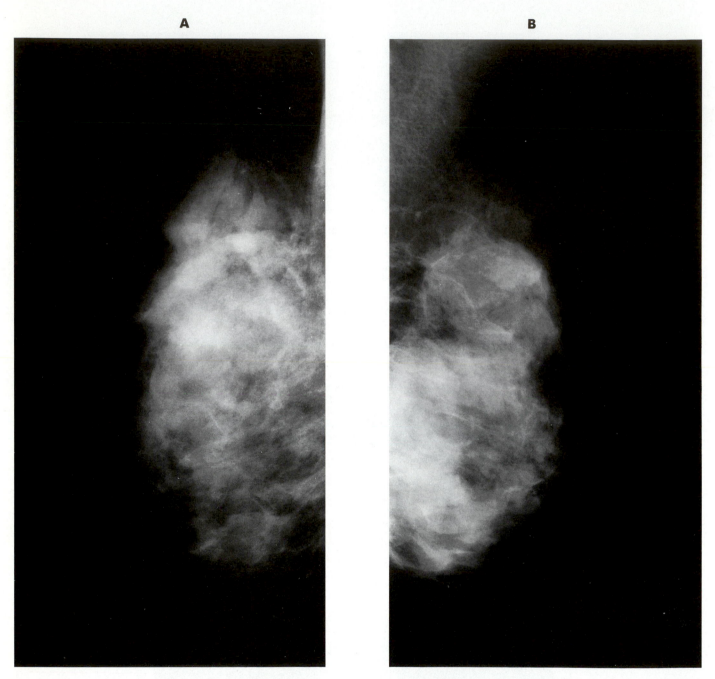

Fig. 11-21. A, Right MLO; **B,** left MLO.

These images (Figs. 11-21 and 11-22) represent a screening mammogram of a 50-year-old asymptomatic woman with very dense breasts.

Fig. 11-22. Left CC.

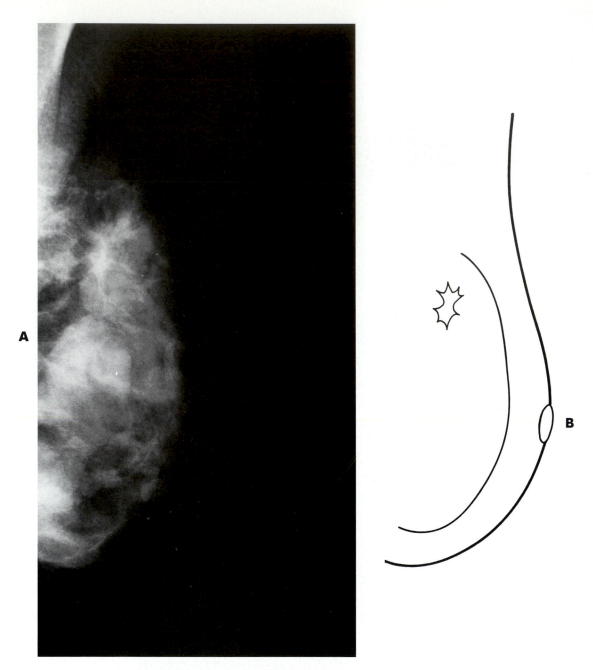

Fig. 11-23. A, Left LM; **B,** left LM (line drawing).

In the left mediolateral oblique projection there is evidence of a suspicious stellate-type lesion (Fig. 11-21, *B*). The lateromedial projection confirms the presence of a dense area of stellate configuration (Fig. 11-23, *A*).

On the craniocaudal view, the position of the lesion in the horizontal plane cannot be seen with certainty (Fig. 11-22). Coned projections were acquired, leaving no doubt that the lesion is present. The mammographic stellate feature is particularly visible on the coned mediolateral oblique projection (Fig. 11-24). This appearance, suggestive of carcinoma, must be further evaluated.

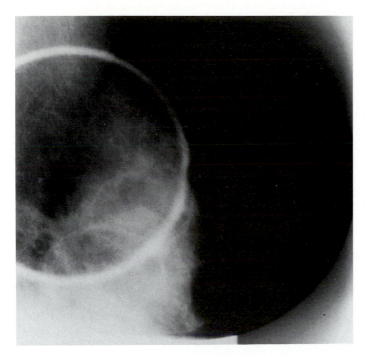

Fig. 11-24. Coned left MLO.

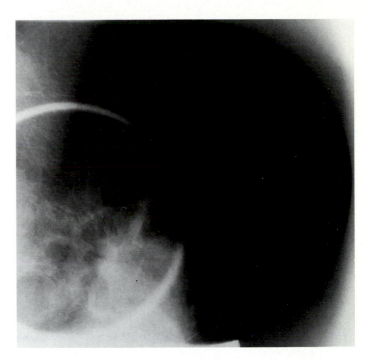

Fig. 11-25. Coned Left LM.

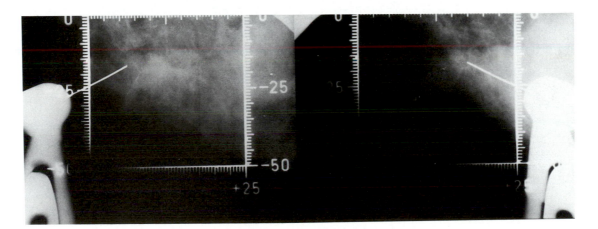

Fig. 11-26. SFNB.

The breasts are extremely dense overall. Usually, additional coned views of any suspicious areas will assist in confirming the presence of true distortion of breast architecture.

SFNB was performed, and cytology revealed abundant malignant cells with atypia (Fig. 11-26). Histology of the lesion confirmed invasive lobular cancer and lobular carcinoma in situ.

Code 5

PATIENT 6

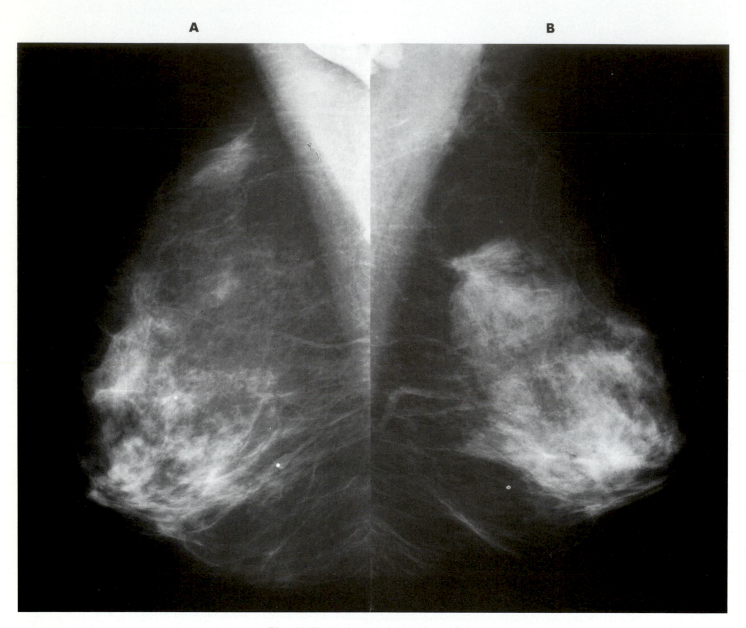

Fig. 11-27. A, Right MLO; **B,** left MLO.

These images (Figs. 11-27 and 11-28) are from a baseline screening mammogram of a 58-year-old woman. Twelve years before the woman had undergone breast surgery in the left upper outer quadrant, as a result of trauma from an auto accident.

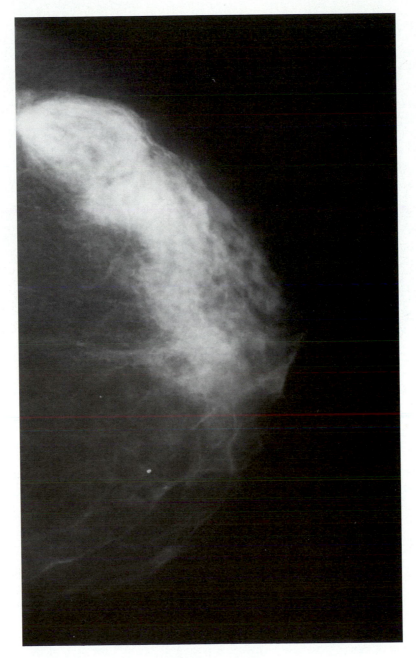

Fig. 11-28. Left CC.

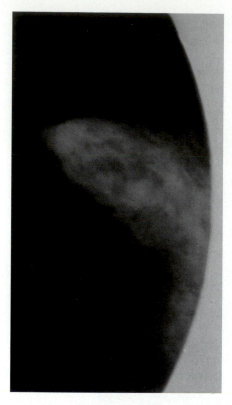

Fig. 11-29. Coned left CC.

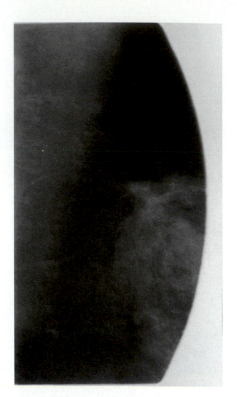

Fig. 11-30. Coned left MLO.

Parenchymal asymmetry of the left breast is seen at the site of previous surgery. In addition, this routine mammography study reveals a stellate-patterned distortion in the same area as her surgical scar (Figs. 11-27, *B,* and 11-28). There were no previous mammograms for comparison and no detectable palpable abnormality.

Further mammographic evaluation confirms the presence of a lesion (Fig. 11-31). The rolled position of the breast in the coned craniocaudal projection shows the lesion to much greater advantage than the conventional craniocaudal position. The importance of appropriately applied compression to the breast with even slight positional change of the breast tissue is demonstrated in this study (see Chapter 3 for the technique for special projections and appropriately applied breast compression and rolled technique). While a portion of the very dense breast tissue is moved in the rolled projection, relieving superimposition of dense breast parenchyma, it does not "relieve" the area of the frank and stellate-patterned tissue (Fig. 11-29). The coned mediolateral oblique projection confirms the exact stellate image as seen on the conventional mediolateral oblique projection (Fig. 11-30).

SFNB was performed, and cytology revealed epithelial cells with gross atypia representing malignancy (Fig. 11-32). Surgery was again performed, and histology of the stellate lesion confirmed moderately well-differentiated ductal carcinoma.

Code 4

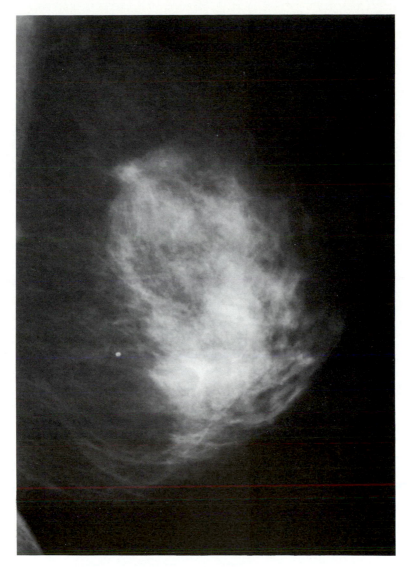

Fig. 11-31. Left LM.

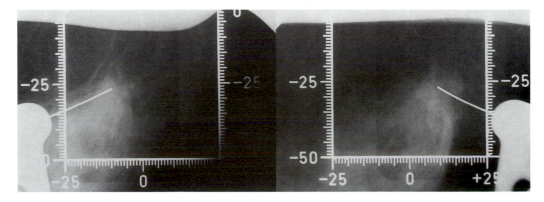

Fig. 11-32. SFNB.

PATIENT 7

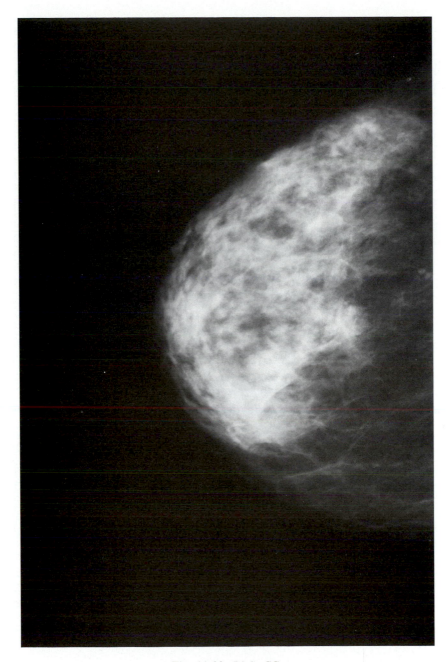

Fig. 11-33. Right CC.

This right breast image is from a screening mammogram of a 49-year-old asymptomatic woman with moderately dense breasts.

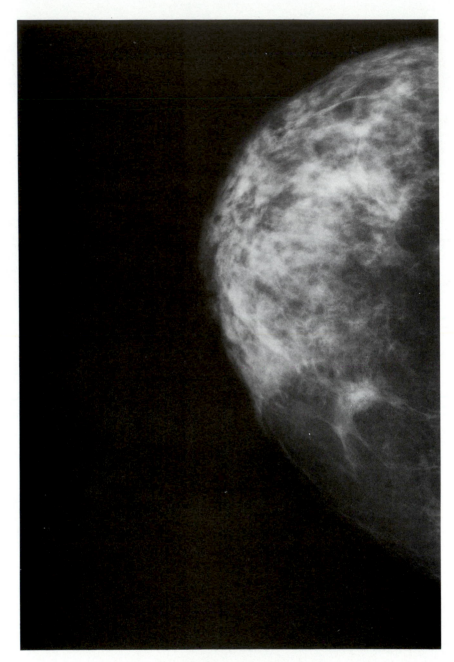

Fig. 11-34. Rolled right CC.

This woman was referred for consultation to confirm the presence of a right breast lesion and the consequent need for stereotaxic biopsy procedure. Her original mammogram was reviewed and returned to a hospital outside our city. Unfortunately, it could not be located for publication. This absence, however, does not preclude the ability to identify the unsharp and ill-defined density approximately 5.5 cm posteriorly from the nipple (Fig. 11-33). It is again demonstrated in rotating the breast tissue and is clearly a mammographic cancer (Fig. 11-34). This right breast lesion is also seen on the rolled coned compression image (Fig. 11-35) (see also case 6).

SFNB produced malignant cells. Histology of the lesion confirmed poorly differentiated invasive ductal carcinoma.

Code 5

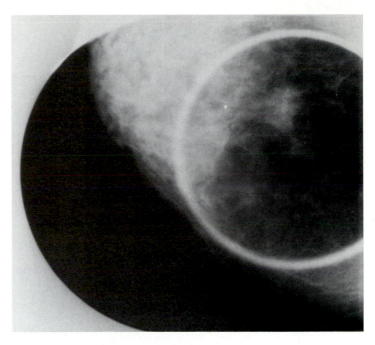

Fig. 11-35. Rolled coned right CC.

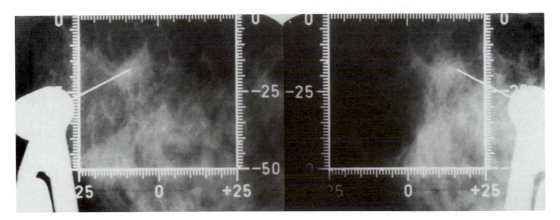

Fig. 11-36. SFNB.

PATIENT 8

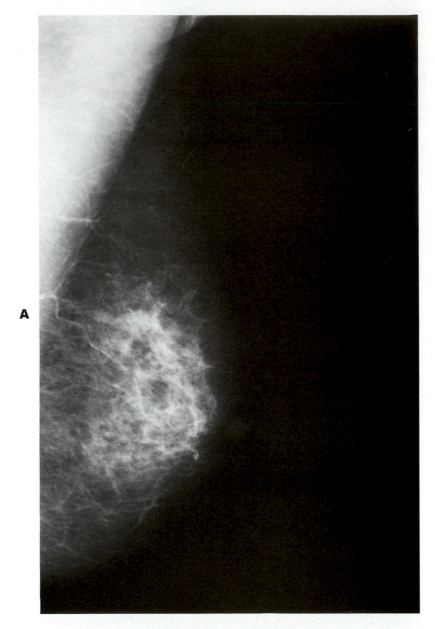

Fig. 11-37. A, Left MLO.

These left breast images (Figs. 11-37, *A,* and 11-38) are from a screening mammogram in a 68-year-old asymptomatic woman.

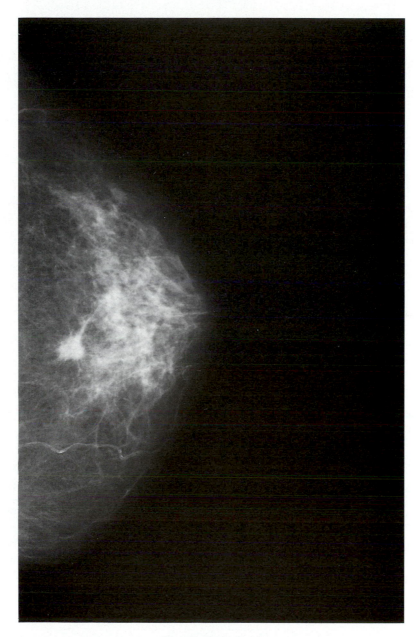

Fig. 11-38. Left CC.

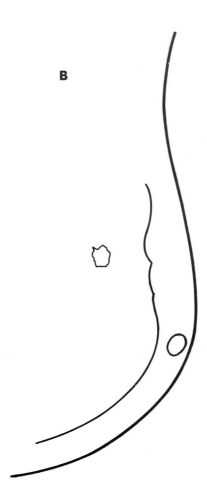

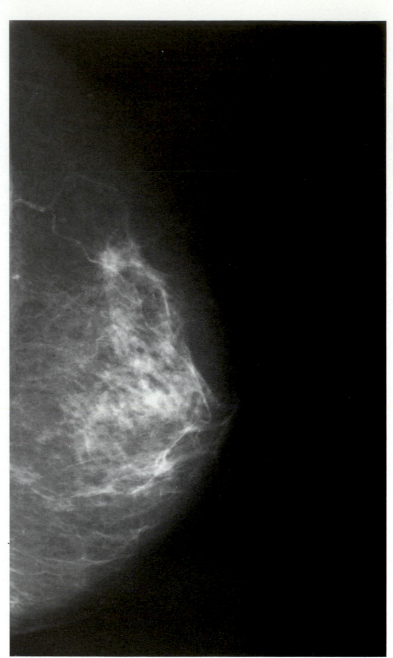

Fig. 11-37, cont'd. B, Left MLO (line drawing).

Fig. 11-39. Left LM.

At clinical breast examination there were no detectable palpable abnormalities. Mediolateral oblique projection of the left breast reveals a dense, but unclear, area of breast tissue (Fig. 11-37, *A*). However, in the craniocaudal projection, a classic stellate lesion, approximately 4 cm from the nipple, can be readily seen (Fig. 11-38). Irregular architecture of the lesion is further demonstrated in both the lateromedial and the coned projections (Figs. 11-39 and 11-40).

SFNB was performed, and cytology of the lesion demonstrated malignant epithelial cells. Histology of the lesion confirmed this to be poorly differentiated invasive ductal carcinoma.

Code 5

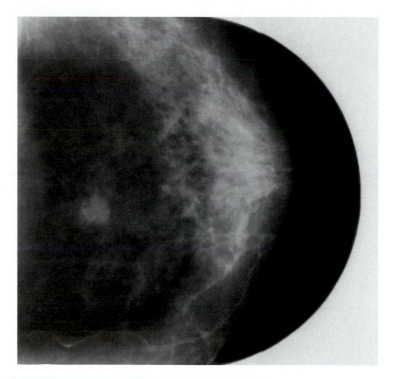

Fig. 11-40. Coned left CC.

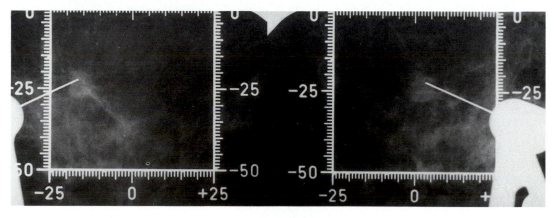

Fig. 11-41. SFNB.

PATIENT 9

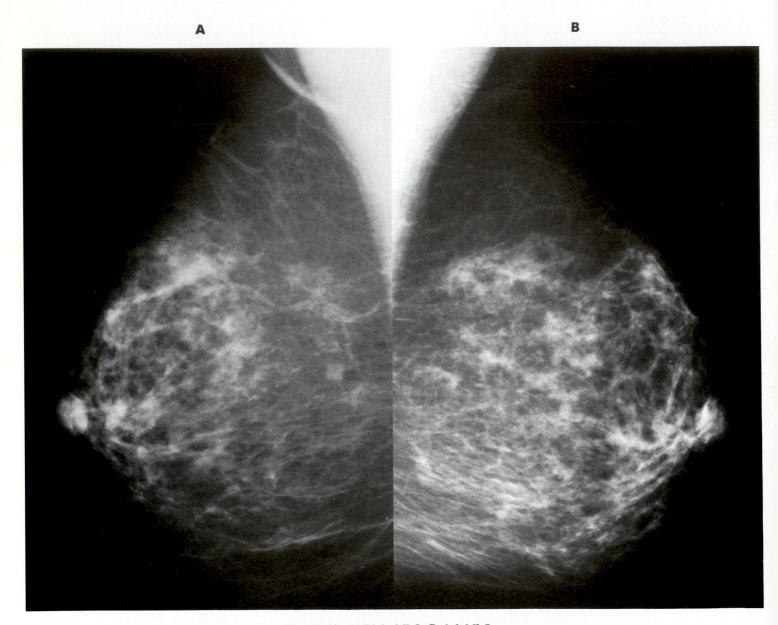

Fig. 11-42. A, Right MLO; **B,** left MLO.

These images (Figs. 11-42 and 11-43) represent a screening mammogram of a 67-year-old asymptomatic woman.

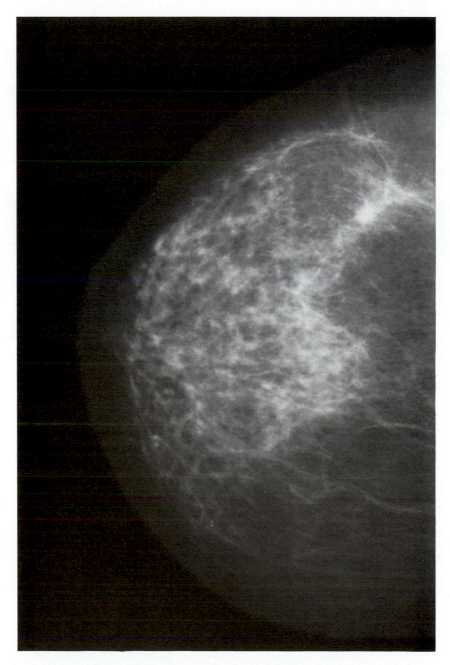

Fig. 11-43. Right CC.

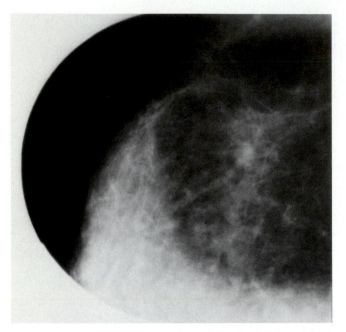

Fig. 11-44. Coned right breast.

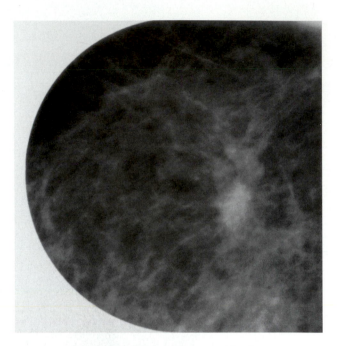

Fig. 11-45. Right coned magnification.

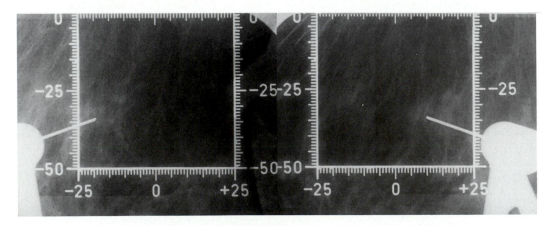

Fig. 11-46. SFNB.

A stellate lesion is seen on the lateral side of the right breast (Figs. 11-42, *A,* and 11-43). This lesion can be studied in further detail in both coned and coned magnification projections (Figs. 11-44 and 11-45). Both demonstrate again a dense, spiculated distorted architecture. Mammographically, this is a carcinoma.

SFNB was performed and cytology proved malignant epithelial cells (Fig. 11-46). Histology of the lesion confirmed poorly differentiated invasive lobular mammary carcinoma of small-cell type.

This woman had a mammography examination 2 years before the study featured here. No evidence of a breast lesion was found on her first mammogram. When she returned 2 years later, rather than appearing for a recommended annual evaluation, the lesion was obvious. While there is not unanimous agreement as to the effectiveness of regular breast screening examination in preventing mortality from breast cancer, the advantages of annual screening of women over 50 years of age are recognized. Mammography evaluation is the only modality to discover the nonpalpable breast lesion. Women must be educated and encouraged in vigilance of their own breast care and not be lulled into a false security with a negative mammogram report.[3]

Code 5

PATIENT 10

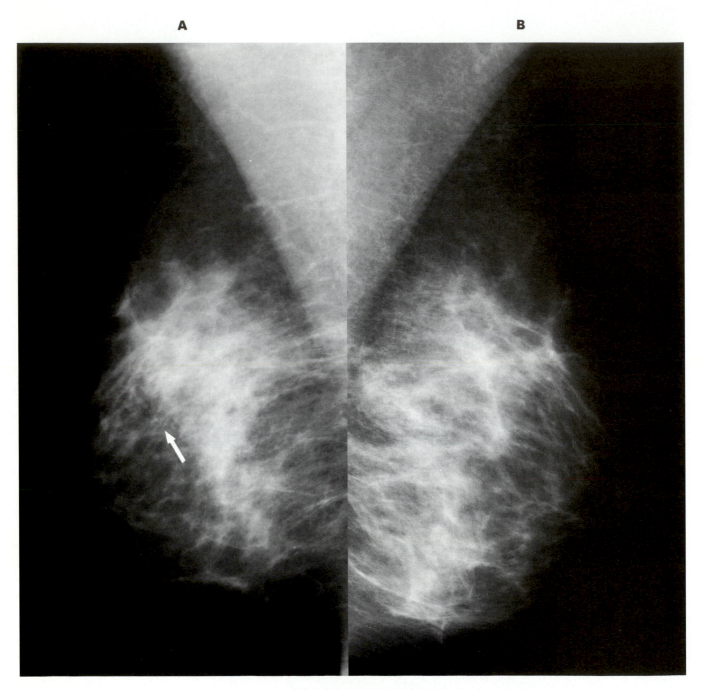

Fig. 11-47. A, Right MLO; **B,** left MLO.

These images (Figs. 11-47 and 11-48) represent a screening mammogram in a 51-year-old asymptomatic woman with dense breasts.

A

B

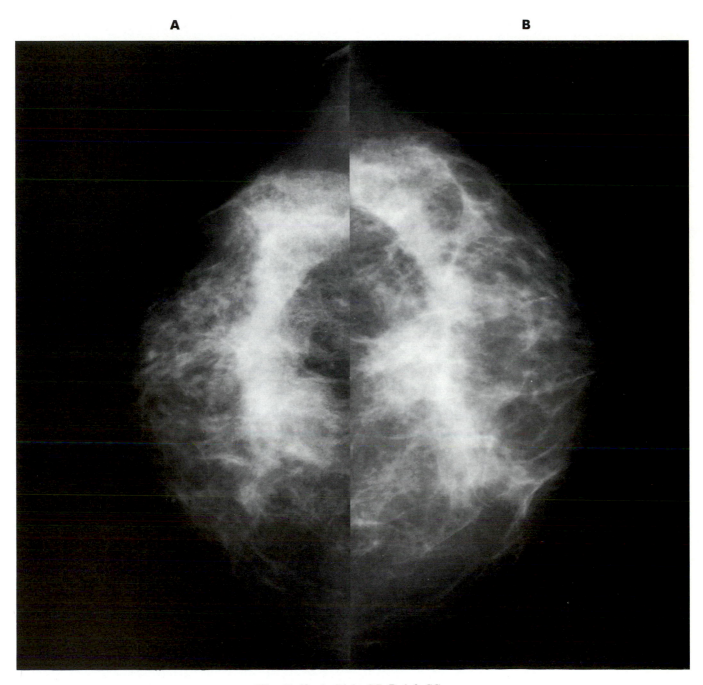

Fig. 11-48. A, Right CC; **B,** left CC.

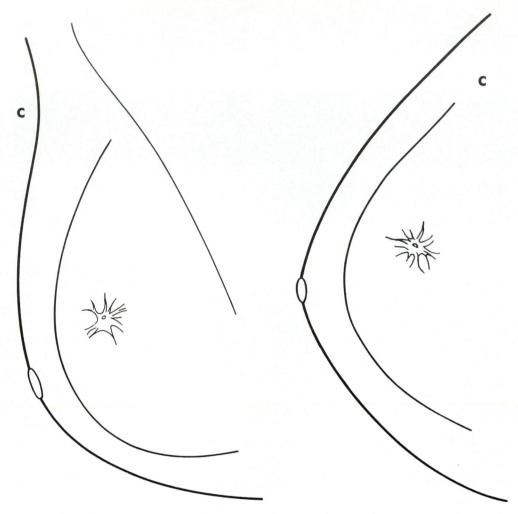

Fig. 11-47, cont'd. C, Right MLO (line drawing).   **Fig. 11-48, cont'd. C,** Right CC (line drawing).

An extremely discrete asymmetric area is noted in the retromammary region approximately 5 cm behind the right nipple. It is essentially "undetectable" on the mediolateral oblique projection. The retromammary area must be studied much more specifically by comparing the right and left craniocaudal projections (Figs. 11-47, *A,* and 11-48, *A* and *B*). Although the core of the lesion is not particularly dense, a "spoke-wheel" configuration remains persistent (Fig. 11-48, *A*). Bilateral lateromedial projections exaggerate the lesion's consistent appearance and location on the right (Fig. 11-49, *A*).

Mammographically, this lesion is very suspicious. SFNB and carbon localization were therefore simultaneously performed. Cytology of the lesion was negative. However, because of the mammographic evidence and resultant suspicion of the spiculated tissue being malignant, surgery was nonetheless carried out. Histology confirmed the lesion to be moderately differentiated invasive ductal carcinoma.

Regardless of negative cytology, in certain instances mammographic patterns support surgical biopsy of an area in question for final confirmation of whether a woman has an otherwise unrecognizable focus of disease.

Code 4

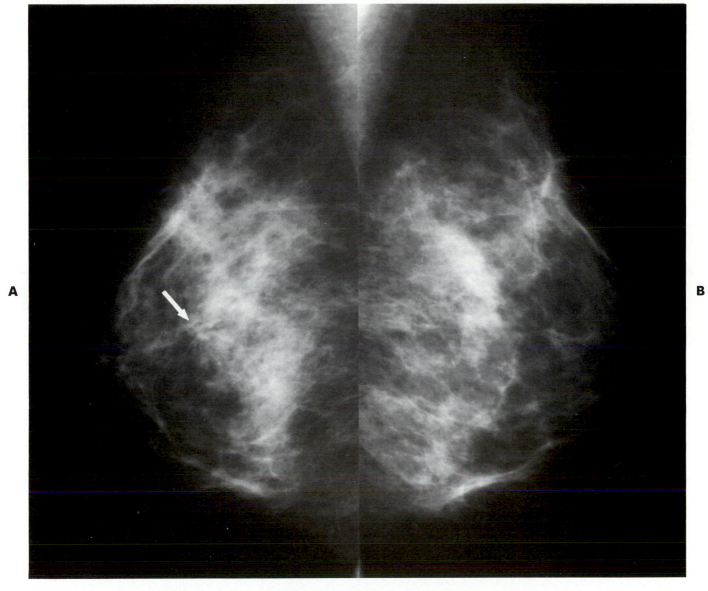

Fig. 11-49. A, Right LM; **B,** left LM.

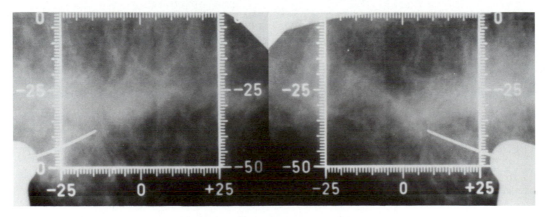

Fig. 11-50. SFNB, right breast.

PATIENT 11

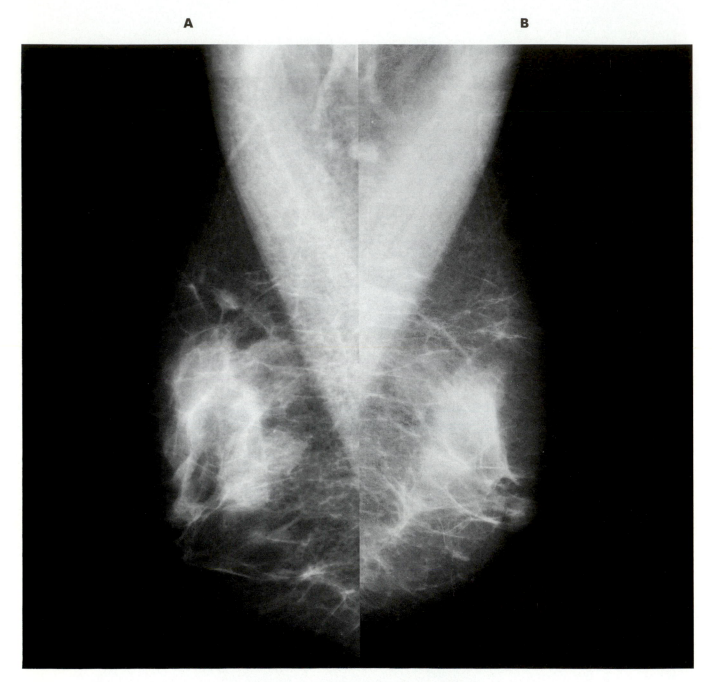

Fig. 11-51. A, Right MLO; **B,** left MLO.

These images (Figs. 11-51 and 11-52) represent a screening mammogram of a 57-year-old asymptomatic woman.

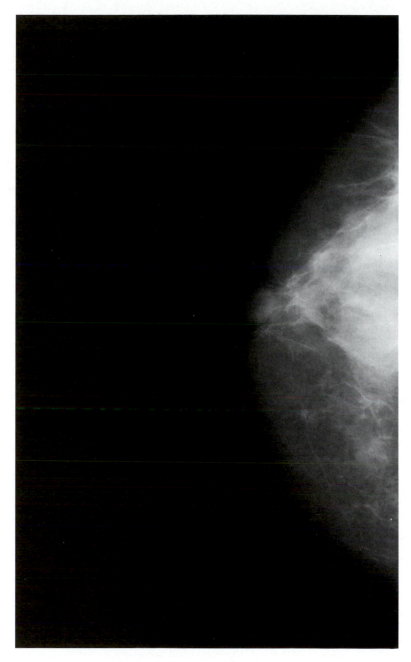

Fig. 11-52. Right CC.

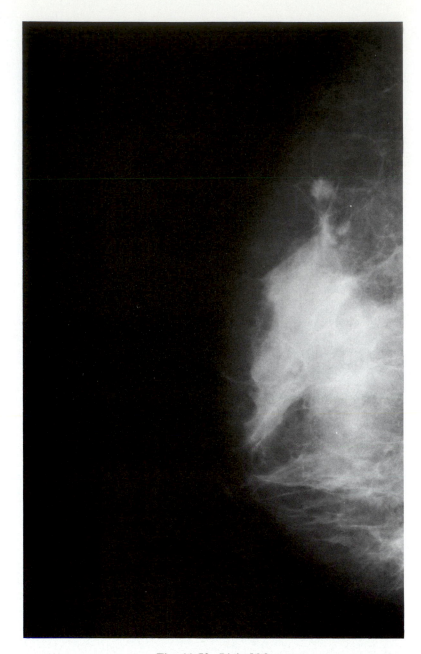

Fig. 11-53. Right LM.

A stellate lesion can be appreciated in the upper inner quadrant of the right breast (Fig. 11-51, *A*). The asymmetry and location of the lesion are much less subtle than in case 10, and its distorted stellate appearance verifies a mammographic cancer. Both the conventional lateromedial and the coned lateromedial projections confirm the lesion's location (Figs. 11-53 and 11-54).

SFNB was performed. Interestingly, the cytology of this lesion was also inconclusive (Fig. 11-55). There is no question, however, that in this case surgery must be performed. Biopsy-proved histology confirmed this lesion to be well-differentiated invasive ductal carcinoma.

Code 5

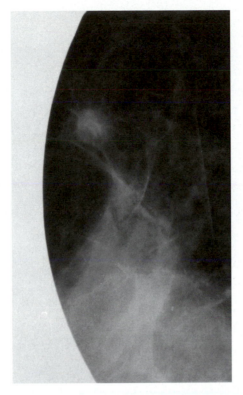

Fig. 11-54. Coned right LM.

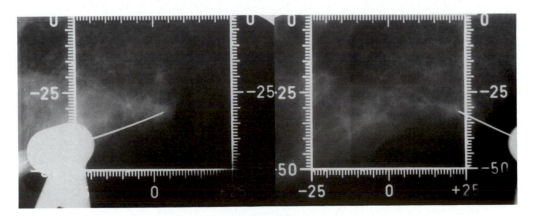

Fig. 11-55. SFNB.

PATIENT 12

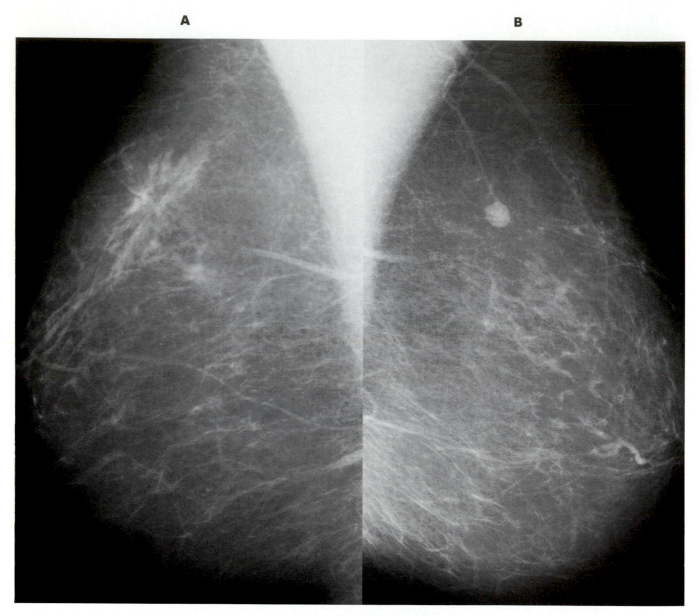

Fig. 11-56. A, Right MLO; **B,** left MLO.

These images (Figs. 11-56 and 11-57) are from a screening mammogram of a 57-year-old asymptomatic woman with lucent breasts.

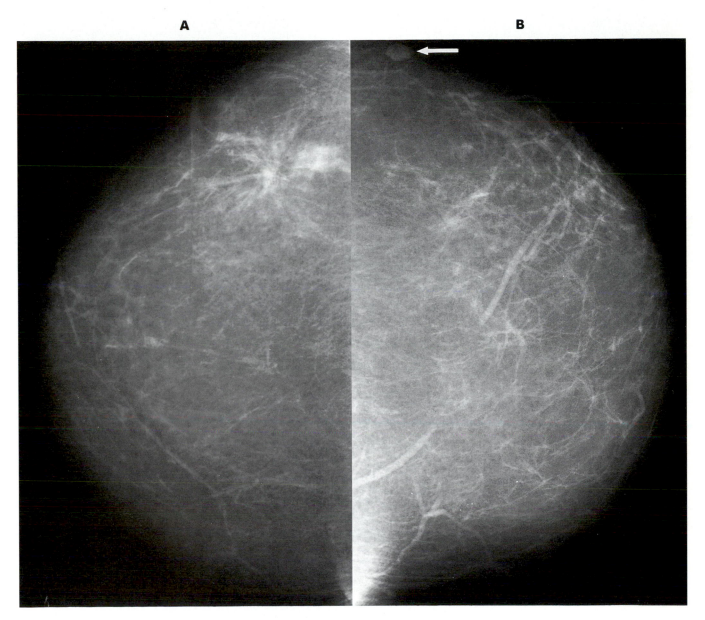

Fig. 11-57. A, Right CC; **B,** left CC.

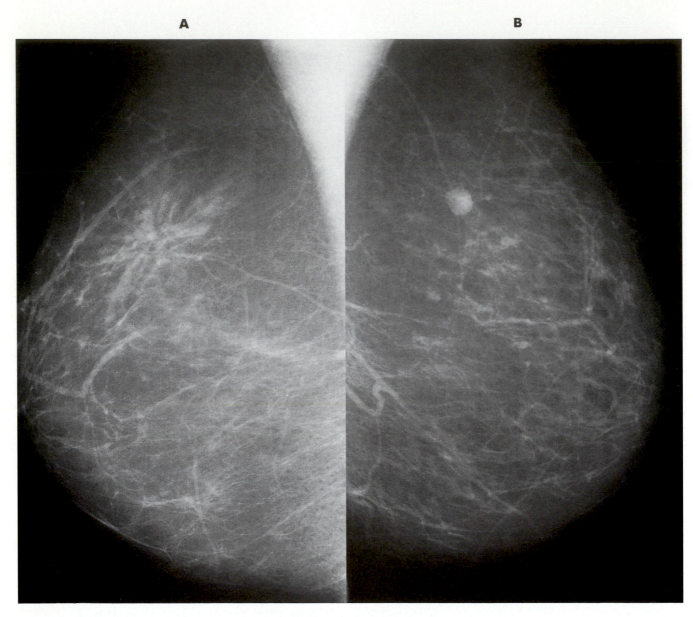

Fig. 11-58. A, Right LM; **B,** left LM.

In the left breast, the visualized dense circumscribed lesion is a benign skin lesion. In addition, a parenchymal distortion with coarse spicula can be seen in the upper outer quadrant of the right breast (Fig. 11-56, *A*). In such lesions, the mammographic differential diagnoses are malignancy versus radial scar.

Preliminary mammography images suggested radial scarring, or streaks, that are apparent and are surrounding a somewhat dense fibrotic-appearing central body.[4]

SFNB was performed. Cytology of the lesion demonstrated malignant epithelial cells. Histology of the lesion confirmed moderately differentiated invasive ductal carcinoma.

Code 3

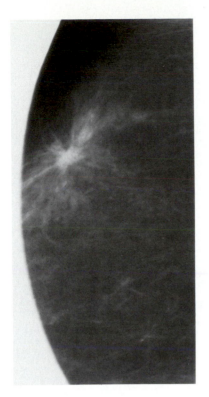

Fig. 11-59. Coned right CC.

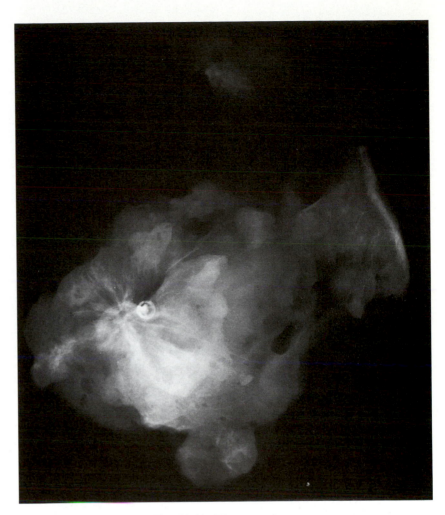

Fig. 11-61. Biopsy specimen.

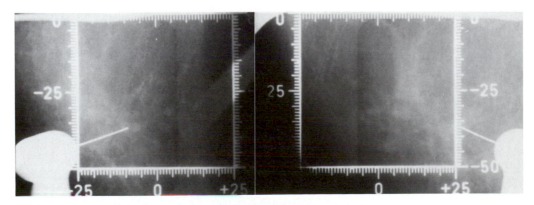

Fig. 11-60. SFNB.

PATIENT 13

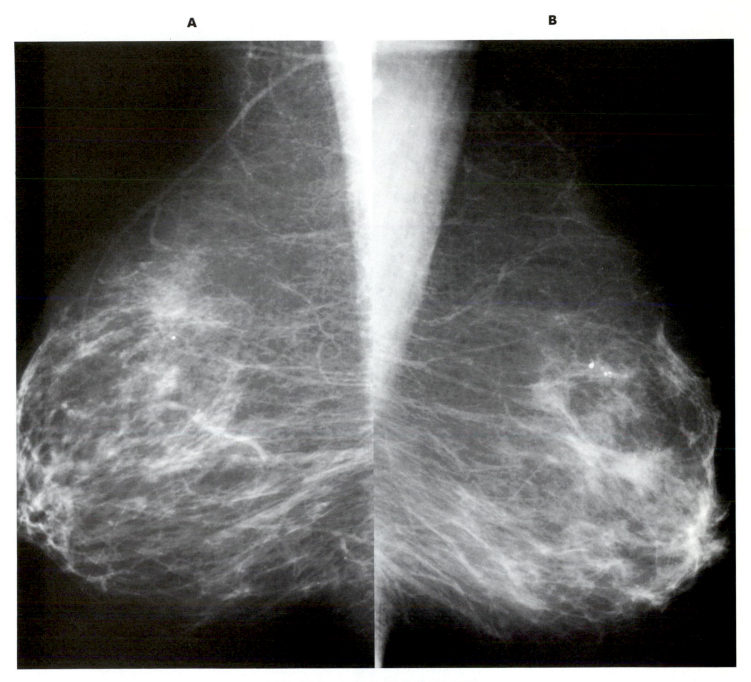

Fig. 11-62. A, Right MLO; **B,** left MLO.

These images (Fig. 11-62) represent a screening mammogram of a 65-year-old asymptomatic woman.

An incidental finding of benign calcifications is noted in the midportion of the left breast (Fig. 11-62, *B*). However, there also are two stellate-appearing lesions in the upper outer quadrant of this woman's left breast, located approximately 2 cm apart (Fig. 11-64, *A*). The lesion closest to the left nipple is mammographically more dense than the lesion more distant from the nipple. Regardless of this subtle difference in density, both lesions are very suspicious for malignancy (Figs. 11-63, *A,* and 11-64, *A*).

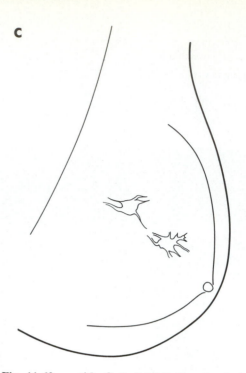

C

Fig. 11-62, cont'd. C, Left MLO (line drawing).

A

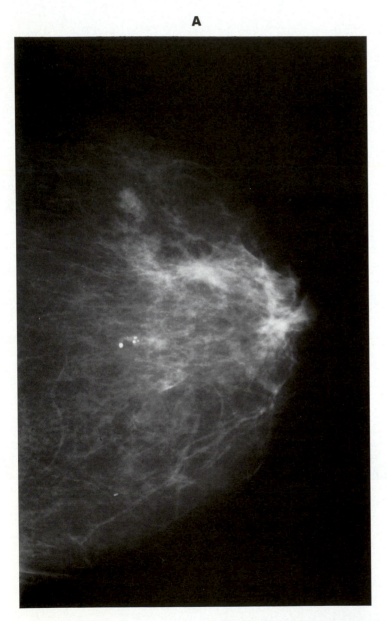

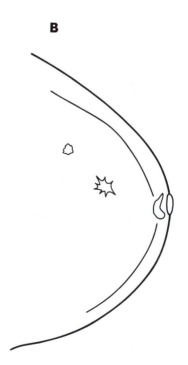

B

Fig. 11-63. A, Left CC; **B,** left CC (line drawing).

A

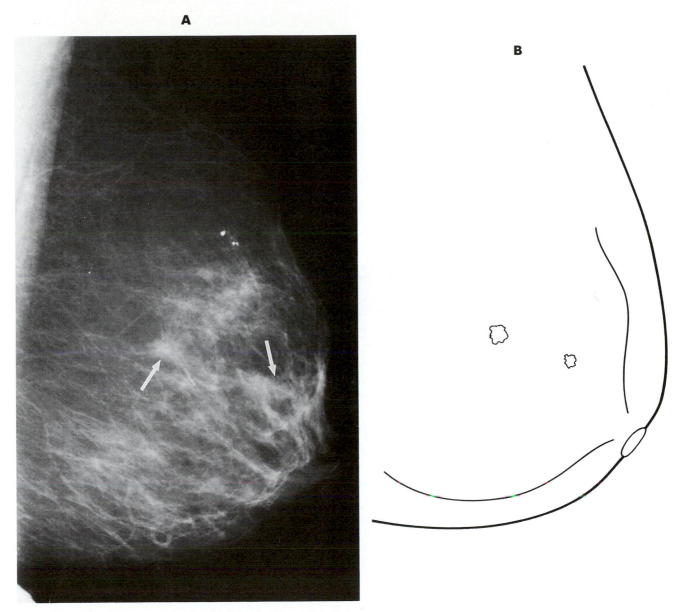

B

Fig. 11-64. A, Left LM; **B,** left LM (line drawing).

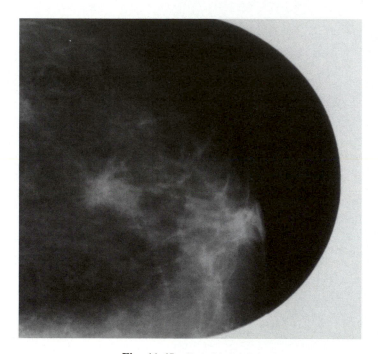

Fig. 11-65. Coned left CC.

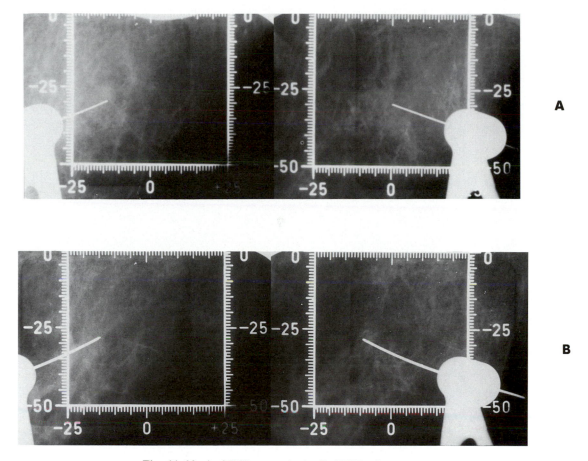

Fig. 11-66. A, SFNB, near nipple; **B,** SFNB, distant.

SFNB was performed at both sites (Fig. 11-66). Cytology of the more dense lesion revealed frank cancer cells, and cytology of the less dense lesion demonstrated gross cellular atypia also representing malignancy. Following carbon localization of both areas, surgery was performed revealing multifocal moderately well-differentiated invasive ductal carcinoma.

PATIENT 14

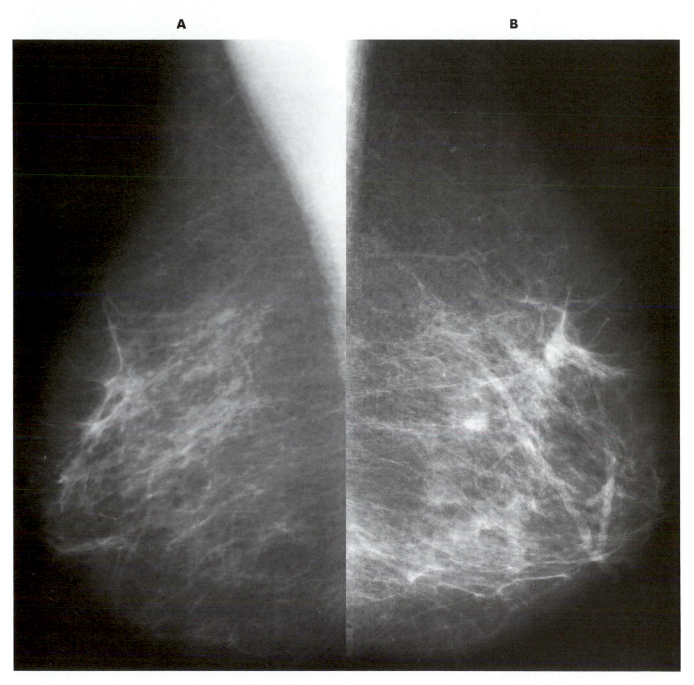

Fig. 11-67. A, Right MLO; **B,** left MLO.

These images (Fig. 11-67) are from a screening mammogram of a 56-year-old asymptomatic woman.

C

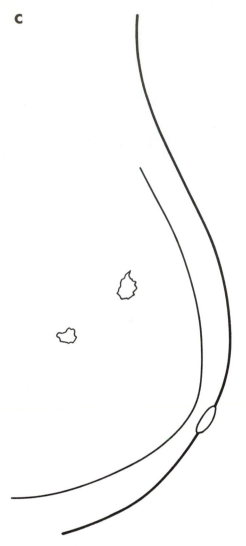

Fig. 11-67, cont'd.   C, Left MLO (line drawing)

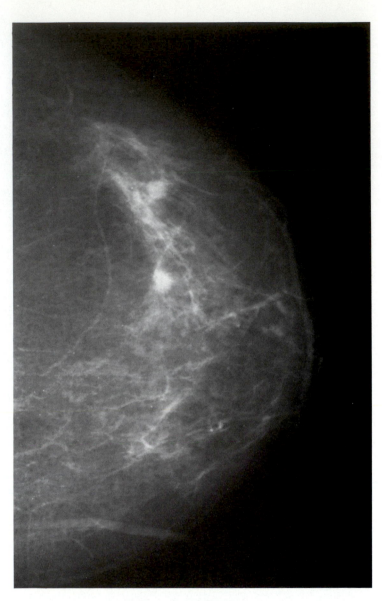

Fig. 11-68. Left CC.

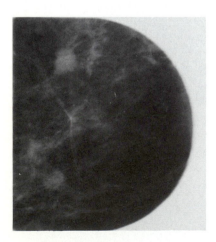

Fig. 11-70. Left coned CC.

Two lesions are identified in the upper outer quadrant of this woman's left breast (Fig. 11-67, *B*). The diameter of each of these lesions is nearly identical, between 5 and 6 mm in size. Depending on the mammographic projections, one or the other lesion can look slightly more dense and can also appear more spiculated (Figs. 11-68 and 11-69, *A*). Clinical breast examination, performed by trained medical personnel, failed to detect any palpable masses. Mammographically, these lesions are suspicious for cancer and are given a code 5 distinction.

Consequently, SFNB was performed at both sites, followed by carbon marking. Cytology of both lesions revealed malignant epithelial cells. Left breast mastectomy confirmed both lesions to be multifocal well-differentiated invasive ductal carcinoma.

Code 5

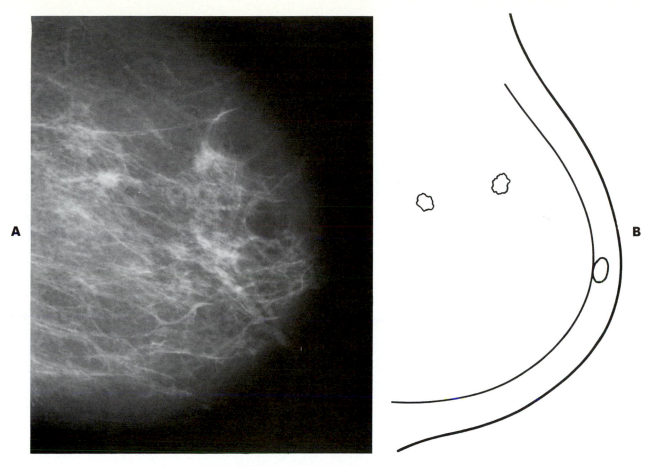

Fig. 11-69. A, Left LM; **B,** left LM (line drawing).

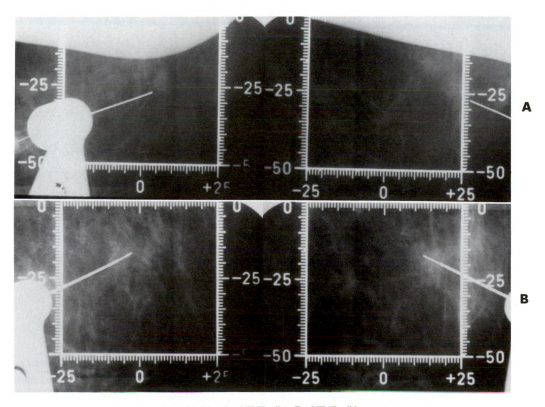

Fig. 11-71. A, SFNB #1; **B,** SFNB #2.

PATIENT 15

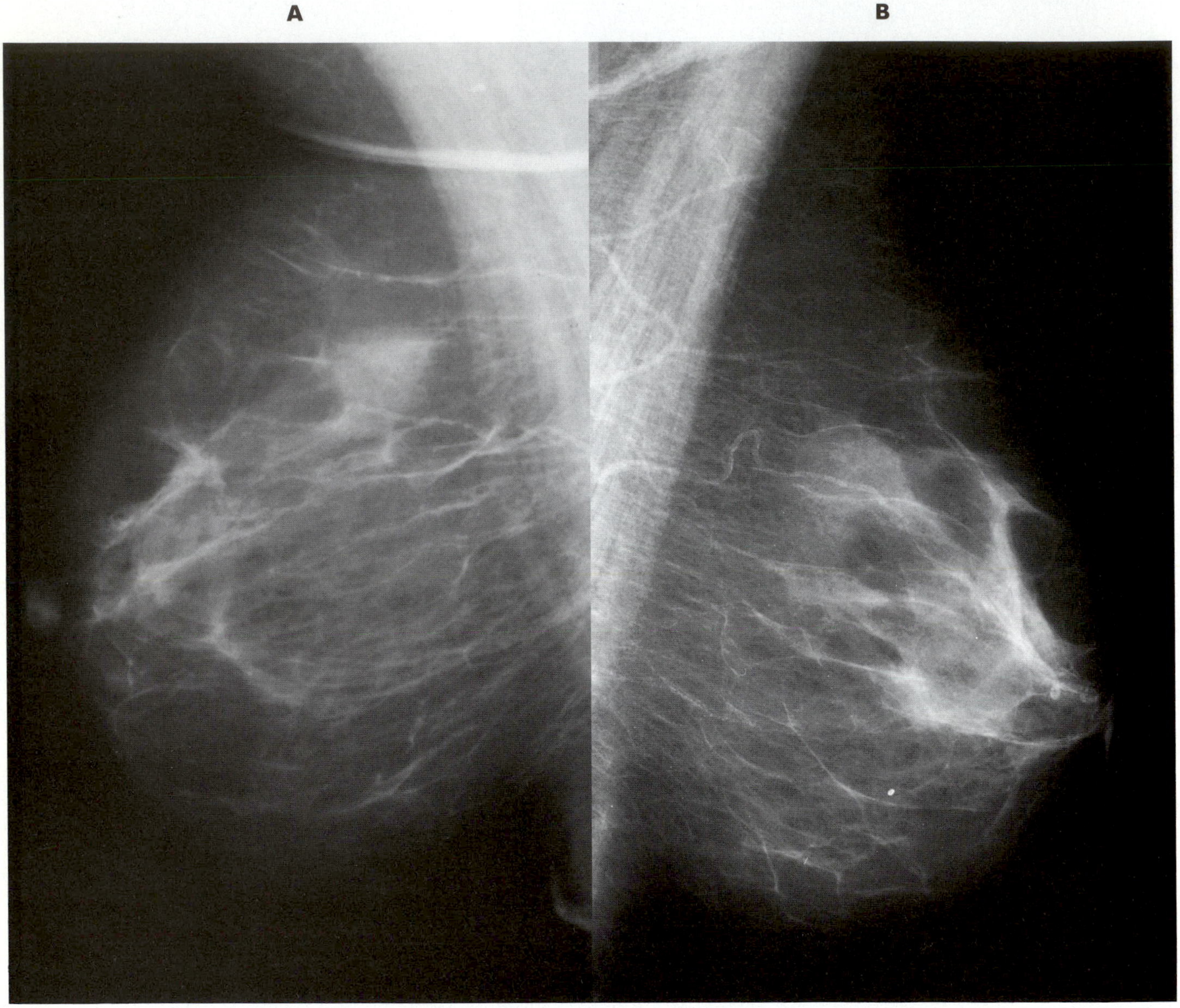

Fig. 11-72. A, Right MLO; **B,** left MLO.

These images (Figs. 11-72 and 11-73) represent a screening mammogram of a 69-year-old asymptomatic woman with rather lucent breast parenchyma.

A

B

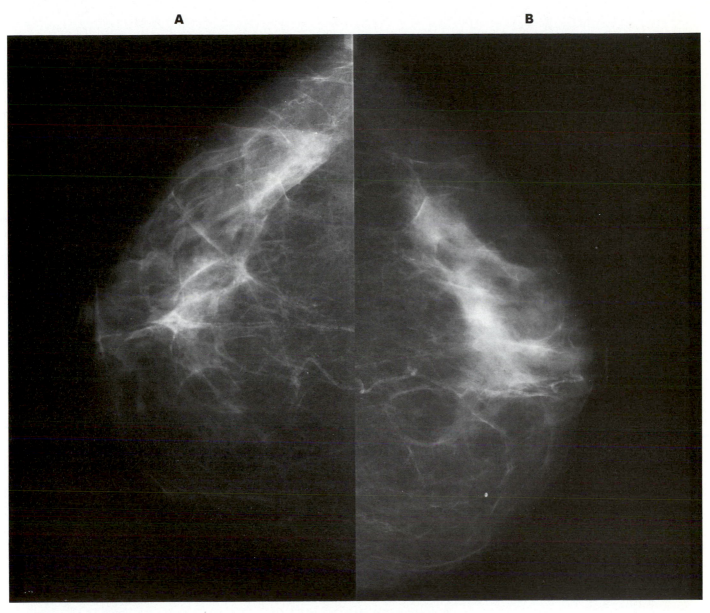

Fig. 11-73. A, Right CC; **B,** left CC.

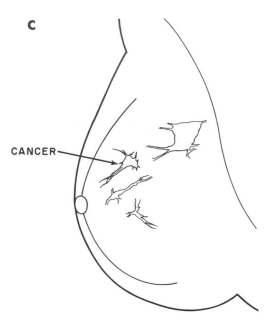

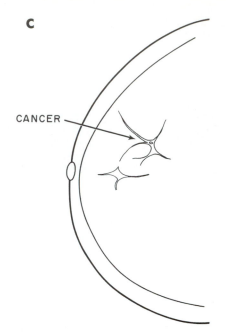

Fig. 11-72, cont'd. C, Right MLO (line drawing).

Fig. 11-73, cont'd. C, Right CC (line drawing).

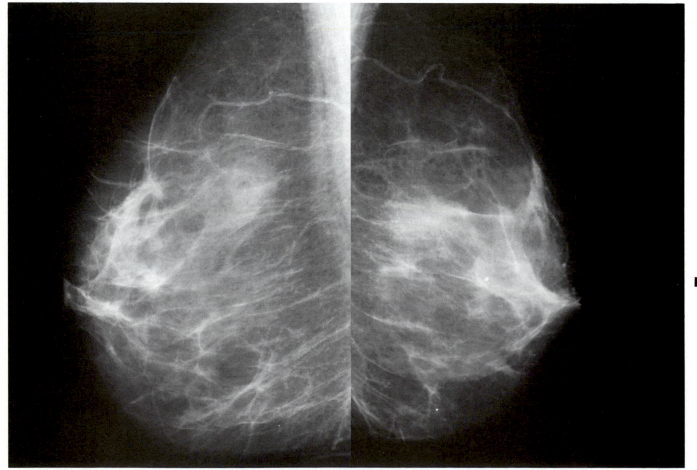

Fig. 11-74. A, Right LM; **B,** left LM.

Bilateral involutional breast change is mammographically obvious. For the most part, its occurrence is strongly symmetric in corresponding regions in the right and left breasts (Fig. 11-72, *A* and *B*). However, in review of both the mediolateral oblique and the craniocaudal projections of this screening evaluation, an apparent area for concern is noted in the right upper outer quadrant of the breast (Figs. 11-72, *A,* and 11-73, *A*).

Lateromedial projections confirm the stellate configuration on the right and raise suspicion for yet another dense area, directly below the stellate lesion and approximately 2 cm behind the right nipple (Fig. 11-74, *A*). Coned compression projection quickly substantiates the superiorly located stellate lesion and dispels concern for a second suspicious dense area (Fig. 11-75).

SFNB and carbon localization were performed (Fig. 11-76). Cytology of the stellate area revealed cancer cells. Histology of the lesion confirmed well-differentiated invasive tubular carcinoma.

Code 5

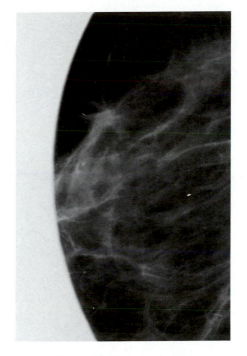

Fig. 11-75. Coned right LM.

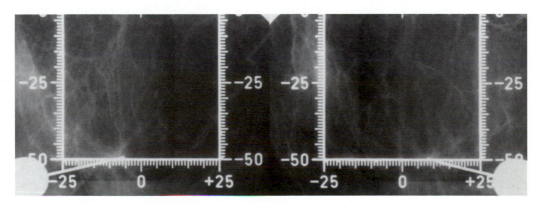

Fig. 11-76. SFNB.

PATIENT 16

A   B

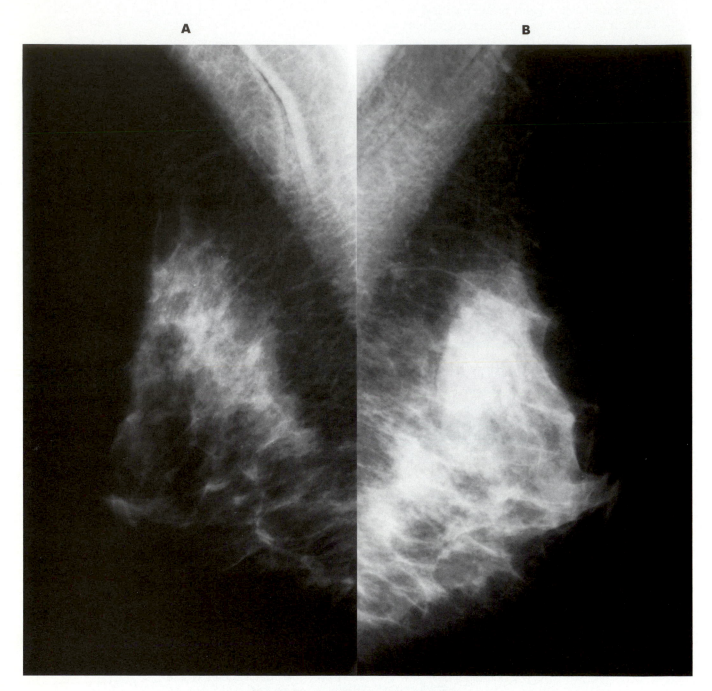

Fig. 11-77. A, Right MLO; **B,** left MLO.

These images (Figs. 11-77 and 11-78) represent a screening mammogram of a 55-year-old asymptomatic woman with dense breasts.

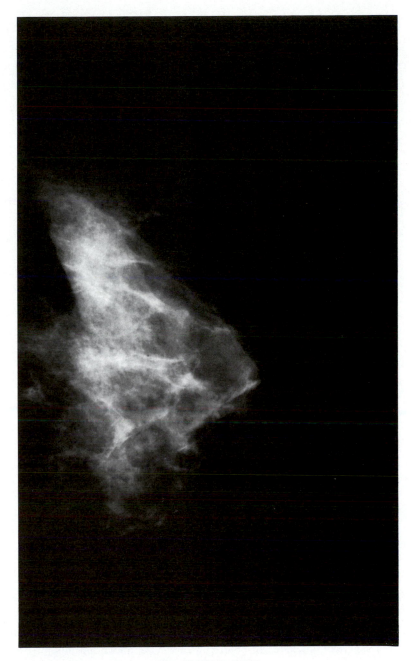

Fig. 11-78. Left CC.

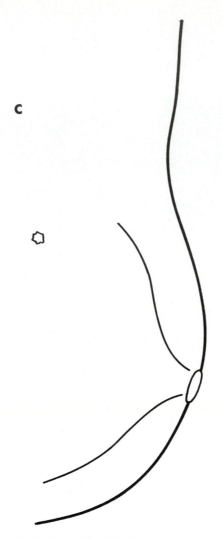

Fig. 11-77, cont'd. C, Left MLO (line drawing).

On the craniocaudal projection of this routine screening mammogram, approximately 7 cm from the left nipple is a small stellate-appearing lesion (Fig. 11-78). Careful evaluation of the mediolateral oblique projection again permits visualization of its location in a superior direction and approximately 7 cm above the nipple (Fig. 11-77, *B*). In the lateromedial projection, this small abnormality is less easily recognized (Fig. 11-79, *A*).

Multiple coned projections clearly locate the lesion and demonstrate slightly varying degrees of density. Coned compression projections in particular often allow for prompt discovery of subtle lesions as well as discovery of classic mammographic features of malignancy (Figs. 11-80, *A*, and 11-81, *A*). This lesion was given a code 4 classification.

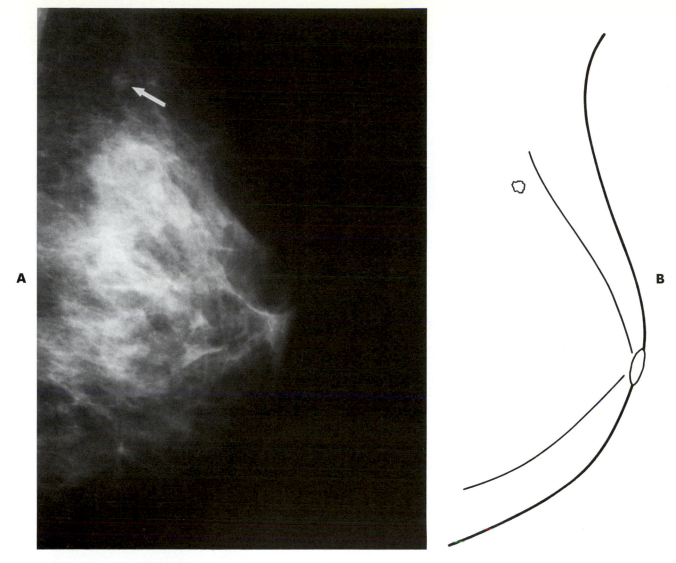

Fig. 11-79. A, Left LM; **B,** left LM (line drawing).

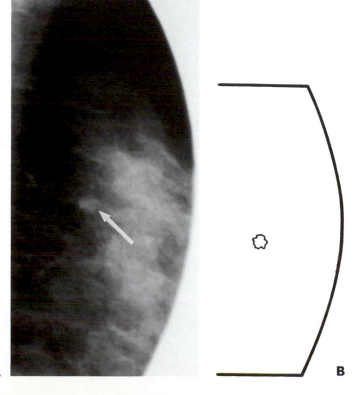

Fig. 11-80. A, Coned MLO; **B,** coned left MLO (line drawing).

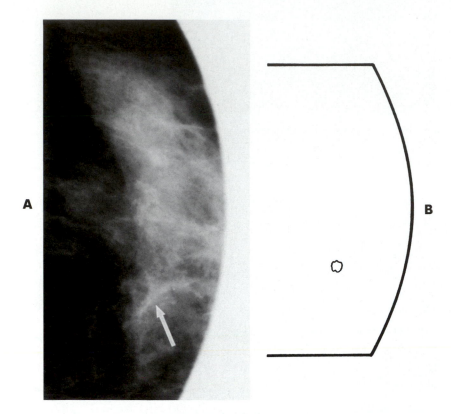

Fig. 11-81. A, Coned CC; **B,** coned CC (line drawing).

SFNB was performed, and cytology confirmed grossly atypical epithelial cells (Fig. 11-82). Histology proved this lesion to be moderately well-differentiated invasive ductal carcinoma.

Code 4

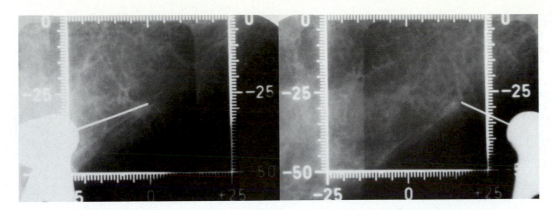

Fig. 11-82. SFNB.

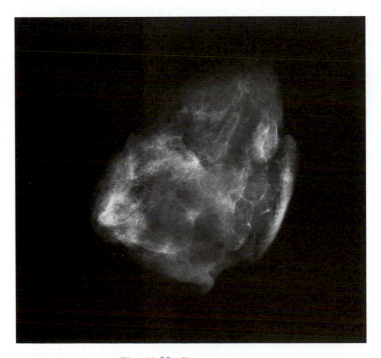

Fig. 11-83. Biopsy specimen.

PATIENT 17

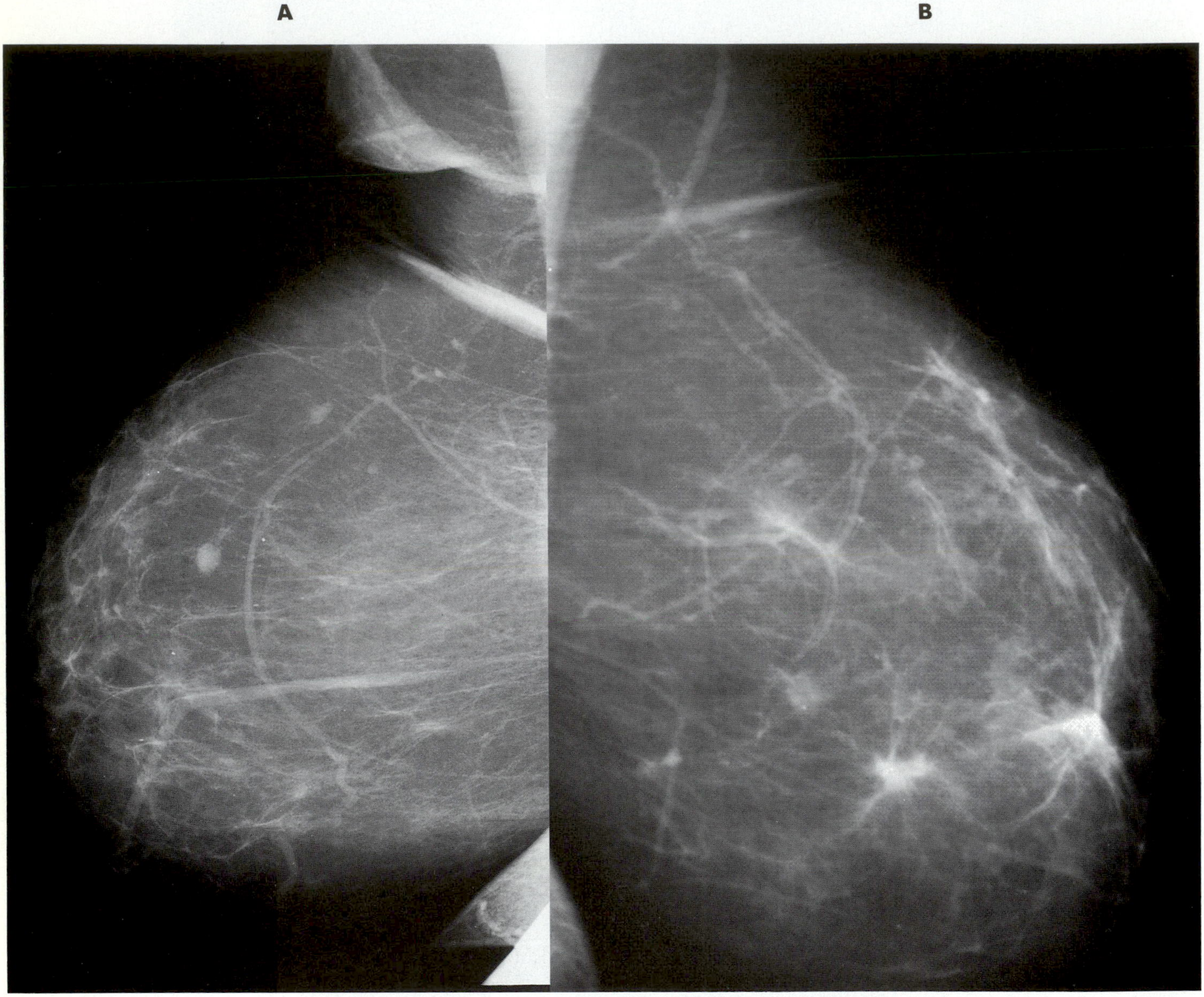

Fig. 11-84. A, Right MLO; **B,** left MLO.

These images (Figs. 11-84 and 11-85) are from a screening mammogram of a 65-year-old asymptomatic woman with lucent breasts.

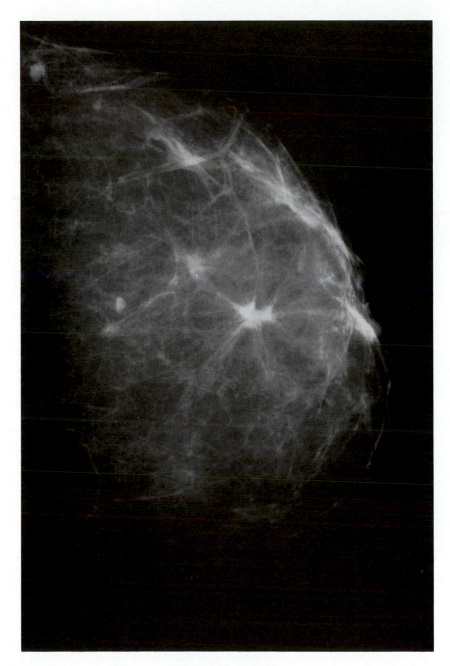

Fig. 11-85. Left CC.

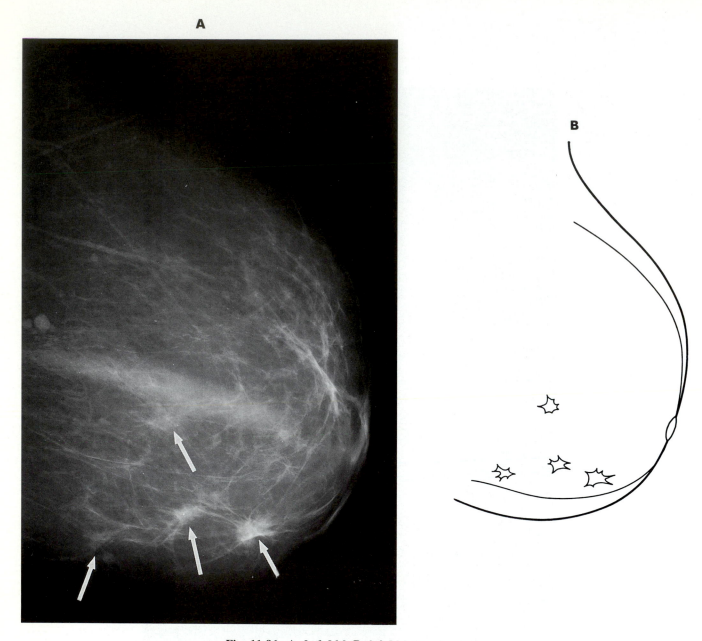

Fig. 11-86. A, Left LM; **B,** left LM (line drawing).

Documented advantages of the detection and treatment of minimal breast cancers are quoted throughout this text. It is remarkable that this asymptomatic woman's mammogram revealed four code 5 lesions, none of which was clinically detectable. Unfortunately, this was a baseline screening mammogram.

In the right breast, two lymph nodes and one small cyst are seen (Fig. 11-84, A). In the left breast, however, while there are several mammary lymph nodes, three stellate lesions of significant proportions are also unmistakably present. Two of the stellate lesions show slightly greater density than the third. All three of these stellate lesions are located in the lower portion of the left breast (Fig. 11-84, B).

In addition to the three obvious stellate lesions, which mammographically represent cancer, a fourth, more diffuse and stellate-type lesion is seen with less certainty. It is

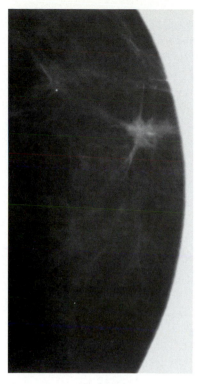

Fig. 11-87. Coned left CC, #1.

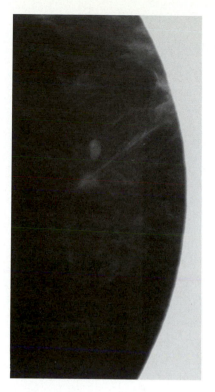

Fig. 11-88. Coned left CC, #2.

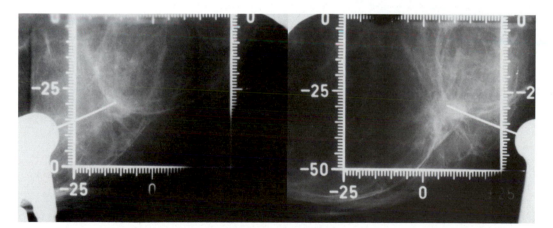

Fig. 11-89. SFNB.

detected only in the mediolateral oblique projection (Fig. 11-84, *B*). The coned views demonstrate the mammographic cancers, which also were verified by SFNB (Figs. 11-87 to 11-89). Histopathology reconfirmed all lesions as cancerous. These four cancers in the left lower breast are moderately well-differentiated ductal carcinoma.

SFNB procedure verified the existence of cancer in three of the four breast lesions. This confirmation of morphologically verified multifocal cancers formed the basis for mastectomy in this case.

Code 5

REFERENCES

1. Arthur JE, Ellis IO, Flowers C, et al: The relationship of "high risk" mammographic patterns to histological risk factors for development of cancer in the human breast, *Br J Radiol* 63:845-849, 1990.
2. Gormly L, Bassett L, Gold R: Positioning in film-screen mammography, *Appl Radiol*, July 1988.
3. Miller AB: Screening and detection. In Bland KI, Copeland EM, editors: *The breast: comprehensive management of benign and malignant diseases,* Philadelphia, 1991, Saunders.
4. Souba WW: Evaluation and treatment of benign breast disorders. In Bland KI, Copeland EM, editors: *The breast: comprehensive management of benign and malignant diseases,* Philadelphia, 1991, Saunders.

Chapter 12

MICROCALCIFICATIONS

PATIENT 1

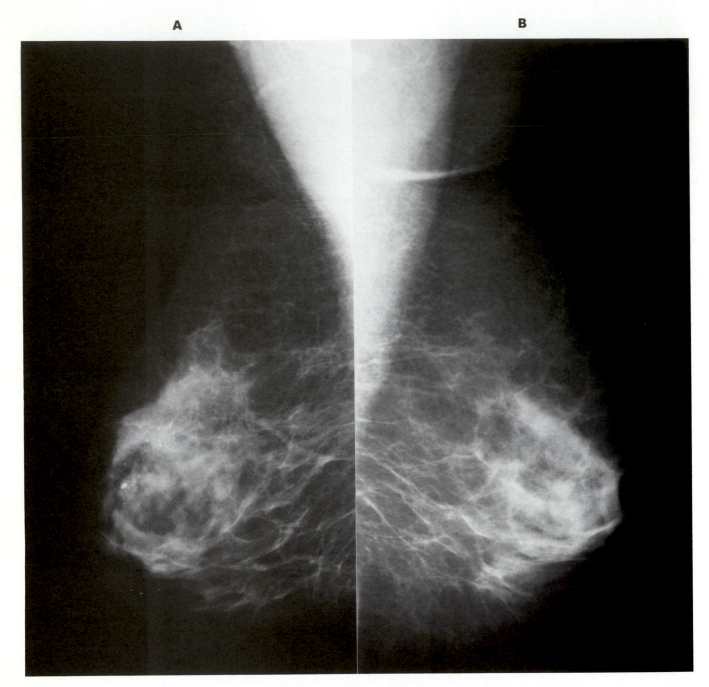

Fig. 12-1. A, Right MLO; **B,** left MLO.

This 63-year-old asymptomatic woman reported for routine screening mammography (Figs. 12-1 and 12-2).

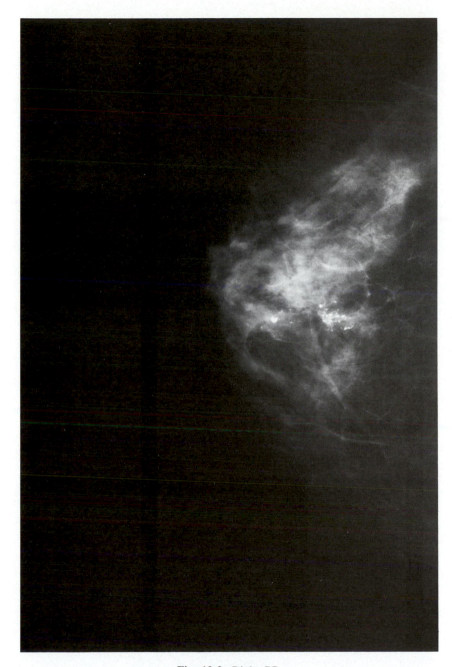

Fig. 12-2. Right CC.

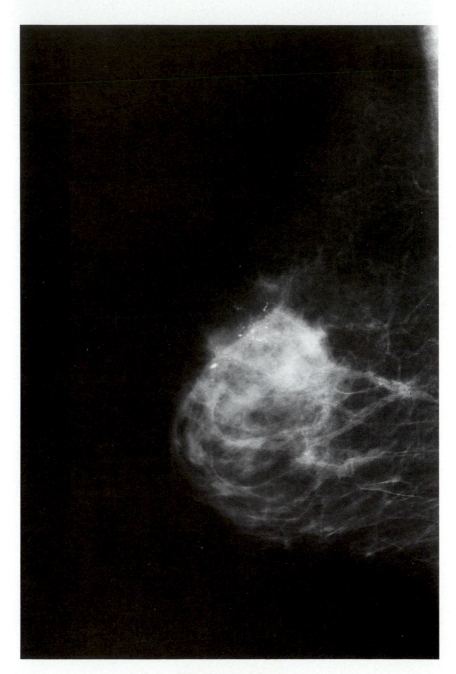

Fig. 12-3. Right LM.

Rather widespread irregular microcalcifications are apparent in the right breast (Fig. 12-1, *A*). There is no increase in breast tissue density or parenchymal distortion. Several coarsely featured, benign-type calcifications are identified along with the mammographically suspicious microcalcifications. Note the intraductal formations of branching and the irregular size, shape, and density of the calcifications (Figs. 12-2 and 12-3).

Ductal calcifications have been characterized as "casts of segments of the ductal lumen."[8] Calcific fragmentation and irregular contouring, as shown in this case, can result from an irregular necrotic process occurring in affected epithelial cell material[8] (Fig. 12-4).

Stereotaxic fine-needle biopsy (SFNB) was performed in the area of the admixture of calcifications to determine the nature of their involvement. Cytology confirmed malignant cells. Surgical biopsy of the lesion confirmed ductal carcinoma in situ.

Code 5

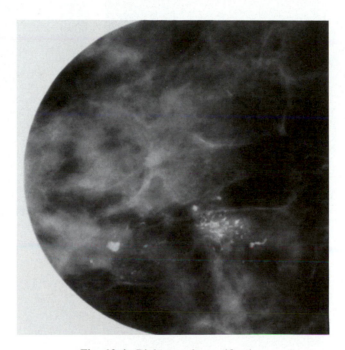

Fig. 12-4. Right coned magnification.

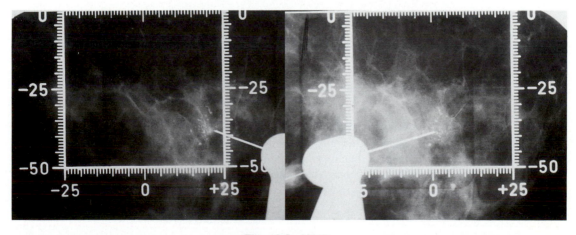

Fig. 12-5. SFNB.

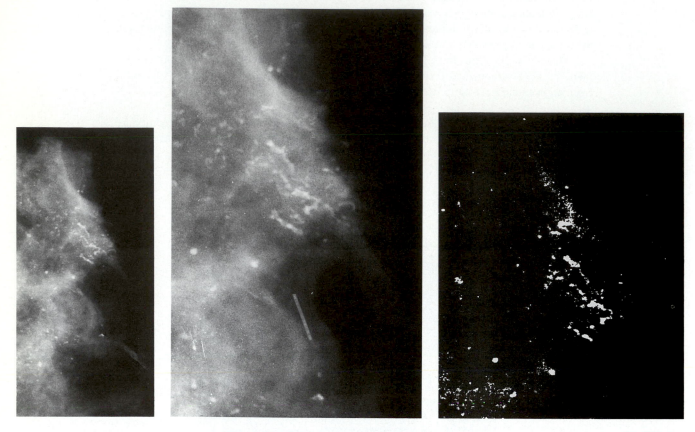

Fig. 12-6. Ductal calcifications of the casting type.

Fig. 12-6 demonstrates the mammographic appearance of ductal calcifications of the casting type. In the magnification image and the high-density photocopy one can see reconfirmed from the original mammographic image the irregular calcific pattern, ranging from microcalcifications to completely filled ductal lumen. Fig. 12-7 reemphasizes the casted segments, as demonstrated in the cytology slide evaluation of the calcific breast tissue.

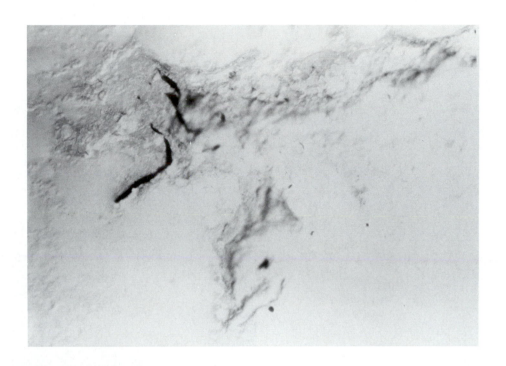

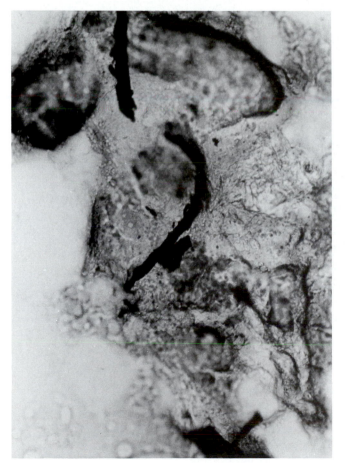

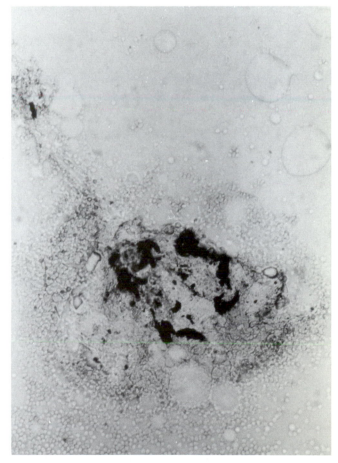

Fig. 12-7. Casted segments.

PATIENT 2

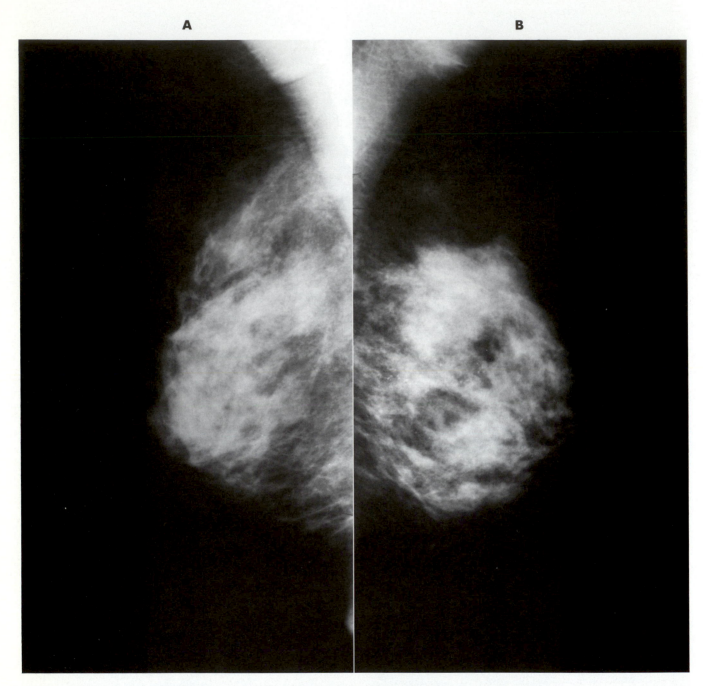

Fig. 12-8. A, Right MLO; **B,** left MLO.

These images (Figs. 12-8 and 12-9) are from a mammogram of a 50-year-old asymptomatic physician who reported for routine screening. Radiographic features reveal dense breasts with asymmetric distribution of parenchyma.

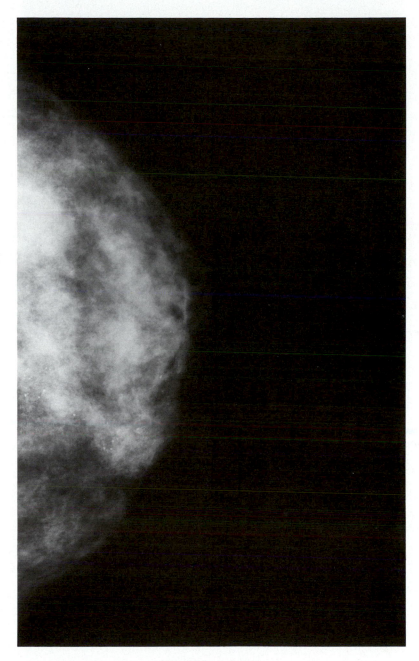

Fig. 12-9. Left CC.

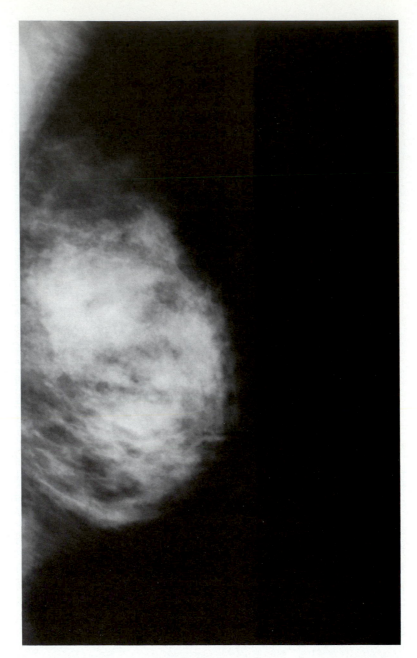

Fig. 12-10. Left LM.

The right breast exhibits asymmetric parenchyma within normal limits but no calcific densities (Fig. 12-8, *A*). Clustered and scattered microcalcifications are apparent on the mediolateral oblique projection throughout the left breast (Fig. 12-8, *B*). Some of the left breast calcifications are of the branching casting-type, depicting intraductal position. This pattern is well known and is said to be characteristic of carcinoma.[8] Calcifications of lunar and semilunar configuration are also apparent, suggesting benign changes (Fig. 12-12).

This mammographic appearance of mixed patterns of calcification is a source of

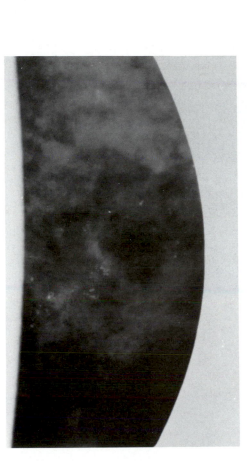

Fig. 12-11. Left coned magnification.

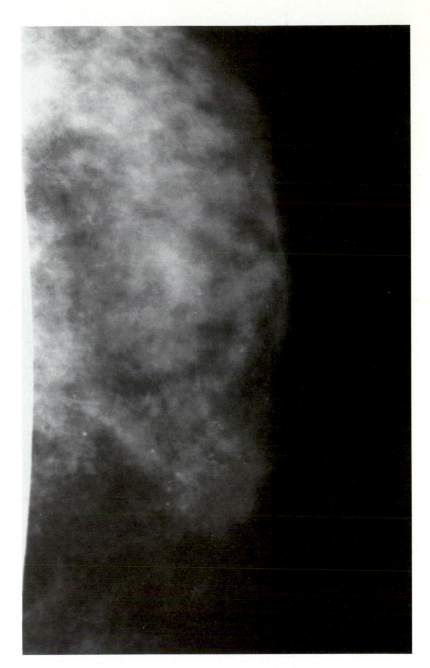

Fig. 12-12. Left coned magnification.

confusion. For patient management, this finding usually leaves no option but surgery, regardless of negative cytology. Using the SFNB technique permits preoperative cell sampling and carbon localization in a single step. In this case, cytology was inconclusive, showing only atypia. Histology of the specimen verified ductal carcinoma in situ of multifocal type. The term "multifocality" indicates foci of the same tumor located close to each other, usually in the same quadrant.[1] The mammographic arrangement of the microcalcific densities substantiates the prebiopsy suspicion of carcinoma.

Code 4

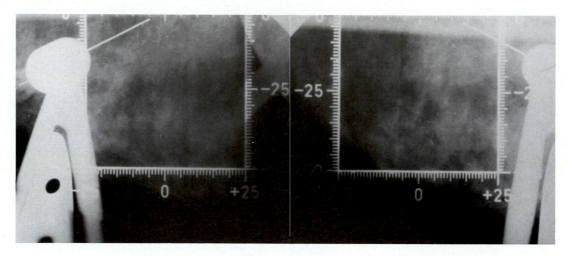

Fig. 12-13. SFNB.

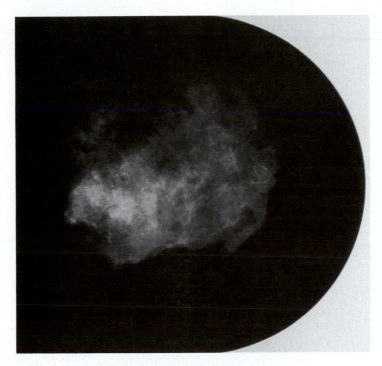

Fig. 12-14. Biopsy specimen.

PATIENT 3

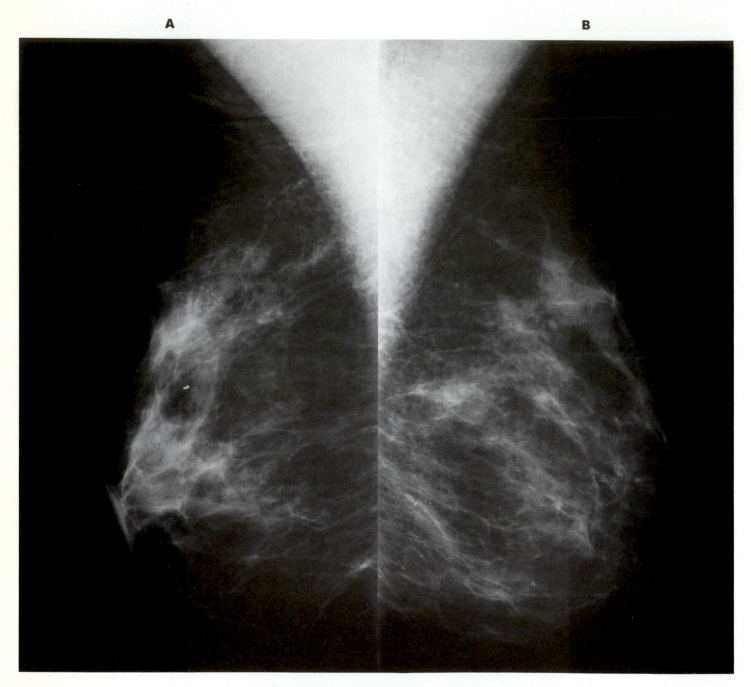

Fig. 12-15. A, Right MLO; **B,** left MLO.

These images (Figs. 12-15 and 12-16) represent a screening mammogram of a 62-year-old asymptomatic woman with a moderate amount of breast parenchyma.

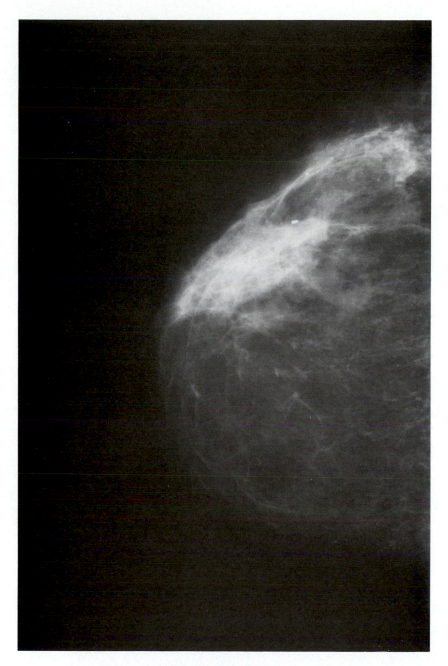

Fig. 12-16. Right CC.

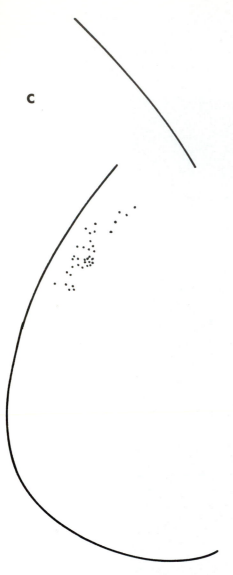

Fig. 12-15, cont'd. C, Right MLO (line drawing).

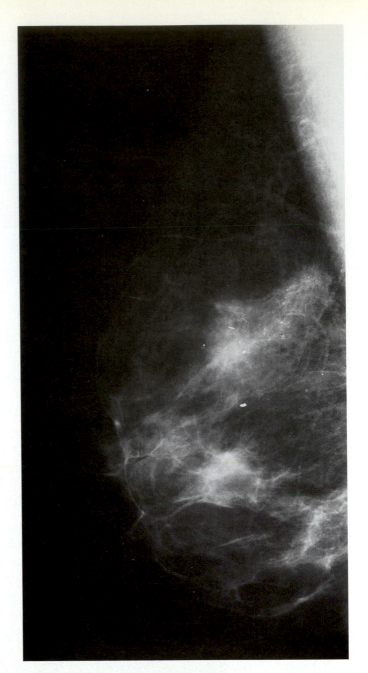

Fig. 12-17. Right LM.

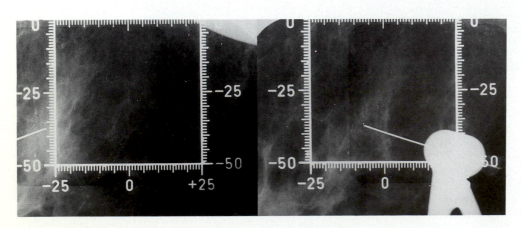

Fig. 12-18. Right SFNB.

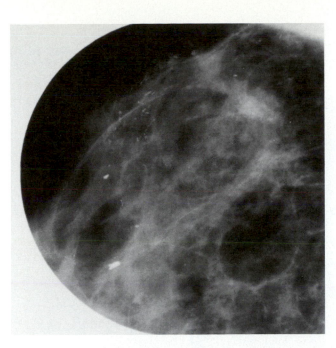

Fig. 12-19. Right coned magnification.

Scattered mixed-type calcifications can be seen in the upper outer quadrant of the right breast (Fig. 12-15, *A*). The calcifications appear linear and branching and consequently have a higher probability of being malignant. The coned magnification projection clearly defines the various patterns of calcification.

SFNB was performed, and the cytologic evaluation demonstrated malignant cells. Histology of the biopsied lesion confirmed ductal carcinoma in situ.

Code 4

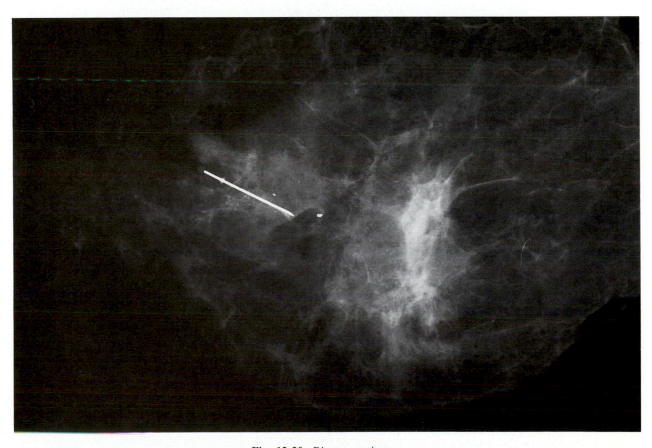

Fig. 12-20. Biopsy specimen.

PATIENT 4

A

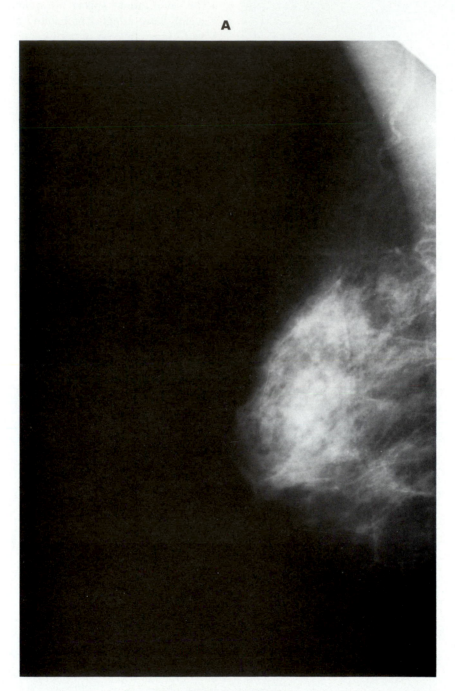

Fig. 12-21. A, Right MLO.

The right mediolateral oblique (Fig. 12-21, *A*) and right craniocaudal (Fig. 12-22) images are from a screening mammogram of a 57-year-old asymptomatic woman with moderately dense breasts.

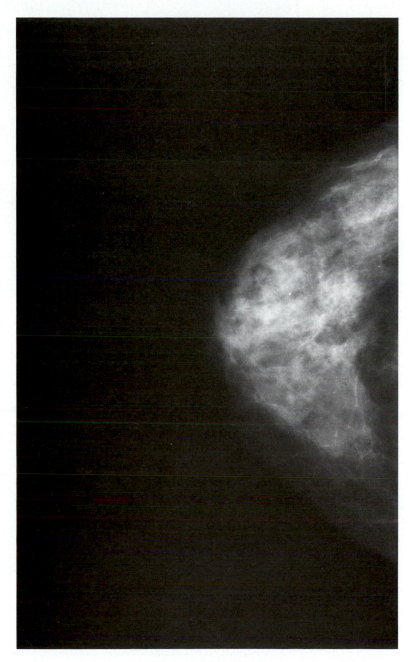

Fig. 12-22. Right CC.

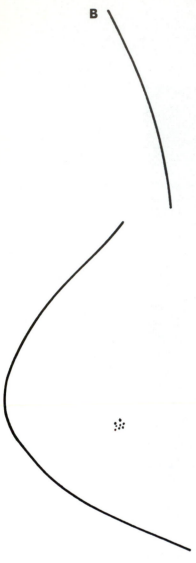

Fig. 12-21, cont'd. B, Right MLO (line drawing).

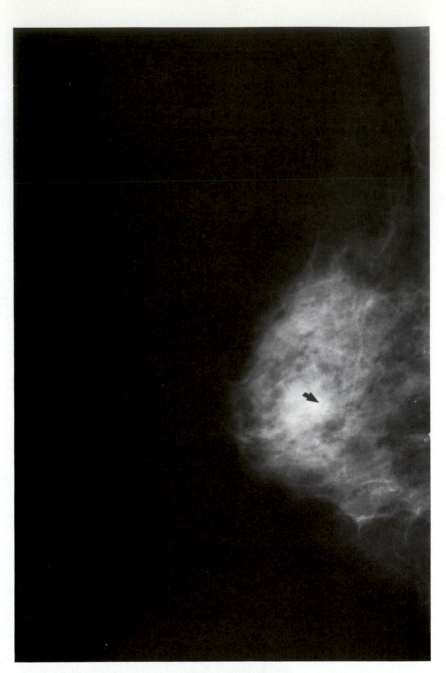

Fig. 12-23. Right LM.

The mediolateral oblique and craniocaudal projections of the right breast reveal a cluster of microcalcifications that require further evaluation (Figs. 12-21, *A*, and 12-22). This small, discrete group of microcalcifications, identified in the medial portion of the right breast, are approximately 4 cm from the nipple. Magnification mammography of the calcifications reconfirms their location and demonstrates their variations (Fig. 12-24). The calcifications are not of a casting type but appear granular and irregular in size, shape, and density (see case 1). This mammographic appearance is very suspicious for malignancy, and biopsy is necessary to determine their exact etiology.

SFNB was performed, and cytology confirmed cancerous cells. Following carbon marking of the calcifications and subsequent surgery, histology of the specimen substantiated both invasive ductal carcinoma and lobular carcinoma in situ (see Chapter 4).

Code 4

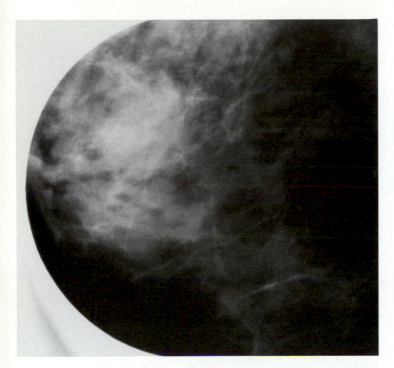

Fig. 12-24. Coned magnification.

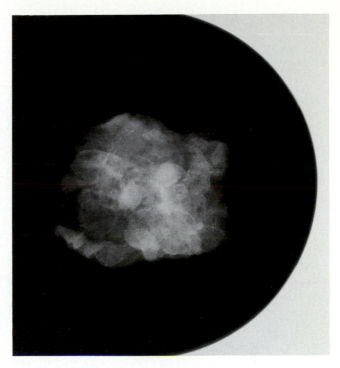

Fig. 12-26. Biopsy specimen.

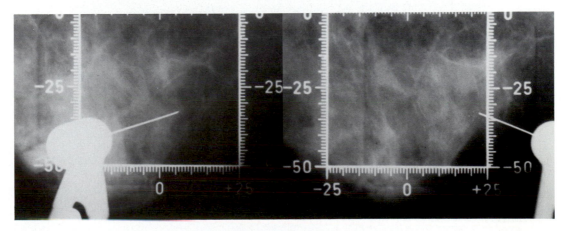

Fig. 12-25. SFNB.

PATIENT 5

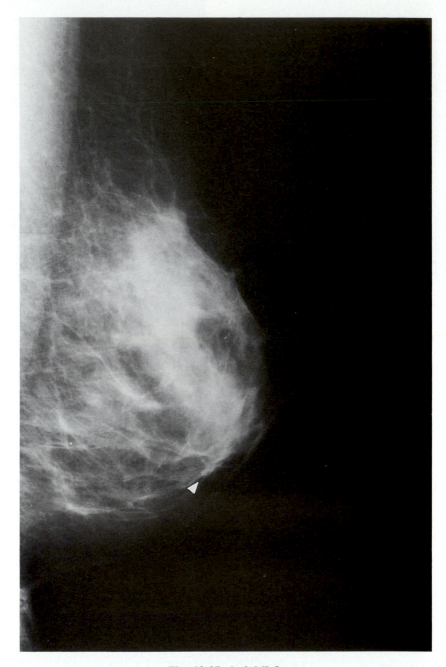

Fig. 12-27. Left MLO.

This 50-year-old asymptomatic woman reported for routine screening mammography (Figs. 12-27 and 12-28).

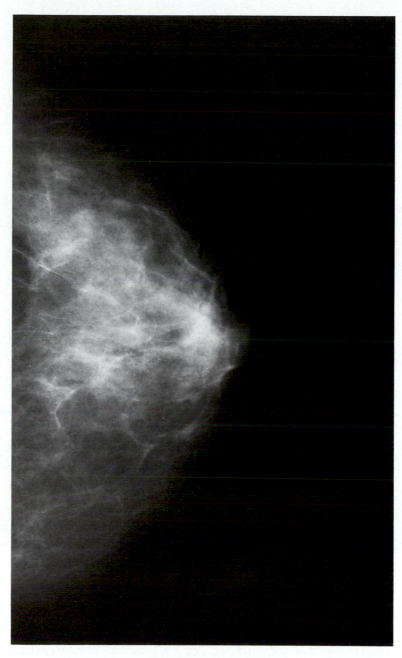

Fig. 12-28. Left CC.

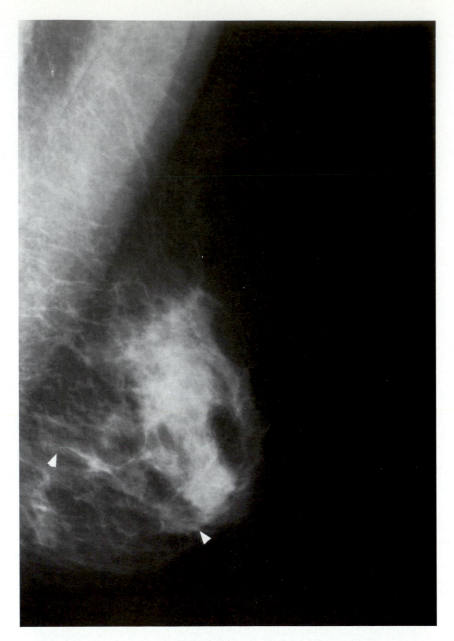

Fig. 12-29. Left LM.

Seen in the craniocaudal projection in the left subareolar portion of the breast is a cluster-like formation of irregular microcalcifications (Fig. 12-28). A similar group of irregular microcalcifications is identified approximately 4.5 mm deeper in the breast (Figs. 12-27 and 12-28). Coned magnification images in both mediolateral oblique and craniocaudal projections are of particular value to aid in confirmation and diagnosis of isolated clusters of microcalcifications (Figs. 12-30 and 12-31).

Using magnification imaging, irregularity in the density, size, and shape of micro-calcifications can be more readily identified. Magnification mammography confirms the presence of microcalcifications by improving on image unsharpness inherent in conventional mammography.[2,6] It is widely appreciated that while there is no direct evidence of

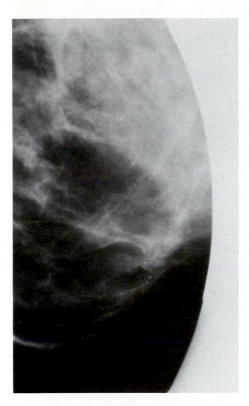

Fig. 12-30. Coned left MLO.

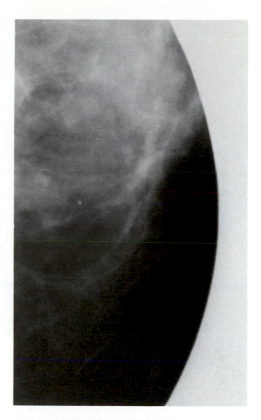

Fig. 12-31. Coned left CC.

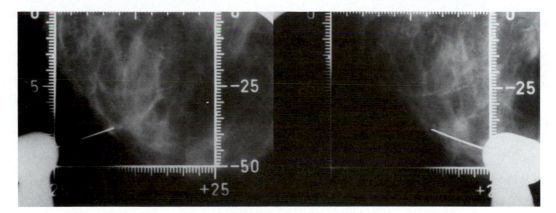

Fig. 12-32. SFNB.

the absolute ability to differentiate benign from malignant calcifications, magnification mammography can demonstrate the nature of calcific patterns, enhancing accuracy and helping to determine the degree of further necessary work-up of a lesion.[7] Regardless of the cytologic outcome, this mammographic pattern of suspicious calcifications requires recommendation for surgical evaluation.

SFNB and carbon localization of both suspicious areas were performed (Fig. 12-32). Cytology proved negative for malignancy. Histology of the lesion, however, confirmed ductal carcinoma in situ in both mammographically suspicious areas.

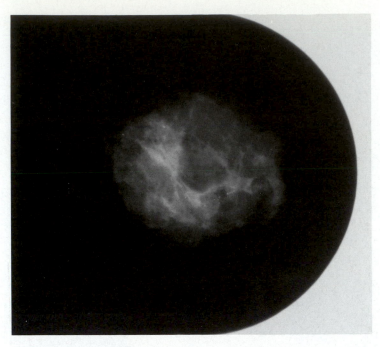

Fig. 12-33. Biopsy specimen.

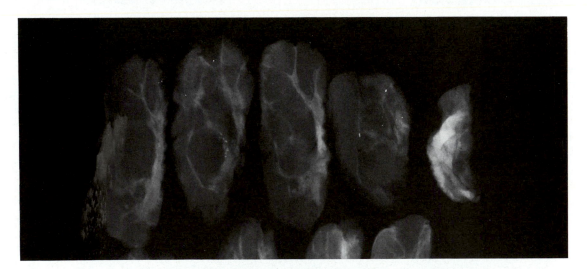

Fig. 12-34. Biopsy specimen slices.

Specimen radiograph of abnormal biopsy tissue is mandatory to assure that calcifications identified at routine mammography are present in the intact breast specimen (Fig. 12-33). If they are not initially detected by specimen radiography, it is incumbent that the radiologist and surgeon insist on specimen serial sectioning to confirm their presence before completion of the surgical procedure (Fig. 12-34).

Code 4

A

B

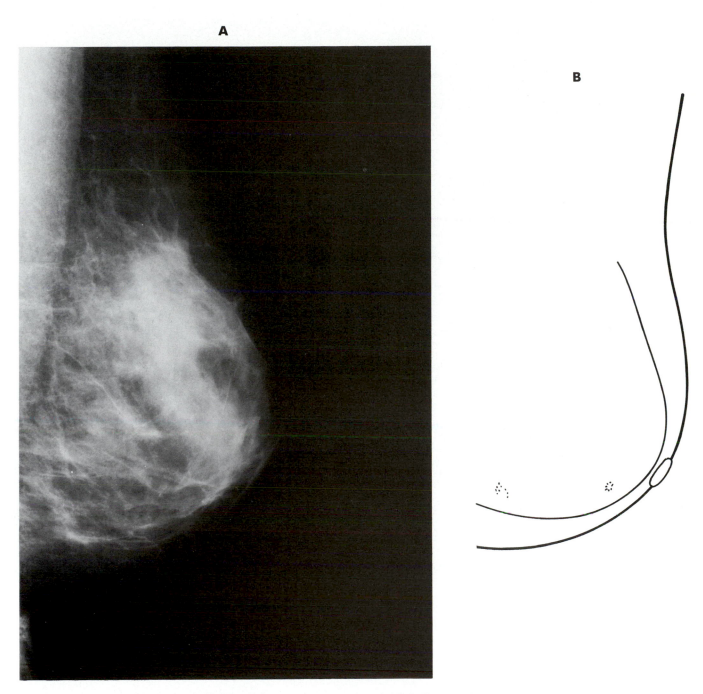

Fig. 12-35. A, Left MLO; **B,** left MLO (line drawing).

PATIENT 6

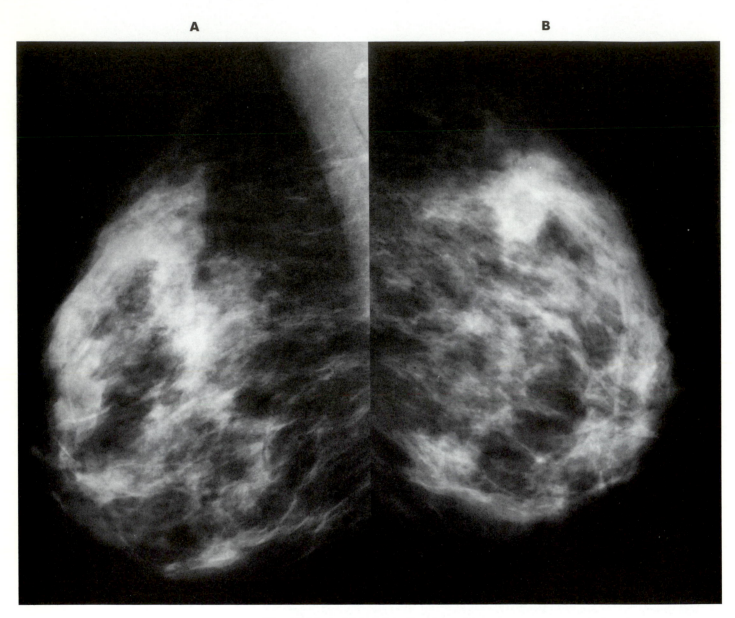

Fig. 12-36. A, Right MLO; **B,** left MLO.

These images (Figs. 12-36 and 12-37) represent a screening mammogram of a 45-year-old asymptomatic woman with dense breasts.

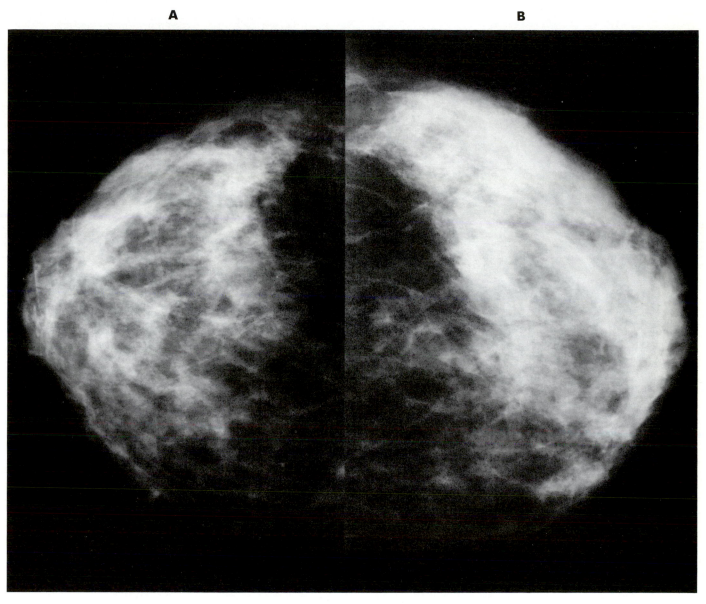

Fig. 12-37. A, Right CC; **B,** left CC.

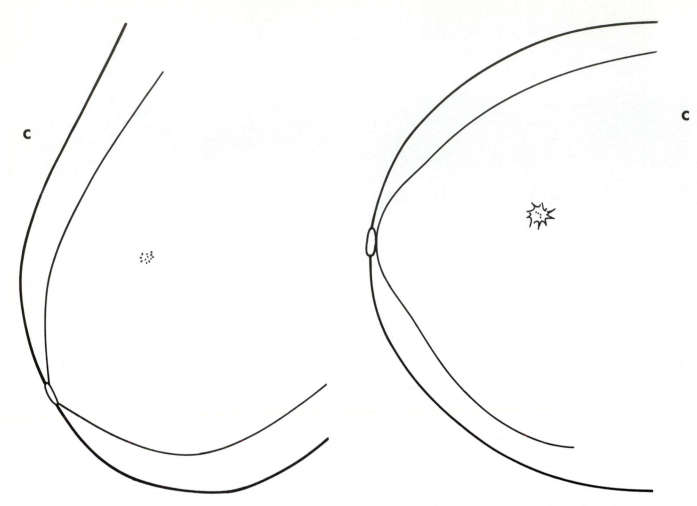

Fig. 12-36, cont'd. C, Right MLO (line drawing).   **Fig. 12-37, cont'd. C,** Right CC (line drawing).

Extreme care in film analysis is always required, particularly when breast parenchyma is as dense as it is in this case. To initially detect microcalcifications, much less determine their size, number, and distribution, is a challenge. Again, the absolute value of magnification radiography becomes apparent to confirm suspicion of their presence and define their variations.

In the upper outer quadrant of the right breast is a small group of calcifications that initially look fairly benign (Fig. 12-37, *A*). Lateromedial standard coned and coned magnification views were obtained (Figs. 12-39 and 12-40). The coned magnification projection demonstrates that the calcifications are associated with a stellate-appearing mass. A closer look confirms an underlying density (Fig. 12-40). This mammographic pattern is highly suspicious for malignancy.

SFNB confirmed malignant cells. Histology of the lesion confirmed fibrosing adenosis and ductal carcinoma in situ.

Code 4

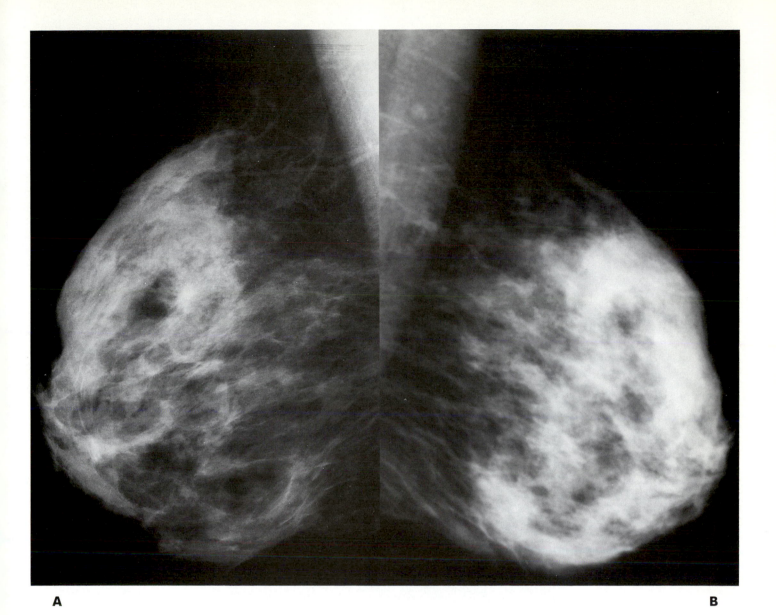

A

B

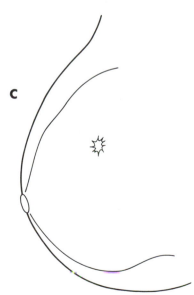

C

Fig. 12-38. **A,** Right LM; **B,** left LM; **C,** right LM (line drawing).

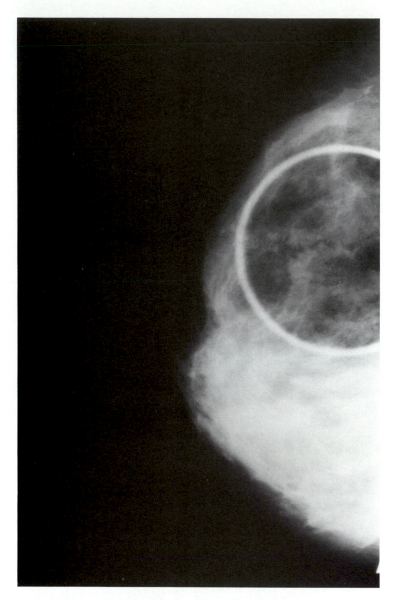

Fig. 12-39. Coned right LM.

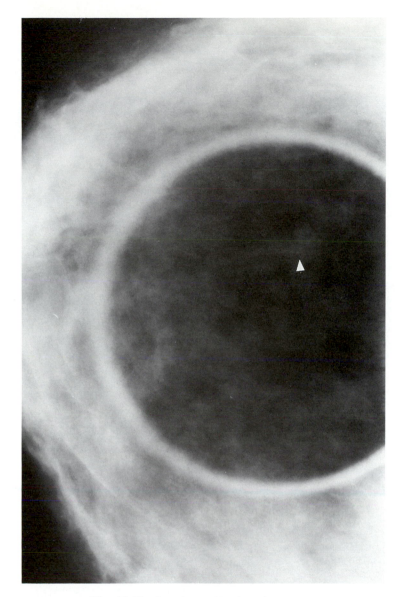

Fig. 12-40. Coned magnification, right breast.

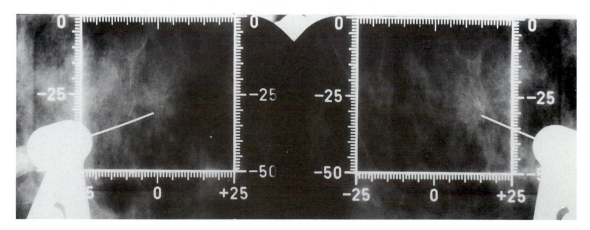

Fig. 12-41. SFNB, right breast.

PATIENT 7

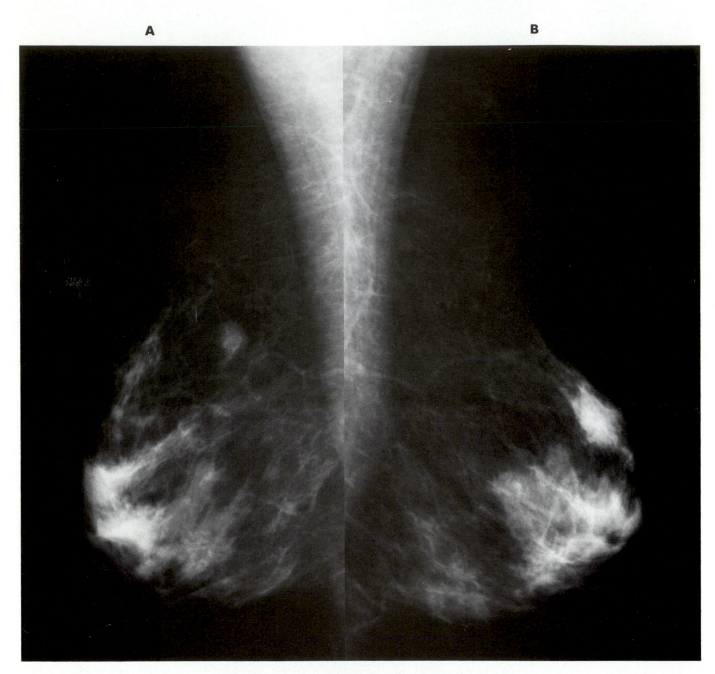

Fig. 12-42. A, Right MLO; **B,** left MLO.

This 46-year-old woman reported for routine screening mammography evaluation (Figs. 12-42 and 12-43).

A

B

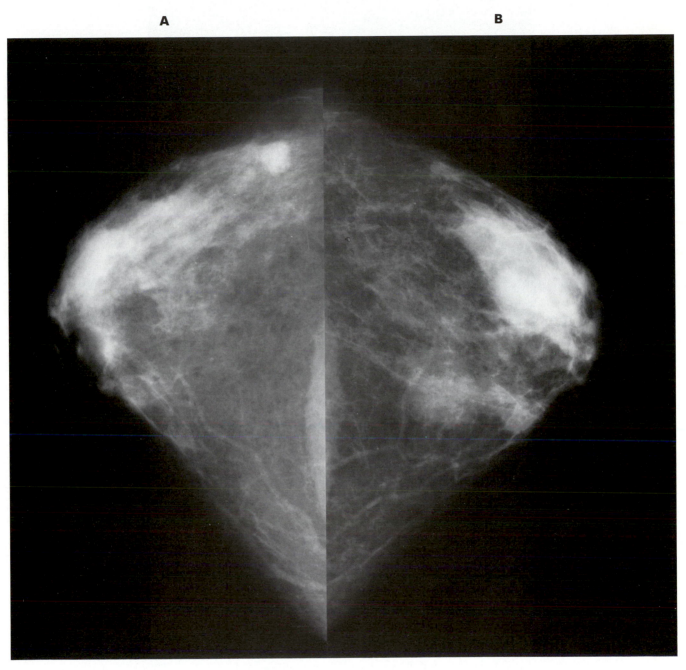

Fig. 12-43. A, Right CC; **B,** left CC.

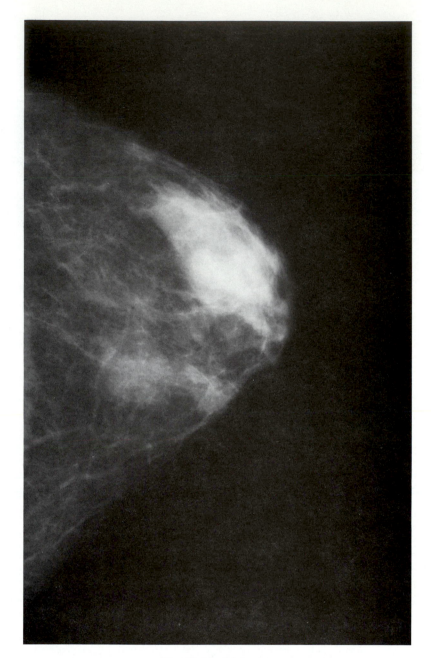

Fig. 12-44. Right CC.

An irregular density is located in the upper outer quadrant of the right breast (Figs. 12-44 and 12-45). The borders of the lesion are moderately lobulated, and while no calcifications are apparent in the craniocaudal projection, they do become apparent in additional images. A partial halo sign is seen in the craniocaudal projection. In the mediolateral oblique projection, the density appears to have a comet-tail sign and the partial halo feature is not evident[8] (Fig. 12-45). A coned magnification provides even better analysis of the density, demonstrating again the lobulated borders and a minute fragment of the comet-tail feature. Most apparent in this projection are the calcifications within the density and the benign-appearing calcifications superimposed on the dense breast tissue (Fig. 12-46). This lesion is suspicious for malignancy.

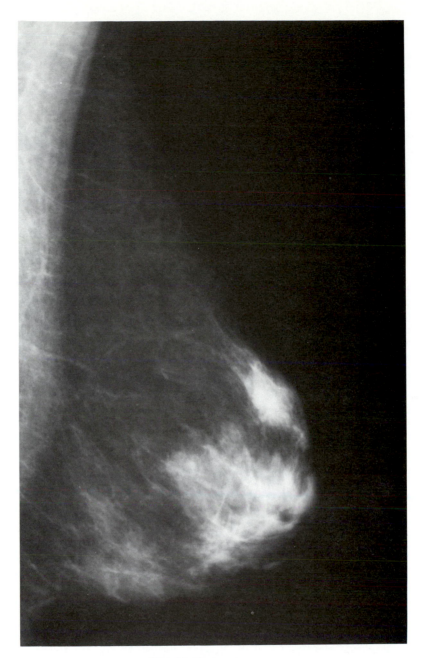

Fig. 12-45. Right MLO.

SFNB was performed and cytology, suspicious for carcinoma, displayed epithelial cells with enlarged and irregular nuclei (Fig. 12-47). Histology of the biopsied lesion confirmed invasive tubular carcinoma with sclerosis and extensive microcalcification. The tumor was confined within the margins of resection.

Code 4

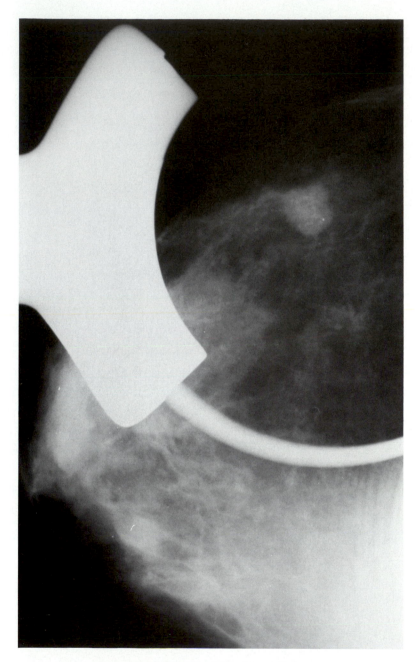

Fig. 12-46. Coned magnification, right breast.

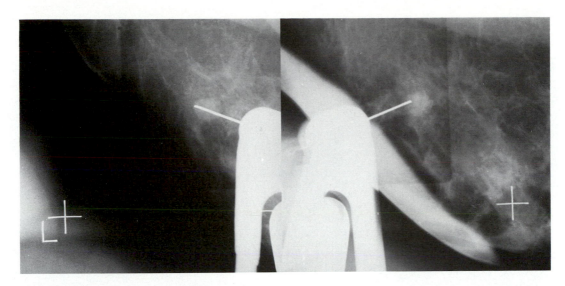

Fig. 12-47. SFNB.

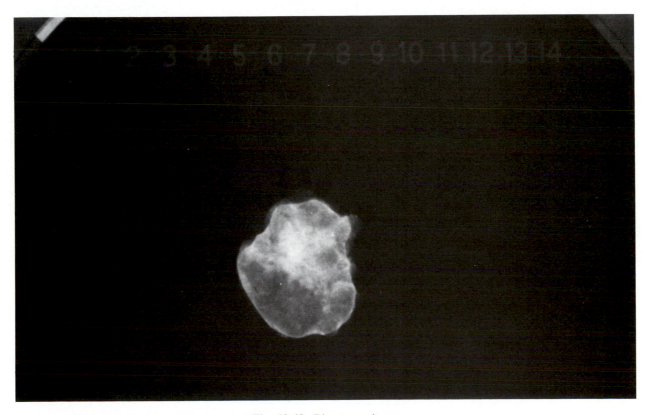

Fig. 12-48. Biopsy specimen.

PATIENT 8

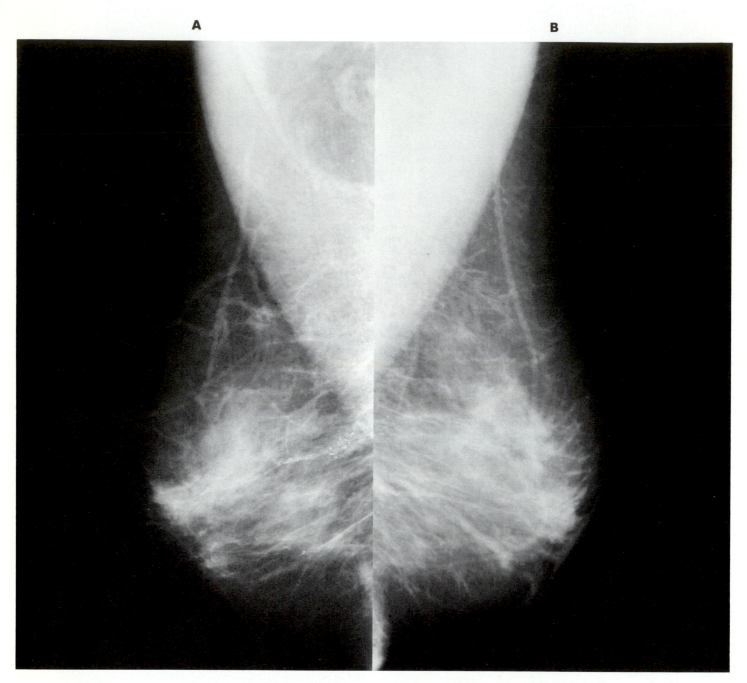

Fig. 12-49. A, Right MLO; **B,** left MLO.

These images (Figs. 12-49 and 12-50) are from a mammogram of a 60-year-old asymptomatic woman with dense breasts.

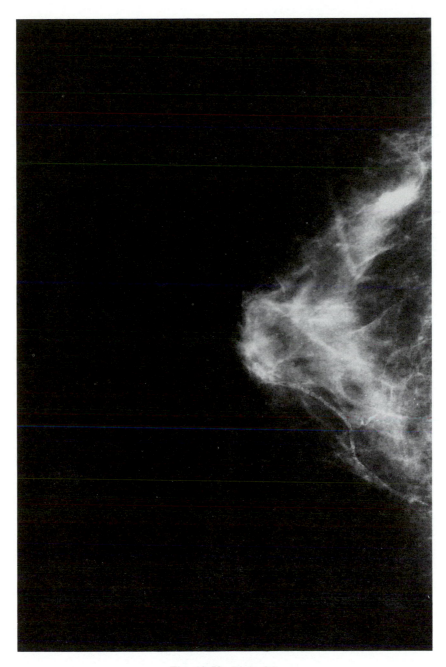

Fig. 12-50. Right CC.

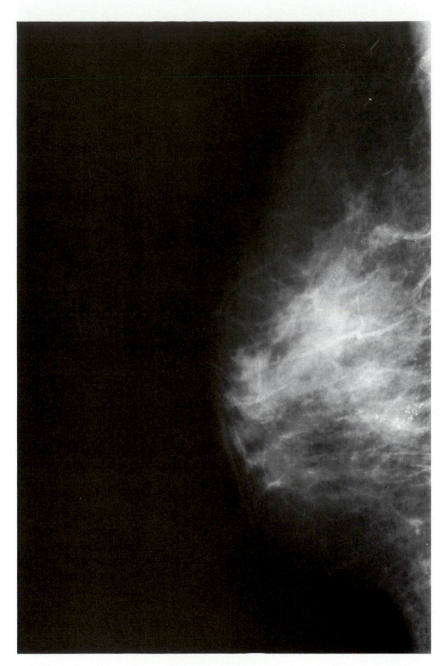

Fig. 12-51. Right LM.

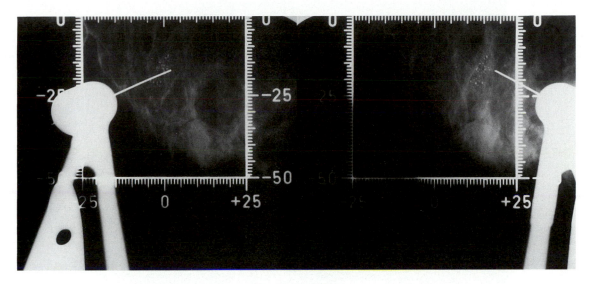

Fig. 12-52. SFNB.

On both the mediolateral oblique and the craniocaudal projections a cluster of microcalcifications is readily identified. Their irregular size, shape, and density warrant a mammographic diagnosis of cancer. While coned magnification images would further demonstrate the obvious pattern of the calcifications, in this case standard images adequately demonstrate their presence and pattern.

SFNB confirmed malignant cells. For this woman, while there is no option except surgical excision of the lesion, surgical management and postsurgical treatment can be discussed.

Histology of the lesion confirmed ductal carcinoma in situ.

Code 4

PATIENT 9

A

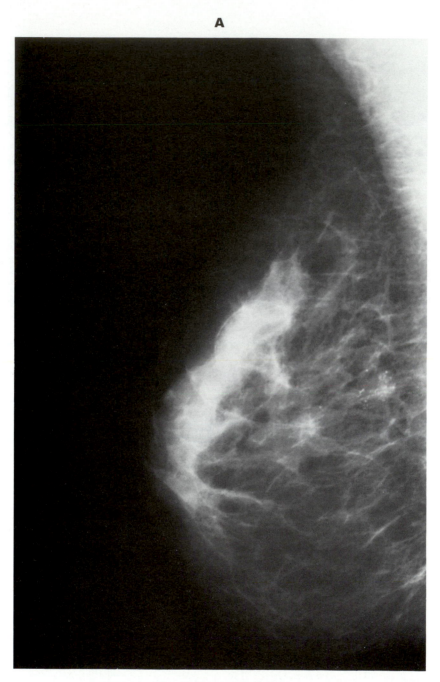

Fig. 12-53. A, Right MLO.

These right mediolateral oblique (Fig. 12-53, *A*) and right craniocaudal (Fig. 12-53, *B*) projections represent images from a screening mammogram of a 67-year-old asymptomatic woman.

B

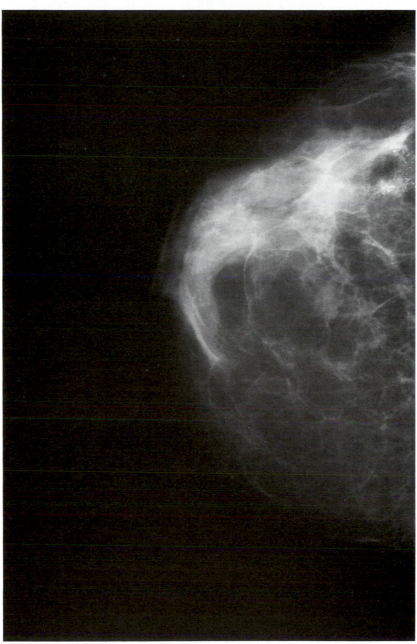

Fig 12-53, cont'd. B, Right CC.

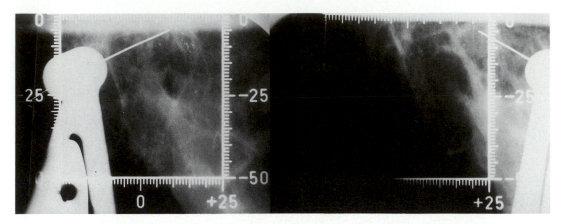

Fig. 12-54. SFNB.

The mammogram of the right breast reveals relatively widespread casting-type intraductal microcalcifications. As previously discussed, this mammographic pattern is considered characteristic of breast cancer (see case 1).[8]

Initially, SFNB was performed and proved negative, with no epithelial cells revealed. When a mammographic appearance characteristic of breast cancer and cytology assessment of a lesion contradict one another, regardless of negative cytology, the breast tissue must be surgically evaluated. A quadrantectomy, performed on the basis of the mammography finding, histologically confirmed ductal carcinoma in situ (DCIS).

To characterize DCIS as a single entity is misleading. Before mammography could detect microcalcification patterns so efficiently and recognize cancerous calcific patterns, DCIS was put in a single group with a single available treatment, mastectomy. Now that microcalcific patterns only millimeters in size can be seen, pathologists have come to recognize many different histologic types of DCIS. Continued improvement in understanding of their complex heterogeneity will offer women treatment alternatives not previously thought available.[4]

Code 5

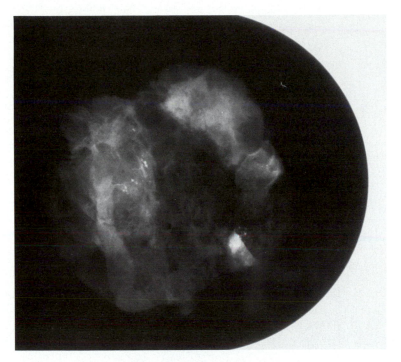

Fig. 12-55. Biopsy specimen.

PATIENT 10

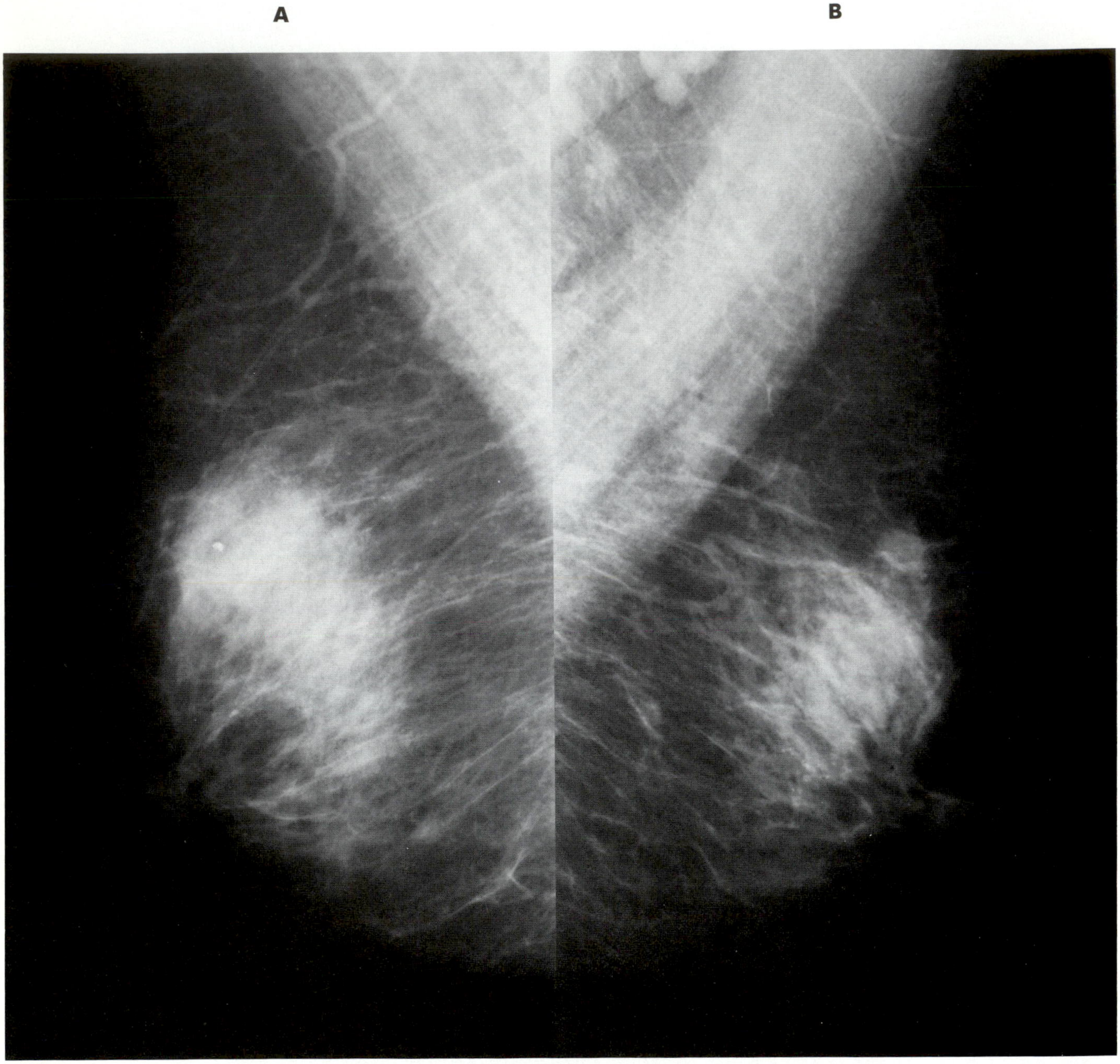

A   B

Fig. 12-56. A, Right MLO; **B,** left MLO.

This 66-year-old asymptomatic woman reported for routine screening mammography (Figs. 12-56 and 12-57). She confirmed a long-term history of bilateral nipple retraction. Observed is abundant bilateral breast parenchyma for a woman this age.

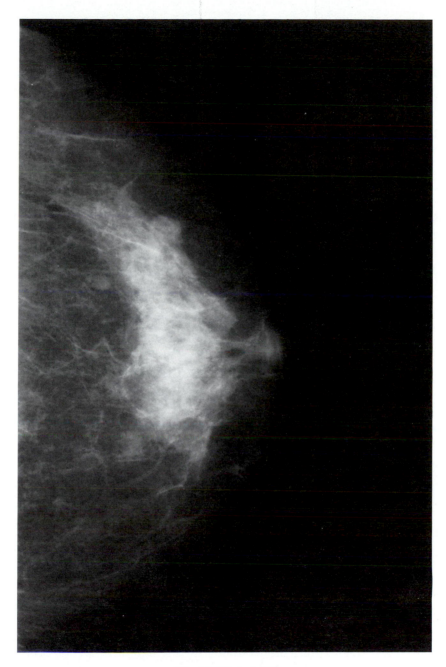

Fig. 12-57. Left CC.

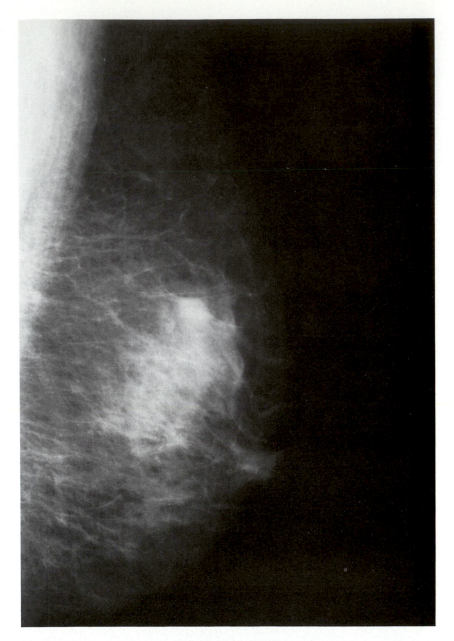

Fig. 12-58. Left LM.

In the right breast several lunar-shaped calcifications and calcified blood vessels can be seen. These calcifications are mammographically benign. There are two separate findings in the left breast. The first is a well-defined, smoothly circumscribed density in the upper outer quadrant, which mammographically is a fibroadenoma (Fig. 12-57). The second finding is the area of scattered microcalcifications that are irregular in shape, form, size, and density. While a few are of the lunar type, the majority are suspicious for malignancy. Coned magnification imaging of the calcifications reconfirms their presence and allows easy recognition of their irregular pattern (Fig. 12-59).

SFNB was performed at both of these areas. Cytology yielded benign epithelial cells and stromal fragments in the left *circumscribed* breast lesion, confirming the mammographic diagnosis of fibroadenoma. Cytology of the left breast *microcalcifications* proved positive for cancer, and histology confirmed ductal carcinoma in situ (Fig. 12-60).

Code 3 —fibroadenoma

Code 4 — microcalcifications

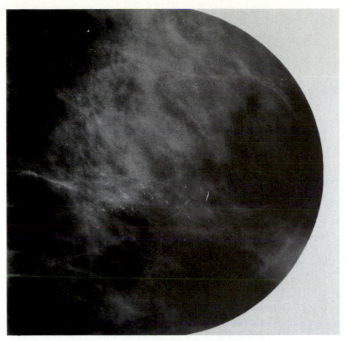

Fig. 12-59. Coned magnification, left MLO.

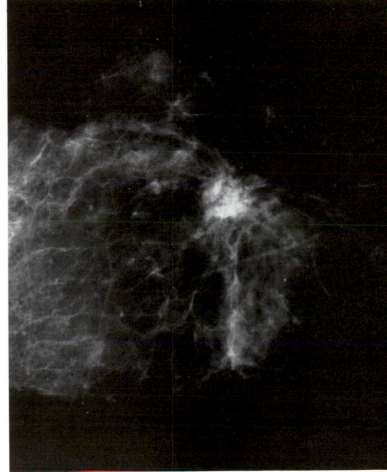

Fig. 12-60. Biopsy specimen.

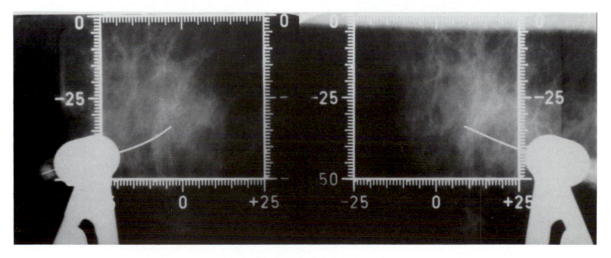

Fig. 12-61. SFNB.

PATIENT 11

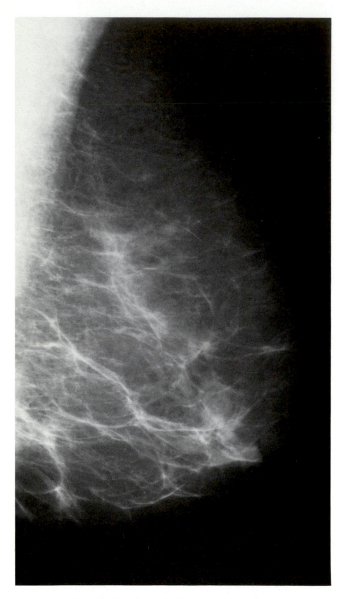

Fig. 12-62. Left MLO, November 1989.

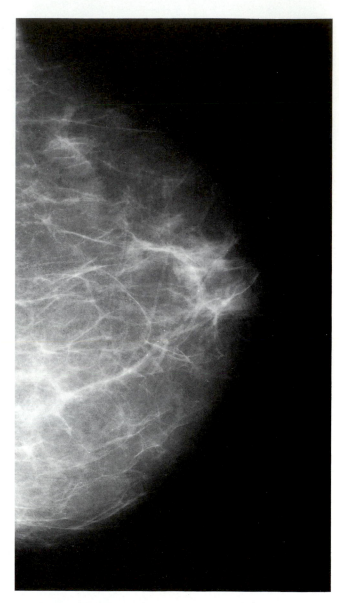

Fig. 12-63. Left CC, November 1989.

This 60-year-old asymptomatic woman appeared for her routine screening mammography evaluation (Figs. 12-62 to 12-65). There is congenital retraction of her left nipple.

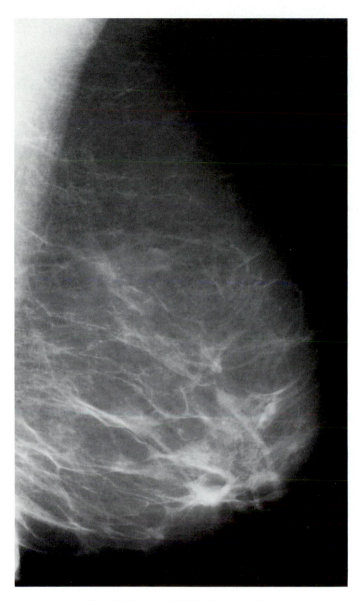

Fig. 12-64. Left MLO, January 1991.

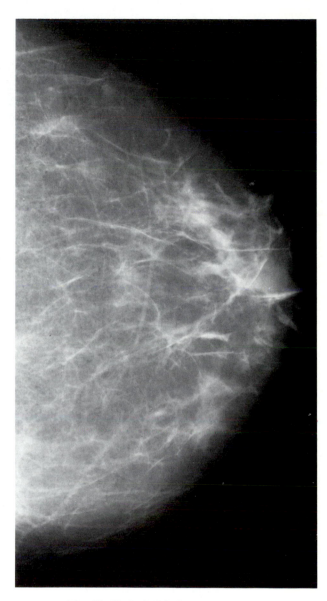

Fig. 12-65. Left CC, January 1991.

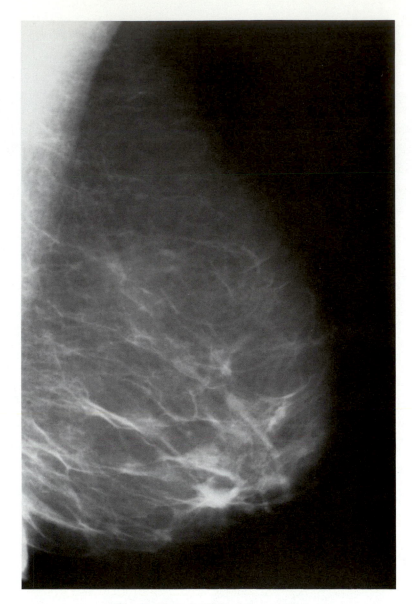

Fig. 12-66. Left MLO, January 1991.

This woman had periodic normal mammograms throughout the 1980s, including her November 1989 examination (Figs. 12-62 and 12-63). In January 1991, the woman phoned to report a skin rash around the nipple area of her left breast. She was urged to return for evaluation.

A clinical breast examination revealed no palpable masses but did reveal an eczematous skin lesion. Mammography was performed and revealed a rather large area of intraductal-appearing microcalcifications near the left nipple that were not apparent on her previous mammograms (Fig. 12-67). Diffuse increased parenchymal densities with calcifications are readily seen in the magnification mammogram (Fig. 12-68).

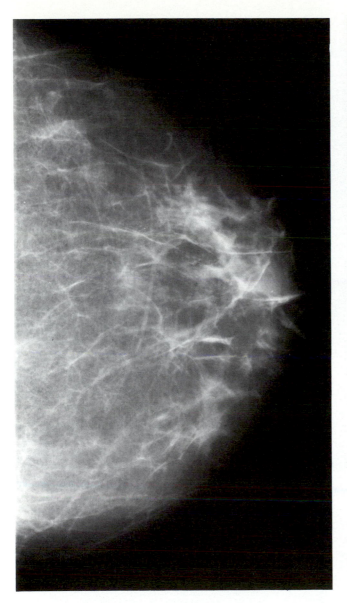

Fig. 12-67. Left CC, January 1991.

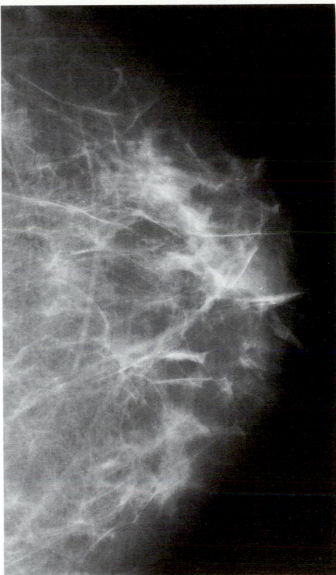

Fig. 12-68. Magnification, left MLO.

Results from exfoliative cytology of the eczematous lesion revealed malignant epithelial cells. This woman went directly to surgery. Histology of the specimen confirmed both microinvasive ductal cancer and Paget's disease. Origin of the Paget cell is controversial. Of importance is that when Paget's disease is not associated with an underlying palpable invasive adenocarcinoma, it is highly curable.[5] Paget's disease of the nipple usually represents carcinoma in situ of the subareolar ducts.[3] In this case, a modified radical mastectomy was performed.

Code 4

PATIENT 12

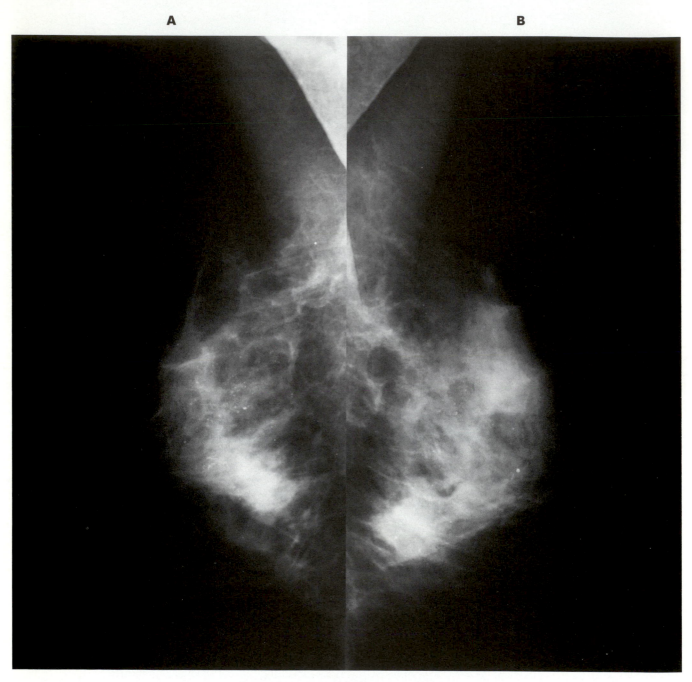

Fig. 12-69. A, Right MLO; **B,** left MLO.

These images (Figs. 12-69 and 12-70) represent a routine screening mammogram of a 56-year-old asymptomatic woman with dense breasts.

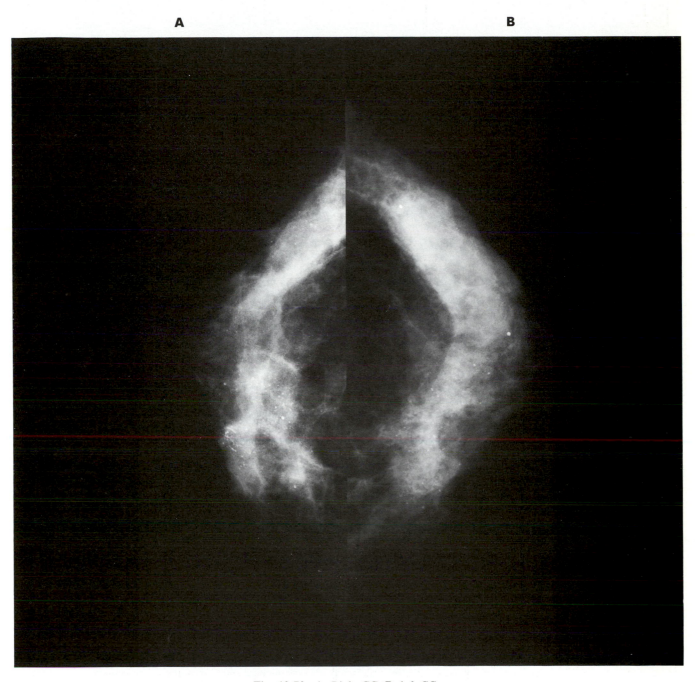

Fig. 12-70. A, Right CC; **B,** left CC.

A   B

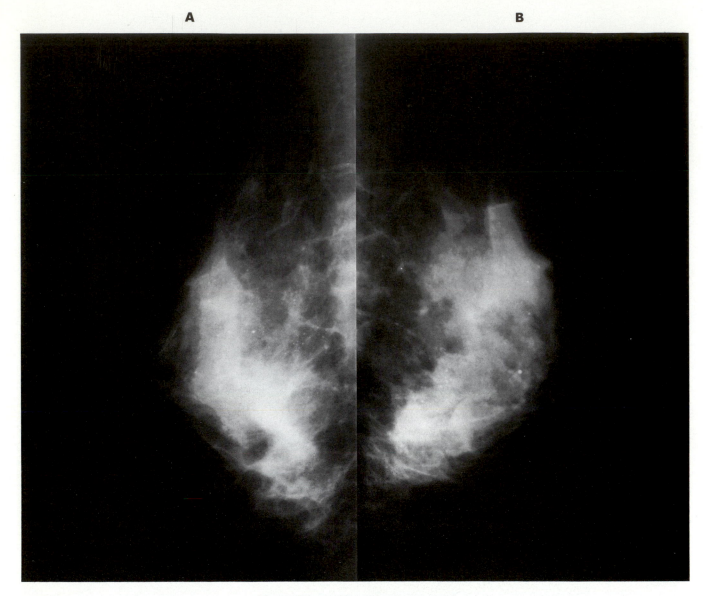

Fig. 12-71. A, Right LM; **B,** left LM.

Microcalcifications on the medial side of the right nipple show typical intraductal pattern of the casting type (Fig. 12-69, *A*). Based on this mammographic appearance this formation is routinely interpreted as suspicious for ductal carcinoma. Lunar and semilunar forms of calcifications are also seen in both the right and left breast, representing benign changes (Fig. 12-70).

Mixed patterns of calcifications demand careful evaluation and action (see also cases 1 and 2). Bilateral SFNB was therefore recommended. Left breast SFNB revealed cytology with no cellular changes suspicious for malignancy and produced benign epithelial cells. Consequently, left breast surgery was unnecessary.

Consistent with the mammographic pattern of the right breast and the mammographic diagnosis of cancer, cytology did reveal cancerous cells (Fig. 12-72). Histology of the lesion further confirmed the diagnosis of right breast ductal carcinoma (Fig. 12-74).

Code 5 — right breast
Code 2 — left breast

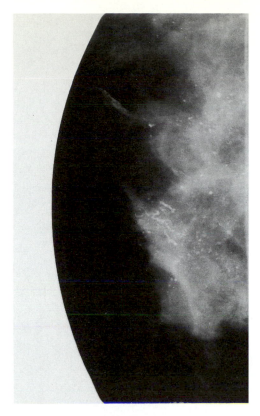
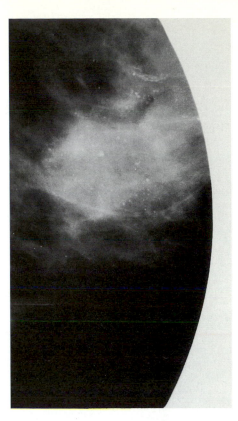

Fig. 12-72. Coned magnification, right CC.

Fig. 12-73. Coned magnification, left MLO.

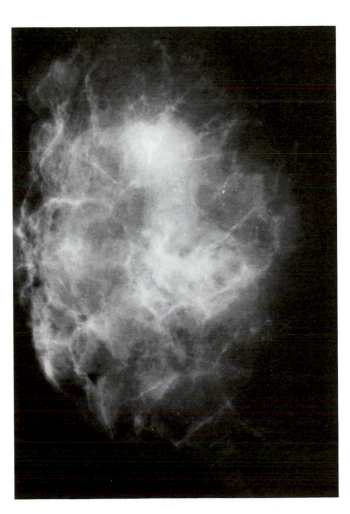

Fig. 12-74. Biopsy specimen, right breast.

PATIENT 13

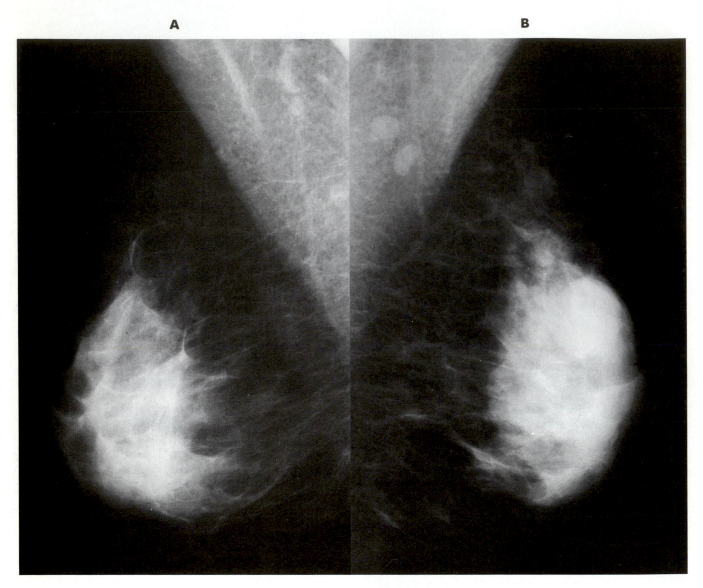

Fig. 12-75. A, Right MLO; **B,** left MLO.

These images (Figs. 12-75 and 12-76) are from a screening mammogram of a 67-year-old asymptomatic woman.

A   B

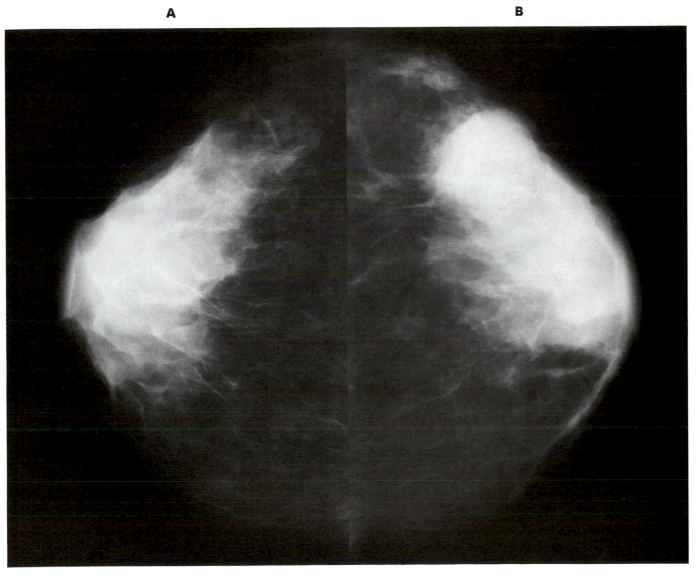

Fig. 12-76. A, Right CC; **B,** left CC.

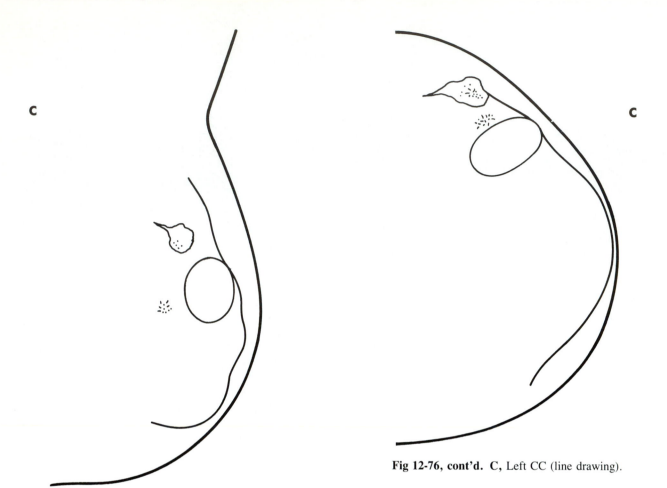

Fig 12-76, cont'd. C, Left CC (line drawing).

Fig 12-75, cont'd. C, Left MLO (line drawing).

Carefully evaluate the multicentric areas of calcification in this woman's mammogram. The mammograms reveal an obvious large, circumscribed density in the upper outer quadrant of the left breast (Figs. 12-75, *B*, and 12-76, *B*). Medical personnel palpated the mass easily, even though the patient denied knowledge of its presence. Unfortunately, she had no way of knowing of two additional, nonpalpable areas of concern surrounding the palpable mass. The first nonpalpable lesion, located directly above the palpable mass, appears as a cluster of microcalcifications. The second lesion, located most laterally in the left breast and adjacent to the first cluster of microcalcifications, appears within an ill-defined mass (Fig. 12-75, *B* and *C*). The lateromedial projection separates the dense breast tissue and defines the border of the palpable mass in greater detail (Fig. 12-77, *B*). The coned magnification projection clearly shows both of the described nonpalpable lesions (Figs. 12-76, *C*, and 12-78).

Fine needle aspiration of the palpable mass and SFNB evaluation of the two nonpalpable areas were all cytology-positive for cancer. Histology confirmed both the palpable mass and the two nonpalpable lesions to be moderately well-differentiated invasive ductal carcinoma.

Code 5

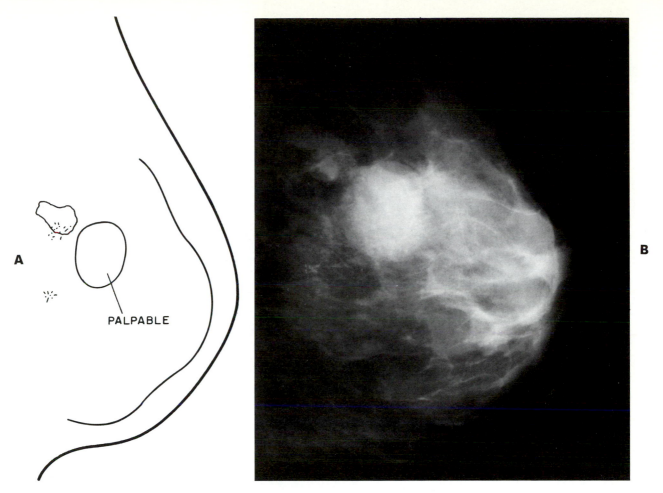

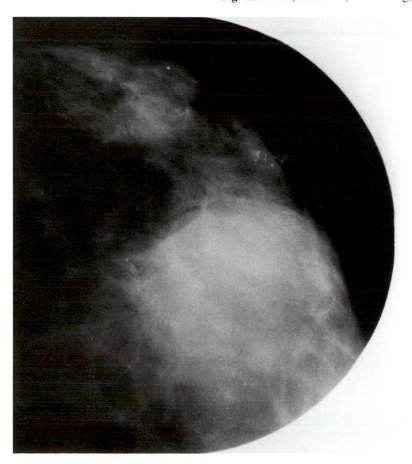

Fig. 12-77. A, Left LM (line drawing); **B,** left LM.

PALPABLE

A

B

Fig. 12-78. Coned magnification, left CC.

PATIENT 14

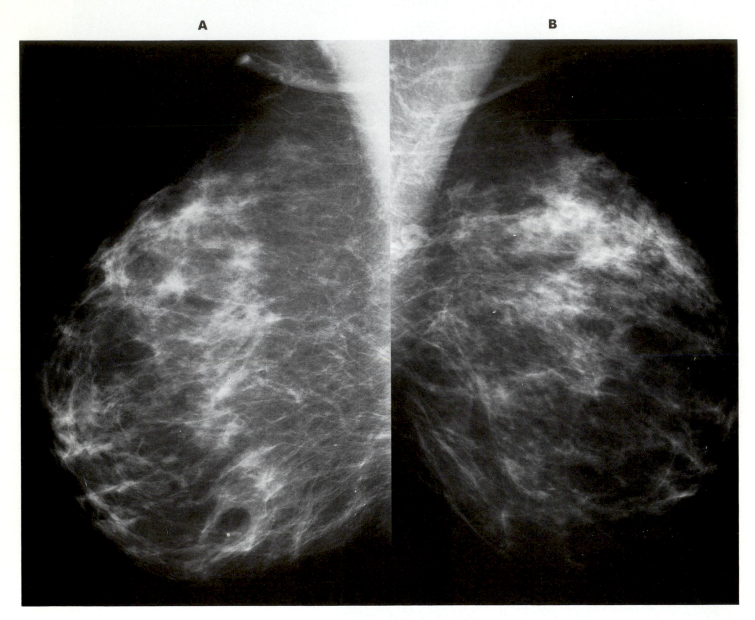

Fig. 12-79. A, Right MLO; **B,** left MLO.

These images (Figs. 12-79 and 12-80) are from a screening mammogram of a 57-year-old asymptomatic nurse with relatively lucent breasts.

A
B

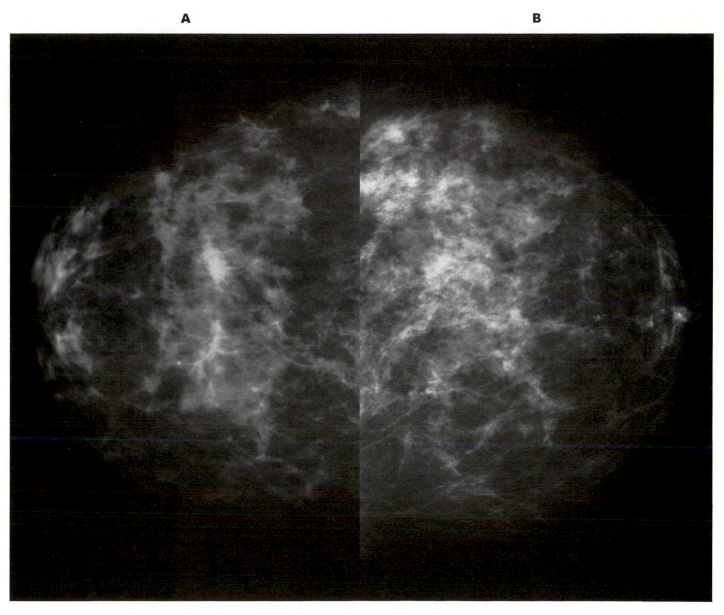

Fig. 12-80. A, Right CC; **B,** left CC.

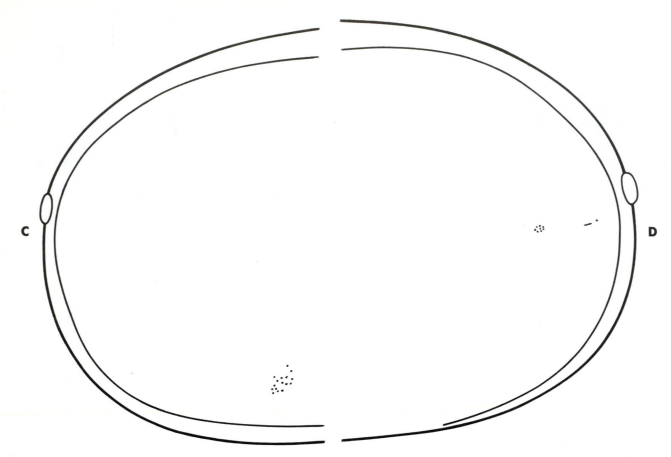

Fig 12-80, cont'd. C, Right CC (line drawing); **D,** left CC (line drawing).

This woman had undergone bilateral breast surgery 15 years before because of palpable breast nodules in the medial lower quadrants of her breasts. At that time, biopsy specimens proved the nodules benign. The patient did not have mammography based on palpable nodules.

Scattered benign-appearing calcifications are now seen bilaterally (Figs. 12-79 and 12-80). Also characteristic of benign-type calcifications are those seen in the lower *inner* quadrant of the right breast, of approximately 15 mm, in both coarse and semilunar patterns (Fig. 12-79, *A*).

SFNB of the right breast was recommended to confirm their benign appearance, based on the woman's history of "palpable lesions." It revealed benign epithelial cells consistent with the benign-appearing mammographic pattern. After correlating this woman's current mammogram with the negative cytology finding, surgery was not recommended for the right breast.

A more suspicious 3 mm group of microcalcifications is detected in the left breast below the nipple (Figs. 12-81, *D,* and 12-83). This left breast finding *is* mammographically more worrisome. SFNB and preoperative carbon localization were performed simultaneously. Despite negative cytology of this lesion, based on the suspicious mammographic pattern, surgery was recommended. Histology of the left breast specimen proved to be noncomedo-type ductal carcinoma in situ.

Considering the result of her left breast surgery, the woman requested right breast surgery also. Histology of the right breast specimen demonstrated benign mastopathy, consistent with the benign-appearing mammographic pattern and with the negative SFNB cytology outcome.

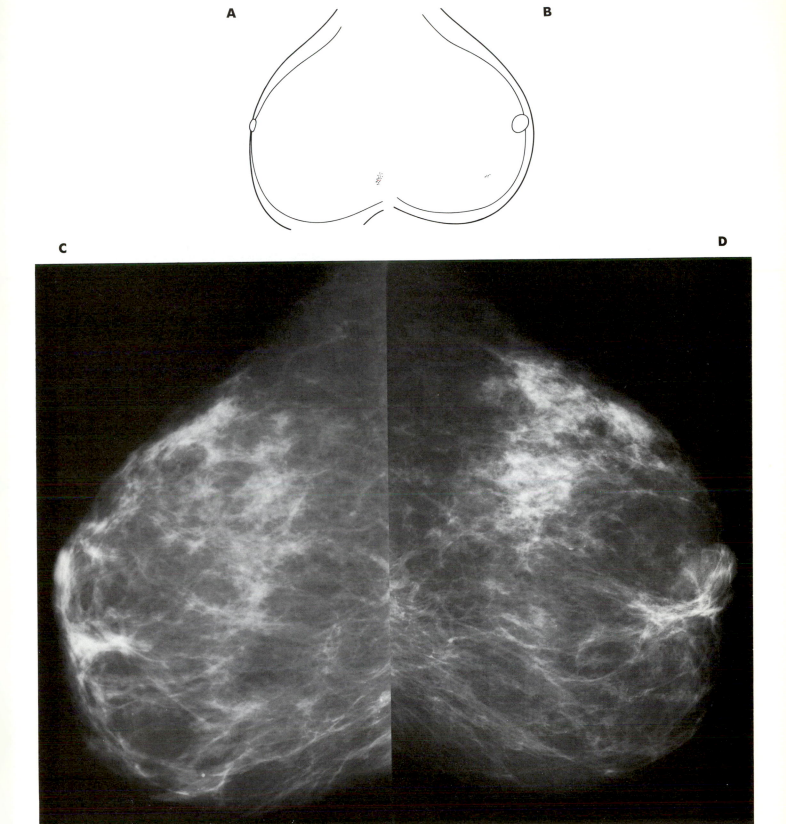

Fig. 12-81. A, Right LM (line drawing); **B,** left LM (line drawing); **C,** right LM; **D,** left LM.

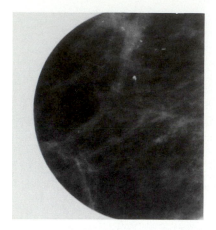

Fig. 12-82. Coned magnification, right breast.

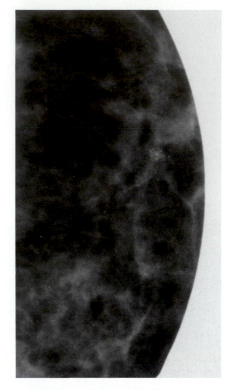

Fig. 12-83. Coned magnification, left breast.

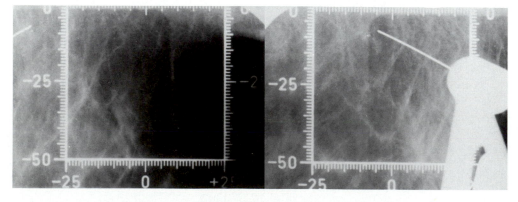

Fig. 12-84. Left SFNB.

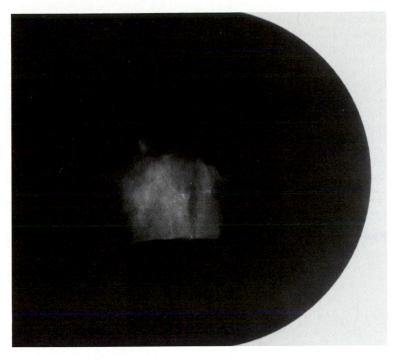

Fig. 12-85. Biopsy specimen, left breast.

This type of complicated and confounding case occurs with greater frequency than radiologists, surgeons, pathologists, and, certainly, women prefer. Routine interdisciplinary discussion of the elements and implications of all mammography test results should provide reliable clinical decisions and optimal patient care. Through continuing multidisciplinary discussion of mammography-detected lesions and subsequent correlation of their pathology, consensus for expanding mammographic criteria may develop. This in turn may improve the ability to distinguish which mammographic lesions and SFNB cytology reports can safely recommend clinical and mammographic follow-up from those requiring immediate surgical biopsy.

Code 2 — right breast
Code 3 — left breast

REFERENCES

1. Dutt PL, Page DL: Multicentricity of in situ and invasive carcinoma. In Bland KI, Copeland EM, editors: *The breast: comprehensive management of benign and malignant diseases*, Philadelphia, 1991, Saunders.
2. Haus AG, Feig SA, Ehrlich SM, et al: Mammography screening: technology, radiation dose and risk, quality control, and benefits to society, *Radiology* 174:627-656, 1990.
3. Page DL, Anderson TJ: *Diagnostic histopathology of the breast*, New York, 1987, Churchill Livingstone.
4. Page DL, Simpson JF: Benign, high-risk and premalignant lesions of the mamma. In Bland KI, Copeland EM, editors: *The breast: comprehensive management of benign and malignant diseases*, Philadelphia, 1991, Saunders.
5. Pierson KK, Wilkinson EJ: Malignant neoplasia of the breast: infiltrating carcinomas. In Bland KI, Copeland EM, editors: *The breast: comprehensive management of benign and malignant diseases*, Philadelphia, 1991, Saunders.
6. Sickles EA: Further experience with microfocal spot magnification mammography in the assessment of clustered breast microcalcifications, *Radiology* 137(11):9-14, 1980.
7. Sickles EA: Mammographic detectability of breast microcalcifications, *Am J Roentgenol* 139(5):913-918, 1982.
8. Tabar L, Dean PB: *Teaching atlas of mammography*, ed 2, New York, 1985, Thieme-Stratton.

INDEX